Jane Brody's
The New York Times
Guide to
Personal Health

Other books by Jane E. Brody

Jane Brody's Nutrition Book
You Can Fight Cancer and Win
(with Arthur I. Holleb, M.D.)
Secrets of Good Health
(with Richard Enquist)

Jane Brody's
𝔗𝔥𝔢 𝔑𝔢𝔴 𝔜𝔬𝔯𝔨 𝔗𝔦𝔪𝔢𝔰
Guide to
Personal Health

By Jane E. Brody

Illustrations by Karen Karlsson

𝔗𝔦𝔪𝔢𝔰
BOOKS

Published by TIMES BOOKS, a division of
Quadrangle/The New York Times Book Co., Inc.
Three Park Avenue, New York, N. Y. 10016

Published simultaneously in Canada by
Fitzhenry & Whiteside, Ltd., Toronto

Library of Congress Cataloging in Publication Data

Brody, Jane E.
    Jane Brody's The New York times guide to personal health.

    Selections from the author's column published in
the New York times since Nov. 1976.
    Includes bibliographies.
    1. Health. 2. Medicine--Popular works.
I. New York times. II. Title. III. Title: New York
times guide to personal health. IV. Guide to personal health.
RA776.B7747   1982   613   82.50050
ISBN 0-8219-1014-1

Manufactured in the United States of America
10 9 8 7 6 5 4 3 2 1

Book Designers: Fay H. Eng and Anthony T. Yee

In loving memory of my mother, Lillian F. Brody, and my grandmother, Bertha Brody, who taught me to love life and treat it with respect.

Acknowledgments

This book would never have happened if not for the wisdom and foresight of Arthur Gelb, Deputy Managing Editor of *The New York Times*. In the fall of 1976, Mr. Gelb decided that The Times should have a weekly column on personal health and he convinced me to write it.

Despite numerous initial misgivings (among others, I anticipated a deluge of queries from hypochondriacal readers and cranky assaults from physicians questioning the right of a journalist to offer health advice), I agreed to give Mr. Gelb's plan a try. That was nearly six years ago, and I've yet to give one thought to quitting.

My weekly "Personal Health" column, which appears in the *Times* and in more than 100 other newspapers throughout the country, proved to be enormously popular with both lay readers and professionals. Many doctors have written to say they use it to educate themselves and their patients. My enthusiasm has repeatedly been bolstered by grateful letters from readers, some of whom were spared considerable pain and expense and, in a few instances, loss of life, for having read my column and heeded its advice.

Thank you, faithful readers, for giving me the encouragement to keep the column going, even during my vacations. Through you, it continues to be its own reward.

Editing, updating, and collating more than five years of columns turned out to be no small undertaking. Hugh Howard, my perceptive editor at Times Books, tolerated many late-night, early-morning, and weekend queries and provided sage advice and support throughout. Thanks, Hugh, for maintaining the perspective and the pace that this project required.

During the eight months that I worked fourteen-hour days six days a week to complete the book, my highly supportive family — husband, Richard Engquist, and sons, Erik and Lorin — kept the household together and minimized demands on me. Though I have sometimes wondered whether they don't prefer me as a part-time wife and mother, I am nonetheless grateful for their forbearance.

Jane E. Brody
June 1982

Table of Contents

IX

XII

Personal Prologue: How I Live

"You will live long and enjoy life."

I know full well that this paper prophecy, which I found in a fortune cookie a few years ago, comes with no money-back guarantee for a good or long life. But while many people are content to accept whatever fate life may have in store, in the seventeen years I have been a medical and science writer I have come to believe that I can and should adopt reasonable measures to help preserve my health and prolong my life.

I know that these measures do not guarantee that I will still be spry at ninety. I also know that many of the recommendations I follow are based on a still-incomplete understanding of the major killing and crippling diseases. Some, in fact, may turn out to be all wrong.

I want to weight the odds in my favor: However long I live, I want to be healthful and zestful, free of disease and disability. I am convinced that my future health largely depends on how I care for myself in the present, and I try to live in accordance with what I consider the best available medical knowledge. It isn't always simple, but I have discovered that it's not a life of misery, deprivation, and self-denial. In fact, it's lots of fun, all the more so because I feel good about my body and my life.

One of the more frequent comments I hear from people I meet is that I am too young to worry about my health. Not so. I turned forty in the spring of 1981, and anyway, I think it is never too early to start taking care of yourself. People also ask whether I practice what I preach. I do. I am slender not by nature, but by design and constant vigilance. I like to eat, and guided by reason and self-control, I eat everything I like. I exercise daily, even though my workday is regularly ten to twelve hours long. I make time for the things I consider important. Most important of all, I enjoy my life.

My guiding principle is moderation. Except for an absolute ban on smoking, I am not a fanatic about anything, unless you think it fanatic that I am determined to try to realize the prophecy in my fortune cookie. Now for the details.

My Diet

I eat pretty much in accordance with the dietary goals spelled out by the Senate Committee on Nutrition and Human Needs.

Carbohydrates account for about 65 to 70 percent of my calories (mostly starches, the complex carbohydrates, consumed in their unrefined, unadulterated form), protein for 10 to 15 percent, and fats, about 15 percent. This is considerably less fat and considerably more carbohydrates than the average American consumes. Contrary to popular belief, starchy foods are not fattening; ounce for ounce, they contain less than half the calories that fat does and no more calories than pure protein. My daily cholesterol intake is usually below 250 milligrams (the amount in one egg yolk), less than half that of the typical adult American.

About half of my protein comes from vegetable sources, particularly grains (breads, cereals, pasta, rice, etc.), dried peas and beans, potatoes. Among the animal protein foods I most frequently consume are skim milk, low-fat cottage cheese, yogurt, chicken (without skin), turkey breast, part-skim hard cheeses, small quantities of very lean beef and pork, boiled ham, shrimp, and fish.

My family of four (husband and thirteen-year-old twin sons) regularly dines on a total of a half pound of slivered meat or chicken, cooked in a soup or sauce for pasta or stir-fried with lots of fresh vegetables and served with hefty portions of rice, bulgur (cracked wheat), or noodles. We rarely (maybe once in three months) have a slab of meat such as a roast, steak, or chops for dinner. The average portion of such cuts of meat would triple the amount of meat each person consumes.

Spaghetti or macaroni with sauce containing small amounts of meat, chicken, or fish and a big salad is a frequent supper favorite (fewer calories than a steak dinner). So is homemade soup — lots of vegetables (including potatoes), small pieces of meat and/or chicken, rice or bulgur and/or noodles in chicken broth. The soup is a great way to use up leftovers, relieving the table clearer of the "obligation" to eat those few hundred extra calories that often remain at the end of a meal.

Another use for leftovers is a favorite breakfast of mine — fried rice or bulgur mixed with whatever's left from last night's supper, perhaps supplemented by a scrambled egg white or slivers of boiled ham or turkey breast. The latter ingredients, incidentally, are usually consumed in sandwiches (on whole grain sandwich or pita bread) for lunch a couple of times a week.

I eat eggs as eggs once a week, discarding one of the two yolks. (If you have a dog or a bird, the yolks you don't eat will give your pet a glossy coat.) My children love pancakes and French toast for breakfast. In both I discard one of every two yolks; pancakes are made with fat-free buttermilk, polyunsaturated oil, and whole wheat flour. I top my serving with sliced banana and a dash of cinnamon sugar instead of syrup. The boys dribble, rather than pour, syrup from a container with a tiny spout.

Rather than buy cakes, I make my own cakelike breads and muffins, laden with nutritious things like fruits, grated vegetables, nuts, whole grain flour or oatmeal, buttermilk or orange juice, and polyunsaturated oil instead of the highly saturated fats used by commercial bakeries. I start with recipes that use relatively little fat, and I automatically reduce the sugar by half. When my sons taste commercially prepared baked goods, they often remark, "Yuk, this is too sweet." The homemade breads and muffins alternate with fresh fruits for desserts and snacks.

Because my diet is well balanced and includes lots of fresh and stir-fried vegetables, salads, whole grains, and fruits, I see no need for vitamin supplements. Even without vitamin C, I went six years without a cold, despite the fact that my sons undoubtedly bring home all sorts of viruses from school.

I don't keep potato chips, pretzels, or other high-calorie, salty, low-nutrient snack foods in the house. When I'm overcome by the urge to nibble, I make unbuttered, unsalted popcorn (high in fiber, low in calories), sometimes lightly sprinkled with grated Parmesan.

I don't worry much about food additives because, other than bread and cereal, I eat relatively few processed foods. The foods with the most offensive additives — like cold cuts and bacon — are too high in fat to be a regular part of my diet anyway. If once a year I want to dress up a fruit salad with maraschino cherries, I do it — despite the suspicions about red dye.

I do drink coffee — about two cups a day with caffeine, another three decaffeinated — with skim milk, no sugar. All told, I consume the equivalent of a quart of milk a day, mostly as a combination of skim milk, buttermilk, low-fat yogurt, and low-fat cottage cheese.

Despite the care I take with my daily diet — or, more accurately, because of it — I don't hesitate to splurge now and again. Once a year, for example, I make blinis (buttery Russian pancakes) served with caviar, sour cream, chopped egg, and melted butter — a fat and cholesterol freak out. Another annual favorite is pumpkin soup made with half-and-half and topped with a dollop of salted whipped cream. Italian sausages are an occasional treat. Ice cream, my undying passion, is a more frequent one, but I keep the flavors I can't resist out of the house.

Weight Control

I once weighed a third more than I do now. I was always on a diet, and after a week of eating library paste and toothpicks, my willpower would run out, and I'd gorge on everything I loved and had missed all week. Or else I would put nothing in my mouth all day, then eat nonstop all night. Eventually I became obsessed with food and weight, and the more obsessed I was, the fatter I got.

Then one day I realized that I had to learn to live more sensibly with food. I stopped dieting and started eating like a normal person:

three reasonable meals a day, with snacks and a preselected "no-no" (such as two small cookies or two tablespoons of ice cream). No more binges, no more whole bags of potato chips or pints of ice cream, and no more going hungry. And, lo and behold, I lost weight. It took two years to reach what I consider a normal weight for my size and bone structure, but I never gained it back. Here's how I do it.

I never skip a meal. That only makes me hungrier for the next meal and increases the likelihood that I'll overeat. Besides, when I'm hungry, I'm irritable and impatient, and I can't write or cope with the kids. I consider breakfast and lunch my most important meals; they provide me with the energy I need to work productively and run around all day. I usually consume two-thirds or more of my day's calories by 2:00 P.M., just the reverse of what most others I know do.

If I've had a big lunch, I eat only a salad (lots of veggies but little or no oil in the dressing) and a piece of bread for supper. Then I may eat the leftover family supper for breakfast or lunch the next day. If I've had only a sandwich for lunch, I eat a small portion of the family dinner plus a salad. If we're planning to have a dinner out, I have a regular breakfast but a smaller lunch.

I don't consume much alcohol — at a dinner party, one drink plus wine with dinner; at home, a small glass of wine with supper. I find that in addition to the calories in alcohol, it diminishes my willpower, and I tend to overeat if I overdrink.

My sweet tooth has subsided greatly with age and lack of dietary encouragement. I keep it pretty well under control by allowing myself one or two moderately sweet things a day, such as a few homemade cookies, a muffin, or a slice of homemade sweet bread (for example, pumpkin, cranberry, zucchini, or banana bread). Many sweets I once loved now taste sickeningly sweet to me.

Exercise

When an injury kept me bedridden for six weeks one year, I discovered that I could, through determination, keep my weight down even without any exercise. But I have a lot more leeway in my diet when I'm active. I nearly always do something vigorous in the morning, and often in the evening before supper as well, for a total of an hour to an hour and a half a day devoted to exercise. Currently I swim a half mile four or five times a week; bicycle ten miles about three or four times a week; jog three and a half miles three or more times a week; play tennis (singles) one to three times week (depending on the season); and walk. Whenever possible, I use footpower instead of cars, taxis, subways, buses, elevators, and escalators.

This activity adds far more to my life than the several hundred extra calories I can eat each day. It is a great tension reliever and relaxer. I find that I get angry and frustrated less often and get over my destructive feelings more quickly than I used to when I exercised less regularly. And I sleep like a baby — six hours a night or less — even though I always have a lot on my mind.

In sum, then, unless you have a chronic illness like diabetes or are genetically prone to an early death from heart disease, you need not become an extremist or an ascetic, nor do you have to give up forever everything you love, to live healthfully and enjoyably. Through the principles of moderation, you can have your cake and eat it, too, as long as it's not too much cake too often. All you have to do is decide it's something you want to do.

Jane E. Brody
June 1982

XVII

Jane Brody's
The New York Times
Guide to
Personal Health

Introduction:
You Can Be Healthy
and Happy

No one needs to be told that good health is important. Without it, the ability to succeed in and enjoy life is greatly diminished. Ninety-nine percent of us are born healthy, but few of us die that way. Contrary to widespread belief, we all don't have to die of "something." Most of us can live out our lives unmarred by chronic disease or disability, and many more of us than now do can succumb not to illness, but merely to old age when our time is finally up.

As Dr. Ernst Wynder, president of the American Health Foundation, so aptly put it, our goal should be to "die young as late in life as possible."

The likelihood of this occurring depends largely on you, on how you live your life and care for your body and mind. Less than 10 percent of the difference in health between any two Americans is determined by the care delivered by physicians. More than 90 percent results from factors beyond medicine's control: your genetic background; the healthfulness of your environment; and, most important, how you live — what and how much you eat, your drinking and smoking habits, how much you exercise, how you relax.

Your genetic heritage may determine your body type and facial features, but it rarely is a direct cause of illness. More often, genes can create a predisposition to illness; this predisposition may never be expressed if you don't give the genes the encouragement they need to do their dirty work. The way you live can greatly influence the chances that an inherited tendency will become expressed as actual illness or premature death.

Thus, someone with a hereditary predisposition to heart disease may live out a full and healthy life despite it, if that life is unmarred by cigarettes, overweight, lack of exercise, a diet high in fat and salt, and a "driven" approach to life's tasks.

Similarly, someone prone to lung cancer will reduce his or her chances of developing this lethal disease by 75 percent if tobacco products are avoided. A person genetically susceptible to high blood pressure is not likely to develop it if he or she maintains a low-sodium diet and a normal body weight. Periodic checkups of a woman predisposed to breast cancer may permit detection of the disease while it is still nearly 100 percent curable. Even a genetic tendency toward depression might be countered by ego-enhancing activities.

We Die As We Live

The "good life" as most Americans now live it has become our way of death. The trappings and temptations of affluence are causing or contributing to three-fourths of the nation's deaths each year. As mainstream America lives it, the good life is causing fat-crippled hearts, fragile bones, alcohol-saturated brains and livers, tobacco-clogged lungs, accident-mangled bodies, and flabby muscles that fatigue on one flight of stairs.

Most of the increase in life expectancy Americans have enjoyed in the twentieth century has been due to fewer deaths in infancy, in childhood, and after childbirth — the result of improved sanitation, immunizations, and antibiotics. Among middle-aged Americans, however, men live only four years longer and women only seven years longer than did their middle-aged counterparts at the turn of the century. Too many of us today succumb to an excessive reliance on physicians and the "miracles" of modern medicine and an insufficient reliance upon ourselves to keep us healthy.

We live in an era of heroic therapies: coronary care units, kidney and heart transplants, antibiotics and other potent drugs. The mass media bring these miracles into the homes of nearly every American. But they obscure the fact that most of medicine is only patch-up, not curative. Doctors may fix the broken plaster on the ceiling, but not the chronic leak that caused it.

The much-heralded coronary care units save only an extra 5 percent of coronary victims (more than half die even before they reach the hospital), and even if all cancer deaths were eliminated, it would add only two years to the average American life-span.

What You Can Do

What *can* make a difference in the length and quality of your life is you, if you take personal responsibility for the good health you were born with. This means that you:

● **Avoid hazardous behaviors,** such as cigarettes, excess alcohol and calories, mind-altering drugs, unsafe driving and recreational practices, misuse of dangerous tools.

● **Pursue health-enhancing activities,** such as regular exercise, a proper diet, and protective health measures such as immunizations and routine checkups.

● **Get proper diagnosis and treatment,** when preventive measures fail or when unavoidable illness strikes. This requires being well informed, alert, questioning, and unintimidated by people with white coats and large black and silver necklaces in their pockets.

It is every patient's right and obligation to participate in his or her own care. The "activated" patient is less likely to be treated in a patronizing manner or suffer an adverse drug reaction or be operated on unnecessarily. Sickness turns most of us into little children who want mommy (i.e., doctor) to make us well. If we are not armed ahead of time with the tools for assuring quality care, we are not likely to be able to call them into play when they are really needed.

Right now American medicine provides primarily "sickness care," not health care. Few doctors are paid to keep people healthy, and most are bored by the healthy patient. Even the routine checkup is designed to find something wrong and treat it, not to instill and reinforce preventive health-enhancing practices. But changes are now taking place. A "wellness" movement is sweeping the land. The future of health care will be marked by a diminishing role of medical care providers (physicians and the institutions where they work) and an increasing role of the health care consumer — you. This book is designed to help make you an into an informed consumer and active participant in your health care.

Your Personal Health Inventory

You can start right now to gain a better appreciation of your health risks and take more responsibility for your own well-being. Following is one of a number of health-hazard appraisal tests recently devised to help motivate people to make health-enhancing changes in their lives. This test determines your health age. It should be no greater than your chronological age, and the lower it is than your chronological age, the better.

Rules: If you are uncertain, leave answer blank. Place scores (given in parentheses) on the lines provided in the + or − columns. In each section, total the columns and subtract the lower number from the higher number to find the section total (+ or −). Follow the instructions for calculating your medical age at the end of the appraisal.

I. LIFE STYLE INVENTORY   +   −

Disposition. Exceptionally good-natured, easygoing (−3); average (0); extremely tense and nervous most of the time (+6).   ____   ____

Exercise. Physically active employment or sedentary job with well–planned exercise program (−12); sedentary with moderate regular exercise (0); sedentary work, no exercise program (+12).   ____   ____

Home environment. Unusually pleasant, better than average family life (−6); average (0); unusual tension, family strife common (+9).   ____   ____

Job satisfaction. Above average (−3); average (0); discontented (+6).   ____   ____

Exposure to air pollution. Substantial (+9).   ____   ____

Smoking habits. Nonsmoker (−6); occasional (0); moderate, regular smoking 20 cigarettes, 5 cigars, or 5 pipefuls (+12); heavy smoking 40 or more cigarettes daily (+24); marijuana frequent (+24).   ____   ____

Alcohol habits. None or seldom (−6); moderate with less than 2 beers or 8 ounces of wine or 2 ounces of whiskey or hard liquor daily (+6); heavy, with more than above (+24).   ____   ____

Eating habits. Drink skim or low-fat milk only (−3); eat much bulky food (−3); heavy (3 times a day) meat eater (+6); more than 2 pats butter daily (+6); more than 4 cups coffee/tea/cola daily (+6); usually add salt at table (+6).   ____   ____

Auto driving. Regularly less than 20,000 miles annually, and always wear seat belt (−3); regularly less than 20,000, but belt not always worn (0); more than 20,000 (+12).   ____   ____

Drug habits. Use of street drugs (+36).   ____   ____

PART I TOTALS _____   ____   ____

II. PHYSICAL INVENTORY

Weight. "Ideal" weight at age 20 was ____. If current weight is more than 20 pounds over that, score (+6) for each 20 pounds. If same as at age 20, or less gain than 10 pounds (−3).   ____   ____

Blood pressure. Under 40 years, if above 130/80 (+12); over forty years, if above 140/90 (+12).   ____   ____

Cholesterol. Under 40 years, if above 220 (+6); over 40 years, if above 250 (+6).   ____   ____

Heart murmur. Not an "innocent" type (+24); with history of rheumatic fever (+48).   ____   ____

	+	−
Pneumonia. If bacterial pneumonia more than 3 times in life (+6).	___	___
Asthma. (+6).	___	___
Rectal polyps. (+6).	___	___
Diabetes. Adult-onset type (+18).	___	___
Depressions. Severe, frequent (+12).	___	___
Regular* medical checkup. Complete (−12); partial (−6).	___	___
Regular dental checkup. Twice yearly (−3).	___	___
Part II Totals	___	___

*Regular refers to healthy people who have thorough medical exams at the following frequencies, according to age: 60 and up, every year; 50–60, every 2 years; 40–50, every 3 years; 30–40, every 5 years; 25–30, as required for jobs, military, etc.

III. FAMILY AND SOCIAL INVENTORY

	+	−
Father. If alive and over 68 years, for each 5 years above 68 (−3); if alive and under 68 or dead after age 68 (0); if dead of medical causes (not accident) before 68 (+3).	___	___
Mother. If alive and over 73 years, for each 5 years above 73 (−3); if alive under 68 or dead after age 68 (0); if dead of medical causes (not accident) before 73 (+3).	___	___
Marital status. If married (0); unmarried and over 40 (+6).	___	___
Home location. Large city (+6); suburb (0); farm or small town (−3).	___	___
Part III Totals	___	___

IV. FOR WOMEN ONLY

	+	−
Family history of breast cancer. In mother or sisters (+6).	___	___
Examines breasts monthly (−6).	___	___
Yearly breast exam by physician (−6).	___	___
Pap smear yearly (−6).	___	___
Part IV Totals	___	___

SCORE	+	-
ENTER TOTALS FROM PART I_____	____	____
PART II _____	____	____
PART III_____	____	____
PART IV _____	____	____
TOTAL _____	____	____

Chart total (+ or–)_____

Enter your current age _____

Divide chart total by 12 and enter with + or – _____

Add or subtract the above figure from your current age to find
YOUR MEDICAL AGE. _____

The table above was adapted by the Center for Health Education, Blue Cross and Blue Shield of Greater New York Center, from *How to Be Your Own Doctor . . . Sometimes* by Keith W. Sehnert, M.D., with Howard Eisenberg, Grosset & Dunlap, 1975.

This book is a collection of columns that have appeared in *The New York Times* and about 100 other newspapers since November 1976. It is not a textbook but rather a series of informative essays. Their accuracy and relevance have been attested to by hundreds of physicians and other health experts who have used them in patient education programs. Each chapter has been edited and updated so that it represents the most reliable and current information available at the beginning of 1982. Of course, medical knowledge continually undergoes modification, and changes will be incorporated as warranted in future printings.

Although not every ailment can possibly be covered in this or any other such work, the book is an all-purpose guide to the most common health problems that confront Americans today. It is also a guide to wise use of medical and other health care resources as well as of resources inherent in you that can enhance your well-being and quality of life. It is not a substitute for medical care, but an adjunct. It should not be used as an excuse to defy "doctor's orders," but to challenge or question them when you have reason to doubt their wisdom. Whenever possible, you are referred to sources of further information and assistance.

This book is meant to be read while you are healthy, not merely used as a ready reference guide when something goes wrong. In many cases it can help you to ward off health problems that might otherwise befall you; in others, it can save you an unnecessary trip to the doctor or needlessly risky therapy. Finally, when illness strikes or threatens, it is a guide to appropriate action, enabling you to be a well-informed consumer and active participant in your own medical care. In other words, this book can help to make you healthier and wiser and may even save your life or the life of someone you love.

For Further Reading

Allen, Robert F., Ph.D., with Shirley Linde. *Lifegain.* New York: Appleton-Century-Crofts, 1981.

Cope, Lewis. *Save Your Life.* Minneapolis: Minneapolis *Tribune,* 1979.

Vickery, Donald M., M.D., *Lifeplan for Your Health.* Reading, Mass.: Addison-Wesley, 1978.

Wynder, Ernst L., M.D., ed. *The Book of Health.* New York: Franklin Watts, 1981.

I.
Nutrition

In the most affluent country in the world, millions of people are nutritionally bankrupt. Even if you can afford the very best, you may have a poor diet — overloaded with animal protein and too high in nutritionally empty fats, sugars, and alcohol. Of the calories in the typical American diet, 60 percent come from fat and added sugars; that means we must get 100 percent of the forty-four nutrients essential to life from just 40 percent of our calorie intake.

There is mounting evidence that this distorted diet, which is also too high in salt and cholesterol, underlies many of the nation's leading killing and crippling diseases, including heart attack, cancer of the colon and breast, high blood pressure, diabetes, osteoporosis, kidney and liver disease.

Eighty million Americans — 40 pecent of the population — are overweight by twenty pounds or more. But instead of adopting a long-lasting, nutritionally sound solution to their weight problem, most grasp at health-damaging straws — fad diets and reducing drugs that nearly always fail in the long run and doom their devotees to a lifetime ride on the weight-gain seesaw.

Most of us have moved far from the simple menus of yore based on readily recognizable elements of the Basic Four — grains, fruits and vegetables, milk and milk products, and animal and vegetable protein. More than half the food we eat today is processed, and most consumers know little of its nutritional virtues and shortcomings. We have also moved far from the menu *Homo sapiens* evolved on: a diet rich in complex carbohydrates and fiber (from starchy food, vegetables, and fruits) and low in animal protein. The high-meat, high-sweet, low-fiber diet we currently eat is overtaxing our metabolic abilities and undermining our health.

Since bad eating habits usually do not take their toll until years later, you may not be sufficiently motivated to make the needed adjustments. The following section is intended to help you get and stay on the right nutritional track. No matter how long you've been eating improperly, it's never too late to benefit from a change for the better.

The RDA:
Guide to a Healthy Diet

In the early 1940's, when wartime food shortages threatened the nation's high nutritional standards and the government had to provide millions of meals for the armed forces, the National Academy of Sciences devised a list of human nutritional requirements to help assess the adequacy of various diets. The list and its accompanying explanations noted, wherever scientific studies allowed, how much of each essential nutrient should be consumed each day to cover the needs of nearly all healthy people.

As new information about nutrition became available, that list, known as the Recommended Dietary Allowances, or RDA, was updated periodically (approximately once every five years) and is now widely used to plan food programs like school lunches, to evaluate the findings of nutritional surveys, and to prepare nutrition information labels on packaged foods and vitamin preparations.

The RDA, the most recent of which were published in 1980 by the academy's Committee on Dietary Allowances, depict the nutritional needs of males and females at various stages of life. Although many uncertainties still exist, especially for the elderly, the RDA represent the latest and best available scientific evidence about what the human body needs nutritionally for good health.

The committee emphasizes that the RDA are designed to be applied to populations of healthy people rather than to the diets of individuals. However, they are used to establish the United States Recommended Daily Allowances (USRDA) used in nutrition labeling on foods and vitamin-mineral supplements and as an overall guide to planning individual diets. The USRDA use only one of the RDA values — usually the highest one — thus taking into account the nutritional needs of nearly all healthy persons, regardless of age and sex. As a general guide, a meal should provide approximately one-quarter to one-third of a day's nutritional needs, but satisfying nutritional requirements over a week's worth of meals is considered adequate by the RDA committee.

Guidelines for Good Eating

The committee's latest report also contains many important nutritional messages to help the average person eat healthfully.

Variety. Everyone's diet, the committee maintains, should be composed of a wide variety of foods. As a general rule, if any one food supplies a quarter or more of your daily calories (especially if that "food" is alcohol or sweet snacks or desserts), chances are you are not consuming all the nutrients your body needs.

The RDA are not intended to be satisfied by your taking nutritional supplements or consuming one or more heavily fortified foods. Contrary to advertisements for certain products, there is no need to obtain 100 percent of the day's requirement for ten vitamins and minerals in your morning bowl of cereal, or in any other single food or pill, unless that's all you will eat for the entire day.

Overreliance on fortified foods or vitamin-mineral preparations can lead to false assurances of nutritional adequacy. No one food or pill contains all the needed nutrients in needed amounts. Nor can such a food or pill be manufactured, since the desirable amounts of several of the twenty-five essential vitamins and minerals have not yet been established. It is also possible that a few essential nutrients have not yet been identified and thus cannot be added to manufactured foods or to nutritional supplements, though they would be present naturally in the foods consumed as part of a varied diet. A daily menu constructed around the Basic Four (see chart, page 7) comes close to assuring adequate consumption of all the essential nutrients.

Taking supplements or concentrating on just a few foods also introduces the risk of overconsuming certain nutrients. Some vitamins and minerals are toxic in large doses, and some can interfere with the body's ability to use other essential nutrients.

Adaptability. The human body is able to adjust to variations in the supply of most essential nutrients. The body can store excess energy (calories) as fat, to call upon when more energy is expended than consumed. It has protective regulatory mechanisms for increasing the absorption and decreasing the excretion of some nutrients when they are in short supply in the diet.

"If the recommended dietary allowance for a nutrient is not met on a particular day, a surplus consumed shortly thereafter will compensate for the inadequacy for normal individuals," the committee states. Thus, though the RDA are expressed as daily amounts, the committee suggests that "in estimating dietary adequacy, it would seem entirely acceptable to average intakes of nutrients over a five- to eight-day period." However, the committee adds, if you consume an inadequate amount of one or more nutrients over a prolonged period of time, your body's ability to cope with trauma and illness may eventually be impaired.

Individual differences. The nutritional requirements of individuals are not known and, for the most part, cannot be practically determined. Therefore, with the exception of energy (calories), the RDA are set high to take into account the varying needs of normal persons. In other words, the RDA contain a built-in safety factor of as much as 45 percent above the expected needs of most people. Thus, just because your diet falls short of the RDA in several nutrients doesn't necessarily mean you are deficient in these nutrients. However, the farther below the RDA you are, the greater the likelihood of nutritional deficiencies.

Furthermore, certain circumstances can increase your nutritional

3

RECOMMENDED DAILY DIETARY ALLOWANCES

Designed for the maintenance of good nutrition of practically all healthy people in the U.S.

	Age (years)	Weight (pounds)	Protein (grams)	Fat Soluble Vitamins			Water Soluble Vitamins							Minerals					
				Vitamin A (rotinal equivalents)	Vitamin D (micrograms of cholesterol)	Vitamin E (mg alpha-tocopherol equivalents)	Vitamin C (milligrams)	Thiamine (milligrams)	Riboflavin (milligrams)	Niacin (milligrams niacin equivalents)	Vitamin B$_6$ (milligrams)	Folacin (milligrams)	Vitamin B$_{12}$ (micrograms)	Calcium (milligrams)	Phosphorus (milligrams)	Magnesium (milligrams)	Iron (milligrams)	Zinc (milligrams)	Iodine (micrograms)
Infants	To 6 mos.	13	kg x 2.2	420	10	3	35	0.3	0.4	6	0.3	30	0.5	360	250	50	10	3	40
	To 1 yr.	20	kg x 2.0	400	10	4	35	0.5	0.6	8	0.6	45	1.5	540	360	70	15	5	50
Children	1-3	29	25	400	10	5	45	0.7	0.8	9	0.9	100	2.0	800	800	150	15	10	70
	4-6	44	30	500	10	6	45	0.9	1.0	11	1.3	200	2.5	800	800	200	10	10	90
	7-10	62	34	700	10	7	45	1.2	1.4	16	1.6	300	3.0	800	800	250	10	10	120
Males	11-14	99	45	1000	10	8	50	1.4	1.6	18	1.8	400	3.0	1200	1200	350	18	15	150
	15-18	145	56	1000	10	10	60	1.4	1.7	18	2.0	400	3.0	1200	1200	400	18	15	150
	19-22	154	56	1000	7.5	10	60	1.5	1.7	19	2.2	400	3.0	800	800	350	10	15	150
	23-50	154	56	1000	5	10	60	1.4	1.6	18	2.2	400	3.0	800	800	350	10	15	150
	51+	154	56	1000	5	10	60	1.2	1.4	16	2.2	400	3.0	800	800	350	10	15	150
Females	11-14	101	46	800	10	8	50	1.1	1.3	15	1.8	400	3.0	1200	1200	300	18	15	150
	15-18	120	46	800	10	8	60	1.1	1.3	14	2.0	400	3.0	1200	1200	300	18	15	150
	19-22	120	44	800	7.5	8	60	1.1	1.3	14	2.0	400	3.0	800	800	300	18	15	150
	23-50	120	44	800	5	8	60	1.0	1.2	13	2.0	400	3.0	800	800	300	18	15	150
	51+	120	44	800	5	8	60	1.0	1.2	13	2.0	400	3.0	800	800	300	10	15	150
Pregnant			+30	+200	+5	+2	+20	+0.4	+0.3	+2	+0.6	+400	+1.0	+400	+400	+150	A	+5	+25
Lactating			+20	+400	+5	+3	+40	+0.5	+0.5	+5	+0.5	+100	+1.0	+400	+400	+150	A	+10	+50

ESTIMATED SAFE AND ADEQUATE DAILY DIETARY INTAKES OF ADDITIONAL SELECTED VITAMINS AND MINERALS

| | Vitamins | | | Trace Elements | | | | | | Electrolytes | | |
	Vitamin K (micrograms)	Biotin (micrograms)	Pantothenic (mg)	Copper (mg)	Manganese (mg)	Fluoride (mg)	Chromium (mg)	Selenium (mg)	Molybdenum (mg)	Sodium (mg)	Potassium (mg)	Chloride (mg)
	Age (years)											
Infants To 6 mo.	12	35	2	0.5-0.7	0.5-0.7	0.1-0.5	0.01-0.04	0.01-0.04	0.03-0.06	115-350	350-925	275-700
to 1 yr.	10-20	50	3	0.7-1.0	0.7-1.0	0.2-1.0	0.02-0.08	0.02-0.06	0.04-0.08	250-750	425-1275	400-1200
Children 1-3	15-30	65	3	1.0-1.5	1.0-1.5	0.5-1.5	0.02-0.08	0.02-0.08	0.05-0.1	325-975	550-1650	500-1500
and 4-6	20-40	85	3-4	1.5-2.0	1.5-2.0	1.0-2.5	0.03-0.12	0.03-0.12	0.06-0.15	450-1350	775-2325	700-2100
Adolescents 7-10	30-60	120	4-5	2.0-2.5	2.0-3.0	1.5-2.5	0.05-0.2	0.05-0.2	0.1-0.3	600-1800	1000-3000	925-2775
11+	50-100	100-200	4-7	2.0-3.0	2.5-5.0	1.5-2.5	0.05-0.2	0.05-0.2	0.15-0.5	900-2700	1525-4575	1400-4200
Adults	70-140	100-200	4-7	2.0-3.0	2.5-5.0	1.5-4.0	0.05-0.2	0.05-0.2	0.15-0.5	1100-3300	1875-5825	1700-5100

NOTE: Because there is less information on which to base allowances, these figures are not given in the main table of the Recommended Daily Dietary Allowances and they are provided here in the form of ranges of recommended intakes. Since the toxic levels for many trace elements may be only several times usual intakes, the upper levels for the trace elements given in this table should not be habitually exceeded.

Adopted from Food and Nutrition Board, National Academy of Sciences-National Research Council Revised 1980.

requirements significantly above the RDA. Though the RDA take ordinary life stresses into account, severe physical and emotional trauma, such as illness, injury, and surgery, can increase the need for protein and certain vitamins and minerals, such as vitamin C, calcium, and iron.

Dietary balance. To diminish the risk of heart and other chronic diseases, the RDA committee endorsed "for individual consideration" a shift in the balance of nutrients to favor complex carbohydrates (starches) and fiber-rich whole grains, beans, fruits, and vegetables as partial replacements for refined sugars and dietary fats, especially saturated animal fats.

To prevent high blood pressure, the 1980 RDA also suggest a halving of the usual intake of sodium (consumed primarily as salt) to a range of three to eight grams of salt a day (five grams of salt equal one teaspoon). This could be accomplished, the committee says, by reducing the amount of salt used in cooking and at the table and by cutting back on consumption of obviously salty foods.

Energy and exercise. The committee recognizes that different people need different numbers of calories to maintain normal body weight. Calories are a measure of the amount of energy supplied by foods, just as BTUs (British thermal units) are used to measure the energy of coal. Calories are released when the body digests and absorbs food and then "burns" or stores it as a source of fuel. Some people who are overweight may actually consume fewer calories than those of normal weight. The amount of energy expended as physical activity accounts for much, though not all, of the difference. Age is another factor, with energy requirements diminishing by 2 percent per decade after twenty-one years of age.

The latest national nutritional surveys have shown that some groups of people — particularly women of childbearing age and the elderly — typically consume too few calories to take in the amounts of essential nutrients in the RDA. Yet obesity is increasing among Americans of all ages.

The only way around this apparent contradiction in energy needs is to increase physical activity, which uses up calories and thus allows you to eat more, and to make nearly all the calories you consume count toward good nutrition. The RDA committee points out that a moderately active person can consume an average of 300 calories a day more than the typical American, whose activity level is described as light to sedentary. "For individuals whose energy needs are relatively low, such as the elderly, it is especially critical that foods of high nutrient density be selected to provide an adequate supply of all nutrients," the committee states.

In other words, if you're eating 1,500 calories a day or less, there's little or no room in your diet for "junk food" (nutritionally deficient, calorically dense foods like fats, sweets, and alcohol). Yet, the committee points out, many Americans derive 30 percent or more of their energy (calories) from foods that provide no or few vitamins or minerals.

Megadoses of micronutrients. The committee found no scientific evidence for the nutritional benefits of vitamins, minerals, or trace elements in doses significantly greater than the amounts needed to prevent obvious deficiency symptoms. In some cases, possible hazards were list-

THE BASIC FOUR FOOD GROUPS

Food	Amount per serving*	Servings per day
MILK GROUP		
Milk	8 ounces (1 cup)	Children 0-9 years: 2 to 3
Yogurt, plain	1 cup	Children 9-12 years: 3
Hard cheese	1 ¼ ounces	Teens: 4
Cheese spread	2 ounces	Adults: 2
Ice cream	1 ½ cups	Pregnant women: 3
Cottage cheese	2 cups	Nursing mothers: 4
MEAT GROUP		
Meat, lean	2 to 3 ounces, cooked	2, can be eaten as mixtures of animal
Poultry	2 to 3 ounces	and vegetable foods or as combina-
Fish	2 to 3 ounces	tion of complementary vegetable pro-
Hard cheese	2 to 3 ounces	teins (see p. 11)
Eggs	2 to 3	
Cottage cheese	½ cup	
Dry beans and peas	1 to 1 ½ cups, cooked	
Nuts and seeds	½ to ¾ cup	
Peanut butter	4 tablespoons	
VEGETABLE AND FRUIT GROUP		
Vegetables, cut up	½ cup	4, including one good vitamin C
Fruits, cut up	½ cup	source like oranges or orange juice
Grapefruit	½ medium	and one deep-yellow or dark-green
Melon	½ medium	vegetable.
Orange	1	
Potato	1 medium	
Salad	1 bowl	
Lettuce	1 wedge	
BREAD AND CEREAL GROUP		
Bread	1 slice	4, whole grain or enriched only, in-
Cooked cereal	½ to ¾ cup	cluding at least one serving of whole
Pasta	½ to ¾ cup	grain.
Rice	½ to ¾ cup	
Dry cereal	1 ounce	

*These amounts were established by the U.S. Department of Agriculture to meet specific nutritional requirements. For the milk group, serving sizes are based on the calcium content of 1 cup of milk. For the meat group, serving size is determined by protein content. Thus, rather than eat 2 cups of cottage cheese (milk group) or 4 tablespoons of peanut butter (meat group), it would make more sense to eat half those amounts and count each as half a serving in its group. If cottage cheese (½ cup) is consumed as a meat substitute, you may count it as a full meat serving and a quarter of a milk serving.
Source: "JANE BRODY'S NUTRITION BOOK" by Jane E. Brody. New York: W.W. Norton, 1981.

ed. [See chapter on micronutrients, page 42.]

For example, large amounts of vitamins A and D are toxic; excessive zinc can aggravate an otherwise-inconsequential copper deficiency; too much phosphorus may interfere with the body's ability to use bone-building calcium; excess vitamin B_6 can induce a dependency on abnormally large amounts; high doses of niacin can cause heart rhythm irregularities and gastrointesinal problems; and too much vitamin C may precipitate kidney stones and interfere with the germ-fighting ability of white blood cells.

However, in more moderate amounts vitamin C can help increase the amount of essential iron absorbed from the diet, and the committee recommends that foods containing vitamin C be consumed along with foods rich in iron. The committee also recommends moderation in increasing fiber intake since plant fibers can interfere with the absorption of certain micronutrients, including iron, zinc, and possibly calcium.

Protein:
Too Much of a Good Thing

Protein is widely regarded as the most important nutrient, and the average American tends to consume far more protein than is really needed for good nutrition. While packing in protein, most people also consume too much fat and possibly too many calories, which are the "baggage" in our most popular high-protein foods. Instead of being good to their bodies, they may really do themselves a disservice.

At the same time many don't realize that the vegetables they commonly think of as starchy (that is, laden with carbohydrates) can actually be good sources of protein without the artery-clogging fats and cholesterol that are in most animal protein foods.

Others who spurn animal protein — whether for religious, moral, or health reasons — and instead rely on vegetable protein may not consume adequate amounts of usable protein because they don't understand the precise demands of the body's protein requirements.

Yet, if vegetarians eat wisely, they may actually preserve their health by avoiding animal protein. A study of 116 young vegetarians in Boston showed that they had far lower blood pressures and much less fat and cholesterol (lipids) in their blood than comparable Americans who ate a regular diet. The vegetarians who ate dairy products and eggs more than five times a week had higher blood pressures and cholesterol levels than those who ate animal products less often or not at all. But all vegetarian groups had lower pressures and cholesterol levels than the meat eaters, but also weighed less than the comparison group.

Many people believe that athletes can't make it without meat protein, yet the ranks of vegetarians include a number of Olympic athletes and gold-medal winners.

The myths and misconceptions about protein date back at least 150 years, when a Dutch chemist coined the name "protein" from a Greek word meaning "to take first place." Perhaps the chemist was acknowledging the primacy of protein's main functions — to maintain body tissues and support growth — and the fact that the body can make protein only from proteins supplied in the diet, whereas fats and carbohydrates can be derived from one another and from proteins as well.

Thinking of protein as the "first place" nutrient overlooks the nutritional value of carbohydrates and the fact that these foods, rather than protein, provide the bulk of calories in a healthy diet. In fact, if the diet does not contain adequate calories from carbohydrates or fats, the body is forced to use protein for energy instead of for building or repairing body tissues.

The main malnutrition problem in developing countries is actually a shortage of calories rather than protein. If more carbohydrates or fat calories were available, in most cases the diets in these countries would contain enough protein to support normal growth and development.

What Your Body Does with Protein

Proteins are made up of chains of building blocks called amino acids, molecules that contain nitrogen. Sometimes as many as 200 amino acid molecules are strung together to make one protein. There are twenty-two different amino acids in nature, and the human body is able to manufacture all but nine of them from carbohydrates and nitrogen, usually derived from dietary proteins. These nine are called essential amino acids; they all must be supplied in the diet for the body to be able to manufacture the hundreds of different proteins it needs.

All protein is originally derived from plants, which, unlike animals, can incorporate inorganic nitrogen from the air and soil into organic compounds (amino acids) that can be used by humans and other animals. But there are important differences between animal and plant (vegetable) proteins. Most animal protein contains all the essential amino acids, whereas the vegetable proteins may be deficient in one or another essential amino acid. To derive complete protein from vegetable sources, different plant proteins that compensate for one another's deficiencies must be consumed. (Protein content listed on package labels under "Nutrition Information" refers to total protein, not necessarily the amount of usable protein the food contains. If the product contains only a single source of vegetable protein, the amount of usable protein will be less than that listed unless you combine the food with other complementary protein sources.)

The protein you eat is broken down, or digested, into its constituent amino acids, which are absorbed into the bloodstream and distributed to cells, where they can be reassembled into new proteins according to the needs of the cells. Every cell in your body contains some protein. Protein constitutes 50 percent of the body's dry weight. Muscle, bone, cartilage, skin, blood, and lymph all contain protein. All enzymes and many hormones are protein. Only bile and urine normally lack protein.

Protein in muscle allows it to contract and hold water. In hair, skin, and nails, the protein is hard and insoluble, giving a body a protective coating. Protein elasticizes blood vessel walls, allowing them to expand and contract to maintain normal blood pressure. And protein provides the rigid framework for the minerals of bones and teeth. Without protein, new tissues needed for growth cannot be formed and old worn-out tissues cannot be replaced. Proteins are also involved in regulating the body's water and acid-base balance and stimulating the production of antibodies.

Getting the Most Out of Protein

Diet factors that affect the body's ability to use protein include the following:

● Whether the diet contains sufficient calories to fulfill the body's energy needs. If calories are inadequate, the body will use protein in the diet for fuel rather than for tissue building.

● The frequency with which protein is supplied in the diet. The body doesn't store protein the way it stores extra fat in fat cells or extra carbohydrates in the liver and muscles. Protein must be consumed daily, preferably at each meal. The body uses protein most efficiently if it is consumed in frequent small meals — for example, six a day — than if it is eaten at two or three big meals. If your diet chronically contains insufficient protein, your body will use the protein of your muscles and organs to perform life-sustaining functions.

● Whether the protein consumed is balanced to supply adequate amounts of essential amino acids plus a healthy supply of the nonessential ones. Because protein is not stored, all the amino acids needed to make new protein must be supplied at the same meal. If the protein you eat comes from animals (for example, meat, milk products, fish, poultry, or eggs), it will be balanced enough to assure efficient utilization. An exception is gelatin, which is missing two essential amino acids. If eaten alone (say, as a bedtime snack), the protein in gelatin can be used only for energy, not to make new protein.

A vegetable protein source that is nearly as well balanced as animal protein is soybeans. However, most vegetable proteins lack adequate amounts of one or more essential amino acids to suffice by themselves as protein sources. For the body to use these vegetables (and gelatin) to make new protein, several different ones — called complementary proteins — must be combined in the same meal or they must be eaten with animal protein so that the amino acid deficiencies in the vegetable are made up for by the other foods eaten. [See chart.]

For example, the Mexicans eat tortillas (corn bread, which is low in the essential amino acid lysine) with beans (which have plenty of lysine but are short on another essential amino acid, methionine, which is plentiful in corn) and thereby derive a balanced protein. A peanut butter sandwich on whole wheat bread is also balanced protein. Some other examples are rice and beans, yams and beans, nuts and beans, macaroni and cheese, cereal and milk, rice or bulgur with meat, fish, or poultry.

When a vegetable protein is supplemented with animal protein, only a very small amount of the animal protein is needed to provide the complementary amino acids for the vegetable protein. In many Asian cultures, for example, rice is the main source of protein, with meat or poultry used as a condiment to balance out the vegetable protein.

Other factors that affect the body's use of protein include inactivity, injury, illness, and emotional stress, all of which lead to an excessive loss of nitrogen in the urine, indicating that protein in body tissues is being used up or that protein in the diet is not being used efficiently and instead is being excreted.

Calculating Your Protein Needs

In general, the amount of protein your body needs is mainly determined by your age and size. Per pound of body weight, the need is greatest during the first six months of life, and except for women who are pregnant or breast-feeding and need extra protein, the protein requirement declines slowly with age.

The Food and Nutrition Board of the National Research Council has prepared a list of Recommended Dietary Allowances (RDA) for protein. [See chart, page 12.] However, the average American eats two to four times the recommended amounts, with the extra protein simply being a source of calories (4 calories a gram), not protein, for the body. This is why you can get fat eating excess protein. It is generally recommended that a third to a half of the needed protein should come from

COMPLEMENTARY VEGETABLE PROTEINS

To obtain complete protein from plant foods, combine any mature legume — soybeans or soy products like tofu or soy milk, peanuts, black-eyed peas, lentils, kidney beans, chickpeas (garbanzos), navy beans, pinto beans, lima beans, etc. — with any of the following:

Corn
Rice (white or brown)
Wheat (bread, pasta, cereal, or grains)
Seeds (sesame, pumpkin, or sunflower)
Barley
Oats

Or combine rice or corn with wheat germ or seeds.

animal sources, and the rest from vegetables, but in this country 60 to 80 percent of the protein eaten is animal protein, and most of that is laden with fat and cholesterol. [See chapter on fats, page 14.]

According to the RDA, an eight-year-old child weighing 60 pounds needs nearly the same amount of protein each day — about 33 grams — as a 100-pound adult woman. A 150-pound adult, whose RDA for protein is about 54 grams a day, could satisfy that need by eating, for example, 3 ounces of cooked beef or chicken (about 24 grams protein), a cup of broccoli (6 grams), two tablespoons of peanut butter (8 grams) and a cup of cooked dried beans (16 grams).

In planning your total diet, nutritionists recommend that protein constitute only 10 to 15 percent of your daily calories; fats no more than 30 percent (and preferably 10 to 20 percent); and carbohydrates, 55 to 70 percent. In cutting back on protein, most Americans will automatically reduce their fat intake, probably to the benefit of their hearts and blood vessels. There is some experimental evidence that too much protein, as well as excess fat, can promote atherosclerosis and cancer. Eating less fatty protein should also help to reduce calorie intake since gram for gram, fat has more than twice the calories that carbohydrates have.

Excessive consumption of protein also taxes the kidneys, which must rid the body of the nitrogen from the protein it doesn't need. For

DAILY RECOMMENDED DIETARY ALLOWANCE FOR PROTEIN

	Age (in years)	Protein (grams per lb. ideal body wt.)
Infants	0-0.5	1.00
	0.5-1	0.90
Children	1-3	0.81
	4-6	0.68
	7-10	0.55
	11-14	0.45
	15-18	0.39
Adults	19 and over	0.36
	Pregnant women	0.62
	Nursing women	0.53

Note: Here are some sample calculations to determine a day's protein needs:
   For a 5-year-old child who weighs 50 pounds: 0.68 X 50 =34 grams.
   For a 160-pound man: 0.36 X 160 =57.6 grams.
   For a 110-pound 12 year old: 0.45 X 110 =49.5 grams.
   For a 125-pound pregnant woman: 0.62 X 125 =77.5 grams.
   According to the Food and Nutrition Board of the National Academy of Sciences—National Research Council, the amounts of protein determined in this fashion should be adequate to meet the needs of virtually all healthy persons.

most people, this is no problem, but for those with actual or potential kidney disease or immature kidneys (such as premature babies), the extra protein may be more than the kidneys can handle, and toxic levels of urea compounds can build up in the blood. Diets very high in protein also promote the loss of calcium from bones and may contribute to bone loss. [See chapter on osteoporosis, page 610.]

Protein is indeed an essential nutrient. But like every other good thing, it is possible and potentially undesirable to get too much of it.

For Further Reading

Lapplé, Frances Moore. *Diet for a Small Planet.* New York: Ballantine Books, 1975.
Sussman, Vic S. *The Vegetarian Alternative.* Emmaus, Pa.: Rodale, 1978.

WHAT COMES WITH THE PROTEIN YOU EAT

When choosing protein to fulfill your RDA, you should have some idea of what else is in the food you eat. Some protein foods contain mostly fat calories, whereas others are primarily starchy carbohydrates, which are more nutritious and less damaging to health.

Food	PERCENT OF CALORIES		
	Protein	Fat	Carbohydrate
I-bone steak	17	82	—
Frankfurter	16	80	2
Bacon	20	77	2
Cheddar cheese	25	73	2
Cottage cheese, creamed	51	35	11
Cod fish fillet	67	28	—
Fish sticks	38	46	15
Chicken with skin	44	53	—
Chicken, white meat without skin	76	18	—
Eggs	32	63	2
Tuna in oil	34	64	—
Tuna in water	88	6	—
Whole milk	22	46	30
Skim milk	40	2	57
Yogurt, low fat	27	31	42
Kidney beans	25	5	70
Lentils	29	—	70
Peanut butter	17	76	13
Bread, whole wheat	17	11	79
Oatmeal	15	16	70
Macaroni	14	3	81
Potato, baked	11	1	90

13

Fats and Cholesterol: Arterial Nemesis

If there is one nutrient that has the decks stacked against it, it's fat. The typical American diet not only is rich in protein, but it also has a higher fat content than nearly any other diet in the world. While agreement on this issue is not universal, many scientists blame this high-fat diet for a number of our chronic health problems and killing diseases, among them heart disease, obesity, and possibly cancers of the colon, breast, and uterus.

Fat is a more concentrated source of calories than any other nutrient and thus is the most "fattening" foodstuff we regularly consume. A gram of dietary fat supplies your body with 9 calories, compared with only 4 calories per gram of either carbohydrates or protein. Even alcohol has fewer calories (7 per gram) than fat. Cutting down on fats is one of the best ways to reduce calorie intake and achieve and maintain a normal body weight.

At the turn of the century fat accounted for about 32 percent of the calories consumed by the average American. Today, more than 40 percent of our calories come from fat. We eat a lot more cholesterol-lowering polyunsaturated vegetable fats than we used to, but we haven't cut back much on cholesterol-raising saturated fats, which come mainly from animal foods.

Although the role of dietary fats and cholesterol in heart disease remains controversial, many independent scientific and medical experts are convinced by existing evidence that switching to a lower-fat diet is sensible and potentially lifesaving. Several recent studies suggest that even a relatively late-in-life switch can at least partly reverse arterial clogging and reduce the risk of premature death from heart disease.

To make such a switch in a nutritionally intelligent fashion, it is helpful to know what kinds and amounts of fats are in the various foods you eat and what effects these fats have on the cholesterol that courses through and eventually clogs your blood vessels.

Kinds of Fats and Their Effects

Most of the fat we eat is superfluous from a nutritional standpoint. To meet basic nutritional needs, we need to eat only one tablespoon of a polyunsaturated oil each day. This supplies the essential fatty acid, linoleic acid, and helps us absorb fat-soluble vitamins. The average American adult eats six to eight times this amount of fat, making fat a major source of nutritionally empty calories for millions of Americans.

There's no denying that dietary fats enhance flavor and texture and make foods more palatable. Fats also help to produce feelings of satiety by turning off gastric juices. Since they are absorbed by the gut over a period of four to six hours — far more slowly than proteins or carbohydrates — they help to reduce hunger between meals.

Fats are made up of three types of fatty acids — saturated, monounsaturated, and polyunsaturated — determined by how many places exist on the molecule for additional atoms of hydrogen. A fatty acid that has no room for more hydrogen is called saturated; one which can take two more hydrogen atoms is monounsaturated, and one that has room for four or more additional hydrogen atoms is polyunsaturated.

Animal fats generally have a high proportion of saturated fatty acids and few polyunsaturates. In addition, all animal fat contains cholesterol (see chart below). By contrast, vegetable oils have no cholesterol,

CONTENTS OF FATS AND OILS
Amounts in one tablespoon

Types of Fats	Calories	P/S Ratio	Chol.	Fatty Acids (as percent of calories)		
				Sat.	Mono-unsat.	Poly-unsat.
Butter	100	0.08	31	64	30	4
Lard	115	0.2	13	40	41	10
Tub margarine						
Liquid safflower oil	101	4.5	0	14	23	60
Liquid corn oil	102	2.2	0	18	41	40
Stick margarine						
Liquid corn oil	102	1.6	0	22	39	35
Stick or tub margarine						
Partially hydrogenated						
or hardened oil	102	1.7	0	20	44	33
Imitation (diet) margarine	49	1.8	0	20	40	37
Mayonnaise	100	2.8	0	18	22	50
Vegetable shortening,						
hydrogenated	110	1.0	0	26	47	24
Corn oil	120	4.6	0	13	25	59
Cottonseed oil	120	1.9	0	28	20	53
Safflower oil	120	7.7	0	10	12	75
Sesame oil	120	2.7	0	16	41	43
Soybean oil	120	3.9	0	16	24	60
Soybean oil, lightly						
hydrogenated	120	2.4	0	15	44	35
Sunflower oil	120	5.9	0	11	22	67
Olive oil	120	0.6	0	14	73	8
Peanut oil	120	1.8	0	17	47	32
Coconut oil	120	0.02	0	91	6	2
Palm oil	120	0.2	0	54	37	10

Source: Based on data from the American Heart Association.

15

DAILY FAT AND CHOLESTEROL FOOD SCORE

How to use this chart: For each portion of fat-containing foods consumed during a day, record the appropriate score. The goal is to keep your daily total score to 10 or less.

SCORE	Fat-containing foods
	Egg and Egg Preparations
5	Egg (1)
2	Waffle (1 piece)
2	French toast (1 slice)
2	Pancakes (two 5-inch)
−1	Egg substitute (¼ cup)
−1	Above items made with egg substitute and 0 or −1 fat or oil
	Fat and Oil Foods
2	Butter (1 teaspoon)
2	French fries (20 pieces)
2	Hash browns (½ cup)
2	Breaded, fried vegetable (½ cup)
1	Regular margarine (1 teaspoon)
1	Bacon fat or lard (1 teaspoon)
1	Bacon (1 slice)
1	Cream or cheese sauce (2 tablespoons)
1	Peanuts or mixed nuts (2 ounces)
1	Shortening (2 teaspoons)
1	Chicken fat (2 teaspoons)
1	Gravy of beef or pork fat drippings (4 tablespoons)
1	Gravy of poultry drippings (8 tablespoons)
1	Potato or corn chips (20 pieces)
0	Margarine with polyunsaturate-to-saturate ratio of 2:1 (1 teaspoon)
0	Salad oils—soy, peanut, olive, or blends (1 teaspoon)
0	Mayonnaise or salad dressing (1 tablespoon)
−1	Margarine with polyunsaturate-to-saturate ratio of more than 2:1 (1 teaspoon)
−1	Salad oil—corn or safflower (1 teaspoon)
−1	Walnuts (8 halves)
−1	Sunflower seeds (1 ounce)
	Dairy Foods and Substitutes
3	Whole milk (1 cup)
3	Cheese (1 ounce)
3	Ice cream (½ cup)
3	Yogurt from whole milk (1 cup)
2	2% milk (1 cup)
2	Yogurt of part-skim milk (1 cup)
2	Creamed cottage cheese (½ cup)
2	Sour cream (1 tablespoon)
1	99% fat-free milk (1 cup)
1	Milk sherbet (1 cup)
1	Ice milk (½ cup)
1	*Cream soups (1 cup)
1	*Chowders (½ cup)
1	Nondairy coffee whiteners (2 tablespoons liquid or 3 teaspoons powder)
1	Pressurized whipped cream or whipped toppings (1 heaping tablespoon)
1	Light cream or light sour cream (1 tablespoon)
0	Skim milk (1 cup)
0	Buttermilk of skim milk (1 cup)

SCORE	Fat-Containing foods
0	Low-fat or uncreamed cottage cheese (½ cup)
0	Nondairy polyunsaturated coffee whitener (2 tablespoons)

Baked Goods, Desserts, and Sweets

4	Cream or whipped cream pastries and desserts
4	Custard, rice, or bread puddings (½ cup)
4	Pies: Cream, custard, pumpkin, chiffon
4	Danish or butter pastries
4	Cheese cake
4	Pound cake or all-butter cakes
4	Sponge cake or jelly roll
2	Doughnut
2	Sweet roll or coffee cake
2	Fruit pies or turnovers
2	Frosted cake or cupcake
2	Puddings (¼ cup)
2	Chocolate candy bar
1	Muffin or coffee breads
1	Brownie or bar cookie (2-inch square)
1	Rich cookie (1 large or 2 small)
1	Pie crust
1	Biscuits (1 large or 2 small)
1	Unfrosted cake or cupcake
1	Fudge or butterscotch sauce (2 tablespoons)
1	Rich snack crackers (1 dozen)
0	Any of above items made with 0 foods
−1	Any of above items made with −1 foods

Meat and Meat Substitutes

6	Highly fat-streaked beef, pork, lamb, ham, or Canadian bacon (2-3 ounces)
6	Hamburger, cold cuts, sausages, frankfurters, tongue (2-3 ounces)
6	Liver or liver spread (2-3 ounces)
4	Slightly fat-streaked beef, pork, lamb, ham or Canadian bacon with visible fat trimmed (2-3 ounces)
4	Lean ground beef, meatballs, or meatloaf (2-3 ounces)
4	*Breaded and fried meat, chicken, or shellfish (2-3 ounces)
4	*Italian meat sauce (2-3 ounces)
2	Very lean, fat-trimmed beef, pork, lamb, ham, or Canadian bacon (2-3 ounces)
2	Boiled shrimp or shrimp salad (2-3 ounces)
2	Ham salad (½ cup)
1	Chicken or turkey (2-3 ounces)
1	Peanut butter (4 tablespoons)
5	Macaroni and cheese (1 cup)
5	Pizza (½ of 10-inch pie or ¼ of 14-inch pie)
5	Lasagna (½ cup)
5	*Creamed main course (1 cup)
5	*Beef hash (1 cup)
5	*Stews (1 cup)
5	*Chili (1 cup)
6	*Spaghetti with meat sauce (1 cup)
5	*American chop suey (1 cup)
5	*Meat pies

*Commercially prepared

Source: Based on data from University of Minnesota Laboratory of Physiological Hygiene.

and most vegetable oils ("oil" merely means fat that is liquid at room temperature, with the word "fat" reserved for those oils that are solid) are relatively low in saturated fatty acids and high in polyunsaturates. In two vegetable oils — peanut and olive — monounsaturates predominate, and coconut and palm "oils" contain mostly saturated fatty acids.

For health reasons, polyunsaturates are preferred because they tend to reduce the amount of cholesterol carried in the blood by enhancing the excretion of cholesterol in the feces. On the other hand, saturated fats (except for stearic acid in cocoa butter) raise blood cholesterol, particularly the type of cholesterol that can become part of the fatty plaques that clog arteries. Ounce for ounce, saturated fats are twice as effective in raising blood cholesterol as polyunsaturates are in lowering it. Monounsaturates have no discernible effect on serum cholesterol and are considered "neutral" as far as heart disease is concerned.

As a nation we have become very fat-conscious in recent years, and many people have switched to leaner cuts of meat and low-fat dairy products and substituted artery-sparing polyunsaturated margarines and vegetable oils for the heavily saturated fats like butter, lard, and bacon fat. Still, most people consume far more fat — and certainly more saturated fat — than they realize. This is because only about a third of the fat we eat is so-called visible fat, such as the hunks or strips of hard fat on meat, the fats and oils we use in cooking and seasoning our foods, and the oil-based dressings we pour on salads.

Cutting Down on Hidden Fat

Most of the fat in our diets is *hidden* fat. It is the hard-to-notice marbling in meat. It is an integral part of hard cheeses and cream cheese, fish, deep-fried foods, nuts, seeds, cream soups, ice cream, and chocolate. It is a major ingredient in a wide variety of factory-prepared products, including baked goods (especially cakes, pies and cookies), processed meats (frankfurters, bologna, and the like), instant meals, coffee whiteners, whipped toppings, snack foods, and granolas. Even one popular diet product, Pillsbury's Figurines, has fat as its main ingredient.

Yet those who advocate more healthful diets that are not overly dependent on red meat often substitute fattier foods than the ones they reject. Examples include the quiches, avocado salads, nuts and seeds, nut butters, sesame paste, and granolas featured in health food restaurants and stores. A quiche is made from cheese in which three-fourths of the calories come from fat that is more saturated than meat fat, cream in which nearly all the calories are fat, and piecrust in which more than half the calories are fat calories.

Similarly, 85 percent of the calories in nuts come from fats, and three-fourths of the calories in seeds (for example, sunflower seeds) and avocados are fat calories. Whereas most breakfast cereals contain little or no fat, granolas derive about a third of their calories from the fat in nuts, seeds, coconut, and added oil.

Don't assume that a label claiming "high in polyunsaturates" means you can eat all you want. High compared with what? It may also be high in saturates and cholesterol. Besides, the idea in the prudent diet is not simply to add polyunsaturates to your current diet. Rather, the goal is, first, to reduce your total fat intake and second, to substitute polyunsaturates for saturates wherever reasonable.

The meals you eat in restaurants also may contain far more fat than you may suspect. You may pass up the butter on your bread, the sour cream for your baked potato, and dishes that are deep-fried. But your soup, gravy, and sauces may be swimming with hidden fat; your steak (already three-fourths fat calories) or your fish may be broiled with butter; your salad may be loaded with a fatty dressing; and your rich desserts may contain far more fat than sugar.

Nutrition and Health, a newsletter prepared by the Institute of Human Nutrition at Columbia University, advises that you avoid certain dishes on restaurant menus: those called creamed, in cream sauce or in its own gravy; sauteed, fried, pan-fried or crispy; escalloped, au gratin, or with cheese sauce; buttery, buttered, or in butter sauce; au lait, a la mode,

CALCULATING FATS ON LABELS

Sun Country Granola

Serving size   2 ounces (½ cup)

	Per serving
Calories	260
Protein	6 grams
Carbohydrates	40 grams
Fat	8 grams

To calculate the percentage of calories from fat in each serving, multiply the number of fat grams (8) by 9, which is the number of calories in one gram of fat. Divide the result, which is 72, by 260, the number of calories per serving. Multiply the result, 0.277, by 100 to obtain the percentage of fat calories, 27.7 percent.

Green Giant Cauliflower in a flavored cheese sauce

Serving size   1 cup

	Per serving
Calories	130
Protein	5 grams
Carbohydrates	13 grams
Fat	6 grams
Sodium	735 milligrams

Percent of calories from fat per serving: 6 x 9 = 54.

$$54 / 130 = 0.415$$
$$0.415 \times 100 = 41.5\% \text{ fat}$$

(Cauliflower without a cream sauce has only 10% fat calories.)

or au fromage; marinated, stewed, basted, or casserole; prime, hash, pot pie, or hollandaise.

Instead, the institute suggests that you choose dishes described as pickled, in tomato sauce or with cocktail sauce, steamed, in broth, in its own juice, poached, garden fresh, roasted, or stir-fried.

Here are some other tips for reducing your consumption of hidden fats:

Meats, fish, and poultry. Avoid the heavily marbled prime cuts of meat and all processed meats. Lean boiled ham or sliced turkey are much lower in fat than bologna, salami, or other luncheon meats. Buy lean hamburger (especially if you prefer your burgers rare). Flank steak, sirloin tip, and London broil are among the leaner cuts of beef. Leg of lamb and veal are also lean.

Broil or grill, rather than fry, meats, fish, and poultry. Prepare stews and soups in advance, chill them, and remove the fat that hardens at the top. Discard the skin of poultry before or after cooking. Avoid gravies and cream sauces in restaurants; make gravy at home after skimming off the fat.

Tuna and salmon are among the fattier fish. Sardines packed in oil and many forms of smoked fish are also high in fat. Fillets of flounder, cod, haddock, halibut, perch, and sole and shellfish have considerably less fat. Canned tuna packed in water has two-thirds less fat than tuna packed in oil.

Substitute vegetable sources of protein — dried beans and peas (for example, kidney beans, split peas, lentils, and bean curd) — and low-fat dairy products (cottage cheese and yogurt) for meat in some of your meals.

Dairy products. Use skim milk or low-fat (1 to 2 percent) milk, yogurt, cottage cheese, and ricotta cheese. Buttermilk (contrary to its name, it contains little or no butterfat) adds richness but little fat to pancakes and baked goods. Avoid sour cream and sweet cream, both light and heavy. If you prepare pudding from a packaged mix, use skim milk to reduce the fat — and calorie — content.

Ice milk and frozen yogurt have less fat than ice cream, and "thick" shakes have less fat than milk shakes, but there is usually no calorie saving because they contain considerably more sugar than ice cream does. Soft ice cream (frozen custard) and soft-serve ice milk contain more fat than the hard varieties.

Parmesan cheese and mozzarella cheese made from part-skim milk have less fat than other hard cheeses. Many markets now also carry reduced-fat "imitation" cheeses in which the saturated dairy fat has been replaced by polyunsaturated vegetable oil.

Fats. Whipped butter and margarine and diet or imitation margarines contain less fat per serving than regular butter and margarine (air or water replaces some of the fat in these products). Many margarines, especially the cheaper brands, contain large amounts of vegetable oils that have been partially saturated during processing. The best margarines list a "liquid" vegetable oil as the first ingredient. Also check the nutrition information listed on the label. The product should contain at least two grams of polyunsaturates for every one gram of saturates, and the higher the poly-to-saturate ratio, the better. The highest ratios are found in soft tub and bottled liquid margarines.

A tablespoon of oil or mayonnaise has as many fat calories as a tablespoon of hard fat; however, the softer fats are less saturated.

Baked goods. Most commercially prepared sweetened baked goods contain a lot of fat, and it is usually saturated fat. An exception is angel food cake. A graham cracker crust can be made with less fat than ordinary pie crust. Slightly sweetened toasts, gingersnaps, fig bars, and vanilla wafers have less fat than cookies made with chocolate, cream filling, or nuts.

In place of fat-rich biscuits, muffins, croissants, and butter rolls, choose sandwich bread, hard rolls, pita bread, English muffins, or French or Italian bread. Matzos, toasts, breadsticks, and crisps are low-fat substitutes for fattier crackers. Popcorn without butter or margarine (especially if hot-air popped) is an excellent low-fat, low-calorie snack food.

Soups. Use skim milk to prepare cream soups. In restaurants, choose clear consommé or broth, madrilene, or clear soup prepared with noodles, rice, or vegetables.

Salads. In restaurants, order your salad dressings on the side. At home, experiment with low-fat dressings made with herbs and spices, yo-

THE FAT IN PACKAGED FOODS

It is difficult to know how much fat might be contained in most processed foods. Check the list of ingredients on the label; ingredients are listed in order of their prominence by weight. If a fat is listed among the first few ingredients — especially if it is listed ahead of other main ingredients (such as butter in pound cake, which precedes the flour) — it is likely to be high in fat.

To determine the fat content of a product that has nutrition information listed on the label, multiply the number of grams of fat in a serving by 9. Then divide this total by the number of calories per serving. Multiply the result by 100, and you will have the percent of fat calories in the product. For example, 8 ounces of whole milk contain 165 calories and 9 grams of fat. Multiplying 9 grams by 9 calories per gram yields 81 calories from fat. Dividing by 165, then multiplying by 100 gives 49 percent fat calories.

If the nutritional label says one gram of fat or less per serving, consider the food acceptable for a low-fat diet. However, if the label lists "vegetable oil," with its kind unspecified, or if it lists coconut or palm oil as a major ingredient, avoid it. Some products, including many cake mixes, are made with the cheapest oil available at the time (often coconut oil, which is far more saturated than any animal fat), and, therefore, the label is nonspecific. If you don't know the kind of fat in a processed food, it's better to make your own.

THE AMOUNT OF FAT IN FOOD

Percent of Calories from Fat	Type of Food
	Dairy Products
More than 75%	Butter
	Cream — half-and-half, heavy, and sour
	Cream cheese
	Whipped cream
50 to 75%	Rich ice cream
	Hard cheeses — cheddar, Swiss, American, etc.
40 to 50%	Regular ice cream
	Whole milk
	Whole-milk yogurt
30 to 40%	2% milk
	Creamed cottage cheese
	Ice milk
	Low-fat yogurt
20 to 30%	Thick shake
	1% milk
	1% fat cottage cheese
Less than 20%	Skim milk
	Buttermilk
	Uncreamed cottage cheese
	Farmer's cheese
	Frozen yogurt
	Fish
More than 75%	(none)
50 to 75%	Fried perch
	Tuna with oil
	Tuna salad
40 to 50%	Sardines, drained
	Mackerel
	Canned salmon
30 to 40%	Fried flounder or haddock
	Broiled halibut
	Tuna in oil, drained
	Scallops and shrimp, breaded and fried
20 to 30%	Broiled cod
	Raw oysters
Less than 20%	Broiled ocean perch
	Scallops and shrimp, steamed or boiled
	Tuna in water

Percent of Calories from Fat	Type of Food
	Red Meats
More than 75%	Bacon
	Choice sirloin
	Regular hamburger
	Cold cuts (bologna, salami, etc.)
	Frankfurters
	Pork sausage
	Spareribs
50 to 75%	Corned beef
	Rib lamb chops
	Pork loin
	Ham
40 to 50%	Lean T-bone
	Lean hamburger
30 to 40%	Flank steak
	Lean chuck pot roast
20 to 30%	Sirloin tip
Less than 20%	(none)

Percent of Calories from Fat	Type of Food
	Vegetable and Grain-based Foods
More than 75%	Avocado
	Coconut
	Cole slaw
	Nuts and peanut butter
	Olives
50 to 75%	Pound cake
40 to 50%	Chocolate cake with icing
30 to 40%	Yellow or white cake without icing
	Granola
	Pizza
20 to 30%	Corn muffin
	Pancakes
	Wheat germ
Less than 20%	Angel food and sponge cake
	Dried beans, peas, and lentils
	Bread
	Grains — bulgur, couscous, rice, millet, etc.
	Pasta
	Breakfast cereals (except granola)
	Vegetables and fruits (except those listed above)

gurt, and buttermilk, perhaps with just a small amount of mayonnaise. Treat avocados with the same discretion you bestow upon bacon, butter, and margarine; they all are high in fats.

The Cholesterol Controversy

Probably no other aspect of nutrition confuses people more than cholesterol, a waxy alcohol found only in animal foods that has long been labeled a primary culprit — along with its usual companion, saturated fats — in the national epidemic of heart disease.

Every other week, it seems, conflicting evidence is reported that alternately blames and absolves cholesterol and the foods, such as eggs, in which it is most prominent. In 1980 the prestigious Food and Nutrition Board of the National Academy of Sciences, which sets the nutritional standards for normal Americans, contradicted the advice of twenty other organizations concerned with public health by stating that healthy people need not restrict dietary cholesterol and saturated fats since such a cutback has not been proved to have lifesaving benefits.

On the one hand, most of us would love to believe we can eat all the eggs, well-marbled meat, ice cream, cheese, and other rich sources of fats and cholesterol we want without risking a blockage in our coronary arteries. On the other hand, we are nagged by the question of whether it's worth taking a chance. Can all those other scientists be wrong?

There are at least five different categories of evidence to consider, according to Dr. Donald Berwick, pediatrician at the Harvard School of Public Health and coauthor of *Cholesterol, Children, and Heart Disease* (New York: Oxford University Press, 1980). Most of the evidence shows a clear link between how much fat and cholesterol people regularly eat, how much cholesterol can be found in their blood, and how high is their risk of dying of coronary heart disease, the nation's leading cause of death.

Unfortunately, the studies necessary to prove — or disprove — the lifesaving benefits for the average American of eating less fat and cholesterol are unlikely to be done because they are too cumbersome and costly. Besides, it would take decades to obtain convincing findings, one way or another. In the meantime, the issue will become moot for a generation of Americans.

Cholesterol is an essential body chemical used to make cell membranes, hormones, vitamin D, bile acids, and the protective sheath around nerve fibers. The human liver typically produces about 1,000 milligrams of cholesterol a day, and after the first six months of life, cholesterol is not needed in the diet.

Nonetheless, the average adult American consumes about 600 milligrams of cholesterol a day. Though less than that made by the liver, this amount of dietary cholesterol seems to overwhelm the ability of many people to maintain low levels of cholesterol in their blood and to prevent deposits of cholesterol from clogging their arteries.

Far more important than the cholesterol eaten are the total amounts and kinds of fats in the diet. Fats account for about 85 percent of the effect the diet has on blood cholesterol levels.

The Evidence Against Cholesterol

The following kinds of studies have linked dietary fats and cholesterol to coronary deaths:

Biochemical. Cholesterol and substances made from cholesterol are the primary constituents of deposits that clog arteries, producing atherosclerosis, the main cause of deaths from heart disease. Cholesterol consumed as part of the diet has been shown to wind up in these deposits, rendering it guilty by association but not proving its harmful role beyond a reasonable doubt.

Epidemiological. Of seventeen major studies among peoples in various parts of the world, fourteen showed a very strong relationship between the average blood cholesterol level and the incidence of heart disease and coronary deaths. In the famous Framingham Heart Study, elevated blood cholesterol was singled out as one of three major risk factors for coronary heart disease. [See chapter on heart risk, page 628.]

Crosscultural. A comparative study of middle-aged men in seven developed countries showed that the more saturated fat in the typical diet, the higher the level of cholesterol in the blood and, in turn, the higher the death rate from coronary disease. Coronary deaths are uncommon among Japanese living in Japan, where the traditional diet is very low in fat and cholesterol. But when Japanese migrate to the United States and adopt a more Westernized high-fat diet, their coronary death rate rises.

Animal. When many experimental animals, including primates, are fed a typical American diet, they develop atherosclerosis. And when the animals are returned to a low-fat, low-cholesterol diet, the arterial deposits seem to dissolve away. A similar regression of cholesterol deposits has been found in the leg arteries of people who were treated with cholesterol-lowering diets and drugs.

Intervention. Twenty-three studies have shown that blood cholesterol levels can be reduced 5 to 20 percent by changing the diet to one that is lower in total fat and cholesterol, with polyunsaturated fats representing a larger proportion of the fat consumed. Blood cholesterol levels tend to drop more in people who start out with high levels.

More than half a dozen studies have examined the effects of such dietary changes on coronary disease rates among groups of people living either in institutions or in ordinary settings. All the studies have suffered from one or more shortcomings in their design or execution, which make their conclusions scientifically uncertain. However, five such studies suggested that reducing consumption of fats and cholesterol is beneficial to cardiovascular health. Among them is a twenty-year study by the New York Anti-Coronary Club. Those men who faithfully followed the prescribed "prudent" diet were much less likely to suffer heart attacks than those who ate more fat and cholesterol. In another, involving more than 1,200 Norwegian men with high blood levels of cholesterol who were followed for five years, the half of the group that switched to a low-fat, low-cholesterol diet experienced 47 percent fewer heart attacks and sudden coronary deaths than those who continued on their regular high-fat diet.

The average blood cholesterol level in middle-aged Americans is now between 220 and 240 milligrams per 100 milliliters of blood serum. This represents a decline of 5 to 10 percent in the last decade, during which time the nation's coronary death rate has been declining.

CHOLESTEROL CONTENT OF COMMON FOODS

Food	Amount	Cholesterol (mg)
MEAT GROUP		
Red Meats		
Bacon	2 slices	15
Beef (lean)	3 ounces	77
Frankfurter	2 (4 ounces)	112
Ham, boiled	2 ounces	51
Kidney, beef	3 ounces	315
Lamb (lean)	3 ounces	85
Liver, beef	3 ounces	375
Pork (lean)	3 ounces	75
Veal (lean)	3 ounces	84
Fowl		
Chicken, dark (no skin)	3 ounces	77
Chicken, white (no skin)	3 ounces	65
Eggs (whole or yolk only)	1 large	252
Turkey, dark (no skin)	3 ounces	86
Turkey, white (no skin)	3 ounces	65
Fish		
Clams, raw (meat only)	3 ounces	43
Crab, canned	3 ounces	85
Flounder	3 ounces	69
Haddock	3 ounces	42
Halibut	3 ounces	50
Lobster	3 ounces	71
Mackerel	3 ounces	84
Oysters, raw (meat only)	3 ounces	42
Salmon, canned	3 ounces	30
Sardines	3 ounces	119
Scallops	3 ounces	45
Shrimp, canned	3 ounces	128
Tuna, canned	3 ounces	55

In societies, like Japan, where the coronary death rate is very low, the average adult has a blood cholesterol level of about 150 to 180 milligrams. Four out of eight studies that have examined the relationship between low blood cholesterol and deaths unrelated to heart disease have suggested that cholesterol levels below 180 milligrams may be associated with an increased risk of dying of cancer. In addition, several studies have suggested that excessive consumption of cholesterol-lowering polyunsaturates may have cancerous effects.

Further studies are needed to determine whether the association between low blood cholesterol and cancer is valid and, if so, why it may exist. Meanwhile, a moderate position would seem prudent: reducing blood cholesterol levels to 200 milligrams or less by eating fewer fats and

Food	Amount	Cholesterol (mg)
MILK GROUP		
Butter	1 tablespoon	35
Buttermilk	1 cup	5
Cheese, cottage (4% fat)	½ cup	24
Cheese, cottage (1% fat)	½ cup	12
Cheese, cream	1 ounce	31
Cheese, hard	1 ounce	24-28
Cheese, spread	1 ounce	18
Chocolate milk (low-fat)	1 cup	20
Cream, heavy	1 tablespoon	21
Ice cream	½ cup	27
Ice milk	½ cup	13
Milk, skim	1 cup	5
Milk, 1% fat	1 cup	14
Milk, 2% fat	1 cup	22
Milk, whole	1 cup	34
Yogurt (low-fat)	1 cup	17
BREAD GROUP		
Angel food cake	1 slice	0
Chocolate cupcake	2½-inch diameter	17
Cornbread	1 ounce	58
Lemon meringue pie	⅛ of 9-inch pie	98
Muffin, plain	3-inch diameter	21
Noodles, egg	1 cup	50
Pancakes	7 tablespoons batter	54
Sponge cake	1/12 of 10-inch cake	162

Note: Foods made only from plant sources, such as peanut butter, beans, vegetable margarines, grains, fruits, and vegetables, contain no cholesterol.
Source: Based on analyses by the U.S. Department of Agriculture.
Source: "JANE BRODY'S NUTRITION BOOK" by Jane E. Brody, New York: W. W. Norton, 1981.

less cholesterol and by substituting polyunsaturates for some of the saturated fats remaining in your diet.

For Further Reading

Hausman, Patricia. *Jack Sprat's Legacy.* New York: Richard Marek, 1981.

Starches:
Not Fattening and Good for You

There's one simple way to save calories and money in your daily food budget: Eat the potatoes. Also the rice, pasta, corn, beans, and bread. Strange advice, coming in a book on healthful living? Aren't these the starchy foods, high in calories and low in nutrients, that our forefathers were forced to live on but that we, in our late-twentieth-century affluence and abundance, can afford to pass up or merely sample now and again?

The answer is yes — and no. Yes, these are starchy foods, laden with so-called complex carbohydrates (as opposed to sugars, which are simple carbohydrates). No, they are not high in calories. Ounce for ounce, they have no more calories than pure protein, and they have fewer than half the calories in fat.

A five-ounce potato, without butter or sour cream, has 110 calories, whereas a five-ounce T-bone steak has about 550. That's because the steak has more fat than protein, and fat is our most calorie-laden nutrient. [See chapters on protein, page 8, and fats, page 14.] Yet, those watching their weight are likely to leave the potato on the plate and down every morsel of the meat. Dieters also pass up the rice (154 calories in five ounces) and the pasta (210 calories). Even five ounces of bread, at 390 calories, are less fattening than the steak.

In addition to saving you calories, the starchy carbohydrates can save you money if you eat them in place of some of the more costly fat-rich protein foods that most Americans consume to great excess.

Experiments with high-carbohydrate diets have shown that they can produce painless weight loss because the dieter feels satisfied without eating too many calories. In one such study, overweight college students consumed twelve slices of bread a day as part of their regular meals and lost, on the average, sixteen pounds in eight weeks. Those eating a high-fiber bread lost the most. The bulk provided by many complex carbohydrate foods, particularly fruits, vegetables, and whole grains, can fill the dieter far better than calorie-dense fats and sweets.

And no, starchy foods are not necessarily low in nutrients. Most starchy foods, particularly those made from whole grains and beans, are rich sources of vitamins, minerals, and trace nutrients. The potato, for example, is a nutritional bargain in terms of its calories. It supplies, among other nutrients, nearly 5 percent of the protein, 5 percent of the iron, 8 percent of the phosphorus, 10 percent of the thiamin, 11 percent of the niacin, and 50 percent of the vitamin C needed in an adult's daily diet, but only 4 to 5 percent of the calories. Starchy foods also contain fiber, or roughage, the noncaloric, undigestible plant materials that are important aids to digestion and may help prevent various diseases of the colon, including cancer. [See chapter on fiber, page 36.] And like the potato, most starchy foods contain small but significant amounts of protein. The protein content of some beans, in fact, is on a par with meat.

The Body's Main Fuel

Carbohydrates, both simple and complex, are the body's main source of energy. They are readily digested and converted into the blood sugar glucose, which fuels the brain and muscles. Without carbohydrates, the body must rely on fats and protein for energy. Fats burn inefficiently in the absence of carbohydrates and leave the kidneys with the burden of excreting large amounts of toxic metabolic chemicals called ketone bodies. These can build up in the blood and cause nausea, fatigue, and apathy, a common effect among those who adhere to the faddish low-carbohydrate diets.

When protein is used for energy, the body is deprived of this crucial nutrient for building and replacing tissues, and the kidneys have to get rid of the unused nitrogen that's left over. That's why on high-protein diets you must drink lots of water to help flush out your kidneys.

Athletes and exercise enthusiasts need a diet rich in carbohydrates to fuel their hardworking muscles. If you exercise vigorously, a high-protein, low-carbohydrate diet can actually be dangerous because it's hard to take in enough water to meet the needs of your kidneys. Tests of athletic performance have clearly demonstrated an advantage to a high-carbohydrate diet before prolonged exercise. Athletes eating mostly protein and fat scored only half as well as those on a high-carbohydrate diet. Many runners have discovered that pasta is the best supper to eat the night before a race.

Since the turn of the century Americans have cut way back on their consumption of carbohydrates, particularly the "low-prestige" items like flour and cereal grains and potatoes. The falloff has been greatest for the more nourishing complex carbohydrates. It was accompanied by an increase in refined sugars, usually found in foods that are high in calories and low in nutrients.

The net result is that whereas Americans once ate mostly complex carbohydrates laden with important nutrients, now their carbohydrates are mainly the relatively "empty" calories of highly refined and sweetened foods like cakes, cookies, soft drinks, and sugar-coated cereals. (In some of these cereals, sugar is the leading ingredient.) If not for our habituation to the sweet taste, our bodies have no need for sugar, as long as they're provided with starch for fuel. [See chapter on sugar, page 32.]

In 1977 the Senate Select Committee on Nutrition and Human Needs recommended a sizable increase in our consumption of carbohydrates — particularly the complex starches and naturally occurring sugars in fruits and vegetables. These should claim a 60 percent share of our daily calorie intake, the committee recommended. Other experts go

A SIMPLE GUIDE TO COMPLEX CARBOHYDRATES

Here is a dietary guide to the good carbohydrates.

Potatoes. As they come from the ground, potatoes are relatively low in calories (150 for a large baking potato) and high in nutrients, including some protein. An adult could derive nearly all needed nutrients from potatoes. Baked, steamed, or boiled, they are an excellent food. But a single pat of butter or margarine increases the calorie content of a medium-sized potato by a third.

Deep-frying destroys some vitamins and adds astronomically to calories. Of the calories in french fries, 70 percent are from fat. Potato chips are also mostly fat (and high in salt) — 150 calories per ounce, 90 of them from fat. About nine chips add up to 100 calories.

Flours. Grains consist of three parts: the starchy endosperm containing the nutrients needed to sustain a seedling, including 70 percent of the kernel's protein; the vitamin-rich germ, which will form the first leaves and roots; and the bran, the protective outer coat that provides undigestible roughage for the human diet.

Milling techniques used in the United States to produce white flour remove the bran and germ, leaving mostly starch behind. In enriched flours, only four of the twenty-six removed nutrients and none of the fiber are added back. Bleaching of flour destroys all the vitamin E. Whole wheat flour (particularly if stone-ground) retains most of the original nutrients and has more B vitamins, vitamin E, and trace nutrients such as copper and manganese, than enriched white flour.

Bread. You'll get the most nutrients for your money from whole grain (unrefined) bread made from stone-ground flour; the next best is 100 percent whole wheat or whole grain, which can be so called even though 5 percent of the kernel, particularly some of the wheat germ, is lost. It's impossible to know how much rye flour may be in rye bread and the flour used is often refined. Brown breads may contain little or no whole grains, merely molasses for coloring. If you buy white bread, be sure it's enriched.

The recently introduced high-fiber breads are lower in calories because a large percentage of their bulk is undigestible fiber (usually cellulose, which is what bran is). One popular brand, Fresh Horizons, uses wood fiber as its source of cellulose. There's no known harm in that, so long as you know that what you're paying for isn't grain. A slice of bread, depending on the type and thickness, ranges from 50 to 80 calories.

Cereals. Here again, the most nutritious are the whole grain cereals. If you buy farina, be sure it's enriched. Steel-cut or rolled oats (not the instant, but the old-fashioned kind) give the best food value since oats are the highest in protein of the commonly consumed grains and these milling techniques do least damage to the natural nutrients. Cooking hot cereals with milk as part of the liquid greatly improves their nutritional value.

Among cold cereals, shredded wheat is made from whole grain, without added sugar. Grape-Nuts and the new Nutri-Grain cereals also rely on the inherent sweet flavor derived from grains. Puffed cereals provide more air than nutrition, though they are low in fat, sugar, and calories. Sugar-coated cereals, some of which contain more sugar than any other ingredient, teach children bad nutritional habits and leave deposits on even higher — to 70 or 80 percent carbohydrates. Currently carbohydrates represent 45 percent of the calories in the typical American diet, and more than a third of those calories come from low-nutrient refined and processed sugars. Most Americans eat their weight in sugar every year.

The committee suggested that we replace some of the animal fats in our current diet, which have been linked to a high risk of heart disease

teeth that may encourage tooth decay and decay-causing bacteria.

Granolas, which swept the market in the wake of the health food revolution, are high in calories, fats, and sugars, although they do have more protein and vitamins than most other packaged cereals. If granola is keeping you away from bacon and eggs for breakfast, you might try making your own, using fewer sweeteners and less oil than the commercial granolas and leaving out the cholesterol-raising coconut and coconut oil. Or try just a handful of commercial granola to add crunch to some other packaged cereal.

Before the milk is added, most cold cereals provide 110 to 140 calories a serving, which ranges from one-fourth cup to one and a fourth cups, depending on how dense the cereal is.

Rice. Brown rice contains nearly all the nutrients in the original rice grain. Polishing removes the brown coat and the germ that contains most of the B vitamins and minerals, but it renders the protein in the grain more digestible. A better buy is parboiled or converted white rice; the process forces many of the nutrients into the white kernel. Instant and minute rices are least nutritious. Avoid washing rice unless it's coated with talc, since some vitamins may wash away. A cup of cooked rice contains 223 calories.

Pasta. Spaghetti and noodles of all sorts can be purchased enriched. Many are now readily available in a high-protein form, in which protein-rich soy flour or artichoke powder has been used. You should also be able to get whole wheat spaghetti; some people prefer it mixed half and half with the regular kind. There are also spinach pastas (green noodles), which have more vitamins and minerals than white enriched. A cup of cooked pasta has 198 calories; home-made pasta somewhat more.

Legumes and seeds. Dried peas and beans, seeds, and nuts are rich sources of protein, vitamins, and minerals. Seeds and nuts contain considerable amounts of fat, albeit polyunsaturated vegetable oils, which bolster their calorie count. The beans and peas vary in fat content, with soybeans containing more fat than lentils, for example. A cup of soybeans contains 234 calories; lentils, 212; and kidney beans, 218. There are 322 calories in 10 large walnuts. A tablespoon of sesame or sunflower seeds has about 50 calories.

Fruits and vegetables. Although most are not high in starch, these carbohydrate foods are vital sources of vitamins and minerals and excellent sources of fiber. Many contain small but significant amounts of protein as well. Their fiber and water content add satisfying bulk and volume to the diet and help ward off overeating.

Fruits and many vegetables contain simple carbohydrates (sugars), but since these are "packaged" in a nutrient-laden edible that is relatively low in calories, nutritionists do not consider them empty calories. One medium apple contains 80 calories; a carrot, 30.

Milk products. Skimmed milk, buttermilk (which, despite its fatty name, is really made from skimmed milk), and yogurt prepared from low-fat milk are also nutrient-laden foods in which simple carbohydrates provide the bulk of calories. They are excellent sources of protein. In whole milk products, however, fat calories predominate.

and certain cancers, with more innocuous and nutritious carbohydrates. Since the average American already eats twice as much protein as is really needed, and since most of that protein comes laden with saturated animal fats and cholesterol, many nutritionists believe we would be better off if we replaced some of those protein foods with complex carbohydrates.

In most countries where heart disease is rare, the people derive between 65 and 85 percent of their calories from carbohydrates, mainly whole grains and tubers. Contrary to popular belief, diets high in complex carbohydrates have been shown to reduce the insulin requirements of diabetics and may help stave off the artery-clogging diseases to which they are especially prone. [See chapter on diabetes, page 660.]

Complex carbohydrates and fruits can also replace processed sweets, such as baked goods, candy, and soft drinks, which contribute to tooth decay and obesity and add little of nutritive value to the diet. Alcohol, which the body processes as a carbohydrate (yielding 7 calories to the gram, as opposed to 4 per gram of regular carbohydrates), is another source of nutritionally empty calories.

The complex carbohydrates are the only major nutrients *not* associated with any long-term health risks. The foods described in the box on pages 30-31 should form the bulk of calories in any healthful diet.

Sugar:
Too Much of a Bad Thing

Sugar proponents call it quick energy, opponents say it's empty calories. To the average American, who consumes a third of a pound of it each day, sugar is mostly an irresistibly good taste. Human societies have long equated sweetness with goodness — sweet mystery of life, sweet smell of success, sweetheart — and that enhances the attraction.

People seem to have an innate "sweet tooth." If saccharin is injected into the womb, the fetus will increase its swallowing of the sweetened amniotic fluid. Newborn rats given a choice will consume sugar water in preference to a nutritious diet, even to the point of malnutrition and death.

Cited for such evils as distracting youngsters from more nutritious foodstuffs, enhancing obesity, ruining teeth, and possibly contributing to diabetes and heart disease, sugar has become the most maligned of the main components of the American diet. Since many of the more vocal accusers and defenders of sugar have links to industries that stand to benefit from their views, the public is hard put to sort fact from fiction, evidence from opinion.

Sugar, like starch, is a carbohydrate. The many types of sugars include sucrose (table sugar refined from sugarcane or beets), lactose (milk sugar), fructose (fruit sugar), glucose (blood sugar), dextrose, maltose, and galactose.

Seventy percent of the sugar in today's American diet is "hidden" in processed foods. Check the labels of the packaged soups, cereals, salad dressings, soft drinks, ketchup, sauces, peanut butter, dessert mixes, and what-have-you in your pantry and see how many list sugar (or corn syrup) as a main ingredient.

At the turn of the century the average American consumed about 77 pounds of sugar a year (65 of them as sucrose), and starches formed two-thirds of American dietary carbohydrates; today sugar consumption hovers around 128 pounds per capita (98 of them as sucrose), and sugar represents more than half the carbohydrate calories and about 20 percent of the total calories eaten by Americans — 500 calories of sugar each day. Even the widespread use of artificial sweeteners has done little to curb Americans' appetite for sugar.

In relying on processed sucrose-sweetened foods as a main carbohydrate source, Americans may miss the bulk, satiety, and essential nutrients found in other carbohydrate foods like fruits, vegetables, grains, breads, and pasta, which contain fiber, water, vitamins, and minerals as well as calories. Refined sucrose, as such, is nothing but calories (and unrefined sugar doesn't contain enough trace nutrients to make a difference), and the foods in which it is used most heavily rarely contain enough other nutrients to counter the pejorative label of "empty calories."

The body has no physiological need for sucrose that cannot be satisfied by other more nutritious foods. The body can convert starches to sugar or use the sugar in fruits and vegetables for energy. In fact, experts in carbohydrate nutrition say that even the purported need for sugar as quick energy is a myth except in a few rare situations, such as a diabetic in insulin shock.

If you eat a concentrated source of sugar on an empty stomach, the level of glucose in the blood rises within half an hour and insulin is rapidly released to move the glucose out of the blood and into storage as glycogen in the liver or fatty acids in the fat depots. The blood glucose level falls rapidly, and in two hours it is back to normal.

During exercise the body calls upon its reserve of glycogen (and, if that runs out, fatty acids) to supply the muscles with needed energy. If you eat sugar before exercising, your body simply stores it. Only if "slugs" of sugar were consumed intermittently during prolonged, strenuous exercise would they help to maintain an elevated blood sugar level to fuel the muscles.

What Harm Does It Cause?

As for sugar's reputed adverse health effects, the following can be

33

said on the basis of available evidence:

Obesity. Sugar supplies 4 calories per gram (113 per ounce) — the same as protein and less than half that of fat, which provides 9 calories per gram. Excess calorie intake, not sugar, causes obesity. But since calories can be highly concentrated in sugar-sweetened foods, you may eat many more calories than you need of such foods before you feel full or even realize how much you have consumed. Compare the satiety value of, say, three bananas with that of a two-ounce candy bar; both have about the same carbohydrate content. Fructose, the primary sugar in fruits, is 50 percent sweeter than sucrose, and so fewer fructose calories are needed to obtain the same degree of sweetness. However, the use of fructose in nutritionally deficient sweet foods does little to improve their health value.

Tooth decay. Sugar definitely promotes the development of dental caries. Bacteria in the mouth digest the sugar on tooth surfaces and produce acid, which etches the protective tooth enamel and fosters periodontal disease. It is the frequency of sugar consumption and the amount of time sugar remains on the teeth, rather than the total quantity of sugar eaten, that makes the difference.

Thus, chewy candies, sucking candies, and sweetened cereals (whether sweetened by sugar or honey) are far more harmful to the teeth than a sweet drink or ice cream. Sweet, chewy granolas, the latest rage in breakfast cereals, are bad actors as far as teeth are concerned. (They also are not sufficiently more nourishing than regular cereals to justify their high calorie and sugar content.) To reduce the risk of decay, dentists recommend that you rinse your mouth or brush your teeth after consuming anything sweet and that you avoid eating sweets between meals.

Diabetes. In diabetes, the pancreas fails to produce adequate amounts of insulin to clear the blood of excess glucose. Thus, diabetics are told to curb their intake of sweets lest their blood sugar rise dangerously high. Eating a lot of starch, however, is not harmful to diabetics. The most important dietary factor in diabetes is controlling body weight.

There is some evidence that a high-sugar diet may promote the development of diabetes in people who are genetically predisposed to the disease. In laboratory experiments, rats prone to diabetes develop the disease on a high-sugar diet, but not on a sugar-free diet. When Yemenites, who ordinarily eat little sugar and have no diabetes, emigrate to Israel and adopt a sugar-rich diet, they frequently develop obesity and diabetes. However, other populations with high-sugar diets have low rates of diabetes, perhaps because they are not overweight. [See chapter on diabetes, page 660.]

34

Heart Disease. The theory that diets high in sugar are an important cause of atherosclerosis and heart disease does not have wide support among experts in the field, who say that fats and cholesterol are the more likely culprits. Although most of the countries that consume a lot of sugar have a high incidence of heart disease, these are the same countries where consumption of animal fats and cholesterol is very high. There is a much stronger correlation worldwide between fat consumption and heart disease.

Well-controlled studies have shown that people who developed heart disease did not consume excessive sugar compared with those free of heart disease. A high-sugar diet does not cause heart disease in experimental animals, whereas a high-fat diet does.

Some people are said to be carbohydrate-sensitive — they have a tendency to develop high blood levels of fatty substances called triglycerides, which may promote atherosclerosis. They are often advised to reduce their intake of sugar, but reducing dietary fat and losing weight are most important to lowering their triglyceride level. Diets free of sucrose can lower abnormally high blood fat levels, but they have been found to have no effect on fat levels that are acceptable to begin with.

SUGAR LABEL

Kellogg's Pop-Tarts, frosted raspberry

Ingredients: Enriched wheat flour, partially hydrogenated vegetable oil (one or more of: cottonseed, coconut, soybean, and palm), *dextrose, sugar,* red raspberry preserves (*corn syrup,* red raspberries, pectin, sodium citrate, and citric acid), apple jelly (*corn syrup,* apple juice, pectin, and citric acid), *corn syrup,* whey, crackermeal, pre-gelatinized wheat starch, water, salt, baking powder, citric acid, baking soda, gelatin, artificial coloring, reduced iron, niacinamide, riboflavin (B2), thiamin hydrochloride (B1), and folic acid. BHA added to preserve product freshness. (Italics indicate added sugar.)

Nutrition Information
Per serving:

Calories	210
Protein	3 grams
Carbohydrates	36 grams
Fat	6 grams
Total	45 grams

Carbohydrate Information

Starch and related carbohydrates	19 grams
Sucrose and other sugars	17 grams
Total	36 grams

Dietary Fiber:
A Feast for Your Body

"Breadde havynge moche branne fylleth the bealye with excrements and . . . shortely descendeth from the stomacke!" wrote a London physician in 1541.

In *Itinerary of a Breakfast*, published in 1920, Dr. J. H. Kellogg, medical director of the Battle Creek, Michigan, Sanitarium and brother of the founder of the Kellogg Company, described the colon as "the source of more disease and physical suffering than any organ of the body." To counter the unhealthy state of colonic affairs, he prescribed an "antitoxic diet" consisting chiefly of fruits, cereals, and fresh vegetables.

Today, more than sixty years later, similar high-fiber diets are being advocated as capable of preventing or curing everything from constipation, hemorrhoids, and colon cancer, to heart disease, obesity, diabetes, and schizophrenia. Although many researchers have been studying fiber for years, the current fad was triggered in 1970 by Dr. Denis Burkitt, a British physician.

He reported that countries where large amounts of fiber are regularly consumed had low rates of colon-rectal cancer, benign diseases of the colon (such as diverticulosis), appendicitis, varicose veins, gallstones, and heart disease. Popular books and articles soon followed, vastly exaggerating the health claims for dietary fiber.

Now supermarkets offer a wide range of high-fiber breads and cereals. People who once described bran as the closest thing to cattle feed are happily eating like their four-legged friends. In the mid-seventies the fiber fad resulted in a shortage of bran in the United States. High-fiber breads and cereals continue to push the overly refined, pasty white stuff off the shelves as millions of Americans discover that those coarse, nutty-flavored grains rejected a century ago in the name of lily-white gentility may actually be good for you.

With the fiber fad in its second decade, scientists and physicians continue to discover healthful new facts — and cautionary refinements on some old facts — about this "nonnutrient." All the necessary data are by no means in, but the available facts show that fiber can have important health-promoting effects and that many of these effects are more prominently associated with the fibers in fruits and vegetables than with those in bran and other cereal grains. At the same time the findings demand that fiber be treated with intelligence and discretion, and not sprinkled indiscriminately on everything you eat.

What Is Fiber?

Dietary fibers come only from plants. They are the chemical substances in the cell walls that give plants structure and stability. Fibers include cellulose, polysaccharides, hemicelluloses, pectins, gums, mucilages, and lignin.

Different kinds of plants contain different fibers. Even within a species, the fiber content may vary according to growing conditions and maturity at harvest. Bran is almost entirely cellulose; apples, grapes, and some other fruits are high in pectin.

Fibers are not digested by human digestive enzymes. However, many are partially or completely digested by bacteria that reside in the gut, resulting in the production of gases.

Some fibers, such as cellulose, hemicellulose, and lignin, are not soluble in water, although most can absorb several times their weight in water. Insoluble fibers predominate in grains. Others, such as pectin (used to make jelly), gums, and mucilages, are water-soluble and can leach out into cooking water. They are found naturally in fruits and vegetables, beans, and whole oats and are used as additives in processed foods.

Old methods of analyzing for "crude fiber" greatly underestimate the actual amount of *dietary* fiber present in a food. Newer, more accurate — but still imperfect — methods of analysis are quite cumbersome and not yet widely used by the food industry, although a few researchers have used them to determine "total dietary fiber" for a number of fresh and processed foods (see chart pages 40–41). Crude fiber listings on food labels are considered useless by fiber experts; some food packages now also list "dietary fiber."

The Health Effects of Fiber

Fiber is hardly the cure-all some have suggested. But neither does fiber belong at the bottom of the nutritional totem pole, where it resided for more than a century as a nonessential dietary ingredient. There is good evidence, for example, that certain dietary fibers can lower blood cholesterol levels and improve the processing of blood sugar by diabetics.

Although the evidence is conflicting, high-fiber diets have been helpful to many patients with chronic intestinal disorders, such as constipation, spastic colon, diverticular disease, and even Crohn's disease (regional enteritis or ileitis). And there is some evidence that fiber can help to lower blood pressure and ward off gallstones.

But many of the more dramatic claims about fiber — such as its purported ability to prevent the development of intestinal disorders, hemorrhoids, appendicitis, varicose veins, obesity, colon cancer, and heart disease — are as yet untested and unproved. Furthermore, excessive consumption of fiber can be harmful, producing painful intestinal gas, flatulence, nausea, and vomiting and perhaps interfering with your body's ability to absorb certain essential minerals (though this is not a problem if your diet is balanced and your fiber consumption moderate).

Fiber is best consumed as an integral part of foods — whole grain cereals and breads, nuts, seeds, fruits, and vegetables — rather than as a dietary supplement. Fiber "pills" are of no known benefit. The different fibrous substances have different — and sometimes even opposing — effects. Pretreatment of a fibrous food — whether, for example, it is coarsely or finely ground, whole or minced, raw or cooked — can change how it affects the person who consumes it.

Therefore, it pays to know what fiber can and cannot do, both good and bad, before you make dramatic changes in your diet. No matter what you hear or read about fiber's benefits, people with diet-related disorders should never attempt self-treatment with fiber without first consulting their physicians.

Gastrointestinal effects. Fiber substances can absorb many times their weight in water, and most pass through the human digestive tract undigested, resulting in softer and bulkier stools.

Bran, which is mostly cellulose, is the best bet for relieving constipation. It holds a lot of water, softening the stool, increasing its volume, and making it easier to pass, and it speeds the elimination of food wastes. Apples (unpeeled), fresh carrots, and cabbage are also useful in countering constipation, as are bulk laxatives like Metamucil (hemicellulose and gum extracted from psyllium seeds).

Dr. Peter Van Soest, nutrition researcher at Cornell University, has shown that although coarse bran and cellulose have a laxative effect, finely ground bran and wood cellulose (which is also a fine fiber) induce constipation. In fact, he has found that eating bread made solely from wood cellulose kills off bacteria normally present in the gut that detoxify potentially harmful chemicals. However, Dr. Van Soest says, commercial breads made with wood cellulose also contain wheat bran and other fibers that probably counter this effect.

Weight control. Before it gets to the large intestine, fiber swells and creates a feeling of fullness that may help you cut back on the amount of food you consume and lengthen the time between meals. Young men on a diet that included twelve slices of bread a day lost more weight eating whole grain (high-fiber) bread than refined white bread.

An apple, with all its natural fiber intact, is more satisfying than applesauce, which in turn is more satisfying than apple juice, a study showed. In another study, volunteers who ate most of their carbohydrates as refined sugars often felt hungry, whereas those fed the like amount of carbohydrates as vegetable and cereal starches complained of being "stuffed."

Many fibrous foods also take longer to chew and thus force you to eat more slowly and give your brain time to register satiety before you overconsume calories.

Diabetes. When placed on a diet high in fiber-rich carbohydrate foods but very low in fat and sugar, diabetics can greatly improve control of their blood sugar, according to studies by Dr. James W. Anderson of the Veterans Administration Hospital in Lexington, Kentucky. Many patients are able to stop using antidiabetic drugs, including insulin, or they can significantly reduce the dosage of such drugs, he reports. Pectins and gums have the most striking immediate effect on blood sugar, whereas wheat bran (cellulose) seems to offer some long-term benefits.

Dr. David J. A. Jenkins of Radcliffe Infirmary in Oxford, England, showed that fiber delays the passage of food from the stomach to the intestine. This slows the conversion of starches to the blood sugar glucose, which in turn reduces the need for a large output of insulin, the hormone that functions improperly in diabetes. This benefit of fiber is obtained only if high-fiber foods are included in a meal, not as a between-meal supplement.

Blood fats. High levels of blood fats are associated with an increased risk of heart disease, and certain fibers can reduce the amount of fatty substances — cholesterol and triglycerides — in the blood. Here again, the soluble fibers — pectins and gums — are most effective, whereas wheat bran offers no benefit.

Blood cholesterol reductions of 13 to 22 percent have been achieved simply by adding foods rich in soluble fibers, such as whole oats, oat bran, carrots, or guar crispbread, to the diet. But the greatest improvement results from simultaneously eating less fats and cholesterol and more starchy carbohydrates. Dr. Anderson got nearly a 60 percent reduction in triglyceride levels in people with abnormally high triglycerides by putting them on a high-carbohydrate, low-fat diet rich in soluble fibers.

The risks. High-fiber diets can also have some undesirable effects. The most common is a temporary increase in flatulence and bloating, usually lasting about three weeks but in some cases for two or more months. Fibrous foods may impair the absorption of other nutrients, including iron and zinc, but this is thought to be no problem among otherwise well-nourished people.

Eating very large amounts of fiber, more than people could, can cause sigmoid volvulus, an enlargement and twisting of the sigmoid colon. Ulcerative colitis or regional ileitis may be aggravated by fiber, and people with these conditions should consult their physicians before

SOURCES OF DIFFERENT TYPES OF FIBER

Source	Types of Fiber
Cellulose	Coarse bran, unpeeled apples nd pears, Brazil nuts, canned peas, fresh carrots
Hemicellulose	Bran cereals, whole grain breads, beets, eggplant, radishes
Lignin	Pears, toasted whole gran breads, fried or browned potatoes
Pectin	Bananas, oranges, apples, potatoes, cabbage, carrots, grapes
Gums	Oatmeal, sesame seeds (cooked or baked), beans, bulk laxatives

increasing their fiber intake. To prevent blockage of the gastrointestinal tract, cereal fibers such as bran are best consumed with liquid.

Those who decide to leap on the fiber bandwagon are advised to proceed with care since the gastrointestinal tract may rebel at a sudden, large increase in fiber. The amount of added fiber to work up to is about two to four grams of crude fiber a day (Americans already eat about four grams of crude fiber daily), or about forty grams of dietary fiber (see the chart).

One cup of all-bran cereal contains two grams of crude fiber. Three raw carrots or three apples a day are good alternatives. Mangoes, turnips, dried beans and peas, and leafy vegetables are other good fiber sources. Because bran has no effect on cholesterol levels, a number of experts

HOW MUCH DIETARY FIBER IS IN YOUR FOOD?

Food	Amount	Weight (grams)	Fiber (grams)
BREADS, CRACKERS AND CEREALS			
All Bran or 100% Bran	1 cup	70	23
Bran Buds	¾ cup	60	18
Bulgur, dry	⅓ cup	50	5.6
Graham crackers	2 squares	15	1.5
Grapenuts	⅓ cup	45	5.0
Grits, dry	¼ cup	45	4.8
Rolled oats, dry	½ cup	50	4.5
Rye bread	1 slice	25	2
Rye crackers	3 wafers	20	2.3
Shredded wheat	2 biscuits	50	6.1
Whole wheat bread	1 slice	25	2.4
FRUITS			
Apple	1 small	90	3.1
Applesauce	½ cup	120	1.7
Banana	1 medium	100	1.8
Cantaloupe, cubes	¾ cup	120	1.4
Cherries, raw	10	70	.8
Grapefruit	½ fruit	200	2.6
Grapes, raw	16	60	.4
Orange	1 small	90	1.8
Peach, raw	1 medium	100	1.3
Peaches, canned	½ cup	120	1.3
Pear, raw	1 medium	120	2.8
Pears, canned	½ cup	125	1.4
Plum, raw	2 small	90	1.6
Strawberries	½ cup	125	2.6
Tangerine	1 medium	100	2.1

recommend putting more emphasis on fresh fruits and vegetables than on grains.

A longtime student of dietary fiber, Dr. David Kritchevsky, associate director of the Wistar Institute in Philadelphia, concludes that increasing the fiber content of the typical American diet "can't hurt and probably will help as long as you pay attention to whatever else you eat."

"Fiber," he says, "is not a panacea — you can't simply add it to a bad diet and expect to get good results."

For Further Reading

Burkitt, Denis, M.D. *Eat Right — to Stay Healthy and Enjoy Life More.* New York: Arco, 1979.

Food	Amount	Weight (grams)	Fiber (grams)
VEGETABLES			
Beans, green	½ cup	50	1.2
Beets, cooked	⅔ cup	100	2.1
Broccoli, cooked	¾ cup	75	1.6
Cabbage, cooked	¾ cup	100	2.2
Cabbage, raw	1 cup	75	2.1
Carrots, cooked	¾ cup	100	2.1
Carrots, raw	1 medium	100	3.7
Cauliflower, cooked	½ cup	100	1.2
Cauliflower, raw	1 cup	100	1.8
Celery, cooked	⅔ cup	100	2.4
Celery, raw	2½ stalks	100	3.0
Corn kernels	⅔ cup	110	4.2
Cucumber	½ of 7-inch	100	1.5
Kale, cooked	½ cup	100	2.0
Kidney beans, cooked	1 cup	75	3.6
Lentils, cooked	½ cup	100	4.0
Lettuce	1 cup	50	.8
Parsnips, cooked	¾ cup	120	5.9
Peas, cooked	½ cup	60	3.8
Potatoes, cooked	⅔ cup	90 (raw)	3.1
Rice, brown, cooked	1 cup	65	1.1
Rice, white, cooked	1 cup	65	.4
Spinach	2 large leaves	50	1.8
Summer squash, cooked	½ cup	100	2.2
Summer squash, raw	1 5-inch	100	3.0
Turnips, raw	1 cup	100	2.2

Based on analyses for total (dietary) fiber by Dr. James W. Anderson, the University of Kentucky Medical Center.

Micronutrients:
Essential in Tiny Amounts

Throughout most of evolution, food was our only source of vitamins and minerals. Today, however, the "one-a-day" multivitamin-mineral tablet is a kind of nutritional insurance policy for millions of Americans, whether they need it or not. In recent years it has been eclipsed by megadose formulations of individual micronutrients supposedly capable of performing health miracles far beyond warding off the well-known deficiency diseases.

PART I: THE LIFE-SUSTAINING VITAMINS

Even as millions down a veritable alphabet soup's worth of vitamin supplements each day, confusion and controversy surround these nutrients. There's only one fact about which there is no argument: Vitamins are essential to good health. But which ones, for whom, and how much?

Vitamins are organic substances that are required in the diet in tiny amounts — altogether, less than an eighth of a teaspoon a day — to assist in your body's processing of other major nutrients, protein, fats, and carbohydrates. In addition, certain vitamins participate in the formation of blood cells, hormones, nervous system chemicals, and genetic material. Most vitamins function as aids to enzymes. When a particular vitamin is missing from the diet or is present in inadequate amounts, characteristic deficiency symptoms develop.

The amount of each vitamin that the federal government recommends for daily consumption is based on how much is required to avoid any signs of deficiency in the average person, plus a substantial safety margin to take into account natural variations in individual needs and abilities to absorb consumed vitamins. However, a number of circumstances, including cigarette smoking, the use of certain drugs, various illnesses, old age, heavy use of alcohol, and pregnancy and lactation may increase a person's need for certain vitamins beyond ordinary recommended amounts.

Users of oral contraceptives, for example, need extra B vitamins — thiamine, niacin, pyridoxine, and B_{12} — and vitamin C. Heavy smokers need additional C, and heavy drinkers require more thiamine, niacin, pyridoxine, and folic acid than other people, even if they eat otherwise good diets. The elderly tend to absorb less of the B vitamins and vitamin C and so may need to consume extra amounts. Persons with obstructive jaundice, bowel diseases, or chronic diarrhea may absorb little of vitamins A, D, E, and K. Prolonged use of antibiotics can destroy the intestinal bacteria that normally produce several of our B vitamins and vitamin K. Following surgery, illness, injury, or extensive burns, the body's need for vitamin C is increased.

It is commonly asserted that anyone who eats a "well-balanced diet" doesn't need additional vitamins. Such a diet is described as including, each day, at least four servings of grain and cereal products, four or more servings of a variety of fruits and vegetables, two servings of dairy products, and two of meat, fish, poultry, or protein-rich legumes (see chart on page 7). Although this particular balance of foods certainly does not offer the only way to consume adequate vitamins, it is considered a reasonable guide for the average person.

Obviously we all don't eat this way. For some people, such as those who eat erratically, those on strict low-calorie diets, those who rely primarily on heavily processed and canned foods, picky eaters, and vegetarians, a diet containing adequate amounts of vitamins may not be consumed. In these cases supplementing the diet with a multivitamin pill may be advisable.

However, improving one's diet is clearly the preferred route to obtaining essential nutrients, since there is no pill that can completely compensate for the deficiencies in an inadequate or poorly balanced diet. And don't assume that you don't have to worry about what else you eat because you start each day with a vitamin-packed cereal. You can't be sure how many of the vitamins in your bowl actually get into your body, and no cereal contains all the required vitamins in the needed proportions.

If you do need a vitamin supplement, with the exception of vitamin E, it matters not (except to the income of the seller) whether you buy "natural" or synthetic vitamins. The body can't tell them apart. A molecule of vitamin C (ascorbic acid) is the same whether it originated in a rose hip or a chemistry lab. For vitamin E, the natural form is chemically different and slightly more active than synthetic versions.

There are thirteen undisputed vitamins — four that are soluble in fat and nine that are soluble in water — plus one to five other substances (including choline and inositol) that some assert are vitamins but that others say are not, since they are produced in the body in adequate amounts and no deficiency symptoms are associated with their absence in the diet.

The *fat-soluble vitamins* — A, D, E, and K — are generally consumed along with fat-containing foods. They are absorbed through the intestines with the aid of bile produced by the liver or fats in the diet. Because they are stored in your body's fat, they do not necessarily have to be consumed each day.

Thus, a cooked carrot every other day, a cup of spinach every five days, or two ounces of beef liver once a week can fulfill an adult's need for vitamin A. But also because they are stored, there is a danger of overdosing yourself with fat-soluble vitamins.

Water-soluble vitamins — eight B vitamins and C — present the opposite problem. The body has no storage depot for most of them, and

43

they are continually being washed out with urine and sweat. Therefore, they should be consumed daily in adequate amounts to meet the body's needs.

Keeping Vitamin Values Intact

Many vitamins are readily destroyed or lost when foods are preserved, stored, and cooked. With the current emphasis on highly refined and precooked convenience foods and the great distances fresh foods must travel before they reach the consumer's table, the modern American diet may shortchange some people.

Much of the following advice on how to get the most vitamins for your food dollar is derived from research cited in *Nutritional Evaluation of Food Processing,* a professional textbook edited by Drs. Robert S. Harris and Endel Karmas (Westport, Connecticut: Avi Publishing Company, Inc., 1975).

● Eat whole grain rather than refined breads and cereals and brown rice instead of white. Enriched breads, pasta, cereals, and rice are second best. Parboiled or converted rice has more vitamins than polished rice.

● Use fresh or frozen fruits and vegetables instead of canned ones. During canning, the amount of many vitamins is reduced by half or more, and further losses occur during storage of the canned goods. Freezing, followed by storage and cooking, also reduces the vitamin content, but much less than does canning. Boil-in-the-bag frozen foods are preferred for their vitamin content. Don't thaw frozen vegetables before cooking.

● Storage of fresh foods in your refrigerator for one or more days leads to considerable vitamin loss. For those who cannot shop often, frozen fruits and vegetables may be as nutritious as the fresh. Foods that are frozen are picked ripe and processed rapidly, whereas days or weeks may elapse before fresh produce is consumed.

● Fruits and vegetables ripened on the plant (except for pineapples) and in the sun have considerably more vitamin C than those picked green or grown in shade. To preserve vitamin C, fruit should be chilled immediately after being picked and kept cold and uncut until eaten. Most of the vitamin C in fruit is in and just under the skin, so paring fruit results in a considerable loss.

● Avoid prolonged soaking of fresh vegetables, or you'll wash the B vitamins and vitamin C down the drain.

● Prepare salads just before they are to be eaten. Delay the cutting up and preparation of foods until shortly before they are to be cooked and eaten.

● Keep all fresh, cut, and cooked foods well wrapped in the refrigerator.

● In cooking vegetables, pressure cooking is least detrimental to vitamins. Steaming is second best. If boiling a vegetable, use as little water as possible — just enough so that nearly all is reabsorbed by the time the vegetable is done. Or use the cooking water, which will be rich in vitamins, in your recipe or to make a soup or stew.

● Toasting bread destroys much of one of the B vitamins, thiamine. Bread crust has less thiamine than the soft crumb.

● Potatoes baked in the skin retain most of their nutrients. Boiling potatoes in their skins is better than paring and cutting them up. In general, the more a vegetable is cut up before cooking, the greater the vitamin loss.

● Glass, stainless steel, aluminum, enamel, and similar pots and pans do not affect nutrient content. But cooking in iron pots, an advantage to those who need extra iron in their diets, can destroy some of the vitamin C. So can unlined copper, brass, and monel (a nickel alloy). Copper also destroys folic acid and vitamin E.

● Don't cook vegetables with baking soda; it destroys thiamine and vitamin C.

● Use the vitamin-rich syrup in canned fruits to make your own gelatin dessert. Make gravy from the defatted juices that drain from meats during thawing and cooking.

● Riboflavin and vitamins A and D are readily decomposed by light. Keep milk and breads in opaque containers.

● Buy milk and margarine that are fortified with vitamin A. Milk should also contain vitamin D.

Essential Facts About Vitamins

Following is a brief discussion of some important facts about each vitamin. The accompanying charts, pages 46–49, depict the recommended amounts, best sources, established roles, and deficiency symptoms for each vitamin.

Vitamin A. A third of American children consume less than the recommended amount of this vitamin. Vitamin A in animal foods is preformed, but plant foods contain the vitamin precursor, carotene, a yellow-orange substance that is converted to vitamin A in the body. Too much carotene can cause a jaundicelike yellowing of the skin, but not vitamin A poisoning.

To avoid damaging excesses, it's best to get needed A from your diet rather than from pills. If supplements are used, the dose should not exceed 10,000 units a day, twice the recommended amount. Too much A can destroy bone and interfere with growth; cause headaches, skin rashes, nausea, jaundice, and abdominal pain; damage red blood cells; and stop menstruation.

Nonpoisonous chemical relatives of vitamin A are currently under study as possible cancer preventives, capable of blocking the damaging effects of cancer-causing chemicals on the body's epithelial cells, includ-

VITAMINS: WHERE TO GET THEM AND WHAT THEY DO

Vitamins	Best sources	Main roles	Deficiency symptoms	Risks of megadoses
FAT SOLUBLE				
Vitamin A	Liver; eggs; cheese; butter; fortified margarine and milk; yellow, orange, and dark-green vegetables and fruits (e.g., carrots, broccoli, spinach, cantaloupe). Vitamin A is preformed in animal foods. In plants, the yellow-orange "provitamin," called carotene, is converted to an active vitamin in the body.	Assists in the formation and maintenance of healthy skin, hair, and mucous membranes; aids in the ability to see in dim light (night vision); needed for proper bone growth, teeth development, and reproduction.	Night blindness; rough skin and mucous membranes; infection of mucous membranes; drying of the eyes, impaired bone growth and tooth enamel.	Blurred vision, loss of appetite, headaches, skin rashes, nausea, diarrhea, hair loss, menstrual irregularities, extreme fatigue, joint pain, liver damage, insomnia, abnormal bone growth, injury to brain and nervous system. Excessive consumption of carotene-containing foods, while not poisonous, can cause yellowing of skin.
Vitamin D	Fortified milk; egg yolk; liver; tuna; salmon; cod liver oil. Made on skin in sunlight, but required in diet by dark-skinned persons in cold climates, babies, and those confined indoors.	Aids in the formation and maintenance of bones and teeth; assists in the absorption and use of calcium and phosporus.	In children, rickets: stunted bone growth, bowed legs, malformed teeth, protruding abdomen. In adults, osteomalacia: softening of the bones leading to shortening and fractures, muscle spasms, and twitching.	In infants, calcium deposits in kidneys and excessive calcium in blood; in adults, calcium deposits throughout body (may be mistaken for cancer), deafness, nausea, loss of appetite, kidney stones, fragile bones, high blood pressure, high blood cholesterol, increased lead absorption.
Vitamin E (alpha-tocopherol)	Vegetable oils; margarine; wheat germ; whole-grain cereals and bread; liver; dried beans; green leafy vegetables.	Aids in the formation of red blood cells, muscles, and other tissues; protects vitamin A and essential fatty acids from oxidation.	Not seen in human beings except after prolonged impairment of fat absorption. Deficiency symptoms in laboratory animals (e.g., reproductive failure, liver degeneration, heart damage, muscular dystrophy) not seen in people, not even	None definitely known. Reports of headache, blurred vision, extreme fatigue, muscle weakness. Can destroy some vitamin K made in the gut.

	...bage; cauliflower; peas; potatoes; liver; cereals. Except in newborns, made by bacteria in human intestine.	Aids in the synthesis of substances needed for blood to clot; helps maintain normal bone metabolism.	Hemorrhage, especially in newborn infants. In adults, loss of calcium from bones (however, this deficiency is extremely rare). Extra K needed by persons on prolonged antibiotic therapy and those with impaired fat absorption, cancer, or kidney disease.	Jaundice in babies; anemia in laboratory animals.
WATER SOLUBLE				
Thiamine (B$_1$)	Pork (especially ham); liver; oyster; whole-grain and enriched cereals, pasta, and bread; wheat germ; oatmeal; peas; lima beans. May also be made by intestinal microbes.	Helps release energy from carbohydrates; aids in the synthesis of an important nervous-system chemical.	Beriberi: mental confusion, muscular weakness, swelling of the heart, leg cramps. Need for thiamin is increased if calories consumed increase.	None known. However, since B vitamins are interdependent, excess of one may produce deficiency of others.
Riboflavin (B$_2$)	Liver; milk; meat; dark-green vegetables; eggs; whole-grain and enriched cereals, pasta, and bread; mushrooms; dried beans and peas.	Helps release energy from carbohydrates, proteins, and fats; aids in the maintenance of mucous membranes.	Skin disorders, especially around nose and lips; cracks at corners of mouth; sensitivity of eyes to light.	None known. See thiamine.
Niacin (B$_{3}$, nicotinafuide, nicotinic acid)	Liver; poultry; meat; tuna; eggs; whole-grain and enriched cereals, pasta, and bread; nuts; dried peas and beans. Body can convert tryptophan into niacin.	Participates with thiamin and riboflavin in facilitating energy production in cells.	Pellagra: skin disorders (especially on parts of body exposed to sun), diarrhea, mental confusion, irritability, mouth swelling, smooth tongue.	Duodenal ulcer, abnormal liver function, elevated blood sugar, excessive uric acid in blood, possibly leading to gout. See thiamine.

Table continues on next page.

VITAMINS: WHERE TO GET THEM AND WHAT THEY DO (Continued)

Vitamins	Best sources	Main roles	Deficiency symptoms	Risks of megadoses
WATER SOLUBLE				
Vitamin B$_6$ (includes pyridoxine, pyridoxal, and pyridoxamine)	Whole-grain (but not enriched) cereals and bread; liver; avocados; spinach; green beans; bananas; fish; poultry; meats; nuts; potatoes; green, leafy vegetables.	Aids in the absorption and metabolism of proteins; helps the body use fats; assists in the formation of red blood cells.	Skin disorders; cracks at corners of mouth; smooth tongue; convulsions; dizziness; nausea; anemia; kidney stones. Mild deficiency caused by oral contraceptives may cause depression. Otherwise, deficiencies rare. Need for B$_6$ is increased by increased protein in diet.	Dependency on high dose, leading to deficiency symptoms when one returns to normal amounts.
Vitamin B$_{12}$ (cobalamin)	Only in animal foods; liver; kidneys; meat; fish; eggs; milk; oysters; nutritional yeast.	Aids in the formation of red blood cells; assists in the building of genetic material; helps the functioning of the nervous system.	Pernicious anemia: anemia, pale skin and mucous membranes, numbness and tingling in fingers and toes that may progress to loss of balance and weakness and pain in arms and legs. At risk: strict vegetarians who eat no animal foods; persons who have had part of their stomach removed; those with a genetic inability to absorb B$_{12}$.	None known. See thiamine.
Folacin (folic acid)	Liver; kidneys; dark-green leafy vegetables; wheat germ; dried beans and peas. Stored in the body so that daily consumption is not crucial.	Acts with B$_{12}$ in synthesizing genetic material; aids in the formation of hemoglobin in red blood cells.	Megaloblastic anemia: enlarged red blood cells, smooth tongue, diarrhea; during pregnancy, deficiency may cause loss of the fetus or fetal abnormalities. Women on oral contraceptives may need extra folacin.	None identified. But body stores it, so it is potentially hazardous. Can mask a B$_{12}$ deficiency.

Nutrient	Best sources	Function	Deficiency symptoms	Excess/Toxicity
Pantothenic acid	In all plants and animals, especially liver; kidneys; whole-grain cereal and bread; nuts; eggs; dark-green vegetables. Also made by intestinal bacteria. Lost in refined and heavily processed foods.	Helps in the metabolism of carbohydrates, proteins, and fats; aids in the formation of hormones and nerve-regulating substances.	Not known except experimentally in human beings: severe abdominal cramps, vomiting, fatigue, difficulty sleeping, tingling in hands and feet.	Increased need for thiamine, possibly causing thiamine deficiency symptoms.
Biotin	Egg yolk; liver; kidneys; dark-green vegetables; green beans. Made by microorganisms in the intestinal tract.	Aids in the formation of fatty acids; helps release energy from carbohydrates.	Not known under natural circumstances. Large amounts of raw egg white can destroy biotin, causing loss of appetite, nausea, vomiting, pallor, depression, fatigue, and muscle pain. (Cooked egg white has no harmful effect.)	None known. See thiamine.
Vitamin C (ascorbic acid)	Citrus fruits; tomatoes; strawberries; melon; green peppers; potatoes; dark-green vegetables.	Aids in the formation of collagen; helps maintain capillaries, bones, and teeth; helps protect other vitamins from oxidation; may block formation of cancer-causing nitrosamines.	Scurvy: bleeding gums, degenerating muscles, wounds that don't heal, loose teeth, brown, dry, rough skin. Early symptoms include loss of appetite, irritability, weight loss.	Dependency on high doses, possibly precipitating symptoms of scurvy when withdrawn (especially in infants if megadoses taken during pregnancy); kidney and bladder stones; diarrhea; urinary-tract irritation; increased tendency for blood to clot; breakdown of red blood cells in persons with certain common genetic disorders (such as glucose-6 phosphate dehydrogenase deficiency, common in blacks); may induce B_{12} deficiency.

SOURCE: "JANE BRODY'S NUTRITION BOOK" by Jane E. Brody. New York: W. W. Norton, 1981.

ing those that line the lungs and the bladder. These substances are available only for experimental use. It is dangerous to use vitamin A itself for this purpose.

B Vitamins. These fragile vitamins are thiamine (B_1), riboflavin (B_2), niacin, pyridoxine (B_6), pantothenic acid, biotin, folic acid, and cobalamin (B_{12}). The B vitamins tend to be interdependent, so that excess intake of any one may create a greater need for others. For the most part, B vitamins consumed in excess of the body's needs are simply excreted in the urine.

Several of the B vitamins are important to carbohydrate metabolism, so the more carbohydrates (sugars and starches) you eat, the more B vitamins you need. The starchy foods supply their own additional B vitamins, but sugary snacks usually don't. Women and girls tend to be deficient in thiamine and riboflavin.

Niacin can be made in the body from the amino acid tryptophan. Contrary to claims, it is not effective in treating schizophrenia. Strict vegetarians who eat no animal foods must rely on nuts and legumes for niacin. The niacin in cereals and some vegetables (for example, corn) may be present in chemically unusable forms.

The need for pyridoxine is increased with increasing amounts of protein in the diet. The requirement for pyridoxine is increased by cortisone and the antituberculosis drug INH, in addition to oral contraceptives.

Pantothenic acid, widely present in foods, is also made in large amounts by intestinal bacteria. Excessive consumption of pantothenic acid increases the need for thiamine and may precipitate thiamine deficiency symptoms.

Biotin is similarly made by intestinal bacteria and consumed in foods. People who eat lots of raw eggs may become deficient in biotin, since a protein in uncooked egg white, avidin, binds the vitamin and prevents its absorption. This protein is destroyed by cooking.

Unlike the other water-soluble vitamins, folic acid is stored in the liver and kidneys, so it needn't be consumed daily. However, deficiencies sometimes result from an inability to absorb the vitamin as well as from failure to eat the fresh green vegetables in which it's plentiful.

Cobalamin, or B_{12}, can only be obtained from animal sources. Strict vegetarians must take a B_{12} supplement (yeast is not a source of B_{12}). Large amounts of folic acid can mask a B_{12} deficiency, and large doses of vitamin C increase the need for B_{12}. To be absorbed, B_{12} requires a special protein that some individuals are unable to produce, necessitating B_{12} injections. However, B_{12} shots are no use, except as a placebo, or "sugar pill," for persons with emotional problems or fatigue that is not caused by a frank B_{12} deficiency.

Vitamin C. Carefully controlled studies have not borne out the assertion that megadoses of vitamin C, also known as ascorbic acid (a popular food additive), can ward off colds and flu, although it may lessen the severity of symptoms in some people.

The hazards of large doses include the formation of bladder and kidney stones, interference with the effects of blood-thinning drugs, possible destruction of B_{12}, a possible increased need for vitamin E, and loss of calcium from bones. It may also result in an abnormal reading on laboratory tests for blood sugar. In addition, the body can become dependent on large doses, with deficiency symptoms developing when the megadoses are stopped.

Excess vitamin C during pregnancy may result in symptoms of scurvy and an abnormally large need for the vitamin in the infant. On the positive side, vitamin C can block the formation in the body of cancer-causing substances called nitrosamines and enhance the absorption of essential iron and calcium.

Vitamin D. The "sunshine" vitamin is made in adequate amounts on your skin if you spend some time outdoors with your skin exposed to ultraviolet light. However, people living in very cold climates, dark-skinned people living in northern zones, babies, and those confined indoors (especially the elderly) require vitamin D in their diets. Excessive consumption of D is highly poisonous; it can cause kidney damage, lethargy, and loss of appetite.

Vitamin E. This readily oxidized vitamin is important as a protector of other nutrients that might otherwise be destroyed by oxidation, such as vitamin A and essential fatty acids. The need for E is increased proportionately with the amount of polyunsaturated fats (vegetable oils and margarine) in the diet. However, most such fats contain adequate amounts of E.

There is some evidence that vitamin E may also protect against the formation of cancer-causing nitrosamines. Other claims for its miraculous effects — including its purported ability to ward off the ravages of age — have not been substantiated. Properly designed experiments have suggested its usefulness in treating fibrocystic disease of the breast as well as a number of rare conditions that must be treated by medical specialists.

Although E is a fat-soluble vitamin that accumulates in the body, possible toxic effects of large doses have not yet been noted in properly designed studies. However, overdoses have been reported to precipitate headache, nausea, extreme fatigue, muscle weakness, and blood clots in individual cases.

Vitamin K. Newborn infants, persons on prolonged treatment with sulfa drugs, and those with impaired fat absorption may need K supplements. Otherwise, enough is produced by intestinal bacteria and consumed in foods to meet human needs. Excessive use of K supplements can be toxic.

51

PART II: THE MACROMINERALS

Even more than the vitamins, the major minerals demonstrate the importance of getting your essential nutrients from a varied and balanced diet rather than from a vial. Increasing your intake of one or another mineral by gobbling pills and potions can distort the physiological ratio between the various minerals and actually result in a mineral deficiency. In some cases an excess of a particular mineral can have direct hazardous effects.

Except for calcium, dietary deficiencies of the major minerals are rare. Minerals are inorganic substances that, unlike most vitamins, are usually not destroyed by cooking, food processing, or exposure to air or acid. However, they can sometimes combine with other substances in food to form insoluble salts that cannot be absorbed by the human digestive tract. Following is a guide to the major minerals, their roles, sources, deficiencies, and idiosyncrasies.

Calcium. Calcium is the major constituent of the structural framework of bone and is the body's most prevalent mineral. About 3 pounds of a 160-pound man's weight are calcium. Male or female, 98 percent of the body's calcium is found in the bones, 1 percent in the teeth, and the remaining 1 percent in soft tissues throughout the body, where it performs a variety of essential functions.

In addition to supporting the growth and continued strength of bones and teeth, calcium helps maintain cell membranes and the "cement" that holds cells together; it is essential to proper blood clotting; it helps to regulate the transport of ions in and out of cells, making possible muscular contraction and relaxation; and it is necessary to the function of several important enzymes.

The bones act as a calcium depot for the rest of the body. Although bones are commonly thought of as fixed, solid objects, in fact they are continually losing and regaining calcium. A network of hormones keeps the calcium level in blood and other body fluids at a constant level, depositing temporary excesses in the bones and removing calcium from the bones if it is needed elsewhere.

If your diet contains inadequate amounts of calcium, your bones and teeth suffer, but not any of the other life-sustaining functions. Thus, the contentions of some writers on nutrition that a dietary deficiency of calcium can result in a host of miseries, including menstrual cramps, muscle spasms, insomnia, bleeding problems, and indigestion, are simply untrue. The body takes care of all needs by borrowing from the bones.

A persistent calcium shortage results in distorted bone growth in children and a softening and deterioration of bones in adults, including osteoporosis, a weakening of the bone that affects one in four women after menopause. [See chapter on osteoporosis, page 610.] An inadequate calcium supply can occur because too little is consumed, too much is lost, or not enough is absorbed.

The richest food source of calcium is milk and dairy products, including yogurt and hard cheeses. Two glasses of milk supply two-thirds of the recommended daily allowance for adults. Sardines and canned salmon eaten with the bones, and green leafy vegetables — collard and dandelion greens and spinach — are also good sources, but oxalic acid in spinach renders much of the calcium insoluble and nonabsorbable.

The recommended daily allowance for calcium is 800 milligrams for adults, obtainable by consuming two cups of milk or its equivalent (fortified soy milk is an adequate substitute for those with a milk allergy) plus one cup of greens. The need for calcium is increased by half during periods of adolescent growth and during pregnancy and lactation. To meet your calcium requirement through pills, you would have to take twelve or more quarter-sized tablets a day, and the calcium in pills may not be absorbed as well as that from foods.

Unless your body has adequate amounts of vitamin D (made on your skin in daylight and found in fortified margarine and milk products), calcium cannot be absorbed through the intestinal tract. Absorption is enhanced by the milk sugar, lactose — another reason milk is such a good source of calcium. But calcium absorption is impaired by excessive dietary fat, and large amounts of animal protein result in an increased loss of calcium through the urine.

A relative shortage of calcium can result if the ratio of calcium to other minerals is distorted, even if the total amount of calcium consumed is appropriate. If a newborn is given too much phosphorus relative to the amount of calcium consumed, a condition called hypocalcemic tetany can result. This is one reason breast milk is better than cow's milk. Similarly, a relative excess of magnesium can have a narcotizing effect, reversible by injections of calcium.

Too much calcium has been shown to depress nerve function and cause drowsiness and extreme lethargy. Large excesses of calcium have also resulted in calcium deposits in tissues where it doesn't belong, producing false X ray signs of cancer.

Several individuals who supplemented their diets with calcium-rich bone meal developed lead poisoning from the lead that contaminated the meal. Lead is just one of many toxic substances that the body stores in bones. One such victim, a forty-six-year-old actress whose career was destroyed as a result, was seriously ill for three years, seeing thirty-two doctors and having more than 340 X rays before her problem was correctly diagnosed.

Phosphorus. Phosphorus, a partner with calcium in bones and teeth, is widespread in foods, including meat, fish, poultry, milk, nuts, legumes, and whole-grain cereals and breads. The recommended daily allowance is 800 milligrams for adults, 1,200 for adolescents and pregnant and nursing women. Most people get more than enough from the large amounts of meat they eat and from the phosphates (phosphorus salts) used in processed foods. If the diet contains too much phosphorus, calcium is not used efficiently.

In addition to helping to form bones and teeth, phosphorus is in every cell as a part of nucleic acids; it is needed for the release of energy from carbohydrates and for the functioning of several B vitamins, and it is used to transport fats around the body. Prolonged use of antacids can lead to a harmful loss of phosphorus, and frequent consumption of carbonated drinks (which contain phosphorus) can distort the crucial ratio of calcium to phosphorus.

Magnesium. Magnesium, also a constituent of bones, is found in nuts (almonds and cashews are highest), meat, fish, milk, whole grains, and greens (eaten fresh as salad). Cooking can wash away some magnesium. Magnesium in the body's soft tissues catalyzes hundreds of metabolic reactions. Among its essential roles are the release of energy from glycogen (stored muscle fuel), the manufacture of proteins, the regulation of body temperature, and the proper working of nerves and muscles.

The recommended daily allowance is 350 milligrams for men, 300 milligrams for women. Deficiencies are rare except in chronic alcoholics and persons with certain neuromuscular diseases. Excessive doses, such as are contained in milk of magnesia and Epsom salts, have a cathartic effect.

Potassium. Potassium, important to the proper working of muscles, including the heart muscle, is plentiful in bananas, orange juice, dried fruits, meat, peanut butter, potatoes, and coffee. Potassium is a crucial regulator of the amount of water in cells, which determines their ability to function properly. It helps in the transmission of nerve impulses, it's a buffer for body fluids, and it catalyzes the release of energy from carbohydrates, proteins, and fats. It may also help to prevent high blood pressure. No recommended allowance has been set. However, too much salt (sodium) in the diet can compromise the body's supply of potassium, and deficiencies can occur following a bout of severe diarrhea and the use of diuretics. People who sweat very heavily may have a larger than usual potassium requirement, though recent studies have indicated that little or no potassium is lost through sweat.

Sulfur. Sulfur also has no set recommended amount. Deficiencies in human beings are unknown, since sulfur is widespread in protein foods. Sulfur can form bridges between protein molecules, and thus, it is a constituent of firm proteins in hair, fingernails, toenails, and skin.

Chloride. Chloride, which enters the body mainly through table salt (sodium chloride), regulates the balance of body fluids and their constituents. Only people on a severely salt-restricted diet need to be concerned about getting enough, perhaps by using potassium chloride, a salt substitute.

PART III: THE MICROMINERALS

Probably no aspect of human nutritional needs is more misunderstood and unappreciated than the so-called microminerals, or trace elements. These are inorganic substances that the body requires in tiny amounts to maintain normal health and growth, but that can be deadly poisons if consumed in large doses.

Many people fail to appreciate this delicate balance and mistakenly assume that if a substance is harmful in large doses, small doses taken over a long period of time may also be poisonous. Others make the opposite, equally incorrect assumption that if a small amount of a substance is good for you, more of it must be better.

As a result, claims have been made that large doses of one or another micronutrient may cure or prevent various diseases, including cancer. While there is some evidence to support such claims, all the important facts are not yet in, and the risk of overdosing oneself with a poisonous substance is always present.

The minerals required in trace amounts include iron, copper, iodine, zinc, fluorine, chromium, and — animal and other evidence suggests — cobalt, manganese, molybdenum, selenium, nickel, tin, vanadium, and silicon as well. Although deficiencies of some of these have never been demonstrated in human beings, dietary shortages of others that may compromise health sometimes occur.

Following is a description of the known and suspected roles of trace elements, the foods that contain them in substantial amounts, and the hazards of overdoses.

Iron. Iron is an essential ingredient in all cells, but it is especially important to the oxygen-carrying cells of the blood and muscles, which use two-thirds of the iron requirement. Hemoglobin, the oxygen transport pigment of red blood cells, and myoglobin, the hemoglobin of muscle cells, cannot be formed without iron. Nor can certain vital enzymes.

Dietary shortages of iron represent the nation's most widespread nutritional deficiency. Iron-deficiency anemia can produce such symptoms as easy fatigue, weakness, pallor, and shortness of breath. The problem most commonly affects infants, young children, adolescents, and women of childbearing age, some of whom may need to take iron supplements to avert a shortage of this essential nutrient. Iron supplements are routinely given to pregnant and nursing women.

However, iron supplements should not be taken without a physician's recommendation that is based on one or more blood tests. Since iron is stored in the body and lost only through bleeding, it is possible to accumulate a toxic overdose that can damage the liver, pancreas, and heart.

The iron in animal foods, such as beef, liver, fish, and poultry, is more readily absorbed than that in milk, eggs, cheese, or vegetables, such as spinach. Eating an iron-containing food along with a food rich in vitamin C (such as citrus fruits, tomatoes, or green peppers) can enhance iron absorption.

Copper. All mammals require small amounts of copper, an element that can be a deadly poison in large quantities. Copper is an essential ingredient of several respiratory enzymes and is needed for the development of young red blood cells.

Deficiency of copper in mammals leads to such problems as anemia; faulty development of bone and nervous tissue; loss of elasticity in the tendons and the major arteries, possibly causing rupture of the blood vessels; abnormal development of the lung's air sacs, possibly predisposing to emphysema; and abnormal pigmentation and structure of the hair.

No specific level of copper required in the diet has been set, but most diets far exceed needed amounts. The richest dietary sources of copper are nuts, cocoa powder, dry tea, beef and pork liver, kidney, raisins, dried beans, bran flakes, and some shellfish.

Milk is very low in copper, but the human infant is born with enough copper to last until other foods are consumed. However, premature infants fed cow's milk exclusively for two to three months may develop a copper deficiency. In adults, even during prolonged malnutrition, a copper deficiency does not develop.

Iodine. Iodine is an integral part of two important thyroid hormones that regulate metabolism. Deficiency leads to a shortage of thyroid hormones and goiter, an enlargement of the thyroid gland. If the deficiency occurs before or shortly after birth, it may result in cretinism. Iodine is also essential for normal reproduction.

The National Academy of Sciences has established a daily recommended dietary allowance for adults of between 100 and 140 micrograms, depending on age and sex. Growing children and pregnant and nursing women may need proportionately greater amounts.

Except for seafood and seaweed, most foods contain precious little iodine. Iodine is added to salt (iodized salt) to help prevent goiter in people living where little seafood is consumed and the soil is deficient in iodine. However, with today's national pattern of food distribution and iodine introduced through food production and processing, few if any parts of the country fail to consume foods containing iodine.

Zinc. This element is essential to plants, animals, and man. It is a constituent of nearly 100 human enzymes involved in major metabolic processes. Deficiency causes loss of appetite and failure to grow. Prenatal zinc deficiency may interfere with the maturation of the brain and cause abnormal behavior later in life.

Soils in three-fifths of the United States contain very little zinc, and some Americans may be marginally deficient in this element. Such people experience more rapid wound healing and improved taste sensitivity when zinc is added to their diet. Otherwise healthy children in Denver were found to have impaired taste, poor appetites, and less than normal growth as a result of a zinc deficiency.

The recommended daily allowance is 3 milligrams during the first six months of life, 10 milligrams for children, and 15 milligrams for adults, with an extra 5 milligrams during pregnancy and an extra 10 milligrams when one is nursing.

The best way to get enough zinc is to eat a varied diet containing animal protein. Meat, liver, egg, and seafood are good sources, followed by milk and whole grain products. Diets that depend heavily on grains, which contain large amounts of phytates that block absorption of zinc, may result in a deficiency.

However, the zinc supplements sold in health food stores are unnecessary except in a few rare conditions, including a hereditary disorder called acrodermatitis enteropathica and patients who are fed entirely by vein. As a drug zinc sulfate may be an effective treatment for acne. However, as little as one 220-milligram capsule can cause nausea and vomiting. Other toxic effects of excess zinc include abdominal pain, fever, and severe anemia.

Fluoride. Small amounts of fluoride, starting before birth and continuing throughout life, are essential for the formation of strong, decay-resistant teeth. [See chapter on tooth decay, page 282.] Fluoride may also help to prevent the loss of bone with age and the debilitating fractures that follow.

Food sources of fluoride include fish, tea, most animal foods, and plants grown in areas where fluoride is present in the water. Drinking water is naturally a good source of fluoride in some areas of the country; in others, low levels of fluoride are added to the water to protect teeth. But many communities still lack fluoridated water because of vehement opposition from small groups of people who regard it as a poison.

Indeed, at high doses, fluoride is toxic just like the other trace elements. However, toxic effects, such as mottling of the teeth, do not appear except after daily intake for many years of amounts far above those commonly consumed in the United States. There is absolutely no reliable evidence to support contentions that water fluoridation causes or contributes to cancer.

Chromium. This element is needed to maintain normal metabolism of glucose (blood sugar) and may be important in preventing diabetes. Some Americans, particularly the elderly, pregnant women, and malnourished persons, may not consume adequate amounts of chromium. Only a small amount of dietary chromium is absorbed by the body. Meat, cheese, whole grain products (chromium is lost during processing), dried beans, peanuts, and brewer's yeast are good sources of chromium. No daily requirement for this element has been established thus far.

The following trace elements are believed to be essential to human nutrition on the basis of two types of evidence: proved necessity in other mammalian species or identification of the element as part of an essential body ingredient, or both. No required levels have been established for human beings.

Cobalt. This element is an essential part of vitamin B_{12}. Ruminant animals use cobalt from plants to make this vitamin, which people obtain when they eat animal foods. In excessive amounts, cobalt can cause goiter (by blocking iodine uptake) and a red blood cell disorder called polycythemia. When added to beer, it resulted in an "epidemic" of heart muscle damage in heavy beer drinkers.

Manganese. Manganese is needed for normal bone structure, reproduction, and proper functioning of the central nervous system. It is also part of several enzymes systems in man. No human manganese deficiency is known. Good sources of the element are nuts and whole grains, followed by vegetables and fruits. The effects of manganese poisoning include a masklike facial expression, difficulty in walking, blurred speech, tremors of the hands, and involuntary laughing.

Molybdenum. This element is a component of an important enzyme called xanthine oxidase. It is an essential nutrient for several species of mammals, but deficiencies in people are not known. Good sources include legumes, some cereal grains, beef liver and kidney, and certain dark green vegetables.

Selenium. Little is known about the importance of selenium to humans. It is believed to serve as an antioxidant, preventing the breakdown of fats, and may be an enzyme catalyst. It can prevent death of liver cells in animals. There is some evidence that diets rich in selenium may lower the risk of developing cancers of the digestive tract. Animal studies also have suggested that selenium may help to prevent heart disease. Selenium is found in seafood, whole grain cereals, meat, egg yolk, mushrooms, chicken, milk, and garlic. Excessive selenium may increase susceptibility to dental problems and cause central nervous system damage.

Nickel, tin, vanadium, and silicon. Deficiencies of these elements have been produced in experimental animals, suggesting that they are essential to good nutrition, but their importance to humans has not been established. Nickel is found in considerable amounts in legumes, tea, cocoa, pepper, and some grains. Tin is found in water as well as foods, especially in canned foods. Vanadium is plentiful in skim milk powder, seafood, oats, rye, and soybean and corn oils. Silicon is found in unrefined cereals and beer. All are poisonous when consumed in excess.

For Further Reading

Herbert, Dr. Victor, and Dr. Stephen Barrett. *Vitamins and "Health" Foods: The Great American Hustle.* Philadelphia: G. F. Stickley Co., 1981.

Food Additives:
Most Good, Some Bad

In this day of aversion to chemicals, few people would be tempted to buy a food product labeled as follows: "Contents: Water, triglycerides of stearic, palmitic, oleic and linoleic acids; myosin and actin; glycogen, collagen, lecithin, cholesterol, dipotassium phosphate, myoglobin, and urea. (Note: Product may also contain steroid hormones of natural origin.)"

Unless you're a vegetarian, you probably eat this food with some regularity and considerable relish. It is nothing but beefsteak, America's most popular main course. As ordinary "natural" foods go, steak is a rather simple collection of chemicals. Milk has 95 chemicals, and potatoes contain 150, including one, solanine, that's an outright poison. The natural flavoring in butter has the breathtaking name of aceton-3-hydroxy-2-butanone.

Many people, when they pick up a package of instant mashed potatoes and read "Dried potato (with color and freshness preserved by sodium phosphate, sodium sulfite, and BHT), mono- and diglycerides, calcium stearoyl-2-lactylate" are repulsed by the list of hard-to-pronounce chemical ingredients that have been added to the natural product. Few realize that many added chemicals are "natural" substances that have been extracted from plants or animals and that among those additives artificially produced there are several that offer nutritional benefits and others that protect against contaminants that might make the food unsafe.

Trying to appeal to consumers who prefer "no additives," some food companies are making irrational changes in their products. For example, some bread manufacturers have stopped adding the mold inhibitor calcium propionate so that they can declare their product free of preservatives. But in fact, calcium propionate is safe, it provides the nutrient calcium, it is naturally present in larger amounts in Swiss cheese, and it inhibits the growth of molds that themselves may produce toxins.

Years ago, sensitive to the public's wariness of anything "chemical," the food industry adopted the name "additives." Several can legally be listed by their initials — for example, BHT, the more forbidding chemical name of which is butylated hydroxytoluene. For some products that are covered by government food standards, certain additives don't have to be listed at all on the package label.

Food additives introduced since 1958 have been subjected to laboratory and animal tests, but more than 600 additives in use before then were designated "generally recognized as safe" and only recently were subjected to careful review by a national group of independent scientists. (Of the 415 chemicals examined, the group declared 73 percent safe, 16 percent all right but in need of more study, 5 percent uncertain and in need of more study, 1 percent warranting restrictions, and 4 percent lacking enough data to be evaluated.)

Why Do We Need Food Additives?

First of all, to make food taste better. No matter how "natural" your diet, if you use salt, pepper, baking soda, sugar, mustard, or other condiments, you're using food additives. A second major reason is to keep foods fresh during their long trek from producer to consumer and to provide a variety of foods the year round. In our society 92 percent of the population is dependent on the remaining 8 percent to produce all its food; without food additives of any kind, the offerings of unspoiled, nutritious, tasteful foods on supermarket shelves would be significantly reduced.

Without food additives, there would probably be no need for supermarkets since the vast majority of the 15,000 items on sale today could not exist without one or more added chemicals. There would be few convenience foods — no canned fruits or vegetables, packaged soups, breads or cakes, pancake mixes or syrups, TV dinners, or frozen pizzas — and few such low-calorie or low-cholesterol foods as diet sodas, margarines, or egg substitutes. Even brown sugar would bite the dust since it is white sugar that has been colored and flavored with caramel (caramelized sugar), a food additive.

Many foods would have to be purchased in small quantities or stored in the refrigerator instead of the cupboard because without added preservatives they would spoil quickly. You would have to shop more often, and since waste caused by spoilage would be extensive, food would cost more.

But none of this means that the thousands of chemicals used by American food processors are all desirable, necessary, or safe. The public confidence in food additives has been shaken badly over the last decade with the banning as possible cancer risks of several additives once considered safe, notably the artificial sweetener cyclamate (now its substitute, saccharin, is also suspect).

Several synthetic food colors have been banned, and the safety of those still used is in doubt. Norway has outlawed them all, and many experts in this country see no reason to go on using questionable chemicals that add nothing but window dressing to food. If all hot dogs were gray, their argument goes, those who like hot dogs would eat them that way.

Other experts are concerned that food additives that are individually safe may add up to a toxic burden in a person who consumes hundreds of different food additives in the course of a day. These experts point out, accurately, that the possible interaction of the various chemicals, even those used in the same food, has not been tested.

It is also true, however, that the interaction of chemicals naturally present in foods has never been tested and that the possible toxic effects of food additives have been much more carefully studied than the natural toxins in foods.

What They Are and What They Do

Before we issue a wholesale condemnation of added food chemicals, it would help to know where they come from, why they're used, and how much of them you really consume.

Many are *natural substances,* including ascorbic acid (vitamin C, from citrus fruits) and its more soluble salt, sodium ascorbate; sorbic acid (from berries); gum tragacanth and guar gum (from trees); lecithin (from plants); gelatin (from bones); glycerol (from fats); carrageenin (from seaweed); caffeine (from coffee and tea); alpha-tocopherol (vitamin E); monosodium glutamate (MSG, the salt of a natural amino acid); and sodium caseinate (casein, the protein in milk).

Other additives are *synthetic chemical copies of natural substances,* such as vanillin, the flavoring from the vanilla bean, which is synthesized so that more of the substance can be obtained at lower cost.

The third class of food additives consists of *entirely synthetic chemicals:* saccharin, sorbitan monostearate, sodium bisulfite, butylated hydroxyanisole (BHA), calcium stearoyl lactylate, ethylene-diamine tetra-acetic acid (EDTA), among many others.

The additives most commonly used are natural substances: sugar (98 pounds a person a year) and other such sweeteners as corn syrup, dextrose, and fructose (28 pounds), and salt (15 pounds). Thirty-three different natural and synthetic additives that are used to flavor, thicken, stabilize, neutralize, emulsify, moisturize, leaven, and preserve processed foods add up to 9 pounds per person a year. These include MSG, pepper, mustard, baking soda, yeast, casein, and caramel. Another 1,800 food additives, half of them consumed in amounts of less than half a milligram a year, add up to a total of 1 pound per person.

All these additives are consumed as part of the 1,500 pounds of food that the average American eats each year. In other words, by weight, added chemicals make up less than 10 percent of the food we eat, and nine-tenths of that 10 percent are added sugars and salt. The chemicals most people think of as food additives represent only 1 percent of our total diet.

Just because a food chemical is "natural" doesn't mean it's necessarily good for you; conversely, all artificial chemicals are not necessarily unhealthy. Caffeine, a natural substance added to colas and other soft drinks, can cause anxiety reactions, sleeplessness, and, possibly, birth defects. Some people have life-threatening allergic reactions to gum tragacanth.

MSG can damage brain cells in baby animals and cause "Chinese restaurant syndrome" (a gripping headache) in sensitive adults. Manufacturers of root beer now use artificial flavoring because the natural flavor, safrole, from the sassafras plant, causes cancer in animals.

Many consumers are agitating for the elimination of nitrates and nitrites from cured meats because they may result in the formation of cancer-causing nitrosamines in the body. But some commonly eaten foods, including spinach, beets, lettuce, celery, carrots, eggplant, and radishes, naturally contain very high levels of nitrate. Some honeys contain cancer-causing chemicals that are naturally present in pollen, and others have been linked to botulism in infants.

On the other hand, EDTA, a safe synthetic, is used in many processed foods to trap metallic impurities that would otherwise cause rancidity and loss of natural color. Iodine, added to salt, prevents goiter among people living in iodine-deficient parts of the country. Added synthetic vitamins and minerals make bread and milk more nourishing, and carotene, used as an artificial coloring, is converted in the body to vitamin A. Sodium benzoate, a preservative, helps prevent the growth of bacteria, yeasts, and fungi that spoil food and cause food poisoning.

Like everything else in life, the rational use of food additives must involve a careful weighing of benefits versus risks. No substance, synthetic or natural, is completely safe under all conditions of use. If used inappropriately, all chemicals are potentially hazardous.

62

Sometimes, when the public is given its say in deciding benefits versus risks, the outcome is surprising. For example, when it was found that saccharin could cause cancer in test animals and a government ban on its widespread use was imminent, consumers who would ordinarily chide the government for failing to protect the public health protested vehemently and continued guzzling saccharin-sweetened beverages. Similarly, health food enthusiasts who deplore the "unsafe" chemicals used by American food processors encourage the consumption of cyanide-laden apricot pits (Laetrile).

If you want to reduce your consumption of added food chemicals, however, there is a very simple solution: Reduce your dependence on processed foods, and instead, eat more unrefined and fresh foods. Fill most of your market basket with the foods sold at the periphery of the supermarket, and venture with care into the center aisles, reading labels all the way.

For Further Reading

Bunin, Greta, and Michael F. Jacobson, Ph.D. *Does Everything Cause Cancer? A Food Safety Primer.* Washington, D.C.: Center for Science in the Public Interest, 1979.
Burros, Marion. *Pure and Simple.* New York: Berkley, 1978. An additive-free cookbook.
Jacobson, Michael F., Ph.D. *Eater's Digest: The Consumer's Factbook of Food Additives.* New York: Doubleday, 1976.

Water:
The Most Essential Nutrient

Though rarely found in a list of required nutrients, water is in fact the single most important substance we consume. While we can survive prolonged fasts with a total absence of all other nutrients, several days without any external source of water usually means death.

Few people realize just how much water the human body requires to function properly, and many fail to consume enough, especially during hot weather or strenuous activity. Thirst, a useful sign that your body is in need of fluid replacement, is not an adequate signal because it tends to shut off before you've consumed enough.

In most cases you need to drink more than is required to satisfy your thirst, especially if you've been perspiring a great deal. Sports medicine specialists urge athletes to "force liquids" in the summer heat. The many roles water plays to keep your body going should convince you to give this vital fluid the attention it deserves.

Although you may think of yourself as a "solid citizen," actually you're mostly water. Newborn babies are 75 to 85 percent water. On the average, a woman's body is 55 to 65 percent water and a man's, 65 to 75 percent. The difference results from the higher proportion of fat in a woman's body; fat holds less water than lean muscle does. Your blood is 83 percent water; your muscles, 75 percent; your brain, 74 percent; your bones, 25 percent; and your body fat, 20 to 35 percent.

What Water Does for You

Water carries nutrients, hormones, disease-fighting cells, antibodies, and waste products to and from body organs through the bloodstream and lymphatic system. Your cells live in a salty sea (reflecting our aquatic origins), which supplies them with essential elements and carries off their products. Water lubricates your joints and mucous membranes. It is also the solvent that enables you to digest and absorb food.

Without water, you would not be able to rid your body of toxic wastes through urine and feces. Nor could your body cool itself to prevent a potentially lethal buildup of internal heat. Water cools primarily through sweat. Sweat evaporates from your skin, using heat from your body to turn the liquid to vapor. Obese people have a harder time cooling off because fat under the skin acts as an insulator, reducing the speed with which heat is lost from the body. In humid weather, your sweat cannot evaporate readily, so you feel hotter than you would on a dry day at the same temperature. Even the slightest breeze can enhance comfort on a hot, humid day because it increases evaporation.

Dr. Helen A. Guthrie, professor of nutrition at the Pennsylvania State University, points out that lack of water has a more damaging effect on work performance than lack of food. "A reduction of 4 to 5 percent in body water will result in a decline of 20 to 30 percent in work performance," she points out in her college textbook *Introductory Nutrition* (St. Louis: C.V. Mosby Company, 1979). She adds that a loss of 10 percent of body water could cause circulatory failure, and a 15 to 20 percent loss almost certainly spells death.

Your body loses water through urine, feces, skin, and lungs. Even if you drank nothing, you would produce about ten to seventeen ounces of urine a day. If your body is dehydrated, your kidneys will cut back on water lost through urine, and your urine will become dark and concentrated.

Under normal circumstances you need about two and a half to three quarts of water a day to replace what is lost. You take in water through the fluids you drink and the foods you eat (most fruits and vegetables are more than 80 percent water; meats and poultry are one-half to two-thirds water; even bread is one-third water). Water is released inside your body by the metabolic breakdown of proteins, carbohydrates, and fats.

Babies need proportionately more water than adults and should be offered bottles of water between feedings during hot weather. Nutrition experts advise adults to drink at least six to eight cups of liquids daily, obtaining the rest of needed water from food and metabolic processes.

WATER CONTENT OF COMMON FOODS
(percent of total weight)

Food	Percent Water	Food	Percent Water
Chicken consommé	97	Blueberries	83
Iceberg lettuce	96	Clams, raw	81
Zucchini, raw	95	Cottage cheese, creamed	78
Watercress	93	Olives, green	78
Watermelon	93	Bananas	76
Cantaloupe	91	Potatoes, baked	75
Green beans, raw	90	Eggs, hard-boiled	74
Cola	90	Noodles, cooked	70
Yogurt	89	Codfish, broiled	65
Strawberries	89	Ice cream	63
Broccoli, raw	89	Ham, lean, baked	58
Farina, cooked	89	Chicken, fried	54
Orange juice	88	Pizza	48
Carrots, raw	88	Lamb, loin chops, broiled	47
Grapefruit	88	Sirloin steak, broiled	42
Apple juice	88	Cheddar cheese	37
Milk	87	Bread, whole wheat	36
Apple	84	Bread, Italian	32
Gelatin dessert	84		

Drinks containing concentrated nutrients, such as milk, sugar-sweetened soft drinks, and salty tomato-based juices, count more as food than drink since they themselves increase your body's water needs.

Contrary to widespread belief (especially among weight-conscious women), drinking water does not cause bloating. If you exceed your body's water needs, the excess is quickly eliminated. What does cause swelling is a holding of water in the body, usually because there is too much salt or sodium in your diet. To reduce bloat, then, cut back on salt and other sodium sources. [See chapter on salt, page 66.]

Replacing Sweat

In hot weather or when you're exercising or working strenuously, the amount of water your body loses through sweat and respiration increases dramatically. You may lose four or more quarts of body water in one workout. Such deficits can cause extreme thirst, giddiness, and a potentially dangerous rise in body temperature. Therefore, it's extremely important to drink lots of water before, during, and after prolonged activity. To determine how much to drink, weigh yourself before you start exercising, and afterward drink enough to bring your weight back to its original level, about one pint of liquid for each pound of weight.

As for what to drink, cold water is the hands-down winner during exercise or whenever you're overheated. Though some claim warm liquids cool you faster because they increase perspiration, that's no help on humid days. Cold liquids cool you from within by absorbing your heat as they warm to body temperature. Cold drinks also leave the stomach faster — and therefore reach your blood more quickly to counter dehydration — than warm liquids do.

Active people should avoid sweet drinks until after exercise. These slow the absorption of water into the blood and draw water from body tissues (where you really need it) into the gut to dilute the sugar. Beverages containing caffeine or alcohol are not the best for supplying needed water, since they act as diuretics and increase water loss through urine.

"Athletic" drinks designed to replace the salts lost in sweat are not necessary unless you lose more than three quarts of water (about six pounds of weight) during your activity. Sweat has a lower concentration of salts than your blood does, so you lose proportionately more water than salts when you perspire. The most pressing need, then, is to replace the lost water.

If you exceed three quarts of replacement fluid, add about one-half teaspoon of salt for each quart thereafter. Salt tablets are not recommended, and concentrated salt should not be consumed unless you drink large quantities of water at the same time.

People not adapted to vigorous activity in hot weather are likely to lose more salt and water than those accustomed to workouts in the heat. Unadapted individuals, therefore, face a greater risk of depleting their bodies of essential fluids and should take extra care to avoid dehydration and its serious consequences.

Salt:
A Crumbling Pillar

For at least 5,000 years salt (sodium chloride) has been an important, indeed revered constituent of the human food supply. Salting and drying were the earliest methods used to preserve otherwise highly perishable meat and fish, making unspoiled food available during lean times.

In ancient days there was such a clamoring for salt that it was used for barter and pay, and battles were fought to capture or protect salt deposits. To the ancient Greeks a prized slave was "worth his weight in salt." The word "salary" was derived from the Latin word salsus, for salt. It is also the root of the word "sausage," which depends in part on salt for defense against microbial decay.

A Blood Pressure Hazard

However, in health circles in recent years salt has become persona non grata. Some doctors refer to it as a killer since the sodium it contains appears to be a major precipitating cause of potentially fatal high blood pressure, or hypertension. This insidious disorder, which afflicts some 60 million Americans and often produces no symptoms until it has done irreparable damage, can lead to kidney failure, stroke, and heart disease.

Many point out that we have overextended our dependence on salt, consuming far more than our bodies were designed to handle. For millions of years human beings and their primate ancestors consumed no salt or sodium except what was naturally present in foods. Those primitive peoples, whose diets were primarily fruits and vegetables, were on what now amounts to a severely restricted low-sodium diet. Even the meat eaters among our forebears consumed at most a quarter of the amount of sodium that the average American eats today.

Throughout the world today, populations that live on low-salt diets never develop hypertension. In fact, their blood pressure does not rise with age, as it does in the typical American. If anything, it drops. On the other hand, a few preindustrial peoples, such as the Gashgai nomads of southern Iran, who consume a lot of salt, also have a lot of hypertension, despite the lack of stress in their society.

Other hazards of a high-salt diet include edema, or swelling of body tissues, and extreme symptoms of premenstrual tension. Some women experience bloating, headache, irritability, weepiness, and even uncontrollable rages just before their menstrual periods. These symptoms are in part due to retention of salt and water, and they may be relieved by following a low-salt diet for ten days before menstruation is expected. [See also chapter on menstruation, page 224.] One headache specialist has found that salt restriction reduces the frequency and severity of migraines.

For athletes and others who indulge in vigorous exercise, a large dose of salt to replace salt lost through sweating can be harmful and even fatal, causing a loss of potassium (needed for muscle contraction, including the heart muscle) and thickening of the blood. Salt tablets are unnecessary and potentially dangerous. In fact, some athletes have been shown to perform better in hot weather if they reduce their salt intake before the dog days of summer set in; over a period of weeks the body learns to conserve salt, and less is lost through sweating.

The elaborate mechanism that regulates the body's internal supply of water and its essential balance of sodium and potassium evolved for a world in which sodium was relatively scarce and in which potassium, a common mineral in fruits and vegetables, was plentiful. Thus, the kidneys and the chemicals that govern their activities are set up to conserve sodium and get rid of excess potassium.

The diet we currently consume is quite the reverse of what the human species evolved on. Today we eat sodium to considerable excess beyond the body's needs, and potassium, while usually adequately consumed, is in relatively short supply. The net result is that excess sodium can accumulate in the body fluids, drawing water to maintain a proper balance. This in turn increases the volume of blood, the blood pressure, and the heart rate.

How the body reacts to this sodium excess is determined largely by heredity. Approximately 15 to 20 percent of Americans have inherited a genetic susceptibility to the effects of excess sodium. Eventually, on the high-salt diet that most of us eat, they develop high blood pressure. There's no way to know in advance who is and who is not susceptible to the damaging effects of sodium, so a wise approach is for everyone to reduce sodium consumption.

A Habit We Can Break

Actually, our taste for salt is acquired. No salt needs to be added to the diet to meet the body's need for sodium, which amounts to only 220 milligrams a day. The Senate Select Committee on Nutrition and Human Needs recommended that instead of the 10 to 24 grams of salt consumed per person each day, Americans should eat at most 5 grams. This supplies 2,000 milligrams of sodium, more than enough for practically everyone under all circumstances. Others recommend even less salt — below 2 grams a day (which supplies 800 milligrams of sodium) — to protect the genetically susceptible from developing high blood pressure. The Food and Nutrition Board of the National Academy of Sciences suggests a range of 1,100 to 3,300 milligrams of sodium daily, with an average consumption of 2,200 milligrams.

Once high blood pressure develops, salt restriction should be the first line of treatment. It is cheaper and less hazardous than taking blood pressure-lowering drugs for the rest of your life, and, as a Melbourne, Australia, research team has shown, salt restriction can be as effective as drug therapy.

Few people realize just how pervasive an ingredient salt has become in the modern American diet. Although with refrigeration and other methods of food preservation we no longer have to depend on salt to keep our food safe and edible, it is the nation's leading food additive after sugar. It is a major additive in most processed foods, and it is the main condiment used in cooking and at the table. The sodium content of 788 common food items and 19 nonprescription drugs is listed in "The Sodium Content of Your Food," a United States Department of Agriculture publication available free as Home and Garden Bulletin 233 from the Human Nutrition Information Service, USDA, 6505 Belcrest Road, Hyattsville, Maryland 20782.

The average American consumes two to five teaspoons of salt a day, a total of fifteen pounds per person a year. On top of that are sodium-containing food additives, including baking soda and baking powder, widely used in our most popular processed foods. Even those who add no salt in cooking or at the table are likely to consume far more sodium than they realize.

Most people are aware of the saltiness of certain foods, such as anchovies, green olives, dill pickles, sardines, salted snack foods, smoked herring, soy sauce, ketchup, and meat tenderizer. But much of the salt and sodium we eat is hidden in foods that none of us would think of as salty — for example, cereals, bread, dairy products, meats, fish, puddings, and pancakes. In fact, some of these foods contain more sodium than obviously salty edibles (see chart pages 70–71).

Other common high-sodium foods include canned soups, tomato juice, canned tuna and salmon, processed cheese, cured meats and sausages, bouillon cubes, sauerkraut, and nearly all canned vegetables. Although some vegetables, such as beet greens and chard, are fairly high in sodium to start with, most vegetables are low in sodium. However, they can become very high in sodium when commercially canned.

Thus, fresh peas contain only 2 milligrams of sodium in a three-and-a-half-ounce serving, whereas the same portion of canned peas has 236 milligrams. And six spears of fresh asparagus have 4 milligrams of sodium, but canned asparagus has 410. And while processing increases sodium, it decreases the amount of potassium, which has some protective effect in warding off high blood pressure.

Processing also increases the sodium content of cereals. Regular Cream of Wheat has 0.6 milligram of sodium in one serving, Quick

Cream of Wheat has 71 milligrams, and wheat flakes have 369.

Salt is added to processed foods for several reasons: to impart a salty flavor, to enhance other flavors (a low level of salt enhances the sweetness of sugar), to mask disagreeable flavors, to make up for the flavor lost through processing, and to repress the growth of food spoilage microorganisms.

Manufacturers insist that eliminating or greatly reducing salt in most products would be commercial suicide because the average consumer is adapted to the taste of salt and regards foods lacking salt as bland. After strong public and professional protest, most of the baby food companies greatly reduced or eliminated salt from their products. But reduction of salt in processed foods for adults requires a public education program and a reconditioning of taste buds. In the 1970s, Campbell's test-marketed a no-salt-added line of soups, but it didn't sell well and was withdrawn. A new low-sodium line was introduced in 1982. Some bread and cereal manufacturers say they are gradually lowering the sodium content of certain products, and a number of major food companies are preparing to introduce low- or reduced-sodium products.

How to Cut Down on Sodium

To lower your own salt intake, start by not adding salt at the table and certainly *never* before you taste your food. At the same time, gradually reduce the amount you use in cooking. There's a world of new taste sensations waiting for you to explore. In place of salt, try seasoning your foods with spices, herbs, garlic (but not with garlic salt), onion, lemon juice, bitters, and fruits. Don't substitute soy sauce, MSG, hydrolyzed vegetable protein, or bouillon cubes, since all are high in sodium.

If you feel uncertain about adapting your present recipes, there are several good low-salt cookbooks to help you. Among them are *Gourmet Cooking Without Salt* by Eleanor P. Brenner (New York: Doubleday, 1981), *The Secrets of Salt-Free Cooking,* a paperback by Jeanne Jones (San Francisco: 101 Productions/Scribner's, 1979), and *Living With High Blood Pressure — The Hypertension Diet Cookbook,* by Joyce Daly Margie and Dr. James C. Hunt (Radnor, Pa.: Chilton Press, 1979). Another, *The Good Age Cookbook,* by Jan Harlow, Irene Liggett and Evelyn Madel (Boston: Houghton-Mifflin, 1979), is recommended highly by James Beard, the gourmet cook who himself had to go on a low-fat, low-salt diet. *Craig Claiborne's Gourmet Diet* is by the food writer for *The New York Times* (New York: Times Books, 1980). Or there's *Cooking Without Your Salt Shaker,* a 145-page spiral-bound cookbook and dining-out guide published by the American Heart Association and available through local chapters.

Cut down on salty foods and others high in sodium, including canned soups and vegetables, prepared dinners, processed cheeses, and cold cuts. Fresh meats and fresh or plain frozen vegetables are best. If

HOW MUCH SODIUM IS IN YOUR FOODS?

Food	Portion	Sodium (in mg)
Beverages and Soups		
Beef broth, from cube	1 cup	1,152
Chicken noodle soup	1 cup	1,107
Tomato soup (with milk)	1 cup	932
Tomato juice	1 cup	878
Thick shake	1 shake	317
Buttermilk, salted	1 cup	257
unsalted	1 cup	122
Chocolate milk	1 cup	149
Milk (whole and low-fat)	1 cup	122
Mineral water	1 cup	42
Club soda	1 cup	39
Diet cola	1 cup	21
Orange juice	1 cup	5
Apple juice	1 cup	5
Cranberry juice cocktail	1 cup	4
Coffee	1 cup	2
Tea	1 cup	1
Dairy Products		
Parmesan cheese	1 ounce	528
Cottage cheese (regular and low-fat)	4 ounces	457
American cheese	1 ounce	406
Bleu cheese	1 ounce	396
Swiss cheese, processed	1 ounce	388
natural	1 ounce	74
Muenster cheese	1 ounce	178
Cheddar cheese	1 ounce	176
Mozzarella, part-skim	1 ounce	132
Ricotta, whole milk	½ cup	104
Gruyere	1 ounce	95
Meat, Poultry, Fish and Eggs		
Smoked herring	3 ounces	5,234
Chicken dinner, fast food	1 dinner	2,243
Shrimp, canned	3 ounces	1,955
fried	3 ounces	159
Fish dinner, frozen	1 dinner	1,212
Ham	3 ounces	1,114
Ravioli, canned	7.5 ounces	1,065
Pizza, frozen with pepperoni	½ pie	813
Corned beef	3 ounces	802
Cheeseburger, fast food	1 burger	709
Salami, beef	2 ounces	649
Frankfurter	1 frank (2 ounces)	639
Bologna, beef and pork	2 ounces	570
Salmon, canned	3 ounces	443
fresh, broiled with butter	3 ounces	99
Turkey roll	2 ounces	332
Egg, frozen substitute	¼ cup	120
fresh	1 egg	59
Beef, cooked lean	3 ounces	55
Grain Products		
Stuffing mix, cooked	1 cup	1,131
Devil's food cake	1/12 cake	402
White cake	1/12 cake	238
English muffin	2 ounces	293

Food	Portion	Sodium (in mg)
Whole wheat bread	2 slices	264
White bread	2 slices	228
Cream of Wheat, Mix 'N Eat	¾ cup	350
Regular (no salt)	¾ cup	2
Wheaties	1 cup (1 ounce)	355
Wheat Chex	⅔ cup (1 ounce)	240
Nutri-Grain, wheat	¾ cup (1 ounce)	195
Shredded Wheat, spoon size	⅔ cup (1 ounce)	2
Puffed Wheat	2 cups (1 ounce)	2
Oatmeal, instant	¾ cup	238
regular or quick (no salt)	¾ cup	1
Popcorn, salted	1 cup	175
unsalted	1 cup	1
Legumes, Nuts and Vegetables		
Kidney beans, canned	1 cup	844
dry, cooked (no salt)	1 cup	4
Cauliflower, frozen, cheese sauce	1 cup	735
frozen plain	1 cup	18
Potatoes, au gratin	1 cup	1,095
instant reconstituted	1 cup	485
baked or boiled	1 cup	8
Green peas, canned	1 cup	493
frozen	1 cup	150
fresh cooked (no salt)	1 cup	2
Peanut butter, smooth or crunchy	1 tablespoon	81
natural (no salt)	1 tablespoon	1
Condiments		
Miso (fermented soybean)	¼ cup	3,708
Salt	1 teaspoon	1,938
Garlic salt	1 teaspoon	1,850
Garlic powder	1 teaspoon	1
Meat tenderizer	1 teaspoon	1,750
Onion salt	1 teaspoon	1,620
Onion powder	1 teaspoon	1
Soy sauce	1 tablespoon	1,029
Teriyaki sauce	1 tablespoon	690
Baking soda	1 teaspoon	821
Baking powder	1 teaspoon	339
MSG	1 teaspoon	492
Ketchup	1 tablespoon	156
Barbecue sauce	1 tablespoon	130
A-1 sauce	1 teaspoon	92
Mayonnaise	1 tablespoon	78
Worcestershire sauce	1 teaspoon	68
Mustard, prepared	1 teaspoon	65
French dressing, from dry mix	1 tablespoon	253
bottled	1 tablespoon	214
home recipe	1 tablespoon	92
Margarine, regular	1 tablespoon	140
unsalted	1 tablespoon	1
Butter, regular	1 tablespoon	115
unsalted	1 tablespoon	2

Source: Based primarily on data in "The Sodium Content of Your Food," Home and Garden Bulletin Number 233, United States Department of Agriculture.

you use canned vegetables, drain off the liquid and heat them in tap water. Use unsalted butter and margarine. Leave out the salt in cake and pastry recipes.

Salt substitutes — salts in which part or all of the sodium has been replaced by potassium — should not be used without a doctor's advice, since they can result in a potassium overload in some people. Many find the taste of potassium chloride less palatable than giving up salt entirely.

There are a number of low-salt and low-sodium products on the market, including low-sodium cheese, bread, cereals, and canned vegetables. Unfortunately, because they are low-volume items prepared for people with special dietary needs, they cost more than their salt-laden counterparts.

In addition to foods, a number of common drugs, including antacids, some cough preparations, analgesics, laxatives, and vitamin C (as sodium ascorbate), contain a lot of sodium. If you have high blood pressure, check with your doctor before taking such medications.

Drinking water is also a source of considerable sodium intake in many communities; the local water district can tell you how much comes out of your tap. In some southern communities it's as much as 400 milligrams of sodium per cup. Avoid softening your drinking water; water softeners exchange the hard-water minerals for sodium, which you then consume.

If you have high blood pressure and are taking drugs to control it, remember that the drugs are most effective when your salt intake is below 5 grams a day (the amount in one level teaspoon). The less sodium you consume, the fewer drugs you need. You may even be able to bring your blood pressure down to normal without any medication at all.

Permanent Weight Control: Forget Fad Diets

The water diet, the grapefruit diet, the Atkins diet, the Stillman diet, the Pritkin diet, the drinking man's diet, the Air Force diet, the Mayo diet, the Scarsdale diet, the Beverly Hills diet, the Southampton diet, the I Love New York diet, the sex diet, the ice cream diet, the rice diet, the low-calorie diet, the calories-don't-count diet, the liquid protein diet. . . .

Did it ever occur to you why there are so many different kinds of diets? It's because no fad diet really works, at least not in the long run. Any diet — even unbalanced, unhealthy ones — can help you lose weight if you eat fewer calories than you have been, but no diet works permanently if all you do is go on it until you've lost a certain amount of weight and then go off it. No matter what diet is chosen, more than 90 percent of dieters regain the weight they lose — only to be ready to try the next weight-loss scheme that comes along.

Actually it's a good thing people can't stick with fad diets, since they are all nutritionally unbalanced and dangerous in the long run. Nearly all shortchange the body on several vitamins and minerals. Some, like the Atkins and Scarsdale diets, are loaded with artery-clogging fats and cholesterol. Others, like the Beverly Hills diet, deprive the body of essential protein. The liquid protein diet fad of the seventies resulted in at least fifty-nine deaths from heart rhythm abnormalities, mostly in young, previously healthy people.

How to Change Your Eating Behavior

To make weight loss permanent, something more than a diet is needed. You need a new way of eating, a change in how and why you eat that you can live with for the rest of your life. Rather than "go on" a diet — which implies that one day you will "go off" the diet — you must make appropriate life-style changes and adopt a permanent eating plan that you can maintain for life.

This does *not* mean that you can never again eat apple pie or ice cream or candy or whatever strikes you as an irresistible high-calorie no-no. It *does* mean that you won't eat a box of candy or a quart of ice cream at a sitting and then, because you feel guilty or disgusted with yourself, chase it with a bag of potato chips. Rather than eliminate your favorite foods, you can find a healthful way to include them in your menu.

Lest this seem like an improbable or impossible achievement, let's look at how some formerly fat people have succeeded in losing weight seemingly forever. The techniques they applied were developed by experts in a field called behavior modification, which has helped people to kick the smoking habit, get rid of irrational fears, and overcome depression as well as overeating.

Behavior modification programs have proved to be more successful in the short run — helping more people to lose more pounds — and in the crucially important long run — helping them to keep the weight off — than other traditional weight-loss schemes, including individual psychotherapy. According to Dr. Albert Stunkard, psychiatrist at the University of Pennsylvania, who developed a behavior modification scheme for weight loss, behavioral techniques can be applied by anyone anywhere — the individual independently, those enrolled in structured programs or self-help groups, and people in psychotherapy.

The first and most important step, Dr. Stunkard says, is to get a clear picture of what, how, how much, and under what circumstances you eat. Do you nibble while watching television or reading or writing? Does an argument with your spouse lead you to the refrigerator? Do you clean off the children's plates?

73

Start an eating diary. Construct a diary in which, for every single thing you eat and drink, you write down the time of day, what you consumed, how much, where you were, who you were with, and how you were feeling. This eating diary will enable you to detect bad eating habits and situations in which you really shovel in the calories and will help you devise effective ways to cut down. If you nibble while watching television, take up something like knitting or wood carving to keep your hands too busy to reach for the peanuts. Keep tempting high-calorie foods out of the house. Your children will survive if there's no ice cream or cookies in the larder.

By keeping a diary, many people (some of them may claim that however little they eat, they don't lose weight) discover that they actually consume more calories than they thought. Others realize that they overeat only when they are angry, disappointed, tired, or bored. The trick, then, is to find better ways to handle those negative feelings — saw wood or take a walk around the block, go to sleep, call a friend, do someone a favor, but don't punish yourself further by overeating.

Dr. Stunkard admits that, at first, keeping the diary seems a terrible annoyance, but gradually it becomes more enjoyable as people discover how revealing it is. The very act of monitoring daily food intake results in a decrease in consumption for most people. When you realize you will have to write down that piece of cheesecake you're about to eat at 11:00 P.M., you just may decide not to eat it.

Recognize your eating signals. The next step in modifying your obesity-inducing eating behavior is to recognize the signals that stimulate it and learn to control them. Obese people often find themselves salivating at the sight or smell of a bakery, unable to resist an offered sweet or pass a candy machine without putting in a coin, or willing to consume a tempting platter of food even though they have just eaten. Rather than respond to such external cues (events outside the body's true need for food), you must learn to recognize the sensation of physical hunger and eat only in response to that.

How and where to eat. Dr. Stunkard has found that it helps to restrict all eating to one room in the house, sitting down at a distinctive place setting and focusing on the process of eating. Make your eating experience meaningful and satisfying. No reading, or watching television, or arguing with your spouse at mealtime. Concentrate on the sight, smell, texture, and taste of your food. Chew slowly, and above all, eat slowly.

Overweight people tend to eat very rapidly, consuming their entire meal before the satiety center in their brains can register satisfaction and a sense of fullness. The signal takes about twenty minutes to reach consciousness, but most people down their food in half that. Thinking they are still hungry, they reach for a second helping. To slow down, count the number of bites you take, put your knife and fork down between each bite, and after every four bites wait two minutes before taking another.

Dr. Michael J. Mahoney of the Pennsylvania State University, coauthor with Kathryn Mahoney of an excellent book called *Permanent Weight Control* (see "For Further Reading" below), recommends eating a small portion, then setting a timer for twenty minutes. If you are still hungry when the timer rings, you can have a second helping. Otherwise, consider your meal finished.

Your reward. A further aid to developing self-control over your eating is to reward yourself for good behavior — not by eating forbidden foods but by giving yourself points or stars or setting aside money with which to buy clothes for your new figure or to donate to a worthy cause (your loss being its gain).

Exercise Is Crucial

The final important ingredient is exercise — not necessarily jogging or tennis or biking every day, but an overall increase in the amount of energy you expend (i.e., calories you use). Simple life-style changes that can help include walking instead of riding short distances, taking the stairs instead of an elevator, using manual appliances (for example, a hand mower), parking your car at the far end of the parking lot, or eliminating extension phones.

You might also consider a moderate exercise program. Brisk walking is possible for nearly everyone and is a very effective calorie consumer and total body conditioner. Contrary to popular opinion, Dr. Mahoney points out that exercise does not increase your appetite and may actually decrease it. Body metabolism and appetite control are "tuned" to work most efficiently and accurately when you are moderately active. [See Part II on exercise, page 85.]

By following such a behavior modification program, you're likely to find that you don't have to live on celery sticks or grapefruit or water to lose weight. You can eat what normal-weight persons eat (only less of it) and still lose weight and keep it off. Dr. Mahoney warns dieters against being in too much of a hurry to reach their desired goal. A slow weight loss, he points out, involves the least disruption in your life and is most likely to be a permanent loss.

For Further Reading

Dusky, Lorraine, and Dr. J. J. Leady. *How To Eat Like a Thin Person*. New York: Simon and Schuster, 1982.

Jordan, Dr. Henry A.; Leonard S. Levitz, Ph.D.; and Gordon M. Kimbrell, Ph.D. *Eating Is Okay*. New York: Signet, 1976.

Katahn, Dr. Martin. *The 200 Calorie Solution*. New York: W.W. Norton, 1982.

Kuntzleman, Charles, Ph.D. *Diet Free!* Emmaus, Pa.: Rodale, 1982.

Lansky, Bruce. *Successful Dieting Tips*. Deephaven, Minn.: Meadowbrook Press, 1981.

Mahoney, Kathryn, and Michael J. Mahoney, Ph.D. *Permanent Weight Control*. New York: W.W. Norton, 1976.

Stuart, Richard, Ph.D. *Act Thin, Stay Thin*. New York: W.W. Norton, 1978.

Nutrition Advice:
How to Get Reliable Information

Nutrition misinformation and outright quackery abound these days. Millions of people are spending billions of dollars on self-styled nutritionists and worthless books, magazines, and products that claim nutrition can prevent and cure a never-ending list of ailments, ranging in seriousness from fatigue to cancer. Others accept without question the testimonials of friends and acquaintances who believe they were helped by one or another nutrient, diet, or food supplement.

Example: A woman in Maine followed the advice of the late Adelle Davis and gave her daughter massive doses of vitamin A, which permanently stunted the child's growth. A damage suit against the Davis estate was settled out of court for $150,000.

Example: The widely touted health food supplement, "B15," doesn't exist and cannot be legally sold in the United States, according to the Food and Drug Administration. Though the agency has won seven out of seven actions against major wholesalers of this nonsubstance — which may actually be anything from milk sugar to a poison that dilates blood vessels or damages genes — it is still being sold in nearly every health food store.

Example: On the advice of a nutritional hair analyst, a woman found to have high levels of selenium in her hair was being treated with a potent chemical to clear the "excess" selenium from her body. In fact, she had no such excess, and the treatment could have seriously depleted her body of essential minerals. The selenium in her hair came from prolonged use of an antidandruff shampoo.

Few people know how to distinguish nutritional quackery from scientifically sound facts and advice. Few realize that under the protection of the First Amendment, claims made in print or on the air need not be true. While a manufacturer is not allowed to make unproved and unapproved health claims on the label of a product or the literature accompanying it, such claims can legally be made in books, pamphlets, and magazines sold in the same store.

Even people who can recognize quackery often have to deal with nutritionally ignorant physicians and may not know where to turn for reliable guidance on what to eat and what, if anything, to take as a dietary supplement.

How to Recognize a Quack

Almost anyone can call himself or herself a nutritionist since licensing is not required. Among those who have assumed this title are chiropractors, holders of mail-order degrees from nonaccredited colleges, holders of "honorary" degrees, proprietors of health food stores, people trained in unrelated fields, people previously convicted of nutritional fraud, book authors, and a few ill-informed or unscrupulous physicians who espouse unproved remedies.

The nutritional quack often cloaks his or her information in scientific language, supported by references in the scientific literature. Most people are in no position to check the accuracy of the claims against the original references. More often than not, the claims are distortions or unwarranted extensions of the true findings.

In seeking advice, most people seem to prefer certainties and the kind of confidence — some would call it blind faith — exuded by nutritional quacks. Unfortunately, while many facts about human nutritional needs and how to meet them *are* known, all the needed data are not yet available. Furthermore, a legitimate scientist rarely speaks in certainties, since tomorrow may yield new information that contradicts today's "facts."

In his illuminating book *Nutrition Cultism* (see "For Further Reading," page 79) Dr. Victor Herbert, chief of the Nutrition Laboratory at the Veterans Administration Medical Center in the Bronx and president of the American Society of Clinical Nutrition, outlines clues for detecting nutrition frauds. Other cautions are given by Betsy McPherrin, research associate for the American Council on Science and Health. They include:

● Advice to buy something you would not otherwise have bought, such as megadoses of vitamins or gadgets, especially if the adviser would gain financially from the purchase.

● A fake specialist bearing imposing "front" titles, including director of some nutrition institute unaffiliated with a well-established univeruniversity or member of an unrecognized "scientific" society (such as the International Academy of Biological Medicine, the Orthomolecular Medical Society, or the American Nutritional Consultants Association).

● A name followed by a string of initials that stand for irrelevant degrees, such as N.D. (Doctor of Naturopathy), C.H. (Certified Herbologist), or C.A. (Certified Acupuncturist), R.H. (Registered Healthologist), or even a legitimate degree in an unrelated field (such as O.D., for Doctor of Optometry, or D.C., for Doctor of Chiropractic).

● Claims that most disease is due to a faulty diet; that most people are poorly nourished; that food processing, prolonged storage, soil depletion, and chemical fertilizers are causing malnutrition; or that chemical additives and preservatives are poisoning people.

● Claims that a bad diet or a health problem can be countered by taking vitamin or mineral supplements, by eating only "organic" or "health" foods, or by taking a phony vitamin like B_{15} (pangamate) or B_{17} (Laetrile).

● Use of hair analysis as the primary method of detecting a nutritional problem. Hair analysis can be highly misleading; blood and urine tests are far more accurate.

- Promises of quick, miraculous cures and the use of testimonials and case histories — rather than properly designed scientific studies — to support claims for the recommended nutritional therapy.
- Claims that the American Medical Association, government agencies, orthodox medicine, or the medical establishment have suppressed the person's work or refuse to investigate the claims.

Where to Get Trustworthy Advice

Many sources offer sound nutritional information and advice, unbiased by the promise of financial gain and based on properly designed scientific research. But unless you have a clear-cut nutritional deficiency, such as iron deficiency anemia, you're not likely to receive a nutrient prescription that will produce a remarkable reversal of symptoms. Rather, you will be guided to the consumption of a well-balanced, nutritious diet that can enhance health and weight control. Here are some trustworthy sources:

Qualified nutritionists. Such persons have completed a four-year curriculum of science, nutrition, and other courses at an accredited college or university. Many have master's degrees in nutrition, which usually involves two years of additional study, again at an accredited institution. A Ph.D. requires still further education and scientific research. According to Betsy McPherrin, most legitimate nutritionists seek professional certification and are likely to be members of the Society of Nutrition Education, the American Institute of Nutrition, or the American Association of Clinical Nutrition, which have strict entry requirements.

Registered dietitians (R.D.'s). These professionals have completed a prescribed course of study in dietetics or nutrition at an accredited college or university, plus an internship in a hospital or other professional setting, or three years of specialized work experience, or a master's degree in nutrition or a related field with six months' work experience. In addition, an R.D. must pass a registration exam and maintain proficiency through continuing education. Most are members of the American Dietetic Association. Though once found almost exclusively in hospitals, schools, and other institutions, more and more R.D.'s today are setting up private practices as consulting dietitians and counsel clients who are self-referred or referred by physicians. Such individuals may be listed in the Yellow Pages or with the nutrition clinic of a local hospital. Or send a stamped, self-addressed envelope to Virginia Bayles, Membership Secretary-Treasurer, Consulting Nutritionists, 5018 Indigo, Houston, Texas 77096.

Health and food organizations. Local chapters of such groups as the American Heart Association, the American Dietetic Association, and the American Diabetes Association can provide nutritional guidance to individuals. Your local health department may have a nutrition bureau, and your county cooperative extension service (operated through land-grant colleges and universities throughout the country) has a staff nutritionist who can give advice by phone and provide useful pamphlets. The United States Department of Agriculture also produces many useful publications, including *Nutrition and Your Health: Dietary Guidelines for Americans* (Home and Garden Bulletin No. 232, available free from the Human Nutrition Information Service, USDA, 6505 Belcrest Road, Hyattsville, Maryland 20782, or through your congressman) and *Ideas for Better Eating,* a menu and recipe guide (available for $2.25 from the U.S. Government Printing Office, Superintendent of Documents, Washington, D.C. 20402).

Newsletters. Nutrition and Health, prepared and published six times a year by the Institute of Human Nutrition, Columbia University College of Physicians and Surgeons, 701 West 168th Street, New York, New York 10032; *Environmental Nutrition,* prepared by registered dietitians and published by Environmental Nutrition, Inc., 52 Riverside Drive, Suite 15-A, New York, New York, 10024; and *Nutrition Action,* published by the Center for Science in the Public Interest, 1755 S Street NW, Washington, D.C. 20009.

For Further Reading

Herbert, Dr. Victor. *Nutrition Cultism.* Philadelphia: G.F. Stickley Co., 1980.
————, and Dr. Stephen Barrett. *Vitamins and "Health" Foods: The Great American Hustle.* Philadelphia: G. F. Stickley Co., 1981.

Breakfast:
The Most Important Meal

Breakfast is a catch-as-catch-can, eat-on-the-run, or skip-it-entirely meal for millions of Americans of all ages. The high school senior washes down a bag of potato chips with a can of pop on his way to class. The third grader gobbles a large bowl of sticky-sweet cold cereal with as little milk as possible, ignoring the juice which now "tastes sour." His older sister runs out of the house with a cookielike granola bar in hand that purports to be the nutritional equivalent of a ham and eggs breakfast.

Adults may carry around a cup of coffee as they rush through their morning routine, then subdue midmorning gastrointestinal growls with a danish and more coffee at the office. Or in an effort to control calories, they may have nothing more than the taste of toothpaste in their mouths until lunch.

Is this the way to start the day? After what amounts to a fast of ten or twelve hours, surely we must need some refueling to fire the activities of the forenoon. Most people are no doubt aware of the admonition to "eat a good breakfast," though the reasons for it may slip their minds as they turn off the alarm and catch another fifteen minutes of sleep or as they race to make the school bus or join the rush-hour hordes on their way to work.

Even those who are convinced that eating breakfast is important may be confused about *what* to eat now that the concern for cholesterol has sounded the death knell for the American standby of bacon and eggs, while its fast-food alternative — ready-to-eat cereal — has crumbled under the criticism that it contains too much sugar, sodium, and additives.

Once you escape the confines of orthodoxy, you will discover that a huge variety of interesting, healthful — and not necessarily time-consuming — breakfasts are possible. But first, eating breakfast must become a priority in your morning.

What Breakfast Can Do for You

Why is breakfast important? Clearly there are some people who claim to have no appetite in the morning and seem to get by on no breakfast without feeling any sense of impairment or deprivation. For most, however, having to function on an empty stomach and a low blood sugar level definitely undermines productivity and sabotages the most pleasant of dispositions.

A ten-year study that followed nearly 7,000 men and women in California showed that skipping breakfast is among seven health risks that increase the chances of an early death. The study, by the University of California, Los Angeles, Center for Health Sciences, found that death rates were 40 percent higher for men and 28 percent higher for women who "rarely or sometimes" ate breakfast, compared with those who ate breakfast "almost every day."

An earlier long-term study conducted by the University of Iowa Medical College showed that eating a nutritious breakfast was associated with better physical and mental performance among children and adults. In particular, the study revealed, those who ate breakfast were more productive during the late morning. They also had a faster reaction time

BASICS OF A GOOD BREAKFAST

Menu Plan	Examples
Fruit or juice with vitamin C.	Orange, grapefruit, tomato, cantaloupe, strawberries, apple.
Bread or cereal.	Oatmeal, whole wheat toast, bran or enriched muffin, kasha, wheat flakes, rice, pasta.
Protein-rich food.	Low-fat milk, cottage cheese, ricotta, yogurt, egg, smoked fish, Canadian bacon, turkey breast, boiled ham, mozzarella.
Beverage.	Coffee, tea, skim or low-fat milk, grain-based beverage.

(which may mean fewer accidents) and less muscular fatigue than those who skipped breakfast. Children who had had no breakfast were more likely to be listless and have trouble concentrating. A study of nine- to eleven-year-old children by the Massachusetts Institute of Technology showed that skipping breakfast reduced the youngsters' problem-solving abilities.

Further, skipping or skimping on breakfast helps not a whit toward weight control. Meal skippers in general are more likely to be obese than those who eat three square. A study of college girls showed that breakfast skippers consumed more snacks — mostly snacks high in calories and deficient in nutrients — than those who ate breakfast. A University of Minnesota study showed that 2,000 calories a day consumed at breakfast helped people to lose weight, whereas on the same 2,000-calorie meal consumed at supper, they gained.

Another risk associated with skipping breakfast is that you're likely to miss some important nutrients, including vitamin C, riboflavin, and calcium, that you might not get enough of in the meals that remain, according to Dr. Helen A. Guthrie, professor of nutrition at Pennsylvania State University. Dr. Guthrie reports that among adolescents who skip breakfast, the amount of calcium and vitamin C consumed during the day is 40 percent less, and the amount of iron and thiamin consumed is 10 percent less, than among breakfast eaters.

Currently the demands that the American breakfast be appealing to the appetites of those with other priorities, quickly and simply prepared (or completely ready to eat) and portable (so that it can be eaten while one dries one's hair or drives the car) have created a nutritionally questionable line of fast breakfast foods: doughy, gooey pies that are popped in the toaster; instant breakfast drinks; breakfast bars (fortified cookies that are mostly sugar and fat); and breakfast sticks (chewy candy that is probably not brushed from the teeth, given the morning rush of the consumer). Food marketing consultants even regard frozen orange juice as too much bother for the modern American family.

Cancer and Diet:
What to Worry About

The proposed ban (now defunct) on saccharin, the earlier bans on cyclamates and red dye No. 2 and the growth stimulant DES, the continuing debate over the safety of food preservatives like nitrates and nitrites, and the discoveries of pesticide residues in foods have prompted a growing concern about the cancer-causing potential of the American diet. Diet sodas, bacon, hot dogs, and other cured meats, maraschino cherries, packaged breads and cereals, even fresh meats and milk have at one time or another contained these suspected carcinogens. Even coffee and tea have been accused of promoting the growth of cancer. Is it safe, people wonder, to eat anything?

Many who no longer trust the mainstream American food supply have stopped eating processed foods and turned instead to so-called natural foods and organically grown fruits and vegetables to avoid the known and suspected risks of added chemicals. Others take large quantities of various dietary substances, particularly certain vitamins and minerals, in the belief that they are protecting themselves against cancer.

What, in fact, is the evidence supporting these concerns, and what modifications of the diet could really reduce the risk of cancer?

Possible Dietary Carcinogens

A number of substances deliberately or inadvertently added to foods have been shown to cause cancer in animals, but their role in human cancers is still uncertain. These include the following:

Nitrates and nitrites. Used as preservatives in cured meats, fish, and vegetables, these substances can be transformed in the stomach of animals into substances called nitrosamines, which readily cause cancer in animals. It is thought that the same reaction can occur in the human stomach. (Nitrates are also naturally present in some vegetables, including spinach, and probably contribute to the amount of nitrosamines formed in your body.)

Food colorings and flavorings. Butter yellow, violet No. 1, and red dyes Nos. 2 and 4 were banned by the Food and Drug Administration (FDA) after they were shown to cause cancer in animal tests. Several other food colorings still in use may also be a cancer hazard. Flavorings for root beer and vermouth and the artificial sweetener cyclamate met a similar fate, and saccharin came close to joining the list, stopped only by mass public protest that prompted an act of Congress to stay the FDA's hand. [See chapter on food additives, page 59.]

Pesticides. Several, including aldrin, dieldrin, DDT, and arsenicals, have been shown to cause cancer in animals. Most of these were banned because residues were repeatedly found in foods sold for human consumption.

Other inadvertent food contaminants that can cause cancer in people as well as in animals include DES, a growth stimulant used in cattle, and aflatoxin, a poison produced by a mold that grows on corn, peanuts, rice, wheat, and other foods stored under humid conditions.

The Main Culprit: A High-Fat, Low-Fiber Diet

By concentrating on food additives and inadvertent contaminants as the main cancer-causing culprits in the American diet, we may be allowing the most dangerous dietary villain to escape. For a growing body of evidence suggests that the very structure of the typical American diet may be cancer-promoting. The studies show that the heavy reliance on meat and dairy products, laden as they are with saturated fats and cholesterol, and the minimal consumption of fibrous foods (grains, fruits, and vegetables) are associated with an increased risk of cancer, particularly cancers of the colon-rectum and breast, two of the leading cancer killers of Americans. [See chapters on breast cancer risk, page 644, and colon cancer, page 652.]

An international study showed that people who developed colon-rectal cancer consumed more meat than those free of this disease. Throughout the world, in countries where the consumption of meats and dairy products is low, the incidence of colon-rectal and breast cancer (as well as heart disease) is also low. In Japan, for example, deaths from these diseases are far less common than in the United States. But when Japanese migrate to this country and adopt a more Western diet, the rates at which these cancers occur increase, and in one or two generations Japanese Americans have the same cancer rates as other Americans.

Native Americans, Seventh-day Adventists and Mormons, most of whom live on vegetarian diets, have much lower rates of cancer of the colon-rectum, breast, and uterus than the average American. Obese people have more cancers of the breast, uterus, pancreas, and gallbladder than people of normal weight. Women who are chronically constipated (and presumably eat a low-fiber diet) may face an increased risk of breast cancer, preliminary studies suggest.

When the diet is high in animal fats and cholesterol, bacteria that live in the gut break down these foodstuffs into substances that can cause cancer. Since such diets are usually low in bulky, fibrous foods, the stool tends to be more concentrated and to stay longer in the colon, exposing colonic tissues to these carcinogens. Some of the substances produced from cholesterol by intestinal bacteria can mimic the action of female sex hormones and may promote the growth of cancers in hormone-sensitive tissues like the breast and uterus.

Cancer Prevention Through Diet

The best dietary approach to cancer prevention is not necessarily avoiding food additives and other chemicals found in minute quantities in foods. Rather, it lies in keeping your weight down and adopting a prudent diet that may protect you from cancer and heart disease at the same time. You don't have to become a total vegetarian; instead, consider reorienting your diet to concentrate more·on fish, chicken, and fiber-rich grains, beans, fruits, and vegetables and less on meats, eggs, and dairy products containing butterfat and cholesterol. [See chapter on fats and cholesterol, page 14.]

You might also eat more vitamin C-rich foods (citrus fruits, tomatoes, peppers) and vegetables in the cabbage family (broccoli, cauliflower, kale, brussels sprouts), since these have been shown to inhibit the formation of carcinogens and people who consume them regularly have been found to have a lower cancer risk. Smokers have a reduced risk of lung cancer if their diets are rich in previtamin A, or beta-carotene. Beta-carotene, found only in plant foods, is the source of the orange color in carrots and a commonly used food coloring (in margarine, butter, etc.); it is also found in deep-yellow fruits and vegetables and dark green vegetables like broccoli, spinach, and turnip greens. Beta-carotene may also protect against cancer of the breast and bladder, among others. Already formed vitamin A, however, confers no such protection, studies thus far indicate.

It would also help to avoid consuming excessive amounts of alcoholic beverages. Heavy drinkers face a much higher than normal risk of developing cancers of the esophagus, mouth and throat, larynx, and liver. [See chapter on alcohol effects, page 240.] However, the role of coffee in cancer is still uncertain. Although one study linked even moderate coffee consumption to an increased risk of cancer of the pancreas, others have found no such relationship. [See chapter on caffeine, page 262.] In countries where large amounts of tea are consumed, this drink has been linked to cancer of the esophagus and perhaps the stomach. Adding milk to tea binds up the tannins and is thought to protect against a possible cancer-promoting effect.

As for the much-touted preventive value of vitamin supplements, none has been shown to protect against cancer unless the diet lacks the normal recommended amounts. However, large doses of certain chemical relatives of vitamin A seem to protect animals against cancers that affect the body's skin and lining cells. The protective effect of these experimental chemicals is now being tested in people who face an unusually high risk of developing bladder and other cancers. But large doses of vitamin A itself are poisonous and should not be used.

Also under test are supplements of vitamin E, a natural antioxidant that may prevent the transformation of nitrites into nitrosamines. Vitamin C has been added to certain foods, such as bacon, to prevent nitrosamine contamination of the meat during storage and cooking. If you consume foods containing nitrates or nitrites, it might be wise to eat or drink something rich in vitamin C (oranges, tomatoes, peppers, etc.) at the same time. [See the chapter on micronutrients, page 42.]

II.

Exercise

We are a species that evolved on the move: hunting and gathering and, later, herding and harvesting, all by the sweat of the human brow. Though many human tribes still pursue such activities on a daily basis, in affluent countries the bulk of the population sits on the way to work, sits at work for eight or more hours, sits on the way home, sits at the dinner table and then in front of the TV, and finishes off the day by lying down in bed.

In between, we do everything possible to use the fossil fuels the world is short of and to conserve the personal fuel (calories) so many of us have to considerable excess. We drive or ride; take elevators and escalators; use power mowers, electric hedge clippers, golf carts, dishwashers, laundromats, food processors, plug-in corn poppers — the list of labor-saving devices could (and does) fill a Sears catalogue.

None of which means you should give up the devices that have taken over life's drearier tasks and freed you to do better things with your time. But if you are not going to get your needed quota of exercise in carrying out the chores of daily life, then you should be programming activity into your days in other ways. Either you must set aside time each day for a concentrated period of exercise, or you must incorporate more activity into your daily routines. Preferably both.

Exercise is the best way I know to get something for nothing (or next to nothing). It is an all-around tonic for body and mind. The physical and psychological benefits of exercise could go a long way toward reducing the need for medical care and improving the quality of life — your life, whether you're eight, eighteen, forty-eight, or eighty-eight.

That doesn't mean, however, that you should plunge right into the activity closest at hand without a further thought. Exercise has risks as well as benefits, and to minimize those risks, you must choose your activities wisely, learn the proper techniques, observe safety precautions, and make sure your body is in shape to handle the stresses involved.

Benefits of Exercise:
The List Keeps Lengthening

Most of us who regularly walk, run, cycle, swim, jump, skate, or what-have-you don't really have long-term health benefits in mind. We get out there and exercise regularly because it makes us feel good — more relaxed and confident, less tired and irritable, trimmer, stronger, even sexier. But it's nice to know that at the same time we may also be preserving our health and prolonging our lives.

If you haven't caught the exercise bug, or if you're in danger of getting over it, you may be motivated to get moving and stay moving by mounting evidence showing the benefits of vigorous physical activity.

How Exercise Keeps You Healthy

Here's what exercise can do, according to the latest evidence:

Heart and blood vessels. Several studies, including one among 16,936 Harvard graduates, have shown that the more physically active you are, the lower is your risk of suffering a heart attack. Various established physiological effects of exercise contribute to this protection. A physically fit person is better able to get oxygen distributed to body tissues, thus increasing the capacity for work. At the same time the heart can pump more blood with each stroke, so it doesn't have to work as hard.

The oxygen supply to the heart muscle itself is increased because the network of tiny blood vessels feeding the heart is larger in an active person. Furthermore, the opening of the coronary arteries is larger, increasing blood flow to the heart. Active people also have fewer irregularities in heart rhythm and lower blood pressures. In fact, exercise therapy is sometimes all that is needed to control high blood pressure, a major contributor to heart disease and stroke.

If you are cardiovascularly fit you have a lower heart rate at a given level of exercise (and therefore, your heart muscle has more time to rest between beats) than someone whose heart is not fit. You can exercise vigorously for a long time without feeling tired and can respond to sudden physical or emotional demands without your heart racing or your blood pressure rising precipitously.

Researchers at several centers have shown that physically active people have higher levels of a cholesterol-carrying blood protein known as HDL, which appears to protect against heart attacks probably by helping to clear arteries of accumulations of cholesterol.

At the same time, levels of potentially harmful blood fats like triglycerides and other forms of cholesterol are reduced through physical activity. Researchers at Duke University report that physical conditioning also enhances the ability of the blood to dissolve clots, which could cause life-threatening obstructions in the heart, lungs, and brain.

Diabetes. Nearly 2,000 years ago the value of exercise for diabetics was promoted by Celsus. Modern physicians have recently discovered that exercise increases an individual's sensitivity to insulin, making it useful in the treatment of diabetes. Further, diabetics who exercise may have fewer blood vessel complications because the "stickiness" of their blood cells is reduced.

Weight control. Exercise uses calories, and studies of runners and swimmers have shown that they consume about 600 calories a day more than sedentary people of the same age and height. Yet sedentary males weighed 20 percent more and sedentary females 30 percent more than the active people. Other studies have shown that obese and normal-weight people don't differ in the amount of food they eat, but rather in the number of calories they expend by activity and exercise. Not only does exercise use up calories directly, but your body burns extra calories for up to fifteen hours afterward.

Even at the same weight, an active person looks trimmer than one who is sedentary because muscle tissue has a smaller volume than the same weight of fat. It is the percentage of fat in your body, not the numbers on a scale, that determines overweight. Muscle tissue also uses more calories to sustain itself than does an equivalent amount of fat, so if you are well muscled, you can eat more without gaining than can a person who weighs the same but has a higher percentage of body fat.

Bone strength. Inactivity leads to a loss of calcium from bones, increasing their susceptibility to fracture. By contrast, continued physical activity throughout life diminishes the risk of osteoporosis, the loss of bone with age, which is a leading cause of disability among people past fifty. [See chapter on osteoporosis, page 610.] Exercise is especially valuable to older women, who are more susceptible to osteoporosis and resulting fractures than men are. Although treatment with estrogens after menopause can counter bone loss, the hormone treatment also greatly increases a woman's risk of developing uterine cancer.

Personality and mood. An exercise program can help to relieve the anxiety and tension common among people in high-pressure jobs and difficult life circumstances, possibly diminishing the psychological factors that increase the risk of heart attack. Several therapists have found that an exercise program is at least as effective as psychotherapy in treating mild to moderate depression. Others have shown that the combination of psychotherapy and jogging is more effective against depression than either approach alone.

In general, says Dr. Edward D. Greenwood, psychiatrist at the Menninger Clinic, exercise promotes a sense of well-being by enhancing ego strength, dissipating anger and hostility, relieving boredom, and resolving frustration.

Miscellaneous benefits. Among other rewards for following a regular exercise program, studies indicate, are improvement in the mental functions controlled by the left side of your brain (with which you learn), healthier skin with fewer wrinkles, and more efficient use of such dietary elements as protein, vitamins C and B$_6$, and iron.

Caution: It's a Drug

Convinced? Great. But before you don those jogging shoes, jump on that bike, or dive into that pool, take heed. Vigorous exercise can also be dangerous if you don't treat it with discretion and respect. Some doctors refer to it as a drug that must be carefully administered in proper dosages, with attention paid to possible adverse effects.

In general, anyone over thirty-five who has been reasonably sedentary in recent years should have a medical checkup before embarking on an exercise program. Regardless of age or previous level of activity, anyone with a chronic illness, such as diabetes, heart disease, or arthritis, should first check with a physician.

Start slowly. There is nothing more discouraging to a would-be exerciser than aching muscles and injuries. Both are likely if you fail to heed certain cardinal rules:

● Work up gradually — over a period of weeks or months — to your ultimate exercise level.

● Look into the proper techniques and equipment needed to pursue your chosen activity safely.

● Be sure to do the recommended stretches and warm-up exercises before you embark on more strenuous activity. [See chapter on stretching and warming-up, page 97.]

For Further Reading

Havas, Dr. Stephen. "Exercise and Your Heart." National Heart, Lung, and Blood Institute, National Institutes of Health. Free copies available from the Consumer Information Center, Pueblo, Colo. 81009.

Zohman, Lenore R., M.D.; Albert A. Kattus, M.D.; and Donald G. Softness. *The Cardiologists' Guide to Fitness & Health Through Exercise.* New York: Simon & Schuster, 1979.

Choosing an Exercise: What to Consider

... You can achieve total fitness in four minutes a day. ... Jogging isn't enough; you have to *run* if you want to be really fit. ... If you're over fifty, you should stick to walking. ... If you can't exercise every day, you'd better not do it at all. ... Swimming is the best exercise. ... If you're thin (or muscular), you don't need to exercise. ...

The list of myths and mistruths about exercise could go on and on.

There are at least as many as there are miles in a marathoner's diary. For the millions of Americans who already have or eventually will succumb to the admonitions to get moving for the sake of their bodies and souls, the prevailing mythology has prompted confusion, anxiety, and inappropriate decisions on when and how to move.

Exercise can serve many purposes. It can enhance skills, improve flexibility, build muscle strength and tone, relieve tension, help you lose weight and maintain the loss, and improve your body's general physiological condition, especially the ease with which your heart can supply oxygen to body tissues. [See chapter on the benefits of exercise, page 86.]

Different types of exercise may serve some of these functions, but not others. For example, bowling and golf can help you become more skillful at the game, strengthen certain muscles, and expend energy (calories), but they rarely involve enough continuous activity to condition your cardiovascular system. Isometric exercises (those which clamp down on muscles), such as weight lifting, water skiing, and arm wrestling, will promote strong muscles but are useless — in fact, countereffective — as cardiovascular conditioners and may actually be harmful to people with heart disease. On the other hand, brisk walking may do little for your athletic skills or muscle strength, but it can be highly beneficial to your heart and figure.

Consider the Health Value

In choosing an exercise, it's important to know what you hope to get out of it and whether that choice will help you achieve your goals.

Any type of exercise — from hanging laundry and scrubbing floors to badminton, skating, football, or long-distance running — can help you control your weight. Weight gain represents an excess number of calories consumed over the number your body uses for energy. With any kind of motion, your body uses more calories than it does at rest. The more you move, the more calories you use. The heavier you are to start with, the more calories it takes to move yourself a given distance.

As an added benefit, moderate exercise improves the accuracy of your body's appetite control mechanism and usually decreases rather than increases appetite. It helps your body better adjust food intake to calorie expenditure.

You don't have to sweat or exercise strenuously to use energy. In fact, walking a mile uses approximately the same number of calories as running a mile. At moderate ranges of activity the difference, as far as calories are concerned, is that running a mile is faster and you may then have time to run a second mile and use up twice as many calories. In addition to the calories used while exercising, your body continues to use calories at a higher rate for many hours after you stop exercising.

Some activities are intense energy guzzlers, using eight or more times the amount of calories your body consumes at rest. These include

VALUE OF VARIOUS EXERCISES

Energy Range (Approx. calories used per hour)	Activity	Benefits
72-84	Sitting Conversing	Of no conditioning value.
120-150	Strolling, 1 mph Walking, 2 mph	Not sufficiently strenuous to promote endurance unless your exercise capacity is very low.
150-240	Golf using power cart	Not sufficiently taxing or continuous to promote endurance.
240-300	Cleaning windows Mopping floors Vacuuming	Adequate for conditioning if carried out continuously for 20-30 minutes.
	Bowling	Too intermittent; not sufficiently taxing to promote endurance.
	Walking, 3 mph Cycling, 6 mph	Adequate dynamic exercise if your capacity if low.
	Golf, pulling cart	Useful for conditioning if you walk briskly, but if cart is heavy, isometrics may be involved.
300-360	Scrubbing floors	Adequate endurance exercise if carried out in at least 2-minute stints.
	Walking, 3.5 mph Cycling, 8 mph	Usually good dynamic aerobic exercise.
	Table Tennis Badminton Volleyball	Vigorous continuous play can have endurance benefits. Otherwise, only promotes skill.
	Tennis, doubles	Not very beneficial unless there is continuous play for at least 2 minutes at a time. Aids skill.
	Many calisthenics Ballet exercises	Will promote endurance if continuous, rhythmic, and repetitive. Promotes agility, coordination, and muscle strength. Those requiring isometric effort, such as push-ups and sit-ups, not good for cardiovascular fitness.
350-420	Walking, 4 mph Cycling, 10 mph Ice or roller skating	Dynamic, aerobic, and beneficial. Skating should be done continuously.

VALUE OF VARIOUS EXERCISES

Energy Range (Approx. calories used per hour)	Activity	Benefits
420–480	Walking, 5 mph Cycling, 11 mph	Dynamic, aerobic, and beneficial.
	Tennis, singles	Can provide benefit if played 30 minutes or more with an attempt to keep moving.
	Water skiing	Total isometrics. Very risky for people with high risk for heart disease or deconditioned normals.
480–600	Jogging, 5 mph Cycling, 12 mph	Dynamic, aerobic, endurance-building exercise.
	Downhill skiing	Runs are usually too short to promote endurance significantly. Mostly benefits skill. Combined stress of altitude, cold, and exercise may be too great for some heart patients.
	Paddleball	Not sufficiently continuous. Promotes skill.
600–650	Running, 5.5 mph Cycling, 13 mph	Excellent conditioner.
Above 660	Running, 6 or more mph	Excellent conditioner.
	Handball Squash	Competitive environment in hot room is dangerous to anyone not in excellent physical condition. Can provide conditioning benefit if played 30 minutes or more with an attempt to keep moving.
*Swimming		Good conditioning exercise — if continuous strokes. Especially good for people who can't tolerate weight-bearing exercise, such as those with joint diseases.

91

*Wide caloric range depending on skill of swimmer, stroke, temperature of water, body composition, current, and other factors.
Adapted from "Beyond Diet . . . Exercise your Way to Fitness and Heart Health." CPC International.

running more than five and a half miles an hour, cycling thirteen or more miles an hour, playing squash and handball, and skipping rope. But you can use as many calories playing Ping-Pong or volleyball for an hour as you would running for half an hour.

This is not to say that Ping-Pong in any amount can be equivalent to running in total all-around exercise value. You are most likely to achieve a conditioning effect (fitness or endurance) if the activity uses the large muscles in a rhythmic, repetitive, continuous motion — so-called isotonic exercises. While the amount of energy (calories) used depends only on the amount of work your body does, conditioning is a function of both the amount of work and the vigor with which it is done.

A cardiovascular conditioning exercise must also be aerobic — that is, it promotes the use of oxygen and is capable of being sustained for at least two minutes at a time without your getting out of breath. Walking, running, cycling, and swimming are aerobic exercises, but sprinting is not.

To condition the cardiovascular system, the exercise should be performed at least three times a week for twenty minutes at a time during which the heart rate is within the individual's target zone (see diagram below). The target zone falls between 70 and 80 percent of the maximum

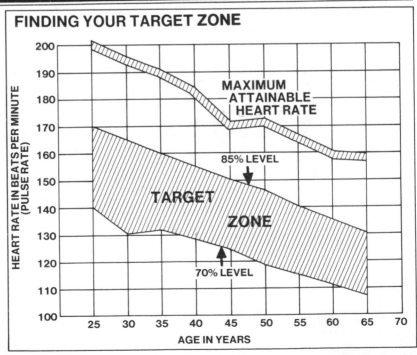

FINDING YOUR TARGET ZONE

The heart rate you should maintain during conditioning exercise is between 70 and 85 percent of the maximum attainable heart rate for your age.

rate your heart can achieve. The maximum heart rate (or pulse rate), counted as beats per minute, can be estimated for the average healthy adult by subtracting his or her age in years from 220; then taking 70 percent and 85 percent of that number. Between the two is the pulse rate range that is the target zone.

Thus, if you are forty-five years old, your maximal heart rate would theoretically be 175, and the pulse rate to aim for — your target zone — in your exercise program would be between 122 and 148 beats per minute. There is little cardiac conditioning to be gained from exercise that falls much below or that exceeds this level.

To determine your heart rate while exercising, stop and immediately take your pulse: Count the beats in ten seconds, and multiply by 6. As you become conditioned to a certain level of exercise, you may have to increase the rigor of your workout to keep your heart rate within the target zone. To avoid undue stress on your muscles and heart, every twenty-minute exercise session should be preceded by a five- to ten-minute warm-up and followed by a five- to ten-minute cool-down period of less intense exercise (if you're a jogger, you might walk briskly during your warm-up and cool-down). Stretching after exercise is important for preventing joint and muscle injuries and stiffness. [See chapter on stretching and warm-up, page 97.]

A conditioning exercise should be done regularly or the benefits are rapidly lost. If you must stop for a week or more, resume at a lower-level workout and gradually build up again.

What Else to Think About

Other factors to consider when you choose an exercise include the following:

Time available. Running or indoor stationary cycling can be done at any time for thirty minutes or more. Organized sports tend to be more time-consuming and restrictive. For those short of time who can take the rigor of the activity, rope jumping for ten minutes can provide a conditioning effect equivalent to thirty minutes of jogging.

Cost and convenience. Tennis, for example, may involve driving miles to a court, paying high fees, searching for a partner, and arranging schedules, all of which may discourage regular participation. The cost of a bicycle (indoors or out) may be prohibitive for some, but a jump rope can be purchased for a dollar or two. For most people, sex is convenient and inexpensive and uses a lot of calories, but to achieve a conditioning effect, the preorgasmic level of activity would have to be maintained for at least twenty minutes.

Your body's capabilities. If you're uncoordinated, ball games or rope jumping may prove very frustrating. If you're tight-jointed, you may need flexibility-enhancing exercises (calisthenics) before you try running or tennis.

Age, health status, and present physical condition. Older people need less rigorous activity to bring their heart rate into the target zone. Beyond the age of thirty-five, you would be wise to check with your doctor before starting a rigorous exercise program. The doctor may recommend an exercise stress test to see what level of activity your cardiovascular system can tolerate. [See chapter on stress testing, page 95.]

Beyond fifty, condition yourself first through a walking program before beginning more strenuous exercises. Beyond sixty, most people would be wise to avoid the more taxing exercises, such as jogging and competitive sports, and stick instead to walking, swimming, and cycling, unless of course they've been engaged in more vigorous activities for years. At any age, if you have been sedentary for years or are out of condition, start slowly and work up to more demanding activities. Anyone with a chronic illness or muscle or joint problems should consult a physician before starting to exercise.

Personal taste. You're more likely to stick with an exercise that you enjoy, but you should give a new activity a trial of a month or two before deciding you don't like it. Dr. Lenore R. Zohman, an exercise cardiologist at Montefiore Hospital in the Bronx, New York, advises that you think back to the activities you enjoyed as a youngster for clues to what you might like today.

94

"If you have an aversion to organized sports or strenuous activity," she says, "brisk walking for twenty to thirty minutes or climbing up twenty-five flights of stairs at a comfortable pace during a day can help you achieve physical fitness."

Dr. Zohman points out that contrary to popular belief, "there is no best exercise for everyone." Others recommend that exercisers hone their skills at more than one activity. This helps to develop muscle strength throughout the body, diminishes the chances of injury that can result when some muscles are developed at the expense of others, and provides alternative exercise possibilities if the main activity can't be done at a particular time. When it rains, for example, someone who usually jogs or plays tennis can jump rope or ride a stationary bicycle.

For Further Reading

Before embarking on a serious exercise program, you might benefit from the descriptions of various activities provided in some popular books. Dr. Zohman's pamphlet, "Beyond Diet . . . Exercise Your Way to Fitness and Heart Health," is an excellent basic primer about exercises of all types and how to go about an exercise program. Single copies may be obtained free by writing to Mazola Nutrition Information Service, Dept. ZD-NYT, Box 307, Coventry, Conn. 06238.

Other useful materials include:

Cooper, Kenneth H., M.D. *Aerobics.* New York: Bantam, 1968.

————, *The New Aerobics.* New York: Bantam, 1970.

————, with Mildred Cooper. *Aerobics for Women.* New York: Bantam, 1973.

Dickman, Irving R. "Listen to Your Body: Exercise and Physical Fitness." Public Affairs Pamphlet No. 599, 1981. Available for 50 cents from Public Affairs Pamphlets, 381 Park Avenue South, New York, N.Y. 10016.

Lance, Kathryn. *Running for Health and Beauty: A Complete Guide for Women.* India-
    napolis: Bobbs-Merrill, 1977.
Zohman, Lenore R., M.D.; Albert A. Kattus, M.D.; and Donald G. Softness. *The Cardiolo-
    gists' Guide to Fitness and Health Through Exercise.* New York: Simon & Schus-
    ter, 1979.

The Exercise Stress Test: What It Can Show

The idea of "being on a treadmill" ordinarily implies a highly undesirable way of living, but today thousands of Americans are choosing
to spend a brief time on a medical treadmill. They are testing the
strength and resilience of their hearts by undergoing a so-called exercise
tolerance test, or stress test. This examination indirectly measures the
heart's ability to deliver oxygen-containing blood to the muscles as they
work harder and harder.

If you're over forty or have a family history of heart disease and
you are planning to take up vigorous exercise, a complete medical examination that includes a stress test is often recommended. Approximately
one in ten middle-aged American men and a smaller percentage of
women are walking around with "silent" heart disease, which at any time
could make itself known in the form of a heart attack or sudden cardiac
death. The stress test can help to identify such individuals in time to institute preventive measures as well as help to set exercise limits for those
already known to have heart disease.

Despite a long-standing controversy over what exercise testing can
and does show, in recent years the examination has become a big business in American medicine. Unfortunately, as with all popular and
potentially profitable procedures that are not restricted to hospitals, the
stress test has attracted the attention of entrepreneurs, some of whom
have set up fly-by-night clinics that may offer bargain tests but may lack
appropriate safety precautions or the ability to interpret the test results
properly or fail to provide necessary follow-up and counseling.

How It's Done

The test basically involves a continuous recording of the heart's
electrical activity — an electrocardiogram (ECG) — plus a check of the
pulse rate, blood pressure, and other possible signs and symptoms of
heart or blood vessel deficiencies while the individual performs increasingly demanding exercise. A stationary bicycle or special two-step stool is
sometimes used in stress testing, but most specialists prefer an automated
treadmill that permits preprogrammed increases in speed and degree of
inclination as the test runs.

Clad in sneakers and shorts or other loose-fitting clothing, the person to be tested is wired to a computerized ECG machine. The treadmill is started, and the individual begins to walk slowly according to its dictated speed as the computer records heart rate, ECG, and the level of a particular portion of the ECG called the ST segment, which can indicate oxygen shortage in the heart muscle. Every three minutes the speed and inclination of the treadmill are increased until the individual's heart rate reaches a preset level that is determined by age. If certain symptoms or signs develop before that level, the test is stopped sooner.

What It Can and Can't Show

Many doctors and patients misunderstand what the test can and cannot do and mistake its results for a definite diagnosis of either cardiovascular health or disease. A negative test result should not lull unconditioned individuals into thinking they can suddenly plunge headlong into rigorous activity without risk to their hearts. A positive test finding should not be taken to mean that the person is or will become a cardiac cripple or that an immediate evaluation for coronary bypass surgery is necessary.

What the test *can* do is identify a group of individuals who face an unusually high risk of developing obvious heart disease, possibly in the form of a heart attack or sudden death. It is much like other heart risk factors — smoking, high blood pressure, and the like — but studies have shown that exercise testing is better able to predict future trouble.

Although an ECG taken at rest may show signs of previously damaged heart muscle, it cannot show abnormalities that develop only when the cardiovascular system must handle increased work loads, such as during activities like climbing stairs, running, cycling, or playing tennis. The heart has to work harder and faster to deliver the extra oxygen needed by the body's muscles during exercise, and the exercise ECG indicates whether this master muscle can do the job without itself becoming short of oxygen.

When the oxygen supply to the heart muscle is deficient, oppressive chest pains called angina pectoris may result, and when a portion of the heart muscle is cut off entirely from its oxygen supply, the result is a heart attack.

By revealing whether the heart muscle becomes short of oxygen when the heart is pumping nearly as fast as it can go, the exercise ECG can indicate the safety of strenuous exercise for individuals who otherwise have no signs or symptoms of heart disease. In patients already known to have heart disease or who have undergone heart surgery, the test can measure just how hard the heart can work before the heart muscle becomes short of oxygen, thereby helping the doctor determine exercise limits and prescribe a safe exercise program for heart patients.

Another use of stress testing is to monitor the accomplishments of an exercise conditioning program. According to the results of sequential stress tests, in the course of a seven-month exercise training program a forty-six-year-old man was able to increase by a third the amount of oxygen that could be delivered to his exercising muscles without putting any additional strain on his heart.

Stress test results can also be used to help motivate people who face a high risk of developing obvious heart disease to make needed changes in their lives to reduce their risk. Such changes might include losing weight; stopping smoking; getting adequate treatment for high blood pressure; reducing fat, cholesterol, and salt in their diets; or starting a regular exercise program.

Necessary Precautions

A stress test should be done only after a physician has done a physical checkup and taken a resting ECG. The test itself should be monitored by the doctor or a trained assistant, who will constantly watch the ECG recording and periodically take the individual's blood pressure and ask how he or she feels.

Emergency resuscitation equipment should be on hand in case serious cardiac problems develop in the course of the test. A review in 1971 of 170,000 stress tests revealed that the test itself may cause one death and necessitate two to three hospitalizations per 10,000 persons tested. In Seattle there were no deaths associated with 17,000 tests done in a six-year period, although nine persons required emergency treatment.

The stress test can be done in a special clinic or medical center or in a well-equipped doctor's office. To avoid slipshod outfits, it is best to get a referral from an internist or cardiologist. In many communities the YMCA provides quality stress testing followed by a prescribed exercise program. The cost of a stress test can range from about $65 to $250, with the usual price at around $125. The fee is covered by many medical insurance policies.

Stretching and Warming Up: Keys to Safe Exercise

Professional pitchers warm up in the bullpen before stepping out to the mound; on-deck batters may be seen swinging a succession of increasingly heavy bats. Hockey players skate up and down the rink, and college football players may do a dozen different calisthenics. Yet thanks to the American desire for instant gratification, enhanced by an undercurrent of impatience and chronic shortage of time, most amateur exercisers impair their performance and invite pain and injury by failing to prepare their bodies for activity and counter the stresses that activity places on the body.

Plunging tight, cold muscles into vigorous activity and failing to stretch out activity-tightened muscles is asking for trouble, including strains and pulls of the involved muscles and injuries to muscles that try to compensate, such as those in the back.

Among people who do take the time to stretch and warm up, many — including a good number of professional athletes — bounce and strain in preparatory exercises that are excessive and counterproductive, adding to, rather than relieving, musculoskeletal tension. The wrong kind of stretching does more harm than good.

Even if you only walk, play golf, or do housework, your body and your mind can benefit from ten or fifteen minutes a day of stretches that relax tight muscles and reduce the stress on supporting ligaments and tendons. If your activities are more vigorous — say, jogging, tennis, cycling, or dancing — preactivity warm-ups and postactivity cool-downs and stretches can make the difference between pleasure and pain and determine whether you will continue to enjoy the activity.

Why Stretch?

If you're interested in improving your performance, gentle pre-activity stretching may be helpful. To prevent soreness and injury, however, stretches should be done after your workout as well. If you are going to stretch only once, after the activity is the more important time. Heavy preactivity stretching of cold muscles is potentially harmful.

Repeated exercise tends to shorten muscles. Unless the activity is followed by exercises that limber up the body and relax and stretch the muscles, the shortened muscles will be more likely to go into spasm. Muscle spasm is a common cause of postexercise pain and stiffness as well as acute, sometimes incapacitating injuries.

Some people are naturally tight, and for them stretching is especially important if injuries are to be avoided. As people age, muscles tend to shorten, so the older you are, the more important it is to stretch. Emotional tension, poor posture, and prolonged sedentary work also can cause muscle shortening that contributes to feelings of fatigue and tension. These feelings can be relieved by relaxed stretching.

"Stretching," says Bob Anderson, author of a detailed book of the same name, "is the important link between the sedentary life and the active life. It keeps the muscles supple, prepares you for movement, and helps you make the daily transition from inactivity to vigorous activity without undue strain." Among the benefits of regular stretching, Mr. Anderson says, are these:

- Reduces muscle tension and makes the body feel more relaxed.
- Improves coordination by allowing for freer movement.
- Increases range of motion.
- Prevents injuries, such as muscle strains.
- Promotes circulation.

- Helps loosen the mind's control of the body.
- Makes strenuous activities easier.
- Feels good.

According to Marshall Hoffman and Dr. William Southmayd, authors of *Sports Health* (see "For Further Reading," page 100), "Stretching lengthens the muscles and tendon units. It also fills the muscles with blood and makes them pliable. The more pliable the muscles and tendons are, the less likely they are to sprain or to strain." An unstretched muscle, they say, is like a tight string, whereas a stretched one is like a rubber band.

How to Stretch

The ruling principle of proper stretching is slow and easy. No bouncing, the experts warn. If a muscle is stretched too fast or too far, the stretch reflex is triggered, and microscopic tears that shorten the muscle occur — exactly the opposite of what you wish to achieve. The stretch reflex is a protective mechanism activated by bouncing or overstretching; it causes muscles to contract to prevent them from being injured. If you are stretching correctly, it should not hurt, nor should your muscles feel stiff and sore afterward.

Dr. Herbert deVries, exercise physiologist at the Andrus Gerontology Center at the University of Southern California in Los Angeles and author of the most authoritative text on the subject, *Physiology of Exercise* (Dubuque, Iowa: Wm. C. Brown, 1981), has shown that so-called static stretching — extending a muscle group and holding it in that position for ten or more seconds — requires less energy and is less likely to injure tissues and cause muscle soreness than calisthenic types of exercises that involve bouncing, bobbing, and jerking movements. In a jogging program in which the 200 participants averaged seventy years of age, Dr. deVries found that easy stretching after each run virtually eliminated postexercise muscle problems.

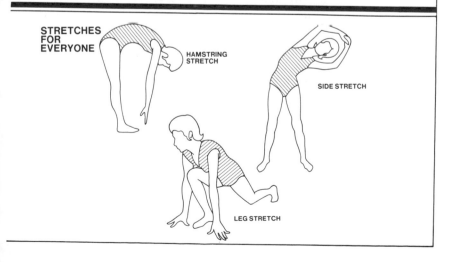

STRETCHES FOR EVERYONE

HAMSTRING STRETCH

SIDE STRETCH

LEG STRETCH

The exact kinds of stretches best suited for you will depend on your particular activity and which muscles it shortens. For example, runners need to stretch the lower back, the muscles in the back of the thighs (hamstrings) and calves (gastrocnemiis), and the inner thighs. [See chapter on jogging, page 101.] A tennis player should stretch the muscles in the upper back, shoulders, and neck as well as the leg muscles used in running. A skier needs both of these, plus limbering stretches for hips. Skating and dancing involve all these, plus waist stretches. Bob Anderson's book is a well-illustrated guide to stretches specifically suited to various activities as well as general stretches helpful to everyone.

After easy stretching (or preferably before) you should warm up the muscles you will be using by starting your activity slowly. Many competitive marathoners, for example, jog for a mile or two just before the race. Tennis players hit back and forth. Swimmers do several laps. Warming up is always important, but especially so in cold weather.

According to Dr. deVries, the warm-up has three purposes: to prevent cardiovascular problems, to prevent joint and muscle problems, and to improve performance. The warm-up increases blood flow and oxygen supply to the muscles and raises their temperature, helping them work better and resist injury. The warm-up acts as a kind of rehearsal for the more strenuous activity to follow.

If you're a jogger, for example, the best kind of warm-up is to start out walking briskly or jogging slowly for about half a mile and then gradually increase your pace.

Similarly, toward the end of your workout it's important to cool down slowly by gradually diminishing the intensity of your activity. The jogger, for example, should slow down for the last quarter to half a mile. Never sprint at the end of a run. If you stop your activity too abruptly, you may pass out because, with your blood concentrated in your muscles, circulation to your brain is impaired, causing dizziness. Too abrupt an end to vigorous activity could also interfere with circulation to your heart and possibly cause it to stop working.

For Further Reading

Anderson, Bob. *Stretching . . . for Everyday Fitness*. New York: Random House and Shelter Publications (P.O. Box 279, Bolinas, Calif. 94924), 1980.
Mirkin, Dr. Gabe, and Marshall Hoffman. *The Sportsmedicine Book*. Boston: Little-Brown, 1978.
Southmayd, Dr. William, and Marshall Hoffman. *Sports Health*. New York: Quick Fox, 1981.

Jogging:
The Benefits and Risks

A man I know in his late forties suffered a heart attack and, within a week the number of joggers on his block had doubled. Spurred by their neighbor's close brush with cardiac death, several men with varying degrees of gray in their hair and fat around their middles joined the large contingent of men and women who each morning leap out of bed before dawn, don old, bleach-streaked clothing, and, chins high and cheeks red, trot breathlessly around the park.

When asked what drives them to pursue with passion a daily ritual that some regard as masochistic, they say such things as: "I feel like a new person. . . . I sleep better. . . . I eat less. . . . I feel sexier. . . . I'm more relaxed. . . . I don't get upset so easily anymore." Beyond such immediate rewards lurks the hope for a long-term gain — that of warding off the dreaded heart attack, currently the leading killer of middle-aged American men.

There is growing evidence that jogging does help to protect against heart attacks. For one thing, it increases the level of a protective form of blood cholesterol known as HDL. For another, it increases the heart's ability to work efficiently — that is, to pump more blood with less effort.

How to Avoid Jogging Injuries

Too often, however, the very activity chosen to enhance health results in injuries that at the least are distressingly painful and at the worst can seriously threaten your ability to function. Injury is a major cause of jogging dropouts, and fear of injury is an excuse often mentioned by those who are reluctant to take up jogging. While every physical activity necessarily entails some risk, most of the jogging injuries are preventable if you treat your body with the respect it deserves and prepare it properly for the stresses you plan to subject it to.

Example: Jerry had been jogging six miles a day for two years when he developed a severe pain down his lower left leg, causing him to limp even when walking. His stress fracture, a fine crack in the bone surface, was cured by rest — that is, no running — for six weeks. The doctor told him that a recurrence could be prevented by the insertion of a support in his running shoes for his high-arched feet.

Example: Kathy was jogging along the edge of a city street with the traffic when she was struck from behind by a car and thrown twenty feet. Her badly bruised leg kept her inactive for two months. Now she runs only on pedestrian paths in the park.

Example: Tess had hurt her kneecap several years earlier. But it caused her no trouble until she tried running more than four miles a day. The pain after running was so severe that she sought medical help. The doctor told her that despite her running, the muscles supporting her knee were in poor shape and needed strengthening. She is now doing exercises daily so she can continue to run.

Example: Sidney was fifty-six years old and, he thought, in excellent physical condition. But within hours of the first time he jogged, he suffered a massive heart attack. He was told that a man his age, no matter how healthy he seemed, had no business taking up so vigorous an activity without first getting a thorough checkup, including an exercise stress test.

Example: I admit that I was lackadaisical about doing the warm-ups that I knew should precede my run and the stretching exercises that should follow it. The price I paid was a severe back injury that kept me bedridden for six weeks. Now, each day, I do exercises to strengthen the abdominal muscles that support my back, I stretch my back and leg muscles after each run, and I alternate jogging with swimming and cycling to balance my muscle tone better.

The most common injuries to joggers involve muscles, tendons, bones, ligaments, and fascia (tissue that surrounds muscles). Nearly all can be prevented. The most important preventive measures involve keeping your body flexible and preparing it adequately for each workout.

Warm muscles are less subject to injury than those that are worked hard from a cold start. Begin your workout with a brisk walk or slow jog for about five minutes. A slow cool-down period at the end of the workout is equally important. While running, your leg muscles help your heart in its job of pumping blood. If you stop too abruptly, your heart may be unable to meet its suddenly increased demand. Therefore, jog slowly or walk at the end of your run.

Tight muscles, tendons, and ligaments are subject to pulls, sprains, and tears. Jogging tends to tighten those tissues along the back of your body, so each workout should be followed by stretching exercises to loosen them up. Stretching cold muscles can be risky, so take it very easy if you do before-run stretches. In fact, some experts advise stretching only after you've done some warm-ups. [See chapter on stretching and warming up, page 97.]

If you regularly combine cycling, skiing, or skating with running, you may further increase the risk of injuring the hamstring muscle in back of your thigh. Therefore, you should spend extra time stretching your hamstrings, using the exercises described on page 103. It's also a good idea to vary your activities, alternating running with, say, swimming.

Some Helpful Exercises

Stretches are done slowly and carefully, and you must hold your body for ten or more seconds in the stretched position. The following flexibility exercises are highly recommended for joggers by orthopedists and sports medicine specialists. However, any exercise that produces pain should not be done without consulting your medical specialist.

Wall push-ups. These are especially good for stretching the Achilles tendon, a common site of crippling athletic injuries, and the muscle in the back of your calf. Stand three or four feet from the wall, and facing it, put your palms on the wall. Keeping your body straight, feet parallel, and heels on the floor, bend your elbows and move the upper part of your body toward the wall. Hold for ten counts, return to starting position, and repeat at least five times.

Lower-back stretch. Lie on the floor on your back, and bend your knees. Then raise one leg, grasp the knee with your hands, and bring it toward your chin. Hold it for ten counts, then release. Then do it with the other leg, repeating the exercise ten times for each leg.

Hurdler's stretch. This stretches the muscles along the backs of your legs. Sit on the floor with legs outstretched. Bend one leg at your side, as you might close a jackknife, but keep your other leg straight in front of you, as if you were leaping a hurdle. Lean forward to grasp the

JOGGING STRETCHES

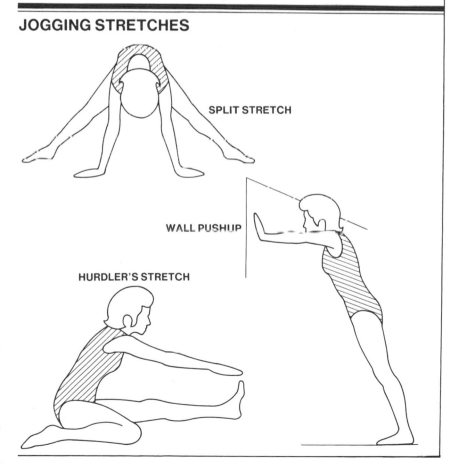

SPLIT STRETCH

WALL PUSHUP

HURDLER'S STRETCH

foot of your outstretched leg. Hold for ten counts, then release. Reverse your position, and repeat the exercise with the other leg outstretched. Repeat five times per leg.

Leg lift. An alternative to the hurdler's stretch is to lift one leg up to a ledge or wall to make a right angle (ninety degrees) with your torso. Keeping your knees straight, lean over toward your raised foot. Hold for ten counts, release, and then do it with the other leg. Repeat five times per leg.

Split stretch. This stretches the inner part of your thighs. Stand with knees straight, and slowly spread your feet apart as far as you can. Then bend over and press your palms against the floor between your feet. Hold for ten counts, and repeat five times.

[See also back-strengthening exercises, page 525.]

The Jogger's Foot

Many joggers' troubles stem from a characteristic of their feet known as pronation, or rolling inward of the foot as it moves forward. Dr. Gabe Mirkin, sports medicine specialist at the University of Maryland and coauthor of *The Sportsmedicine Book* (Boston: Little, Brown, 1978), says excessive pronation — creating an appearance of "flat" feet — is a common cause of injury to runners' ankles, knees, hips, bones, and muscles. Special inserts called orthotics that are fitted into your running shoe can help to prevent this. Orthotics are also useful in preventing stress fractures and knee and hip problems in people with high arches. Orthotics may be purchased ready-made, or they may be custom-made through a podiatrist or orthopedist. Dr. Mirkin says that sometimes a drugstore arch support will do the trick.

It's also a good idea to run on a relatively soft, even surface rather than on concrete or asphalt or through fields of potholes and pitfalls. Properly made running shoes are a must. These have flexible, well-cushioned soles and wide, built-up heels. The average jogger's foot strikes the ground 2,700 times an outing with a force three times his or her body weight. This greatly exaggerates even the slightest abnormality in foot structure or lack of protection by the shoe.

A good running shoe may mean an investment of $25 or more to start with; but that's all jogging need cost you, and it could save you considerable pain and expense later on.

For Further Reading

Fixx, James F. *The Complete Book of Running.* New York: Random House, 1977.
————. *Jim Fixx's Second Book of Running.* New York: Random House, 1980.
Ryan, Allan J., M.D. *The Physician and Sportsmedicine Guide to Running.* New York: McGraw-Hill, 1980.
Sheehan, George, M.D. *Dr. Sheehan on Running.* New York: Bantam, 1975.
Wood, Peter, D.Sc., Ph.D. *Run to Health.* New York: Charter, 1980.
Young Runners' Handbook. New York: Kinney Shoe Corporation, P.O. Box 5006, New York, N.Y. 10150, 1979.

Bicycling:
How to Ride Safely

Cycling is an excellent activity — as an inexpensive means of transportation, an adjunct to a weight-control program, and/or for exercise conditioning — that has become very popular in recent years. There are now more bikes being sold each year than passenger cars, and the Bicycle Manufacturers Association of America estimates that 100 million people — nearly half the population — ride bikes. That's four times more cyclists than in 1960.

While you may not have to be told how to ride a bike (it's an activity you never forget once you've learned it), chances are you were never taught how to ride a bike *safely*.

A thirteen-year-old New York boy whirled around a corner on his bike and was swept up and killed by a street-cleaning machine. A cycling commuter in Washington, D.C., died as a result of head injuries after crashing into a truck door that opened just as his bike approached. A Minneapolis pedestrian was killed when she was struck by a cyclist riding on a sidewalk; the rider survived his injuries.

In any given year well over a million bicyclists in this country are injured, about half of them seriously enough to require emergency room care. For more than a thousand, the accident will snuff out life. Yet studies have shown that the vast majority of these accidents are preventable. Most are due to the cyclist's carelessness — the failure to obey traffic laws, to select a suitable bike and maintain it in good working condition, to observe sensible riding precautions that take none of the joy out of cycling but make the activity far safer.

In the wake of escalating numbers of bicycle accidents, in 1976 the United States Consumer Product Safety Commission issued safety standards for bicycle manufacturers, which all bikes sold today must meet. The standards include protection against sharp edges and protrusions; good brakes; strength requirements for the frame, handlebars, and drive chain; chain guards; strong tires; firmly attached wheels and seats; nonslip pedals; and reflectors on front, back, and sides. The bikes also must pass a road test.

Unfortunately, cyclists don't. While every rider learns how to balance on two wheels, very few school themselves on how to cycle safely once the balancing act is mastered. There is no required driver's license for cyclists. While cyclists are supposed to observe traffic rules, the law is rarely enforced, and many cyclists act as if they were a law unto themselves. They rarely stop at red lights or stop signs, ride the wrong way down one-way streets, ride on the wrong side of two-way streets, ride on sidewalks, tear out of driveways, weave in and out of traffic, and don't signal turns.

Since designated bicycle paths are still uncommon, most two-wheeled excursions occur on roadways frequented by motor vehicles. A California study showed that in 70 percent of bicycle-car accidents the cyclist had disregarded traffic laws. In a collision between a 2-ton auto and a 35-pound bicycle the cyclist has hardly a fighting chance.

Approximately half of serious bicycle accidents involve youngsters between the ages of five and fourteen. In nine out of ten cases, the accident is the cyclist's fault — most commonly, as one detailed study showed, emerging precipitously from a minor roadway such as an alley, driveway, parking lot, or gas station and ignoring stop or yield signs. One-quarter of serious cycling accidents happen to adults, with a third of the accidents the cyclist's fault.

Safe Riding Tips

In addition to learning and obeying basic traffic laws, here are other tips on safe riding:

• Before taking a new bike into traffic, practice riding it in a parking lot or other protected area until you're thoroughly familiar with the equipment and comfortable riding it. This is especially important when you switch from a standard or three-speed bike to a ten-speed one.

• Buy a bike that fits. You should be able to touch the ground with your feet while sitting on the seat. Don't buy a bike for a child to "grow into." Avoid hand brakes and multiple gears for young children. Parents should supervise their child's bike selection and not let the child "customize" the bike in ways that compromise its safety features.

• Teach children that bikes are vehicles, not toys. They should be cautioned against doing stunts (many children have been seriously hurt trying to imitate Evel Knievel on homemade ramps). Except on tandem bikes, only one child should ride at a time. The popular "banana" seats encourage unsafe double riding. Children whose bikes have them should agree to take no passengers.

• If you want to carry a young child while you ride, the child should be securely strapped into a carrier seat that has side panels to prevent his or her feet from getting stuck in the wheel or other working parts. No child should ever be carried on the handlebars, crossbar, or fender, or in a basket. Before attempting to ride with a child, be sure you are an experienced rider secure on your equipment.

• Children under twelve are best restricted to daytime riding, preferably with a high flag on the bike. Older children who ride at night should have reflectors and lights front and back. They should wear light-colored clothing and preferably a reflector vest. Parents should be sure children have mastered both their bikes and traffic rules before allowing them to ride on roadways.

• Pay careful attention to the surface you're riding on. Beware of sewer grates, potholes, large cracks, rocks, sticks, loose gravel, and sand.

Some of the worst skids occur on gravel and sand. It's best to avoid riding in wet weather, when skidding is more likely and brakes may not hold well, if at all.

• Ride with both hands on the handlebars. If you expect to be carrying objects (packages, purse, books, sports equipment), equip your bike with a basket or pannier bag or both. No carrier should obstruct vision or interfere with steering. If you wear a shoulder bag, be sure to put it over your head with the strap across your chest to prevent it from slipping down and jamming the wheel.

• Don't wear loose clothing or pants legs that might get caught in the spokes or chain. If your cuffs are wide, secure them with a pants clip, or roll them up so that they stay up.

• Ride in single file on the right near the curb in the direction of the traffic. When you turn, look both ways first and use hand signals. Always keep alert for turning cars, opening car doors, and vehicles pulling out of parking places.

• Keep your bike in good working condition. Twice a year do a

WHAT IS A SAFE BICYCLE?

1. SEAT: Height should be comfortable for reaching pedals and ground.

2. REFLECTORS: Should be on rear fender, pedals, and spokes of wheels (unless wheels have reflectorized tires). Put reflector tape along metal body.

3. BRAKES: Should stop the bike quickly, without sticking.

4. WHEELS: If they wobble, have bike "trued" or otherwise adjusted.

5. PEDALS: To prevent foot slippage, choose rubber-treaded pedals, or metal pedals with firmly attached toeclips.

6. HANDLEBARS: Should be tight, adjusted to comfortable height, and fitted with handlebar grips.

7. LIGHTS: Headlight and taillight are necessary for riding in the dark.

8. TIRES: Inflate to recommended pressure and replace when worn.

9. FENDERS: Check for sharp or rough edges.

10. CHAINGUARD: Needed on single-speed bikes to prevent clothes from catching in sprockets.

thorough maintenance check of the tires, gears, spokes, steering, brakes, chain (which should be lightly oiled), pedals, reflectors, and tightness of the handlebars and seat. Parents should inspect the bikes of young children.

Motorists, too, have a responsibility for bicycling safety. With so many bikes on the road now, motorists must always expect to encounter cyclists and be ready to pull away slightly or reduce speed when passing them. Unless a cyclist appears about to move into a vehicle's path, don't honk. Needless honking may frighten cyclists enough to cause them to lose control.

For Further Reading and Information

To aid in safe cycling, several organizations offer instructional booklets and kits. The Bicycle Manufacturing Association of America, 1101 Fifteenth Street NW, Washington, D.C. 20005, offers a "Safety Set," including a bike maintenance folder, instructions on safe riding, and a mock driver's license for youngsters. The cost is $1 for fifty sets. The association also has, for 50 cents each, a twenty-four-page booklet on how to set up a bike safety program.

The National Safety Council, Youth Department, 444 North Michigan Avenue, Chicago, Ill. 60611, offers a free "Bicycle Pack," including rules of the road, a maintenance manual, various fact sheets, and a pamphlet for motorists.

The Consumer Product Safety Commission, Washington, D.C. 20207, offers a free "Fact Sheet No. 10" on bicycle accidents, selection, use, and maintenance and *Sprocket Man,* a comic book on bike safety for teenagers.

For biking enthusiasts, three thorough books on the subject are:

Krausz, John, Vera van der Reis Krausz, and Paul Harris, M.D. *The Bicycling Book.* New York: Dial, 1982.

Lieb, Thom. *Everybody's Book of Bicycle Riding.* Emmaus, Pa.: Rodale Press, 1981.

Sloane, Eugene. *The New Complete Book of Bicycling.* New York: Simon & Schuster, 1974.

Swimming: The "Perfect" Exercise

If there is such a thing as the perfect exercise, swimming may come close to being it. It can be done by people of all ages — from three to a hundred and three and beyond — and in almost any physical shape. More people report that they swim regularly for exercise than say they jog. Many find swimming less boring than jogging because by changing strokes and/or doing exercises in the water, they can introduce considerable variety into their activity.

Access to an indoor pool, public or private, can make swimming a pleasurable year-round activity for many millions of Americans. Though the annual cost of pool membership may seem high, when you calculate the cost per swim, it's much cheaper than going to a movie, which exercises only your eye muscles, notes Harvey S. Wiener, a convert to swimming at age thirty-seven and author of *Total Swimming* (see "For Further Reading," page 112).

The Health Benefits

By exercising all the major muscle groups — arms, legs, and trunk — swimming can provide full-body benefits without overly stressing any one part of the anatomy. It can be used to whip the sedentary adult into tiptop form as well as help to maintain fitness in someone already in good shape. Swimming can help you tone up flabby muscles (without making them bulky), increase flexibility, shed excess pounds, relieve tension, condition your cardiovascular system, and counter the mechanical stresses of other activities.

Swimming is very often prescribed as *the* activity for people with back or joint problems or injuries incurred as a result of other sports, like jogging or tennis. Few other activities strengthen the muscles of the back and abdomen, which help to support your back. The backstroke (done lying faceup on the water) is especially helpful for those with chronic backaches.

Swimming is also considered ideal for arthritics. With water providing buoyancy, swimming places few mechanical stresses on the body and actually helps to loosen stiff joints. Drs. Lenore R. Zohman and Albert A. Kattus, coauthors with Donald G. Softness of *The Cardiologists' Guide to Fitness and Health Through Exercise* (New York: Simon & Schuster, 1979), point out that since the water, not your body, bears your weight, the joints of your legs are spared the continuous pounding associated with an activity like jogging.

Further, the cardiologists say, swimming can help counter varicose veins. "The improved muscle tone in the legs from swimming massages the leg veins as the legs move, thus helping to avoid venous distention [swollen veins] and varicosities," they state.

Swimming is also often recommended as a conditioning exercise for heart patients as well as for ordinary healthy individuals, to improve the efficiency of the heart muscle and its ability to withstand the stress of any physical activity. Swimming in a steady, continuous fashion vigorously enough to raise your heart rate to within the so-called target zone can provide aerobic conditioning comparable to the effects of jogging. [See chapter on how to choose an exercise, page 88.]

To calculate your heart's target zone, subtract your age from 220 and multiply the result first by 70 percent and then by 85 percent. The resulting numbers represent the range within which your pulse rate should fall during a conditioning exercise (see diagram, page 92). For swimming to enhance fitness, you should maintain a pulse rate at the lower limit of your target zone for twenty to thirty minutes at a time, three times a week.

For the asthmatic, swimming is far less likely than running or cycling to trigger an asthmatic attack, perhaps because the air near the water is free of dust and other allergy-provoking substances. If anything, swimming seems to counter the tendency of asthmatics to develop spasms in the bronchial tubes during exercise.

Those with weight problems may also find swimming to be the ideal activity. The more body fat a person has, the more buoyant he or she will be, making it relatively easy for someone who is very overweight to move through the water. Since the water helps to cool the body, overheating is far less likely to happen while you swim than, say, when you jog on a hot day.

Swimming — vigorous, continuous stroking, not casual paddling about — also uses a lot of calories, more, in fact, than most other common activities, even though it may seem to require less effort. Depending on the speed, current, water temperature, stroke used, and the skill level and body composition of the swimmer, swimming can use from 300 to more than 1,000 calories in an hour.

In general, the butterfly stroke (not usually used as a conditioning stroke since most people cannot maintain it for long) and the crawl have the highest energy cost. Next come the breaststroke, sidestroke, and backstroke.

According to Jane Katz, swimming is a superb mental tonic. Dr. Katz is an accomplished swimmer, professor of health and physical fitness at Bronx Community College, and author, with Nancy P. Bruning, of *Swimming for Total Fitness* (see "For Further Reading," page 112), a 355-page encyclopedia on swimming that includes instructions on the various strokes and outlines fitness workouts. "Water is a wonderfully

POPULAR SWIMMING STROKES

THE BREASTSTROKE

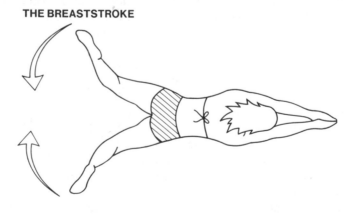

sensuous medium [that] lifts your spirits as well as your body," Dr. Katz says. "It is relaxing and exhilarating at the same time. After a swim, there's a euphoria that permeates your entire existence for hours afterward." Harvey S. Wiener says that for him swimming has produced an unexpected "inner strength and calm."

The Risks

Swimming is less likely than other vigorous activities to result in physical injury, but it's not a free lunch. Those who try to do too much too soon can develop sore muscles from swimming just as with any activity pursued to excess. If you are just starting to swim for exercise, begin with short, leisurely swims and gradually build up to lengthier, more vigorous activity.

In addition, there are some problems uniquely associated with swimming. Probably the most common one is swimmer's ear, an infection of the ear canal, a part of the outer ear. According to doctors writing in *The Physician and Sportsmedicine,* it usually follows the retention of water in the ear canal. Its main symptoms are itching and pain, and it should be treated immediately by a physician to prevent its spread to the middle and inner ear.

Swimmer's ear is best prevented by getting trapped water out of the ear soon after it enters (by shaking the head vigorously or by jumping with the head tilted to one side) and by drying the ear by fanning or with

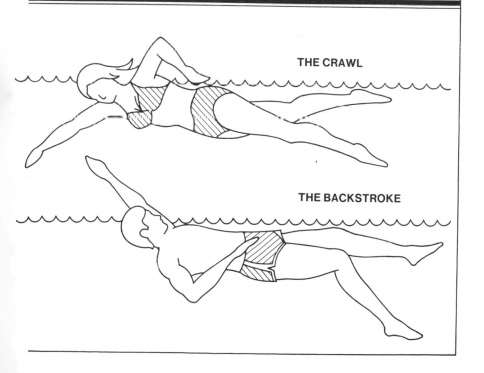

THE CRAWL

THE BACKSTROKE

a hair dryer. Fingernails, cotton swabs, or other objects that can scratch the ear should not be used. After a swim the use of ear drops that contain alcohol, glycol, and boric or acetic acid may also help prevent infections. Unfortunately there is no plug or sealant that is an effective preventive.

Swimmer's knee and swimmer's shoulder are largely problems that afflict the dedicated competitive swimmer. They are caused by sprains or strains that can follow too much hard swimming or an improper swimming stroke. Knee problems may also plague those who use the whip kick during the breaststroke; the older frog kick is less stressful. Shoulder problems may be avoided by alternating the side on which you breathe during the crawl.

Leg or foot cramps may result from fatigue, cold, overexertion, or an inadequate preswim warm-up. Knead the cramped area with your thumbs, and alternately flex and extend the muscles. A five-minute warm-up (with calisthenics or slow swimming) before each swim and a five-minute cool-down of slower swimming at the end will help reduce the risks of injury and other problems.

Minimizing the risks of swimming also means heeding basic safety rules. [See chapter on water safety, page 402.] Never swim alone; preferably a lifeguard should be on duty, or at the least another good swimmer should be nearby. Don't take a sudden plunge into cold water. If you swim in a lake, river, or stream, swim parallel to and near the shore. Never swim in an outdoor pool that has a solar cover (for heating the water) in place; swimmers have gotten trapped under such covers and drowned. Don't swim when you're overly tired or soon after eating a heavy meal or drinking alcohol.

Perhaps most important of all, learn proper swimming and breathing techniques from a qualified instructor. Low-cost swimming lessons are usually available at Ys as well as in schools (many offer adult education classes after school hours) and at municipal pools. Private health clubs also often give swimming lessons.

If your skin and hair are taking a beating from repeated exposures to chlorinated pool water, you might try using soap and hair products called UltraSwim Anti-Chlorine Treatment, made by Eljenn International Corp. in Newton, Massachusetts, and sold at many pools and salons.

For Further Reading

Katz, Jane, Ed.D., with Nancy P. Bruning. *Swimming for Total Fitness.* New York: Doubleday Dolphin, 1981.

Wiener, Harvey S. *Total Swimming.* New York: Fireside (Simon & Schuster), 1981.

Walking:
For Fun and Fitness

Although millions of Americans have taken up jogging and other conditioning activities in recent years, the vast majority remain sedentary resisters to regular endeavors that work up a sweat. For most of them, walking may be the answer. Human beings — the only primates that normally stand erect — were built to walk.

Advantages of Walking

Whereas sitting or standing still for long periods can produce aching backs, tired shoulders and necks, and stiff joints and muscles, walking enhances muscle strength and fluidity of motion. It can improve circulation in your legs, reducing problems with "tired" feet. Although the conditioning effects are slower than with jogging or other more vigorous activities, walking done briskly and frequently can promote physical fitness without risking the injuries common among joggers. [See chapter on jogging, page 101.]

According to a study by Israeli researchers published in the *Journal of the American Medical Association*, a significant improvement in physical fitness can be achieved in just three or four weeks if you walk half an hour a day, five days a week, at a pace of three miles an hour while carrying a six-and-a-half-pound load. Walking is especially suitable for people who are out of shape or unathletic or who have long been sedentary. But it can also help to improve and maintain fitness in people who are well conditioned, the researchers from Tel Aviv University Medical School said. These are some other advantages:

It is easy. Other than a few basic pointers, you need no special training or preconditioning. In fact, walking itself can condition your body for more demanding activities.

It is convenient. It can be done year-round nearly every day and nearly everywhere and can be incorporated easily into your daily routine.

It is cheap. Other than a good pair of shoes, you need no special equipment or facility.

It is accessible. Nearly everyone — even the elderly and those with medical problems such as arthritis, emphysema, and heart disease — usually are able to walk to their health's advantage.

It has variety. While joggers are limited to one kind of running, usually over one or two regular routes, walkers often can follow many different paths to the same end point or can vary their routine.

As Dr. Lenore Zohman, Dr. Albert Kaddus, and Donald G. Softness say in their book *The Cardiologists' Guide to Fitness and Health Through Exercise* (New York: Simon & Schuster, 1979) you "can walk to the job, walk on the job, climb the stairs instead of riding the elevator, pursue walking-type sports, walk the dog, play golf, go hunting, try recreational walking or hiking over gently rolling country, or go back-packing in the high rugged country."

Walking can be done alone or with friends or with the entire family. For those who hate the outdoors, there are indoor tracks in gyms and enclosed shopping malls and treadmills for home use. For more energetic or competitive individuals, there is even race walking (a fast, stylized walk that can be as demanding as jogging).

"Walking is a terrific exercise," says Dr. Zohman, an exercise cardiologist at the Montefiore Medical Center in the Bronx, New York. "It's rehabilitative, it's preventive, and it's simple. But it's underused."

Walking can help you lose weight. On the average, a three-mile walk in an hour's time by a 160-pound person uses about 285 calories. The same activity by a person weighing 120 pounds would use about 215 calories. While this may not seem like much, 215 calories expended four times a week can produce a 13-pound weight loss in a year without any reduction in the calories consumed.

Walking can delay the deteriorating effects of age, such as weakening of the bones and replacement of lean muscle tissue by fat. It can help reduce blood pressure. It can even counter headaches, as a study by Los Angeles exercise physiologist Dr. Herbert deVries showed. Walking is a tonic for the mind as well as the body. It can relieve anxiety and tension and help you unwind at the end of the day or completion of a difficult task. It can help to dissipate anger and lift depression. It can give you uninterrupted time to daydream and work through problems.

Walking Tips

Start slowly. Gradually work up to a pace of three or four miles an hour for at least half an hour at a time. If you are unaccustomed to physical activity, you may want to start with a two-mile-an-hour pace for twenty minutes and increase your speed and distance over a period of weeks.

You should not be huffing and puffing or in pain, but you should be exerting yourself enough to significantly increase your heart rate (to more than about 130 beats per minute if you're a middle-aged person). You can help fitness along by carrying a backpack, shopping bag, or briefcase weighing six to thirteen pounds.

Dress appropriately. Your feet are the most important consideration. Running shoes are best for ordinary walking; hiking boots should be used for rough terrain. Socks should be thick and absorbent — preferably wool or cotton blended with nylon or high-bulk Orlon. Your running shoes should be lightweight and have well-cushioned soles that are flexible across the instep, a firm heel grip, and good arch supports. You should have half an inch of clearance between the end of your toes and the front of the shoe, and the toe box should be high enough to permit you to move your toes freely. Nylon uppers are preferred, but consider getting leather if you expect to walk often in wet weather.

If you walk on the beach on compacted sand, it's best to wear shoes with shock-absorbing soles, Dr. Zohman says. If you plan to walk in hot weather, drink plenty of liquids (water is best), and wear loose, lightweight clothing in fabrics that breathe. In cold weather, layer your clothing (this provides added insulation, and you can shed one or two layers if you get too warm), and be sure to protect your head, ears, and hands adequately. When it's gusty, a windbreaker will protect you against excessive loss of body heat.

Make a plan. Think about how you can fit walking into your life. If you prefer not to set aside a special time to walk (such as before or after work or during your lunch hour), you can build a walk into your day by walking all or part of the way to or from work or by parking a mile or two from your destination and walking the rest of the way. Pick routes that are pleasant and, if possible, relatively uninterrupted by traffic signals and congestion that will slow you down or result in many starts and stops. Check your local bookstore or newsstand for books or maps of walking tours and hiking trails in your area. Hiking clubs, such as the Appalachian Trail Conference in the East and the Sierra Club in the West, can also help you introduce variety into your walk routine.

If you walk at night on a road, walk facing the traffic; wear light-colored clothing, perhaps with reflective tape; carry a flashlight; know the road by day; and avoid looking directly into oncoming headlights.

Check with your doctor. If you have a chronic illness or an orthopedic problem, consult your doctor before you start any exercise program. Although walking is less stressful than nearly all other conditioning exercises, there may be some reason it is ill-advised for you.

Don't forget to stretch. Walking, like jogging, tends to tighten up the muscles, tendons, and ligaments along the back of the legs. Therefore, stretching exercises similar to those done by joggers are best used daily by walkers to guard against injuries caused by inflexibility. [See chapters on stretching, page 97, and jogging, page 101.]

115

For Further Reading

Dreyfack, Raymond. *The Complete Book of Walking.* New York: Arco, 1979.

Gale, Bill. *The Wonderful World of Walking.* New York: Delta, 1979.

Kuntzleman, Charles T., and the editors of *Consumer Guide. The Complete Book of Walking.* New York: Simon & Schuster, 1978.

Rowen, Lilian, and D.S. Laiken. *Speedwalking.* New York: Putnam, 1980; Ballantine, 1980.

Stutman, Fred A., M.D. *The Doctor's Walking Book.* New York: Ballantine, 1980.

Sussman, Aaron, and Ruth Goode. *The Magic of Walking.* New York: Fireside/Simon & Schuster, 1980.

Exercise for Children:
Why and How to Start Young

While tens of millions of American adults have shed their sedentary ways in favor of regular physical activity, another sitdown generation is growing up right under our running, kicking, and pedaling feet. Too many of America's children, after a day of sitting in school (to and from which they ride in buses or cars), go home to watch television, listen to tapes, play electronic games, or read books. One expert has observed that suburban children, who often have to be driven to friends' houses, are even less likely to play outside after school than city kids who usually have several playmates on their own blocks.

When school budgets get too tight, physical education programs are often the first to go. Except for the elite athletic youngsters who play on school teams, most schoolchildren get little fodder for developing those sound bodies in which sound minds are supposed to thrive. Yet, as Lawrence Galton notes in *Your Child in Sports* (see "For Further Reading," page 118), a number of studies have suggested that a person's ability to learn may be increased by physical fitness.

In the elementary grades, as soon as outdoor temperatures drop below 50 degrees Fahrenheit, recess in the schoolyard (which, though rarely inspired, at least involves movement for most of the children) is often replaced by auditorium or library programs. Not that the children mind the cold, but the teachers — who just stand around watching — do!

An alternative approach is to fight the cold by working up some body heat. In Sauk Prairie, Wisconsin, Dr. John A. McAuliffe has got teachers and pupils alike jogging during daily recess. Parents or caretakers who must watch preschool children when they play outdoors might try jogging in place, calisthenics, or jumping rope instead of shivering on a park bench. Or play ball, skate, or go sledding with the children. Why should they have all the fun?

In addition to the logistical problems that discourage youthful exercise, many parents face the dilemma of the "nonathletic" child who shuns team sports and is in turn excluded from them. Yet there are available many noncompetitive or solo activities — such as swimming, skating (roller and ice), dancing, jogging, cycling, rope jumping, gymnastics, skiing, hiking, or just plain walking — that such children might enjoy (and at which they may even excel) and at the same time condition their bodies. Check your local Y for instructional programs. For youthful joggers, you might consult the *Young Runners' Handbook,* available for $3.85 (postage and handling included) from the Kinney Shoe Corporation, P.O. Box 5006, New York, New York 10150.

Children with diabetes need not be excluded from sports activities and endurance exercise, says Dr. Willibald Nagler, physiatrist at the

New York Hospital-Cornell Medical Center. For asthmatic children, who may "clutch" under the stress of competitive sports, swimming is an ideal activity that actually helps them breathe more easily, Dr. Nagler says.

What Fitness Does for Children

Why is physical fitness so important for children? For the very same reasons it is important for adults, plus one additional reason: because physical fitness should be a lifelong goal, and lifetime habits are easier to develop and maintain if started in youth. Here are some other reasons:

Weight control. If calories consumed exceed calories burned, you gain weight — one pound for every 3,500 unused calories. This fact is especially important to youngsters because overweight in childhood often leads to a lifelong weight problem. Study after study has shown that overweight children move far less than children of normal weight — even when both are engaged in the same activity. Among girls swimming at camp, for example, the obese girls stood around in the water, splashing and paddling occasionally, while the lean ones raced one another. A study by Harvard researchers showed that the overweight schoolgirls ate fewer calories than the lean ones, but they also spent two-thirds less time being physically active.

Physical stamina. People who exercise regularly tire less readily than those who are usually sedentary. To the parents of seemingly indefatigable youngsters, this may not always seem an advantage, but for the child it almost certainly is. Physical strength and knowing that your body won't let you down can have important ego-enhancing effects for a child. Physically active people also sleep better, getting more rest from fewer hours of shut-eye.

Psychological strength. Vigorous exercise has a pronounced relaxing effect. It is just as important for a child to be able to shed the stresses and tensions of school as it is for the adult to unwind after work. In fact, excess tension is one of the major causes of fatigue. Exercise, especially when it involves the long muscles of the arms and legs, also has a well-documented antidepressant effect, and depression is a far more common problem in children than most people realize. [See chapter on depression in children, page 149.]

Health benefits. Dr. Thomas B. Gilliam, professor of physical education at the University of Michigan, found that nearly half of 400 high school students he studied had at least one risk factor for heart disease — high blood pressure, high cholesterol level, or overweight — all of which could be reduced by increasing the students' physical activity. Prevention of heart disease is really a problem of youth, since adolescent arteries are already partly clogged with the fatty deposits that can eventually lead to a heart attack. Some specialists have found that through physical conditioning, diabetic youngsters can often significantly reduce the amount of insulin they require.

In toting up the benefits of exercise for children, it's important not to overlook the risks. A major potential hazard is pushing the child too hard too fast. Some call it the Little League syndrome, in which parental goals for the child's athletic achievements exceed the child's ability and replace the joy of participation with tension and anxiety. Exercise should be its own reward; if it's not fun, it will soon be abandoned.

Another important matter is to try to match the child's physical and mental constitution to the sport or sports he or she is best suited for. Trying to succeed at basketball if you're short and stubby is likely to produce nothing but frustration. A child with poor hand-eye coordination is not likely to get much satisfaction from bat-and-ball or racket sports. If a child's body is ill-suited to the sport, injury is far more likely to occur.

Similarly, if a child does not enjoy competition, team sports can be an emotional nightmare. If a parent or older sibling excelled in a sport, it might be wise not to encourage a child who lacks self-confidence to pursue the same activity.

For Further Reading

Galton, Lawrence. *Your Child in Sports.* New York: Franklin Watts, 1980.

Jackson, Douglas W., M.D., and Susan C. Pescar. *The Young Athlete's Health Handbook.* New York: Everest House, 1981.

Lorin, Dr. Martin I. *The Parents Book of Physical Fitness for Children.* New York: Atheneum, 1978. Dr. Lorin reviews the various activities, their benefits and risks, and offers guidelines to matching the child to activities appropriate to his or her age and abilities.

118

Exercise for the Elderly: Keeping Active Throughout Life

Americans spend fortunes trying to ward off the ravages of age with such surface improvements as makeup, hair dyes, toupees, face-lifts, and smart clothes. But once again it turns out, as that old twenties tune put it, "the best things in life are free."

Would you believe that one of them is exercise? Regardless of your age, accumulating evidence indicates that you can delay or reverse many of the deteriorating effects of age through exercise. The benefits can be experienced even by the those confined indoors or to wheelchairs or otherwise limited in physical ability.

Several leading exercise physiologists have devised special programs for the healthy aged and for those with various degrees of incapacitation. They have also put together some well-illustrated exercise manuals that can be used by senior citizens on their own and in nursing homes and community groups as well as by younger persons who are physically disabled or recovering from an illness or injury. Many of the sit-down exercises are also useful for persons who spend their days in a sedentary state.

The Effects of Age

Exercise is certainly not the illusory fountain of youth. But to appreciate some of its demonstrated benefits, it helps to understand what happens to your body as you age. Dr. Herbert A. deVries, director of the exercise laboratory at the Andrus Gerontology Center at the University of Southern California in Los Angeles, says the following changes occur:

• The heart's ability to pump blood declines about 8 percent each decade after adulthood. Blood pressure increases with age, as fatty deposits clog the arteries (atherosclerosis). By middle age the opening of the coronary arteries is 29 percent less than in the twenties.

• As you get older, lung capacity decreases and the chest wall stiffens, reducing the amount of oxygen available to your body tissues.

• The skeletal muscles (such as those in your arms and legs) gradually lose strength, and endurance for muscular activity is reduced. With the passage of each decade, 3 to 5 percent of muscle tissue is actually lost.

• At the same time the percentage of your body that is fat increases. To retain the same proportion of fat to lean body mass, you have to weigh less and less as you get older.

• Your body's capacity to do work, as measured by the maximum amount of oxygen it can use, declines by age seventy-five to less than half of what it was at twenty.

• Reaction time and speed of movement slow down as nerve cells age.

• Bones gradually lose minerals, soften and shrink, and fracture more easily.

How Exercise Counters Them

"So many people rust out before they wear out because they fail to realize that the human body was made to be used for as long as a person lives," notes Dr. Robert E. Wear, exercise physiologist at the University of New Hampshire. Using your body can mitigate and delay — not hasten — the ravages of age.

Perhaps the most dramatic example was the famous marathoner Clarence De Mar, who ran twelve miles a day throughout his adult life and was still running twenty-six-mile marathons at age sixty-eight, two years before he succumbed to cancer. He died with the heart of a young man, with a well-developed heart muscle and coronary arteries two to three times normal size.

Studies of groups of older people have shown that exercise can significantly enhance vigor by increasing the body's work capacity. This means that the person's heart can deliver more oxygen to body tissues for longer periods. Exercise can also slow the loss of muscle tissue and the conversion of lean body mass to fat.

Research conducted by Dr. Everett L. Smith at the University of Wisconsin among people who averaged eighty-four years of age showed that exercise can halt the loss of bone and even increase the size of bones, thereby strengthening them. German studies have indicated that the more nerve cells are used, the less likely they are to age. Animal studies have shown that contrary to popular belief, exercise prevents joints from wearing out. Indeed, older people who exercise were found to have less arthritic changes in their hips than older sedentary people.

When the aged exercise, says Dr. Wear, who has developed exercise programs for people in nursing homes, "their appearance improves, they feel better, their energy reserves increase, they eat better, their peripheral circulation improves, and their range of motion increases. There's a tremendous difference in their vigor and vitality, and they're much less likely to suffer the catastrophic falls that old people are prone to."

Lawrence Frankel of the Lawrence Frankel Foundation in Charleston, West Virginia, has put together a physical fitness program for older persons that can be adapted for those confined to beds, wheelchairs, or walkers. He reports that participants benefit socially, psycho-

EXERCISES FOR THE OLDER PERSON

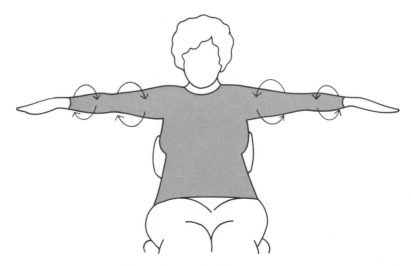

(1) Arm twirl, for arms, chest, and upper back.

logically, and economically as well as physically from the exercises, which help to increase self-confidence, mobility, independence, and work endurance and to diminish physical discomforts.

Dr. deVries reported that among 200 healthy people between the ages of fifty-six and eighty-eight who participated in a jog-walk program at least three times a week for forty-two weeks, oxygen transport, lung capacity, and arm strength all improved significantly when compared with a group of people who did not exercise. The participants also lost body fat and weight, and their blood pressures dropped. Furthermore, exercise had a relaxing effect, as measured by their degree of muscle tension, greater than that induced by the tranquilizer Miltown.

What to Do

Assuming you're now convinced and ready to start flexing those atrophying muscles, how do you go about it? Before any previously sedentary person over thirty-five begins vigorous exercise capable of conditioning the heart, the first step is a thorough physical examination, preferably with an exercise stress test. [See chapter on exercise stress testing, page 95.] These are usually given by cardiologists in private offices, hospital clinics, and preventive medicine institutes and at many YMCAs.

For older people, a regimen of short bursts of low-intensity exercise

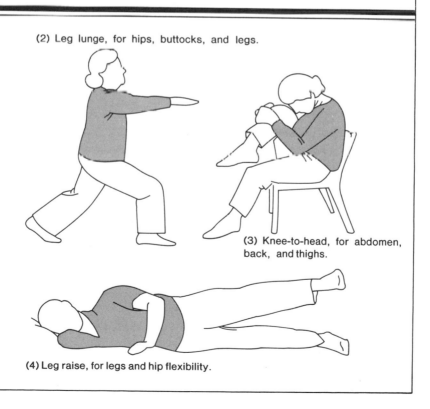

(2) Leg lunge, for hips, buttocks, and legs.

(3) Knee-to-head, for abdomen, back, and thighs.

(4) Leg raise, for legs and hip flexibility.

done over a relatively long time is preferable to the concentrated high-intensity exercise prescribed for the young. Dr. deVries prescribes a fifteen- to twenty-minute jog-walk regimen that starts out with an equal number of running and walking steps and gradually — over a period of ten weeks — progresses into mostly running. If this regimen, which is done three times a week, is too strenuous, it can be cut back to more walking and less or no running.

Before every workout, Dr. deVries insists on fifteen to twenty minutes of calisthenics, and each session ends with fifteen to twenty minutes of yogalike stretching exercises to prevent muscle and joint injuries. The workouts themselves should start with a slow warm-up and end with a slow cool-down (a period of lighter exercise) to prevent heart problems. [See chapter on stretching and warming up, page 97.]

Alternatives to jogging include swimming (a minimum of a quarter

JOG-WALK REGIMEN
(Based on 3 Workouts a Week)

Phase	Days	Run (Steps)	Walk (Steps)	Number of Sets
I	1	50	50	5
	2	50	50	6
	3	50	50	7
	4	50	50	8
	5	50	50	9
	6	50	50	10
II	7-12	50	40	5 sets on Day 7, add 1 set for each workout day
III	13-18	50	30	Same as Phase II
IV	19-24	50	20	Same as Phase II
V	25-30	50	10	Same as Phase II
VI	31-36	75	10	Same as Phase II
VII	37-42	100	10	Same as Phase II
VIII	43-48	125	10	Same as Phase II
IX	49-54	150	10	Same as Phase II
X	55-60	175	10	Same as Phase II
XI	61-66	200	10	Same as Phase II
XII	67	Individualized program		

Adapted from *Geriatrics* magazine; programs developed by Dr. Herbert A. DeVries.

mile done briskly without stopping), hard cycling, dancing, and even horseback riding. Any activity that a person has done for many years, including tennis and skiing, can be continued into old age, Dr. deVries says. But the elderly should not take up rigorous sports that they've never done before or had abandoned years ago, he adds.

For those unable to do vigorous outdoor exercise, there are activities that, although not strenuous enough to condition the heart, can do a great deal for the body and spirit in general. Bonnie Prudden, who at nearly seventy years of age heads the Institute for Physical Fitness in Stockbridge, Massachusetts, recommends the "ten-penny trick":

Put ten pennies on the floor, and, bending from the knees with the back straight, pick them up one by one and put them on the highest shelf; then take them down and put them back on the floor. Gradually the number of pennies can be increased. This builds muscle strength in the thighs, useful for getting out of chairs.

Another of Bonnie Prudden's techniques uses a pet rock weighing one or two pounds that's kept next to the phone. While on the phone, hold the rock in your free hand and swing it over your head, down to your side, up and around. On the next call, switch hands.

For those confined to a wheelchair, Dr. Wear suggests cutting a broomstick into two-foot lengths and, holding a piece in both hands, swinging it up, back of the head, wringing it like a wet towel, and bending over with it. Even without the stick, a person in a wheelchair can do arm swings, side and forward bends, and body rotations. All this is more fun if done to music.

For Further Reading

Among the illustrated exercise guides for the elderly are:

Frankel, Lawrence J., and Betty Byrd Richard. *Be Alive as Long as You Live.* A 256-page, hardcover, spiral-bound book, obtainable for $10.95 from Preventicare Publications, 106 Brooks Street, Charleston, W.Va. 25301.

Smith, Dr. Everett L., and Dr. Karl Stoedefalke. *Aging and Exercise.* A 115-page unbound booklet, obtainable for $4 from Dr. Smith at the Department of Preventive Medicine, 504 Walnut, University of Wisconsin, Madison, Wis. 53706.

Wear, Dr. Robert E. *Fitness, Vitality, and You.* An 81-page soft-cover, spiral-bound pamphlet, obtainable for $5 by writing to Lionel E. Mayrand, Jr., Gerontology Department, New England Center for Continuing Education, University of New Hampshire, Durham, N.H. 03824.

123

III.
Emotional
Health

Our feelings, thoughts, actions, and reactions have a far greater influence on our health, happiness, and success in life than most of us are willing to acknowledge. You don't have to be medically defined as "emotionally disturbed" to be impaired by stress, anxiety, or depression. Since mind and body are really two aspects of the same organism, what happens to one inevitably affects the other.

Thus, the Type A personality, a victim of "hurry sickness" who reacts with hostility to anything and everything that seems to cross his or her path, may be setting the stage for premature death from a heart attack. Someone under the stress of profound grief may develop high blood pressure, and feelings of hopelessness may be the antecedent to cancer. By the same token, a physical ailment can have emotional consequences that seriously interfere with treatment of the disease and with the person's ability to get as much out of life as possible.

Too often those troubled by emotional problems are pessimistic about the possibility of overcoming them. You may not realize that much can now be done — in some cases through self-help — to counter negative emotional influences as well as to treat such major psychiatric problems as serious depression and anxiety. Needed treatment can be obtained, regardless of your ability to pay. Although not all mental illnesses can be cured, treatment can often remove crippling emotional obstacles and pave the way to a fuller, happier life.

Understanding Mental Illness: Burying the Myths

Despite the recent explosion of books and articles about emotional problems and treatment, myths and misunderstandings about mental illnesses and their victims prevail. The result is often social stigmatization and discrimination, avoidance of needed therapy, and undue pessimism about the prospects for recovery. According to the National Association of Private Psychiatric Hospitals, "One-quarter of a population recently surveyed would not want people who have had mental health problems as neighbors, while 60 percent would not have them as tenants. Former psychiatric patients often have trouble getting housing, credit, insurance, and licenses."

Yet, the association suggests, many of these attitudes and fears are unjustified — based not on facts, but on widely believed myths about the mentally ill and their prospects for effective treatment or cure. While few believe that all mentally ill people are raving maniacs, "many people still characterize the mentally ill as unpredictable, erratic, unstable, and dangerous," the association says.

In fact, however, "there are only a few dangerous people, and most of them are not in mental hospitals," notes Dr. Shervert H. Frazier, psychiatrist in chief at McLean Hospital in Belmont, Massachusetts. "Even among mental hospital patients, 98 to 99 percent are not dangerous."

What Is Mental Illness?

Mental illness is not a single, simple entity. In its milder forms it involves underlying emotional conflicts that produce symptoms and thought disturbances that may interfere with a full, happy life. The more severe, less common forms of mental illness — the psychoses — involve extreme changes in mood or personality or major distortions in perception and thought.

Many of the symptoms of emotional problems afflict mentally healthy people from time to time. We all occasionally get depressed, feel unduly tense, anxious, fearful, or overwhelmed by life's demands. The healthy person readily weathers such difficulties and pulls out of them before long. In someone who is mentally ill, however, the emotional distress tends to be prolonged or precipitated by factors that other people cope with easily.

Most of us would quickly realize that a person who has completely lost touch with reality is mentally ill. However, bizarre behavior and speech patterns are characteristic of only a small proportion of mentally ill people. The more common symptoms of emotional problems may go unnoticed. Prolonged withdrawal from the normal pleasures of life, a loss of self-confidence, sleep problems, undue pessimism, feelings of helplessness or hopelessness, and a lack of caring about things or people are signs of profound depression that warrants treatment. [See chapters on depression, page 146, and childhood depression, page 149.]

Some people suffer from deep-seated, persistent anxiety or fear that may be attributed first to one cause and then to another. [See chapter on anxiety, page 155.] In other forms of mental illness, moods or behavior may undergo an abrupt transformation. Mental illness may also be masked or disguised in ways that make it especially hard to recognize. An emotionally disturbed person may complain persistently of physical ailments, although no organic cause for the complaints can be found. [See chapter on hypochondria, page 163.] In other people, emotional problems precipitate actual physical disorders. Some mentally ill people are perfectionists who place unrealistic demands upon themselves or the people or institutions around them. Still others habitually fall far below their potentials in school or at work.

Many people with emotional disorders function well despite their problems; some have even accomplished great work while under the burden of mental illness. There is no question, though, that emotional problems take their toll and destroy much of the joy of life for victims and often for their families as well.

A Common Problem Needing Treatment

Mental illness is far more common than most people realize. A Louis Harris poll conducted for Pacific Mutual, a life and health insurance company, revealed that a third of American adults have experienced emotional problems that affected their physical health, and that twenty million adults have suffered from prolonged mental health problems.

On the average, the hospital association says, 10 percent of the general population is mentally ill, and in large urban areas the incidence of serious emotional problems is as high as 23 percent. Mental illness afflicts children as often as adults. An estimated 10 million people under the age of eighteen have psychiatric problems, with at least 1.4 million suffering from disorders serious enough to require immediate professional attention. Childhood emotional problems include hyperactivity, autism, schizophrenia, and depression.

The mentally ill need treatment. In a society like ours that values self-determination and personal fortitude, people tend to resist asking for help and instead pride themselves on their ability to correct whatever might be wrong without assistance. Those who cannot cope with the stresses of life are often looked down upon and even blamed for their troubles.

For many people, there is an unquestionable stigma attached to needing help for emotional problems. As a result, professional treatment of these problems is often delayed until they are so severe that extended treatment is required and the chances for cure are greatly diminished. Studies have shown that the prognosis for effectively treating a mental disorder is far better when help is sought early.

Contrary to the common belief that few recover from mental disorders, the association points out that "about two-thirds of psychiatric patients show significant signs of recovery, and of these, half will never need treatment again." In some cases the underlying cause of the problem may not be eliminated, but the symptoms can be brought under enough control to permit the patient to function well in society.

Just as physical medicine does not rely on only one method of coping with organic diseases, the treatment of mental illness involves many different approaches. Treatment is usually tailored to the disorder in question since what works best for one type of mental problem may be totally ineffective for another. Only a small percentage of patients are treated with classical Freudian analysis, a prolonged and costly therapy that is not suitable for many types of emotional problems.

Among the modes of therapy available today are traditional psychotherapy, in which patient and therapist exchange ideas aimed at uncovering the roots of the problem; behavior modification, in which patients are taught new behavior patterns that help them overcome emotional obstacles; drug therapy, especially useful in treating depressed or anxious patients as well as those with more severe psychiatric disorders such as schizophrenia and psychosis; and group therapy, in which individuals who share similar problems discuss them together with a therapist.

In addition, there are a variety of newer treatments, including family therapy involving the whole family unit; humanistic therapies that use techniques like sensitivity training and counseling to help patients realize what kind of people they really are, and transactional analysis, a form of group therapy that helps patients understand their unconscious motivations. [See chapter on choosing a psychotherapist, page 129.]

Hospitalization is usually unnecessary. Most treatment for mental disorders can be given in independent or hospital-based clinics or in therapists' offices. As the hospital association says, "Of the 5.5 million episodes of care given by all mental health facilities in 1973, over two-thirds were handled on an outpatient or day-care basis." Thanks largely to psychotherapeutic drugs, many mental patients who would have required hospitalization in the past can now be treated as outpatients. When hospitalization is necessary, it is usually brief.

Not all psychiatric treatment is prohibitively expensive. In many cases it is partly covered by medical insurance policies.

Despite community opposition and an overwhelming list of bureaucratic difficulties, more than 900 federally supported community mental health centers currently exist.

For Further Reading

Mental Illness: Its Myths and Truths. A 32-page pamphlet available for $1 from the National Association of Private Psychiatric Hospitals, 1701 K Street N.W., Washington, D.C. 20006.

Ogg, Elizabeth. *Help for Emotional and Mental Problems.* Public Affairs Pamphlet No. 567, 1979. Available for 50 cents from Public Affairs Pamphlets, 381 Park Avenue South, New York, N.Y. 10016.

How to Choose A Psychotherapist

Psychotherapy is at last coming out of the closet. Prompted by the stresses of family and social upheavals, the narcissism of the "me" generation, publicity about new treatment approaches, and a plethora of popular books prescribing do-it-yourself emotional inventories, many more people than formerly are now seeking help in unraveling the intricacies of their psyches and improving their potentials for happiness.

But the smorgasbord of available approaches to psychological problems would confuse even the most stable of potential clients. To someone who is emotionally troubled, the staggering number of choices can be paralyzing.

In addition to traditional talk therapy and psychoanalysis, there are therapies called Jungian, gestalt, Adlerian, Rogerian, group, reality, cognitive, integrity, drug, sex, family, marital, shock, hypnotic, drama, poetry, and primal scream. These have been joined in recent years by biofeedback, behavior modification, orthomolecular psychiatry, rolfing, transactional analysis, and bioenergetics, not to mention such aprofessional approaches as est, rebirthing, and various "anonymous" self-help groups. *The Psychotherapy Handbook* (see "For Further Reading," page 136) describes more than 250 therapies now in use.

Although every therapist has his or her own opinion about the best therapy or therapist for each client, experts have distilled some useful guidelines.

Which Therapy?

Certain treatment approaches are clearly less appropriate for some patients than others. Behavior modification, for example, emphasizes gaining awareness of undesirable behaviors and changing them rather than gaining insight into their causes; thus, it is of little use to a woman who wants to know why she always chooses men who punish her. She would do far better with a "talk" therapy, such as traditional analysis (à la Freud, Jung, or Adler), analytically based psychotherapy (involving conversations with the therapist), cognitive, or group therapy.

By the same token, psychoanalysis is not the preferred treatment

129

for a man suffering from premature ejaculation, who would get faster and far less expensive help through behaviorally oriented sex therapy and perhaps marital counseling. Psychoanalysis, aimed at unearthing and modifying internal conflicts that cause emotional distress, would not be suited for someone who has difficulty verbalizing thoughts and feelings. It usually means a commitment to four or five sessions a week for several years and thus is not appropriate for any patient lacking the time or financial resources. However, other talk therapies are now placing more emphasis on short-term psychotherapy.

Traditional analysis or psychotherapy may help someone with a phobia understand the basis for his or her fear, but it would not necessarily eradicate the phobia. Behavior therapy can often rapidly extinguish the phobic response, though the patient may never fully understand its origins.

Tension headaches may be relieved by gaining insight into stress reactions in addition to making life changes to reduce stress. But the headaches may respond faster to a more mechanical therapy like biofeedback, in which the patient learns not to translate stress into a tightening of head muscles. A combination of insight, life changes, and mechanical therapy might be the ideal route to permanent relief of stress and its physical and emotional consequences.

130

Group therapy, with or without individual therapy, can be very helpful for persons who think they are alone in their suffering. It is also valuable for those with little self-esteem who think they have nothing to offer, since their contributions to others in the group are ego-enhancing. Sometimes criticism or guidance offered by group members is more readily accepted than when it comes from a therapist. However, a group can be very threatening to someone who is overly sensitive to criticism or who has difficulty talking to people.

Drug therapy (psychopharmacology) is often used as an adjunct to talk or other modes of therapy, especially for patients with severe anxiety or depression. The drugs are primarily intended as short-term aids, not chronic therapies, to alleviate a patient's symptoms enough to reduce suffering and make other approaches to therapy more successful. For patients with severe anxiety or chronic depression, drug therapy, sometimes prolonged, is often essential to successful therapy. For one common disorder — manic-depressive illness — and for some cases of cyclic depression, a drug called lithium is used indefinitely, presumably to correct a chemical imbalance in the brain.

Which Therapist?

The specific therapeutic technique used is often less important than finding the right mix of patient and therapist. The ideal therapist is warm, empathetic, nonjudgmental, and genuine, able to inspire hope and trust in patients. But it is the patient's reaction to the therapist that counts the most. Since the patient has to do far more than half the work in therapy, a congenial relationship with the therapist is most conducive to success. Psychotherapy is ineffective unless the patient is committed to trying to make it work.

A therapist's training, credentials, experience, and skill are also important. Along with the explosion in treatment techniques, there has been an enormous growth in self-styled therapists, many of whom have had no more training than to have become a "graduate" of the therapy themselves. While usually innocuous and occasionally helpful, at least for the short term, sometimes lay therapies like est unleash powerful emotional forces that destroy a person's emotional stability. Without proper training, the lay therapist is unable to prevent such disasters or assist the victims.

As Elizabeth Ogg points out in her illuminating Public Affairs Pamphlet "The Psychotherapies Today" (see "For Further Reading," page 136), "there is nothing to stop rank amateurs from setting up as therapists or from founding pseudo-schools of their own." Further, the terms "psychoanalyst," "psychotherapist," and "counselor" have no legal definition — anyone can claim to be one.

Fortunately the major types of professional psychotherapists must qualify for licenses in most states. The wise consumer will ask about the therapist's training and licensing *prior* to making the first appointment. The main sources of help are:

Psychiatrists. These are medical doctors who have completed a three-year residency in psychiatry in addition to four years of medical school and a year of internship. Psychiatrists are the only psychotherapists permitted to prescribe drugs (though other therapists may suggest that the client's physician write a prescription). But don't assume that because a psychiatrist is a physician, he or she will perform a physical examination or would be more likely to detect a physical cause for emotional symptoms. Ask about a valid state license and certification by the American Board of Psychiatry and Neurology or board eligibility.

Clinical psychologists. These therapists have Ph.D. degrees in psychology plus a year of supervised clinical training and should have passed a state licensing examination. Though clinical psychologists are not medical doctors, the care they offer — as with psychiatric care — is accepted for reimbursement by most medical insurance policies. Psychologists generally charge less than psychiatrists, and studies indicate they are just as effective as psychiatrists. Ask about a state license and certification by the American Board of Examiners in Professional Psychology or a listing in the National Register of Health Service Providers in Psychology.

Social workers. These professionals, who provide more psychotherapy than any other professional group, have master's and sometimes Ph.D. degrees in mental health. They complete at least two years of graduate study and two years of internship in a clinical setting. Most work in hospitals or clinics, but some have private practices. Many are eligible for insurance payments. Ask about a listing in the *National Registry of Health Care Providers in Clinical Social Work.*

Psychiatric nurses. These therapists have master's degrees in psychiatry or mental health nursing. While a few are in private practice, most psychiatric nurses practice in hospitals, community mental health centers, and other agencies. Check for accreditation by the American Nurses Association Division in Psychiatric and Mental Health Nursing Practice.

Psychoanalysts. Athough most are psychiatrists or clinical psychologists who have undergone years of training at an accredited psychoanalytic institute, a person with little or no training may assume the title of analyst. Be sure to check credentials. Other psychotherapists, including social workers and psychiatric nurses, may also undergo analytic training. Only California currently licenses psychoanalysts. Check for a listing in the *National Registry of Psychoanalysts.*

Pastoral counselors. These are members of the clergy with special training in psychology or social work, who may have degrees in such fields. They can be highly effective sources of inexpensive counseling, but be wary of those with little or no training in psychotherapy. Look for certification by the American Association of Pastoral Counselors.

How to Find a Therapist

There are many possible sources of referral: your family doctor, your clergyman, a friend or relative who has had a positive personal experience with a particular therapist, the psychiatry department of a nearby university or community hospital, or local schools of psychotherapy or social work. Check your phone book for the Mental Health Association of your county, which maintains an information and referral service.

If immediate assistance is needed, a crisis center hot line may help. Check your phone book under the name of the crisis: rape, suicide, drug abuse, etc.

If the cost of therapy is a consideration, treatment given at community mental health centers, public hospitals, and clinics is usually far less expensive than private psychotherapy. Group therapy and treatment given by psychologists, social workers, or psychiatric nurses usually cost less than individual therapy by a psychiatrist.

Be wary of any therapist who guarantees success. Psychotherapy is still an art, not a science. Don't be impatient if improvement comes slowly or if there are occasional setbacks or plateaus. However, if months go by with no improvement, it may be wise to see another professional, at least as a consultant.

Regardless of whom you choose as a therapist, be sure to ask in advance about fees, frequency of therapy, projected length of therapy, and how missed or canceled appointments are handled. Check your medical insurance to see if the type of care you are considering is covered.

You might also ask that your first appointment be used as an interview to see if you and the therapist are suited for each other. If you don't

WHO NEEDS HELP?

An estimated 34 million Americans are currently receiving professional psychotherapy or counseling, and millions more are believed to be in need of such help. Part of the problem in obtaining care for those who could benefit from it is the difficulty many people have in recognizing and acknowledging the existence of an emotional problem.

Life is normally a series of emotional ups and downs, with feelings of depression, anxiety, fear, inadequacy, or guilt troubling most of us from time to time. It is only when such feelings dominate our existence or interfere with life at work, at home, or at play and with our potential for happiness that they signify trouble.

Here are some of the more common signals of trouble deserving of professional attention:

● Prolonged feelings of depression, whether lacking any clear cause or precipitated by a specific event, such as a professional setback, death of a loved one, or end of a marriage; inability to bounce back from a crisis or setback within what others consider a reasonable length of time. [See chapter on depression, page 146.]

● Feelings of hopelessness or great confusion; growing demoralization; overwhelming feelings or boredom or meaninglessness of your existence; thoughts of suicide.

● A sense that your life is out of control; erratic mood shifts; inability to concentrate or make decisions.

● Fears that people or institutions are out to get you; feelings that people, places, or events are bizarre or unreal.

● Difficulty getting along with other people; prolonged marital difficulties.

● Compulsive self-destructive behaviors, such as inability to stop gambling, drinking, eating, or using drugs; a compulsive ritual like repeated hand-washing; phobic fears like an extreme fear of heights, elevators, airplanes, or dogs. [See chapters on curing phobias, page 158, and compulsive eating, page 270.]

● Emotional difficulties dealing with a chronic or life-threatening physical illness or disability.

● Frequent sexual difficulties, insomnia, or nightmares.

● In children, chronic disruption of home and classroom; repeated senseless destruction of objects; inability to get along with other children; school failure or work falling far below native potential; delinquency; flagrant criminal acts or violations of the law; frequent physical complaints like stomachaches, sore throats, or headaches for which no medical cause can be found.

In adults, too, emotional problems sometimes first show up as physical ailments, such as chronic headaches, intestinal disorders, or asthma. And sometimes a neurological disorder — for example multiple sclerosis or a brain tumor — first appears as an emotional or behavioral disturbance.

Thus, if a physical disorder does not respond to the usual medical treatment or recurs repeatedly without apparent cause, a psychotherapeutic consultation may be advisable. Similarly, if an emotional problem does not respond to treatment in a reasonable length of time, a thorough physical examination is warranted. Some experts say that such a checkup is wise for anyone in need of prolonged or repeated treatment for an emotional problem.

133

MAJOR TYPES OF PSYCHOTHERAPY *Used by permission from the Public Affairs Committee.*

The following table is adapted from *The Psychotherapies Today*, a Public Affairs Pamphlet written by Elizabeth Ogg. The prices quoted represent an overall national range at the end of 1981; they may be higher in certain parts of the country; for example, in New York City.

Psychotherapy	Description	Frequency	Duration Cost
TRADITIONAL PSYCHOTHERAPIES			
Psychoanalysis.	Using Freud's techniques with client lying on a couch, uncovering unconscious conflicts through free associations to dreams, fantasies, and early memories, and transference of deep feelings associated with those memories onto the analyst.	3 to 5 sessions a week for 2 to 6 years or more.	$40 to $125 per session.
Analytically oriented psychotherapy.	Though based on Freud's theory of unconscious conflicts, involves more direct patient-therapist dialogue than classical analysis.	1 to 2 sessions a week for 1 to 3 years.	$30 to $100 per session (less with analysts in training).
Jungian analysis.	More personal involvement by therapist, who is often supportive in a practical way. Patient involved in imaginative amplification of dreams and artwork as means of getting in touch with unconscious.	2 or 3 times a week at first, then once a week for few months.	$60 to $100 per session. $15 to $25 at training to several years. Institute clinics.
Adlerian therapy.	A reeducation process stressing conscious approach to problems and a reordering of goals to reflect realistic options and self-acceptance.	Weekly sessions for a few months to up to 10 years.	On sliding scale from $18 to $40 per session.
HUMAN POTENTIAL THERAPIES			
Client-centered (Rogerian) therapy.	Building self-esteem through therapist's empathy and unconditional regard for client, with client participating in setting terms for the therapy.	Occasional sessions or 2 times a week, with total of only a few sessions or regularly for years.	Individually negotiated, based on client needs.
Gestalt therapy.	Promotes awareness of moment-to-moment experiences of patient as a whole person, body and mind, and acceptance of full responsibility for them as a condition for	Weekly session for 10 weeks to two years.	$25 to $65 for private sessions, $12 with therapists in training, $15 to $30 for workshops.

Bioenergetics.	Releasing emotional blockages through physical manipulations and movement, together with discussion.	1 session every week or two for few months to 5 years.	$25 to $100 per session.
GROUP THERAPIES			
Psychodrama.	With therapist as director, group member enacts problem situation, with other group members assisting, followed by group discussion.	1 to 2 sessions a week for a few months to 2 years.	$15 to $30 per person per session.
Traditional group therapy.	Discussions among a group of six to ten clients, with members giving feedback on how each comes across, aimed at exposing maladaptive attitudes and behaviors and learning better ways of relating to others.	Once a week for few months to 2 years, sometimes combined with individual therapy.	$20 per person per session, less in clinics.
Family therapy.	Promoting family understanding and cooperation by improving communication among family members and freeing them to express full emotions.	Once a week for few weeks or months.	$40 to $70 perfamily per session, less in clinics.
Transactional analysis.	Based on therapy that people interact in terms of one of three ego states — parent, adult, or child — and seeks to make clients aware of their behavior as overstrict parents or irresponsible children and helps them to behave as adults.	Weekly 2-hour groups sessions for about 2 years; also individual 1-hour sessions available.	$20 per group session; $35 for individual.
COGNITIVE-BEHAVIORAL THERAPIES			
Cognitive therapies.	Assuming habitual errors in perception and thinking cause psychological disturbances, seeks to correct these errors through understanding.	Once a week for 6 to 40 weeks; sometimes followed by 6 months to year of weekly group therapy.	$20 to $50 per session, $12.50 per person in group.
Behavior therapy.	Considers symptoms to be learned bad habits and seeks to eliminate them by teaching new adaptive skills.	1 to 2 sessions a week for up to several months, depending on nature and severity of problem.	$20 to $120 per session, $20 to $30 per person in groups.
Biofeedback.	Patients are trained to modify automatic body processes through deep relaxation and feedback about bodily states from electronic monitoring equipment.	10 to 15 weekly individual sessions of 75 minutes each, exercises at home between sessions.	$130 per two intake with daily sessions, $55 to $75 for therapy sessions.

like the therapist, don't hesitate to try another. And don't be put off if a therapist suggests that you see someone else who may be better qualified to treat your problem.

For Further Reading

Herink, Richie, ed. *The Psychotherapy Handbook*. New York: New American Library, 1980.
Ogg, Elizabeth. "The Psychotherapies Today." Public Affairs Pamphlet No. 596. Available for 50 cents from Public Affairs Pamphlets, 381 Park Avenue South, New York, N.Y. 10016.

Happiness: You Can't Buy It in a Book

If you are to believe the recent dogma, happiness is getting rid of your erroneous zones, looking out for number one, asserting yourself, taking charge of your life and learning to love every minute of it. It is clearing your psyche by screaming, esting, rolfing, encountering, hallucinating, meditating, and levitating; tuning into your biorhythms, following your stars, getting in touch with your feelings, letting it all hang out; and teleporting yourself into an extrasensory universe.

If any of these remedies actually brought people real, lasting happiness, there would hardly be the need for so many. It's very much like diets for weight reduction — the number of cures proposed is inversely proportional to the effectiveness of any one of them. Like diets, each of the happiness formulas may work for a short while, giving people a temporary lift, only to be followed by an inevitable letdown. And then on to the next formula.

"Most of the pop psych books make it seem as if there's an easy answer to finding happiness," says Dr. Jonathan Freedman, Columbia University psychologist who has studied happy people. "This is misleading and grossly oversimplifies the problem. Life is very complicated. You can't find happiness by following some simple recipe." Dr. Willard Gaylin, a New York psychiatrist, adds, "There are recipes for cookies, but not for people."

Undoubtedly many of the psychological self-help books and pop therapies help some people at least some of the time. As Dr. Gaylin points out, "A book may make you aware of a problem that can be treated. A lot of people don't know that what they suffer from is an illness." It is also reassuring to realize that what you feel is shared by others, Dr. Gaylin adds, and that this feeling is either normal or abnormal but potentially treatable. However, he emphasizes, the most helpful and enriching books are not ones that offer do-it-yourself prescriptions, but rather those that bring insight and enlightenment.

Hazards of Simplistic Formulas

Rather than help, Dr. Gaylin and others believe, the barrage of simplistic remedies that are attacking the consumer's psyche these days can do many people real harm. As Dr. Gaylin notes in his book, *Feelings: Our Vital Signs* (see "For Further Reading," page 138), the seemingly endless flow of how-to books "guide the perplexed and despairing to inner peace via conflicting and contradictory pathways." These popular prescriptions can actually be counterproductive, turning people away from the very things that might lead to lasting happiness and perpetuating unrealistic expectations that stand in the way of their prized goal.

The phony formulas encourage people "to kick over the traces, because they think something else, something more, should be happening," notes Susan Dickes Hubbard, a psychotherapist in Boulder, Colorado. The result may be a divorce, or frenetic job search, or frantic therapy-shopping in pursuit of the misleading notion that things should be getting better and better all the time.

As Mrs. Hubbard wrote in the *The Humanist,* the harm done by telling people they can find happiness by following a blueprint of thought and behavior is that "people become overly self-critical when things do not go well for them. If their prospects for happiness and success are entirely in their own hands, then there is never an opportunity to attribute failure to circumstances beyond their control."

Furthermore, many of the books and therapies foster unrealistic expectations of how people should feel and what life should be all about. Mrs. Hubbard says people are likely to compare themselves unfavorably to what they read in half a dozen books and consequently turn their small unhappiness into a much bigger issue. Their expectations are unnaturally inflated, and they are "misled into expecting magical changes."

Dr. Herbert Holt, a New York psychoanalyst and author of *Free to Be Good or Bad* (see "For Further Reading," page 138), calls it "magic-think." The pop therapies, he suggests, create magical expectations, fantasies of happiness. "There's nothing wrong with fantasy happiness as an occasional escape from daily life, as long as it's not confused with reality," he notes. Dr. Gaylin adds that the prescriptions propose an idyllic, romantic stage that can never match reality and that "depresses people as much as New Year's Eve does."

In fact, according to Dr. Gaylin, a common aspect of unhappiness is the persistent clinging to infantile, magical expectations. A major goal of traditional psychotherapy is to help people grow up through the realization that there are no easy solutions. But the pop therapies suggest to people, "If I do this or that, I will be happy." It is an adult version of the child's belief that if only he were cute or did well in school, his mother would love him. Each time a recipe fails to produce lasting happiness, it can compound the person's incipient depression, Dr. Gaylin says. "It's a magic that fails."

Tips for a Happier Time

The real issue, according to Dr. Holt, is "not to drive people into fantasy happiness but to get them to concentrate on what they can do in their daily lives to give life meaning. Happiness grows out of commitment, responsibility. It's the product of meaningful relationships with other human beings. This, however, is not a best-selling notion."

Ironically, Dr. Freedman, the Columbia psychologist, points out, "most of the advice in the pop psych books and therapies is dangerously egocentric. It teaches people just to look out for themselves. Yet the studies of happiness show that people are happiest in a good relationship with someone else."

If you want to be happy, he adds, "you have to care, to take responsibility. Egocentric, narcissistic types don't form relationships easily nor maintain them very well." In fact, Christopher Lasch, a cultural historian at the University of Rochester, notes in his book, *The Culture of Narcissism* (New York: W.W. Norton, 1979) that the current emphasis on looking inward to attain "the feeling, the momentary illusion, of personal well-being, health, and psychic security" is but a symptom of the society-wide narcissism that besets our times.

Mrs. Hubbard further points out that it's a disservice to hand people a burdensome load of "shoulds" to finding their identities. "People just naturally have different emotional styles. Two emotionally healthy adults are not going to experience comparable amounts of joie de vivre, or comparable amounts of anything else, for that matter."

Dr. Freedman's studies showed, for example, that one need not be an optimist to be happy, although that certainly makes happiness easier to attain. There are happy pessimists and cynics as well. Besides, says Mrs. Hubbard, people "should be unhappy now and again. The irony is that everyone could feel a lot happier if you learn to accept who you are. Happiness is the byproduct of being yourself, whoever you are. And you may be nothing at all like what these books describe."

For Further Reading

Freedman, Jonathan. *Happy People.* New York: Harcourt, Brace, Jovanovich, 1978.
Gaylin, Willard, M.D. *Feelings: Our Vital Signs.* New York: Harper & Row, 1979.
Holt, Herbert, M.D. *Free to Be Good or Bad.* New York: Basic Books, 1976.

Stress:
Some Good, Some Bad

Stress is a factor in every life, and without some stress life would be drab and unstimulating. Too little stress can produce boredom, feelings of isolation, stagnation, and purposelessness. Stress in and of itself is not bad; rather, it's how you react to the different stresses in your life that matters.

Many people thrive on stress. They find working under pressure or against deadlines highly stimulating, providing the motivation to do their best. And they rarely succumb to adverse stress reactions. To slow such "racehorses" down to the pace of a turtle would be as stressful as trying to make the turtle keep up with the horse. Yet others crumble when the crunch is on or the overload light flashes. Some take life's large and small obstacles in stride, regarding them as a challenge to succeed in spite of everything. Others are thwarted by every unexpected turn of events, from a traffic delay to a serious illness in the family.

What Stress Does

All stress, positive or negative, stimulates a basic biological reaction called fight or flight. This is a hormonally stimulated state of arousal that prepares you to face whatever challenge is at hand, be it your daughter's wedding, a job interview, an argument with your spouse, or the assault of a would-be mugger. The chemical reaction influences your heart, nervous system, muscles, and other organs, preparing them for action.

Problems arise when the stress reaction is frequently called into play for inappropriate circumstances, such as a missed bus, long line, or reservation mix-up, or when the circumstances of your life result in more stress than you can handle at any one time.

When most people talk about stress, they mean the negative reactions: a churning gut, aching back, tight throat, rapid heartbeat, elevated blood pressure, mental depression, short temper, crying jags, insomnia, impotence, viral infections, asthma attacks, ulcers, heart disease, or cancer. [See chapter on Type A behavior, page 142.]

My stress reaction was headaches. I got them often: when I was writing on deadline, doing a lot of sewing, preparing for a dinner party, driving in heavy traffic. For years I had attributed them to a variety of causes, including eyestrain and allergic reactions to my colleagues' tobacco smoke and to the fumes from my gas stove. But not until I awoke one morning from a bad dream with my teeth tightly clenched did I get a hint of the real reason — a reaction to stress.

Over the next several weeks I realized that whenever I was concentrating hard on something (even opening a stubborn package or chopping an onion) or feeling tense or anxious, I clenched my teeth. After a while the strain on the supporting muscles would result in a headache.

It was an unconscious reaction, a habit that I was finally able to break — with the aid of my dentist — by becoming acutely aware of it and making a conscious effort to relax my jaw when formerly I would have tightened it. Now tension headaches, which account for 80 percent of the head pains that afflict Americans, rarely sneak through my surveillance. [See chapter on headaches, page 518.]

Dr. Donald A. Tubesing, psychologist from Duluth, Minnesota, and author of *Kicking Your Stress Habits* (see "For Further Reading," page 142), likens stress to the tension on a violin string — you need "enough tension to make music but not so much that it snaps."

Whereas some stress reduction programs offer only techniques to induce relaxation, Dr. Tubesing's simply written self-help guide helps you get to the roots of your stress reactions and modify them. He points out that most stress is not the result of great tragedies, but rather an accumulation of minor irritations that "grind us down over the years." He tells you how to recognize the sources of those irritations and what to do about them.

For example, he points out, stress is inherent not in an event but rather in how you *perceive* that event; by modifying your perceptions, you can reduce your stress. Let's say you just missed your bus. You could focus on the fact that you'll be late for work (stressful) or on the fact that you'll now have time to read the paper (not stressful).

He cautions against spending "10 dollars worth of energy on a 10-cent problem." Before you gear up for a battle, stop and think: is the threat real? Is the issue really important? Can you make a difference? Dr. Tubesing's guide helps you to identify your beliefs, values, and goals, which in turn will enable you to focus on what really counts and stop worrying about irrelevant events or concerns.

"There are millions of 'want to's' and 'have to's' in life," he notes. "Ultimately, these pressures create stress only when your time-and-energy spending decisions aren't consistent with your goals, beliefs, and values."

There are many ways to cope with excess stress, and some methods are better than others. Too often people turn to the wrong solutions for stress relief, such as tranquilizers, sleeping pills, alcohol, and cigarettes, and end up further impairing their health while doing nothing to gain an upper hand on the causes of their stress reactions. Others resort to short-term solutions — shouting, crying, taking a hot bath — that help for a while. More lasting, "low-cost" relief could be obtained through regular exercise or talking with friends, Dr. Tubesing says.

How to Cope with Stress

Everyone should have a repertoire of stress-reducing techniques. Here are some that Dr. Tubesing and others have found helpful.

Set priorities. Divide your tasks into three categories — essential, important, and trivial — and forget about the trivial. Hire others, including your own children, to do the tasks that can be farmed out. Learn to say no when you're asked to do something that overloads your time or stress budget or diverts you from what you really consider most important. Be satisfied with a less than perfect job if the alternative is not getting a job done at all. Identify the activities you find satisfying in and of themselves, and focus on enjoying them, rather than on your performance or what rewards the activities might bring.

Organize your time. Identify the time wasters. Figure out when in the day you are most productive, and do your essential and important tasks then. Pace yourself by scheduling your tasks, allowing time for unexpected emergencies. If at all possible, leave your work at the office to reduce conflicts with the demands at home and give yourself time to recharge your batteries.

Budget your stress. The Metropolitan Life Insurance Company recommends taking a periodic glance at your schedule for the next three months to see what events may be coming up that may cause you to overdraw your stress account. Try to avoid clusters of stressful events by spreading them out.

Try "clean living." Be more consistent in your living habits by trying to eat, sleep, and exercise at about the same time every day. Don't overindulge in alcohol or rely on pills to induce sleep (they're counterproductive). Be sure to get enough sleep and rest because fatigue can reduce your ability to cope with stress. Eat regular, well-balanced meals with enough variety to assure good nutrition and enough complex carbohydrates (starchy foods) to guarantee a ready energy reserve. Reverse the typical American meal pattern, and instead, eat like a king for breakfast, a prince for lunch, and a pauper for supper; you'll have more daytime energy and sleep better at night. [See Part I on nutrition, page 1.]

Listen to your body. It will let you know when you are pushing too hard. When your back or head aches or your stomach sours, slow down, have some fun, take time to enjoy the world around you. Set aside some time each day for self-indulgence. Focus on life's little pleasures.

Choose fight or flight. Don't be afraid to express anger (hiding it is even more stressful than letting it out), but choose your fights; don't hassle over every little thing. When fighting is inappropriate, try fleeing — learn to fantasize or take a short break (do a puzzle, take a walk, go to a concert, or away for the weekend) to reenergize yourself. You can also give in once in a while, instead of always insisting you are right and others are wrong.

Learn relaxation techniques. These include deep breathing exercises, transcendental meditation, the relaxation response (a demystified form of meditation formulated by Dr. Herbert Benson, a Harvard cardiologist), religious experiences, yoga, progressive relaxation of muscle groups, imagery, biofeedback, and behavior modification. The last four may require professional help. On a tightly scheduled day, take a minute or two between appointments or activities for a relaxation break — stretching, breathing, walking around.

Revitalize through exercise. A body lacking in physical stamina is in no shape to handle stress. An exercise tune-up can increase your emotional as well as your physical strength. Exercise enhances, rather than saps, your energy; it also has a distinct relaxing effect. [See chapter on the benefits of exercise, page 86.]

Talk it out. Problems often seem much worse when you alone carry their burden. Talking to a trusted friend or relative or to a professional counselor can help you sort things out and unload some of the burden. If things are really bad, don't hesitate to seek professional counseling or psychotherapy.

Get outside yourself. Stress causes people to turn into themselves and focus too much on their own problems. Try doing something for someone else. Or find something other than yourself and your accomplishments to care about. Be more tolerant and forgiving of yourself and others.

Finally, Drs. Robert L. Woolfolk and Frank C. Richardson, psychologists and authors of *Stress, Sanity and Survival* (see "For Further Reading" below), caution against "waiting for the day when 'you can relax' or when 'your problems will be over.' The struggles of life never end. Most good things in life are fleeting and transitory. Enjoy them; savor them. Don't waste time looking forward to the 'happy ending' to all your troubles."

For Further Reading

Benson, Herbert M.D. *The Relaxation Response.* New York: William Morrow, 1975; Avon, 1976.

Carrington, Patricia. *Freedom in Meditation.* New York: Anchor /Doubleday, 1977.

Madders, Jane. *Stress and Relaxation.* New York: Arco, 1979.

McQuade, Walter, and Ann Aikman. *Stress: What It Is, What It Can Do to Your Health, How to Fight Back.* New York: Bantam, 1975.

Norfolk, Donald. *The Stress Factor.* New York: Simon & Schuster, 1977.

Selye, Hans, M.D. *The Stress of Life.* New York: McGraw-Hill, 1956; rev. ed., 1976.

———. *Stress Without Distress.* New York: Lippincott, 1974.

Steinmetz, Jenny; Jon Blankenship; Linda Brown; Deborah Hall; and Grace Miller. *Managing Stress.* Palo Alto, Calif.: Bull, 1980.

Tubesing, Donald A. *Kicking Your Stress Habits.* Duluth: Whole Person Associates, 1981. Available for $10 plus $1 for postage and handling from Whole Person Associates, Inc., P.O. Box 3151, Duluth, Minn. 55803.

Woolfolk, Robert L., and Frank G. Richardson. *Stress, Sanity and Survival.* New York: Sovereign Books (Simon & Schuster), 1978.

Type A Behavior:
Don't Rush Your Life Away

The man who got on the elevator was obviously impatient and tense. One hand was clenched in a fist; the other held two packs of cigarettes. He pushed the button for his floor not once, not twice, but six times. Then he spotted another elevator across the hall and dashed out just as the doors closed on the one he had been on.

Watching him, I couldn't help thinking he was a sitting duck for a heart attack. In one minute's time he clearly showed that he was what cardiologists call a Type A personality, suffering from "hurry sickness."

Then I remembered what I had been like just five years ago — worried about every wasted moment, anxious about every missed train or bus, hostile in every traffic jam, unable to wait in any line. I must have said, "hurry up," to my young sons at least a dozen times a day. I pushed ahead of people without even seeing them. I would start sprinting when I came within a block of the subway station, earning me the nickname Roadrunner from my husband. I regarded busy signals, overly protective secretaries, and slow-moving salespeople as deliberate obstacles to my attempts to get more and more done in less and less time.

Then one day I realized I was rushing my life away. While preparing an article on stress and heart disease, I read a book called *Type A Behavior and Your Heart* (see "For Further Reading," page 146) by Drs. Ray H. Rosenman and Meyer Friedman, two San Francisco cardiologists. I saw myself coming and going in the descriptions of the heart attack-prone person: hurried, aggressive, controlling, impatient, and easily angered. Though then a thirty-five-year-old female not worried about heart disease, I didn't like what I saw. My easily provoked tension and anxiety could not have made me fun to be around. Nor did they make life pleasant for me.

I vowed to make some changes, taking one stressful situation at a time and finding alternative ways to handle it. Once I became aware of the problem, I found that recognizing the trouble spots and making the changes were easier than I had expected. Though there have been numerous lapses back to my more frantic self, I continue to progress toward being a more relaxed person. I may be doing fewer things, but I certainly am enjoying everything I do a lot more. Oddly enough, no one seems to have noticed a decline in my productivity perhaps because most of what I cut out of my life was time-consuming trivia.

Probably no Type A person would be able to — or would even *want* to — convert completely to being a more contemplative, laid back Type B personality. However, most who can recognize the extent of their Type A-ness would agree that many of their typical behavior patterns are counterproductive as well as personally and socially undesirable.

How to Change Your Approach

Changing Type A behavior is probably best done in a group setting with a trained counselor. However, few such groups currently exist (and most involve organized studies of persons who have already suffered heart attacks), and many useful changes can be made on your own. The following tips are derived from ongoing programs that attempt to reform Type As: from the Rosenman-Friedman book, and from my own experience.

Start out by taking stock of your life's goals, how you spend your

143

time, and what is really important to you. Concentrate on what is worth being, rather than on what is worth having.

• Stop measuring your life in quantities, such as number of clients or patients, number of committees on which you serve, number of accomplishments. Begin to think more in terms of quality. Then rid yourself of trivial obligations, be they committee memberships or household duties, that serve your vanity rather than your economic or spiritual well-being. You'll probably find that doing a few things really well is more ego-enhancing — and more likely to be noticed by others — than doing a lot of things less effectively.

• Give up trying to be a superwoman who, despite a demanding career, insists on being Superwife and Supermom, retaining control of everything at home, entertaining lavishly, participating in community affairs, and rearing children. This can be done only at the expense of your health, your marriage, and your relationship with your children. Forget perfection. At home and at work decide what it is you and you alone must do and delegate the other responsibilities. Wherever feasible, pay someone to relieve you of time-consuming chores.

• Spend some time alone with yourself. Sit quietly and contemplate the sky or stare blankly out the window instead of constantly scurrying about "doing things."

• Cultivate your spiritual side. Set aside time to attend a concert or play, visit a museum, read a difficult book. Once or twice a week, walk through the park at lunch instead of dining at your desk or over a business deal. Become really good friends with someone, instead of just having a string of casual acquaintances.

Curing Hurry Sickness

The sense of time urgency is probably the most common of the Type A characteristics and also the one most easily modified. If you've already shed your life of unessential activities, you'll have an easier time fitting in the essentials with minimal stress.

• Leave yourself more time than you'll think you need to get somewhere or accomplish something. Then, if something should delay or interrupt you, you'll have less reason to become anxious. Even if it looks as if you will be late, reassure yourself that worse things can happen — for example, you might not have gotten there at all.

• Take something to read or do whenever you might have to wait around or stand in line.

• Another approach is to practice standing in lines doing nothing. Study the people around you. Fantasize. Think about someone you love. Think about your life. Or wait with your spouse or a friend and have a pleasant conversation.

• Try allowing people to get ahead of you in line, or give other drivers the right-of-way. You may soon learn that no disaster ensues, and through your more relaxed attitude, you end up earning back the time you give up and then some.

● Don't clutter up your calendar with appointments that even Superman couldn't meet. Don't hesitate to break an appointment when more urgent matters get you in a bind. Wherever possible, don't create unnecessary deadlines by making appointments for a narrowly specific time. Say, "I'll be there between 11 and 11:30," rather than "precisely at 11."

● Leave your watch at home for a week, or if you can't quite do that, put it in a pocket or under your sleeve so that you can't easily glance at it many times a day.

● Instead of rising just in time to dress, eat breakfast, and catch a train, get up fifteen minutes earlier in the morning so you won't have to start your day in such a rush. Your body will appreciate the calm much more than the extra sleep.

● Sort your mail each morning into three piles: that which must be done immediately, that which can wait awhile, and that which can be filed or discarded. Take care of the "immediate" pile, and clear the rest from your desk, so you're not constantly reminded of how behind you are. Don't waste your time with mail that someone else can handle for you.

● Instruct your secretary, if you have one, and colleagues not to interrupt with trivial matters and phone calls that are not urgent. Have them take messages and then treat the messages as you do your mail. Let a subordinate or colleague handle matters that don't absolutely demand your attention.

● Stop interrupting the conversations of others or finishing their sentences for them. Practice being a good listener; concentrate on what is being said instead of thinking of something else at the same time.

● Don't take over from someone who is doing a job slowly, unless he or she cannot do it at all. Walk away if you can't stand to watch.

● Even when working against a deadline, take a break periodically to walk about, chat with a neighbor, stare out the window — anything that will help to relieve the tension.

Conquering Hostility

The Type A characteristic of having a short fuse seems to be most closely associated with heart attack risk. It also makes you an unpleasant person to be around. Think about what situations seem designed to upset or annoy you, and try calling upon your intellect and sense of humor to get you through.

● Don't waste your anger on trivial matters, most of which you can do nothing about anyhow, such as a delayed train or plane, an inept waiter, or an abrupt salesperson.

● Avoid contact with people who always raise your hackles. They are probably also Type As who are constantly competing with you. As for those, such as family members, whom you must continue to see, let them do most of the talking, and don't take them so seriously.

● Stop focusing on your "ideals" and how many people fall short of them. This only fosters disappointment in and hostility toward others.

● Go out of your way to do something nice for someone each day. It can be as simple as stopping to give directions, holding a door, or carrying a heavy package. Smile at people — even strangers — as often as you can.

● Make friends with a Type B person, who may not say much but listens well and can serve as a model of more relaxed behavior.

For Further Reading

Friedman, Meyer, M.D., and Ray H. Rosenman, M.D. *Type A Behavior and Your Heart.* New York: Fawcett, 1976.

Depression: Breaking the Bonds of Sadness

146

The feeling is familiar to most everyone: nothing seems satisfying, things don't work out, you can't get yourself to do much of anything, and your mental landscape is bleak. It's called depression, and few of us get through life without experiencing it at one time or another.

Many things can get a person "down," including the weather (midwinter doldrums are an annual event for some), the letdown after the excitement and activity of the holidays [see chapter on holiday blues, page 166], insufficient sleep, too much work and too little time in which to get it done. The ordinary everyday blues are usually brief and self-curing and, although they take the edge off life, are not terribly incapacitating.

However, for millions of Americans, depression is a far more serious, sometimes even life-threatening situation. Most serious depressions are reactions to stressful life events: loss of a job or a spouse, serious financial setback, a serious illness or injury, the end of a love affair. After a reasonable number of weeks or months, most such depressions usually lift, and the world and life begin to seem brighter.

But for some people, depression is a recurring phenomenon that is provoked by events that others seem to weather with little difficulty or get over very quickly. For others, depression happens "out of the blue," unrelated to any particular situation, and totally incapacitates them. Many accomplished people — including Sigmund Freud, Abraham Lincoln, Nathaniel Hawthorne, Winston Churchill, and the astronaut Edwin E. Aldrin — have suffered from severe depression. The National Institute of Mental Health estimates that each year between 4 and 8 million

Americans suffer depressions severe enough to keep them from performing their regular activities or compelling them to seek medical help. Perhaps 10 to 15 million others have less severe depressions that interfere to some extent with the performance of normal activities. All told, depression is the nation's number one mental health problem.

Some experts say the social tensions of the times — the erosion of trust, diminished personal impact, unrealistically high expectations of success, disintegration of the family, social isolation, and loss of a sense of belonging to or believing in some stable, larger-than-self institution — foster a society especially prone to depression.

How to Recognize Depression

Recognizing depression, should it strike you or someone you know, can sometimes be very difficult. In its classic, undisguised form, depression has three main characteristics:

● Emotional: a dull, tired, empty, sad, numb feeling with little or no pleasure from ordinarily enjoyable activities and people.

● Behavioral: irritability, excessive complaining about small annoyances or minor problems, impaired memory, inability to concentrate, difficulty making decisions, loss of sexual desire, inability to get going in the morning, slowed reaction time, crying or screaming, and excessive guilt feeling.

● Physical: loss of appetite, weight loss, constipation, insomnia or restless sleep, impotence, headache, dizziness, indigestion, and abnormal heart rate.

Often the symptoms of depression are masked, disguised in a form that makes recognition by the depressed person, the person's family, friends, and even physician difficult. "The exhausted housewife, the bored adolescent, and the occupational underachiever are often suffering from depression just as truly as the acutely suicidal patient or the one who refuses to get out of bed," according to Dr. Nathan Kline, a New York psychiatrist. Depression in children is usually masked, presenting symptoms like restlessness, sleep problems, lack of attention and initiative. [See chapter on depression in children, page 149.]

Patients with disguised depression may complain of headache, backache, or pains elsewhere in the musculoskeletal system. They may have a gastrointestinal disorder, such as chronic diarrhea, a "lump" in the throat, chest pain, or a toothache. Or their depression may be disguised as sexual promiscuity, overeating, excessive drinking, or various phobias.

In addition to stressful events that cause depression (called reactive or exogenous depression), and unknown internal, probably biochemical causes (called endogenous depression), depression can result from organic diseases, including viral and bacterial infections, such as hepatitis, influenza, mononucleosis, and tuberculosis; hormonal disorders, such as

147

diabetes and thyroid disease; and such conditions as arthritis, nutritional deficiencies, anemia, and cancer.

Certain drugs — including alcohol, barbiturates, estrogens and progesterone, digitalis, cortisone, some blood pressure medications, and amphetamines — may produce depression as a side effect. Serious depression can also follow childbirth, the completion of an exhilarating creative effort, or the loneliness and increasing disability of old age.

The struggle against depression can lead some people to seek relief through excessive drinking (which simply aggravates the problem since alcohol is a central nervous system depressant), marital infidelity, gambling, or compulsive overwork.

Treating Depression

Experts estimate that only one in ten people suffering from depression who could benefit from treatment actually receive it. Many people, Dr. Kline says, don't realize that depression is treatable. Others don't recognize or acknowledge their depression. Still others consider themselves too worthless to warrant treatment.

Mild, self-limited depressions can often be managed effectively without professional help. Doctors advise such "techniques" as compensating yourself with a special treat, keeping busy, keeping congenial company, trying a change of scene or pace, helping others with their problems, or doing difficult but satisfying work. Exercise that uses the long muscles, such as sawing or chopping wood, running, bicycling, or playing tennis, is also helpful.

Family and friends can help by showing a reasonable amount of interest and concern. Be willing to listen, but don't "bug" depressed people by telling them to "snap out of it" (if they could, they most certainly would, and this kind of remark merely intensifies their guilt). Try to keep them busy and active, and avoid arguments or recriminating remarks.

If the degree or length of the depression is inappropriate to its cause, if suicidal thoughts have been expressed, or if depressive symptoms last longer than a month, medical attention is warranted. Simplistic measures by patients and their families rarely work against severe depression. However, a number of drugs can be prescribed by a physician to relieve serious depression and the anxiety that often accompanies it. Drug treatment may take three weeks or more to begin to work, and the patient should be told what side effects to anticipate.

Psychotherapy and psychoanalysis are not considered the most effective treatments for depression, although they may be used to help the patient change life patterns that precipitate recurrent depressions. Sometimes behavior therapy and other modern psychiatric techniques are able to reverse a severe depression rather quickly. For patients who are suicidally depressed or for whom other treatments fail, electroconvulsive (shock) therapy may be used. Mild depressions can usually be treated well by the family physician, but more serious and chronic cases are best referred to a psychiatrist. [See chapter on choosing a psychotherapist, page 129.]

For Further Reading

DeRosis, Helen A., M.D., and Victoria Y. Pellegrino. *The Book of Hope.* New York: Bantam, 1977.

Kiev, Ari, M.D. *The Courage to Live.* New York: Crowell, 1979; Bantam, 1982.

————. *Recovery from Depression.* New York: E.P. Dutton, 1982.

Kline, Nathan S., M.D. *From Sad to Glad: Kline on Depression.* New York: Putnam, 1974.

Sturgeon, Wina. *Conquering Depression.* New York: Cornerstone Library, 1981.

Weiss, Carl, and Ray Weiss. *How to End Mental Depression.* New York: Arco, 1978.

Depression in Children:
Never Too Young to Be Sad

Depression, an emotional disturbance well known to adults, is just now being recognized as the cause of a wide range of developmental and behavioral problems in children as young as three months. The masks of childhood depression are varied and often misleading and differ with the age and circumstances of the child. Too often they are not recognized for what they really are, and the child receives no treatment or the wrong treatment.

Example: Maria was nine months old but the size of an infant half her age. She rarely smiled, paid little attention to her surroundings, slept a lot, and ate poorly. When approached by a stranger, she lowered her face, covered her eyes with her hands, and tightened her lips.

Example: Doris, twelve, was also depressed, though it was hard to see that through her devil-may-care, effervescent behavior. She was wild and rebellious and forever hurting herself accidentally. When she began to calm down through treatment, her underlying depression became more obvious.

Example: Bill, depressed at age four, was a constant problem in his nursery school class. When he wasn't bullying smaller and younger children, he was off in a corner by himself, refusing to participate in any activities.

A child whose underlying problems with depression are not resolved often grows up to be an adult with similar problems. Sometimes a child's depression takes a devastating turn, culminating in suicide attempts. Although often unrecognized as such and poorly reported, suicides among youngsters have been surging in recent years. Children as young as six have succeeded in taking their own lives, although such youthful suicides are frequently recorded as accidents. The precipitating circumstances of youthful suicides may seem trivial to adults, but to the

149

child whose experience in life is limited, they may seem to make life worthless or hopeless.

Recognizing the Depressed Child

To prevent such tragedies, it is essential to recognize the signs of depression in children. Depressed infants may be withdrawn and apathetic and fail to gain weight normally. Preschoolers may have trouble separating from their parents, appear hyperactive, and show learning disabilities. In the elementary grades depressed children commonly complain about a host of physical and emotional hurts. They tend to be self-deprecating and overly sensitive and have trouble forming relationships with their peers. They may become the class clowns or daydream in school, appear lazy and uncooperative, fail to realize their scholastic potential, or refuse to go to school at all. Some have difficulty getting up in the morning and plead to stay home from school; at night they may become obstinate and impudent and resist going to bed.

Adolescents may show more classic signs of depression, such as loss of appetite or sudden overeating, sleep disturbances, neglect of schoolwork and personal appearance, extreme uncommunicativeness, and avoidance of social interactions. Or, as with younger children, their depression may be masked, for example, as extreme hostility and aggressiveness, serious risk taking, or promiscuous sexual behavior. Some have hallucinations or obsessions about death, guilt, hopelessness, failure, humiliation, or worthlessness.

The masks of adolescent depression are often merely exaggerated forms of the "odd" behaviors that are typical of normal adolescent turmoil [see chapter on the normal adolescent, page 151], but experts emphasize that they should be taken seriously, especially if the child has mentioned a wish to die or has made a suicide attempt, however half-hearted it may have been. Three out of four successful suicides by adolescents have been preceded by suicide attempts or threats.

Researchers at the University of Nebraska Medical Center and Creighton University School of Medicine have discovered that many so-called accidental poisonings among children and adolescents are actually suicide attempts. Dr. Matilda McIntire and Dr. Carol Angle, who studied 1,103 self-poisonings among children, report that each year there are 100,000 cases of intentional self-poisonings among children five to fourteen, five times more than the number of meningitis cases that occur in that age-group. Although usually not successful in killing themselves, these children are definitely crying for help, the researchers say.

Causes and Treatment

A major cause of childhood depression, experts believe, is the lack in infancy of a secure relationship with the parent or parent substitute. Many mothers of depressed children are themselves prone to depression.

150

Even if they can meet the physical demands of child care, they may still be absent emotionally. Without a responsive, helpful person to help the child become self-reliant, he or she may fail to learn how to deal with alarming situations or to seek help without hesitation, anguish, or humiliation, says Dr. Irving Philips, director of child and adolescent psychiatry at the University of California Medical Center in San Francisco.

Instead of helping to build a secure personality, the emotionally disturbed parent may shame the child or threaten abandonment. Other factors that can precipitate childhood depression include loss of parental support through separation, divorce, or death; birth of a "rival" sibling who "steals" parental love and attention; lack of affection and cooperation between the parents; excessive expectations by the parents of their children; failures in school; and disappointments in adolescent love relationships.

The treatment of depression in children is a matter of much debate and nearly always requires some form of psychotherapy by a specialist. Some doctors prefer to try mild antidepressant medications for several weeks, particularly if the child is very depressed or has expressed suicidal wishes. Other physicians prefer not to use drugs except as a last resort, noting that children often do not have the same responses to psychoactive drugs that adults do. Thus, an antidepressant medication may make a child more, rather than less, depressed. In either case, if the depression does not lift in a few weeks, psychotherapy and often family therapy are necessary. A child who is actively suicidal may require temporary hospitalization. In some cases foster care is the only solution to a difficult and unresolvable parental problem.

For Further Reading

MacKenzie, Dr. Richard. *Coping with Teenage Depression.* New York: New American Library, 1982.

The "Normal" Adolescent: How to Cope

Margie had never been a very talkative child, but as she entered adolescence, she became practically speechless, at least at home. Days would go by during which she said only two or three short sentences to her mother and not much more to her father. Except for meals and piano practice, she spent nearly all her time at home alone in her room, slamming the door each time she entered it.

For about two years her achievements in school fell short of her ability. She seemed uninterested and disorganized, just managing to get from day to day.

"I thought she was terribly unhappy, and I felt so helpless because she wouldn't share her problems," her mother recalls. "I viewed her refusal to talk to me as a sign of hostility — though now I realize it wasn't — and when we finally did talk on occasion, there was usually hurt, anger, and hostility in my replies."

Now, at sixteen, Margie is beginning to open up. She seems happier with herself, and her schoolwork has improved greatly in the last six months. Though there are still some one-sided conversations with her mother, she seems more accepting of parental comment and now apologizes when she accidentally slams her bedroom door.

What's Normal?

Margie is a normal adolescent, going through the normal pangs of growing up — learning to know, like, and trust herself; seeking her own directions; adjusting to the rapid changes in her body and psyche. Though for many, and perhaps most, teenagers the transition to adulthood is less agonizing than it appears to be for Margie, it is rarely smooth sailing for either child or parent. A teenager may be warm and loving one minute, hostile and rejecting the next, flexible and cooperative today, obstinate and self-centered tomorrow.

Deliberate baiting and temperamental outbursts of "you don't understand me," "you don't understand anything," "get off my back," even "I hate you" are common during this often volatile stage of life. Teenagers can tax the most tolerant and patient of parents. Making it all the more difficult is the fact that most adults have little or no recollection of their own behavior and feelings as adolescents and are likely to be shocked, angered, and hurt by their youngsters' attitudes and actions. This reaction may be compounded by guilt among parents who think they ought to be "more competent and comprehending," note Dr. Barry Lauton and Arthur Freese, in their illuminating book *The Healthy Adolescent: A Parents' Manual* (see "For Further Reading," page 155).

In fact, however, teenagers who are perennially amenable, who accept parental direction and dominance, and totally lack signs of rebellion and inner turmoil are often cause for worry since they may not be taking the necessary steps toward becoming independent adults. Parents who understand and appreciate the parameters of normal adolescence will be better able to cope with their own teenaged children and to recognize which children may need outside help.

This doesn't mean, of course, that it is normal to be *abnormal* as an adolescent. In a questionnaire survey of 1,300 "normal" teenagers by a Chicago research team, 85 percent said they were happy most of the time. The majority harbored no bad feelings toward their parents and generally believed their parents were satisfied with them. Seventy percent said they liked the changes in their bodies. Participants in the survey were physically and psychologically healthy high school students.

Trials and Tribulations of the Teen Years

Still, one in five reported "feeling empty emotionally, being confused most of the time, or hearing strange noises." Anxiety was a common — though rarely chronic — emotion, usually precipitated by a specific event or situation. Girls were more likely to report feeling lonely, sad, confused, and ashamed than were the boys surveyed. More than 40 percent of the girls said they often felt ugly and unattractive.

During adolescence, which commonly starts between the ages of ten and twelve, a youngster must establish an identity separate from his or her parents, relinquish childhood dependencies, adopt a personal value system, establish goals, learn social responsibility, and how to deal maturely with authority. All this is going on at a time of rapid physical changes and emotional shifts that may challenge a teenager's self-image and self-esteem. Adolescence is a time of rejection of parental standards in favor of those of the youngster's peers, whose manner of dress, taste in music, and choice of activities and friends may be abhorrent to parents.

How to Live with Your Teenage Child

By the way they respond, parents may either help or hinder their children's passage through this transitional period. Even when they can do little or nothing to influence the child's behavior, parents may be able to ease their own way over the rough spots of their youngster's adolescence. Here are some tips offered by Dr. Lauton and other experts on adolescent development.

Be loving. Also compassionate and understanding. No matter how outrageous teenage behavior may be, repeated reassurance of parental love is important to the child's sense of security and self-esteem. Often adolescents test their parents' love, consciously or otherwise. Don't fail the test. You may withhold approval, but not love.

Keep communications open. Even though Margie rarely said anything, her mother made certain she knew she could talk over problems anytime she wanted. When there was something important to get across to Margie, her parents said their piece, even though the reply was just a grunt. Being willing to communicate is an important antidote to adolescent isolation. But Dr. Stuart Alan Copans, a child psychiatrist at the Dartmouth Medical School, warns in *The Parents' Guide to Teenagers* (see "For Further Reading," page 155), don't insist on intimacy. If your adolescent child won't talk to you, perhaps you can help him or her find another adult — teacher, coach, aunt, uncle, etc. — with whom to discuss personal matters.

Assure privacy. "Teenagers want and need privacy," write Dr. Lauton and Mr. Freese. "It's important for them to have their own rooms and possessions, their own private thoughts, their mail, phone calls, and diaries untouched by others. Intrusions incite anger, insults, and complaints." Always knock before entering an adolescent's room (or anyone's, for that matter), and don't enter if you're not invited in.

Set limits. Every child needs and deserves parental control. If parents are too liberal, the child will be insecure. Firm discipline is an essential foundation for developing one's own inner controls. A teenager should know exactly what his or her parents expect — for example, curfews on weekdays and weekends, sharing meals with the family, the performance of certain household chores — as long as the demands are reasonable and negotiable to fit in with the child's schedule and quest for independence. If parents are too strict, it merely incites rebellion.

Take adolescent problems seriously. The matter (a bad haircut, a poor grade, no date for a party) may seem trivial or transient to you, but it can be very disruptive to an adolescent with a shaky self-image. Listen carefully, don't argue, and don't belittle. Show respect for adolescent thoughts and feelings. Be sympathetic and understanding, and, if possible, offer constructive advice or alternatives. But don't expect your advice to be followed.

Keep your sense of humor. Always remember that "this too shall pass." Most adolescents emerge from this phase of life unscathed and with renewed respect for the people who reared them. If you're having trouble "keeping your cool" about your teenaged children, you might

HOW TO RECOGNIZE A TEENAGER IN TROUBLE

Since so much of adolescent behavior seems bizarre to adults, it's sometimes hard to recognize when a teenager is really in trouble and in need of outside help. These are some of the signs:

● Schoolwork takes a nosedive from previous levels of achievement and no longer approaches what you believe to be the child's ability.

● The turmoil at home is constant, with frequent explosive fights between parent and child or smoldering anger that lasts for days.

● The teenager has difficulty making friends and seems to be increasingly isolated.

● The teenager is experiencing prolonged boredom, particularly if it is associated with a lack of extracurricular activities or a lack of direction, interests, or goals.

● The teenager engages in serious antisocial or self-destructive behavior, such as repeated accidents, drug abuse, sexual promiscuity, suicide threats or attempts, stealing, destroying property.

● There are numerous physical complaints, such as headaches, stomachaches, intestinal disorders, sleep disturbances, ulcers, and loss of appetite, or more direct signs of emotional disturbance, such as chronic anxiety, depression, and tension.

Given the opportunity, one in five teenagers seeks psychological help. It is important, however, that the therapist be attuned to adolescent emotional problems and able to establish a good rapport with the youngster. Sometimes family therapy is recommended. The school guidance counselor or psychologist may be able to recommend a therapist, or you might contact the local medical society, health department, or psychiatry department at a nearby medical school for a referral to a specialist (psychiatrist or psychologist) in adolescent psychotherapy.

pick up a copy of Carol Eisen Rinzler's perceptive and amusing guide *Your Adolescent: An Owner's Manual* (see "For Further Reading" below). Dr. Harvey A. Rosenstock, a Houston psychiatrist, suggests ending arguments with teenagers by deliberately introducing a non sequitur, which is irrelevant and unanswerable and usually provokes a smile. For example, when you've reached an impasse, suddenly say, "What do you think of the government of Australia?"

For Further Reading

Ginott, Haim G. *Between Parent and Teenager.* New York: Avon, 1973.
Gross, Leonard, ed. *The Parents' Guide to Teenagers.* New York: Macmillan, 1981.
Lauton, Barry, M.D., and Arthur Freese. *The Healthy Adolescent: A Parents' Manual.* New York: Scribners, 1981.
Rinzler, Carol Eisen. *Your Adolescent: An Owner's Manual.* New York: Atheneum, 1981.

Anxiety:
It Assumes Many Guises

Example: Jean's husband was about to be promoted and relocated, good news to both of them. But Jean was not feeling well and was having trouble sleeping. She was easily upset and jittery and worried about her persistent abdominal cramps.

Example: Although Robert's office is on the seventh floor, he always takes the stairs. He tells people it's good exercise, but in fact, even if he had to walk thirty two flights, he wouldn't take an elevator. The mere thought of being in an elevator sends him into a small panic. His heart races, his breathing quickens, and he feels faint.

Millions of Americans experience the symptoms of anxiety. Virtually everyone has them at one time or another. Anxiety is not a disease, but rather a state of feeling. It is a signal that something is not quite right, a kind of vague, unfocused fear, a sense of uneasiness.

There are many symptoms of anxiety, and they often masquerade as genuine physical ailments. Among them are rapid or pounding heartbeat, difficulty in breathing or breathlessness, tremulousness, sweating, dry mouth, tightness in the chest, sweaty palms, dizziness, weakness, nausea, diarrhea, cramps, insomnia, fatigue, tension headache, loss of appetite, and sexual disturbances.

Most feelings of anxiety require no specific treatment. An explanation of the probable cause of the feelings may be all that is needed to dissolve them or make them more bearable. Unfortunately many people and their physicians instead reach for Valium or some other tranquilizer for relief of mild anxiety. In fact, it's usually better not to mask mild anxiety, but rather to treat it as a signal of the need to uncover what may be really bothering you.

As Dr. Willard Gaylin, a New York psychotherapist, points out in his book *Feelings: Our Vital Signs* (New York: Harper & Row, 1979), anxiety frequently serves useful purposes. Anxiety about a forthcoming exam gets students to study hard. The anxiety generated by an impending deadline will often put an end to writer's block. Anxiety can alert us to an impending disaster or to the need for change and adaptation.

Anxiety is closely related to fear, but while the cause of fear is usually apparent, the circumstance that precipitates anxiety is hidden and unknown to the person. When the cause of anxiety becomes known but the feeling of apprehension remains, it is called worry.

Causes and Expressions of Anxiety

We live at a time when so little is stable and the future is so unpredictable that anxiety in one form or another has become a part of everyday life. Many call this the Age of Anxiety. We all have ample opportunity to experience in many forms again and again what psychoanalysts call separation anxiety and castration anxiety.

Separation anxiety is normal for growing children, who depend on their parents for security and love but who periodically must part from these comforts and eventually must leave them forever. Separation anxiety has its counterparts in adult life, appearing in the guise of a need for approval and acceptance. When we feel rejected, criticized, unloved, or unworthy, we become anxious and insecure.

Castration anxiety is related to competitiveness, strength, and power, our basic ability to "make it." When these are threatened, such as through loss of a job, looks, money, or social position, anxiety results.

Sometimes anxiety has an organic basis, such as anxiety attacks precipitated by excessive drinking of caffeinated beverages (coffee and tea) or the abuse of other stimulant drugs.

Although they usually don't realize it, most people have found ways to alleviate anxious feelings. Among those that Dr. Gaylin delineates are spending money (proving yourself both potent, i.e., solvent, and lovable, i.e., worthy of a gift, albeit from yourself); stuffing something into your mouth, such as food, drugs, or cigarettes (forms of self-reward and reassurance); seeking sexual gratification, either with a partner or by yourself (again, proving your worth and lovability); and performing trivial but useful tasks such as polishing the car, shining shoes, straightening bookshelves, and scrubbing floors to induce relaxation and produce a sense of accomplishment. Practically everyone has built up one or more defenses against anxiety, and there is nothing wrong with that so long as they don't have destructive effects on one's life.

Sometimes, however, the degree of anxiety or the method chosen, however subconsciously, to relieve it takes on unhealthy characteristics. People may attempt to drown their anxious feelings in alcohol or obliterate them with drugs or excessive sleep. Others immerse themselves in work.

Rather than live with a vague, undefined dread, some people assign a cause to it, whether true or not. They replace unstructured anxiety with a seemingly rational fear, such as a fear of flying in airplanes, which, after all, do sometimes crash and kill people. Carried to an extreme, such fears become life-limiting phobias. [See chapter on phobias, page 158.] As Dr. Gaylin explains, a person who is afraid of elevators is rarely actually worried about the elevator's breaking down. Rather, he or she has displaced a less avoidable terror, such as a fear of interacting with people, with a more controllable activity.

Other times a person may resolve anxious discomfort by creating a delusion that would appear to justify it. For example, rather than live with an irrational fear, an anxious man may decide that his colleagues are trying to sabotage his work and that's why he feels so anxious.

Like Jean, some anxious people fail to recognize their feelings for what they really are because they are subconsciously converted into physical symptoms. These people may be ashamed of their emotional problem, but physiological distress is easier for them to accept and express. The result may be gastrointestinal disorders, such as chronic diarrhea, with no discernible organic cause, or "anxiety heart attacks" which mimic all the signs of a real heart attack but don't involve any heart damage at all. Such persons may go from doctor to doctor with their complaints and have many tests over and over, seeking a physical explanation for their ill health.

Sometimes it is not how the anxiety is expressed but rather the degree of anxiety that makes it pathological. Some people are chronic worriers, fretting constantly over trivial problems and things that are unlikely to become problems. Since they are anxious much of the time, they get little pleasure from life and give little joy to others, who must constantly offer them reassurance.

An anxiety reaction can sometimes border on or actually become panic. The person may become frantic or immobilized by his overwhelming diffuse fears. Anxiety heart attack is one form of an acute panic reaction.

How to Treat It
Treatment of anxiety depends on its degree, its cause, and the nature of its expression. Simply telling an anxious person with physical symptoms that there is nothing organically wrong with him or her may provide temporary reassurance, but it will not alleviate the underlying anxiety. Similarly, trying to talk someone out of a severe anxiety reaction, such as a fear of heights, does little good because the fear is based on something irrational or subconscious to begin with.

For severe symptoms, tranquilizers may be prescribed while psychotherapy is undertaken. Transient anxiety precipitated by a particular crisis may respond best to talking through the problem, with a tranquilizer prescribed for a brief period only if the symptoms are severe. Phobias can often be treated effectively by behavior therapy using relaxing techniques, among others, but sometimes there is a risk that the anxiety reaction will reemerge in a different form.

Phobias: When Fears Dominate Life

Sheila, a social worker, was afraid of rats. Actually she was more than just afraid. She was positively phobic. Her heart would race, her legs would turn to rubber, she would break out into a profuse sweat and become paralyzed with fear if she even thought she might encounter a rat. As a result of her phobia, Sheila had to change jobs. She stopped visiting friends in the country. She would not take the subway. After reading in the newspaper that rat droppings were found in some restaurant kitchens, she refused to eat out. She was even afraid to open the kitchen cabinets unless her roommate first checked to be sure they harbored no rats.

Sheila's problem, described in *Phobia Free* (see "For Further Reading," page 160), is shared by an estimated 20 million Americans who suffer from one or another phobia. Like Sheila's, the lives of about half a million phobiacs are severely disrupted by their crippling fears. Until recently the few who sought professional help were usually disappointed. After costly psychotherapy or analysis seeking to determine the origin of the phobia, the panic attacks were often worse than ever.

When Fear Becomes Phobia

Everybody has fears, some more rational than others. Fear has survival value, triggering a fight-or-flight reflex when your well-being is threatened. But fear can also occur out of proportion to the reality of a threat, or it can occur in response to an imagined threat.

A phobia is a severe, disabling fear disproportionate to the object or circumstance that evokes it. It is an involuntary reaction that cannot be explained away, and it prompts the individual to avoid the feared object or situation and anything that may be associated with it. Before long the phobiac begins to fear the *possibility* of a panic attack as much as the provoking stimulus itself and may go to ever greater lengths to avoid a phobic response. Many phobiacs are most afraid of losing control, fainting, or doing something ridiculous or extremely embarrassing when confronted by the stimulus of their phobia.

Although phobic individuals may seem to others to be mentally deranged and may themselves think they are going crazy, recent studies and treatment programs have demonstrated that phobias are rarely anything more complicated than an inappropriate conditioned response. In other words, a phobia is a form of learned behavior, just as you might learn to to be afraid when the phone rings unexpectedly in the middle of the night after you have previously had an upsetting call at a similar hour.

However, according to James Ascough, psychologist at Purdue University, certain anxiety-prone people seem more susceptible to developing phobias than others. "These were individuals who pushed for achievement — often perfectionists who were extremely neat, well-groomed, and hyperresponsible," Dr. Ascough says.

People can have highly specific phobias, such as those involving airplanes, freeways, dogs, or spiders, or their phobias may be more generalized, such as a fear of heights; small, enclosed places; or large, open, unfamiliar places. Phobias usually start suddenly, with an unexpected panic attack that may then be repeated when the same or a similar circumstance arises again. Often a particular anxiety-provoking event starts the phobia, but in other cases no such direct cause can be found.

The disruption a phobia causes depends in part on how easy it is to avoid the subject of the phobia. A person phobic about elevators is not likely to have much trouble on a farm in Kansas but would encounter frequent triggers of the phobic response while living in New York City.

159

Another factor in measuring the severity of a phobia is how broadly the fear has been generalized. For example, in Sheila's case it would have been easy to avoid encountering a rat, although she might indeed have had to change jobs. But Sheila extended her phobia by finding reasons to think rats might be almost anywhere. For someone with a diffuse problem like agoraphobia (literally "fear of the marketplace"), anything outside the safety of home may set off a panic attack.

Finally, there is the severity of the actual phobic response, which can range from mild anxiety, damp palms, and increased heart rate to overwhelming feelings of suffocation and impending death.

New Treatments

A growing number of behavior therapists and phobia clinics are taking a new and seemingly paradoxical approach to curing phobias: exposing the victim to the very cause of the panic and waiting it out until the anxiety subsides. Sometimes deep relaxation or antidepressant drugs are used initially to help the individual control the phobic response. Group therapy with other current and former phobiacs is often part of the treatment program.

With such treatment, called desensitization, flooding, or exposure therapy, even people who have spent years virtually confined to their homes by their phobia can be cured, often within a few weeks or months.

Some experts believe phobiacs can cure themselves, with the aid of a nonprofessional helper. Drs. E. Ann Sutherland and Zalman Amit, recognizing that there aren't enough therapists and clinics to treat all who need help, outline specific programs for self-treatment in their book (see "For Further Reading and Information" below).

But no matter how severe the symptoms, therapists have found, the treatment can work if the person really wants to conquer the problem. At Western Psychiatric Institute in Pittsburgh, a twelve-week program produces significant improvement or cure in about three-fourths of patients with agoraphobia, the most common phobic condition for which therapy is sought. The institute is now following up patients to see how long-lasting the results are.

Dr. Manuel Zane, who heads the Phobia Clinic at White Plains Hospital in New York, has achieved 90 percent success in selected patients who undergo systematic desensitization, in which they are exposed in gradual doses to their phobic stimulus and learn to overcome their panic through confrontation. In such therapy, a person with a fear of rats might start by imagining rats, then progress to looking at pictures of rats, seeing an actual rat, and finally perhaps touching a rat. In each case the exposure lasts until all feelings of panic subside.

For Further Reading and Information

For additional information about treating phobias, contact the psychology department of the nearest university, the local health department, or the community mental health center, or write to the American Psychiatric Association, 1700 Eighteenth Street NW, Washington, D.C. 20009, or the American Psychological Association, 1200 Seventeenth Street NW, Washington, D.C. 20036.

The following reading matter may prove helpful:

Kent, Fraser. *Nothing to Fear.* New York: Doubleday, 1977.

Milt, Harry. "Phobias: The Ailments and Their Treatment." Public Affairs Pamphlet No. 590, 1980. Available for 50 cents from Public Affairs Pamphlets, 381 Park Avenue South, New York, N.Y. 10016.

Sutherland, E. Ann., Ph.D., and Zalman Amit, Ph.D., with Andrew Weiner. *Phobia Free: How to Fight Your Fears.* New York: Jove/HBJ, 1977.

Daydreams:
Idle Thoughts Are Useful

Daydreams, those thoughts that leap unbidden into your mind, have long been disparaged as signs of hidden hostility, repressed sexuality, and neurosis or as simply a waste of time. But recent studies of daydreams have shown them to be an extremely useful — perhaps essential — human phenomenon.

● You get into bed, turn out the light, and suddenly remember your mother's birthday is tomorrow and you haven't yet sent a card.

● You are plodding to work through snowy streets, and your mind wanders to that Caribbean vacation you'd love to take and how you might pay for it.

• Stuck in a long line at the airport, you while away the endless minutes wondering what you'd say or do if your old boyfriend were on the plane.

Daydreams are not just the idle fluff of an empty mind. They can help you solve current problems, prepare for future events, ward off tension, relieve boredom, dispel fear, dissipate anger, and lift depression. They can help to build self-esteem and may even increase your chances for success. Many sports figures spur themselves on to victory by imagining the act of winning.

Even those daydreams that might be described as bizarre fantasies can be useful, perhaps changing bad moods to good or enhancing self-image. Children who daydream a lot tend to be happier, more cooperative, and have longer staying power than those who don't often let their imaginations run wild, according to studies by Dr. Jerome Singer, a Yale University psychologist.

Many artists, writers, and scientists have their most creative insights through daydreams. Archimedes realized how to use water to measure an object's density while immersing himself in a bathtub. Gazing at the sun setting on the river Seine inspired many of Debussy's impressionistic compositions.

Yet, Dr. Singer points out, many people are embarrassed by their daydreams or are afraid to let their fantasies unfold. Some repress their daydreams as useless wanderings. Others are so busy they don't take the time for mind wandering. Still others click on the television to escape through someone else's fantasies, which are not necessarily relevant to their own personal situations.

Daydreams Fill a Basic Need

Daydreams, the studies have shown, are a nearly universal experience that reflect a basic need of the human mind to fill itself with thought. "Many of the things we do are automatic," explains Dr. Eric Klinger, a psychologist at the University of Minnesota. "When we're not using our full thinking capacity, the mind works over other aspects of life. This is an efficient use of our thought spaces." His studies showed that 30 to 40 percent of our waking moments are typically spent daydreaming. Most daydreams are just passing thoughts lasting five to fourteen seconds, such as wondering what to wear to a party. Interspersed are shorter scraps of thought — "I must remember to buy toilet paper" — and longer reveries, lasting perhaps a minute or two.

Research by Dr. Leonard M. Giambra of the National Institute on Aging has shown that contrary to what you might think, elderly persons do not while away their hours immersed in idle daydreams, mulling over might-have-beens, or reliving the past. Men aged seventy-five to ninety-one daydream as often about the present and future as they do about the past, his studies show. In fact, the frequency of daydreams decreases with age, with men over seventy-five reporting that they daydream only one-fourth as often as do males aged seventeen to twenty-three.

As you might expect, the leading subject of daydreams among young men is sex. For young women, sexual daydreams occur less often. In both men and women, sexual daydreams are most common among those who are most active sexually. Only after about age thirty do the sexual daydreams of men yield to those of a problem-solving nature. Females apparently daydream more often than males, with problem-solving daydreams the most common type at all ages. According to Dr. Klinger's studies, only about one in five daydreams contains weird or distorted images, and far fewer represent bizarre flights of fancy.

Making Daydreams Work for You

Dr. Singer points out that there are many ways in which you can make daydreams work to your advantage. The most important use is to playact your way through problems, rehearsing solutions or reactions to possible future events or situations or carrying out a mental argument until the matter seems settled in your mind. Other possibilities suggested by Dr. Singer include the following:

162

● You can use them simply to fill up time, to amuse yourself, for example, when you have to wait and can't do anything else or when you're driving long distances on a boring road. Since daydreams are associated with a relaxed state, they help to reduce restlessness and tension that could raise your blood pressure or produce other unwanted signs of stress. Dr. Singer cites studies in which people were enclosed in a booth for a long time and given a "mindless" boring task to do. Those who daydreamed didn't realize how much time had passed.

● You can often reverse unpleasant moods and counter feelings of depression with "positive" fantasies, especially those that enhance self-esteem, such as daydreams in which you imagine yourself winning an Oscar or the U.S. Open or being named president of the company you work for. Daydreams about happy events, joyful feelings, or peaceful scenes can relax the muscles of your head and perhaps even ward off tension headaches.

● Bizarre fantasies can help to diminish anger. Let's say you're angry with the boss for not giving you a raise and you're about to confront the matter head-on. Since anger may not be the best emotion for such a confrontation, you could dissipate it by imagining the boss opening a bottle of champagne and giving you a promotion and a raise, or by picturing the boss standing up to shake your hand and losing his pants (or her skirt).

● Athletes and musicians who engage in fantasy practice (in addition to actual physical practice) of their skills do better in carrying them out. Daydreams about your own activities may help you perform them better.

• If you have phobias, you can use daydreams to diminish your fears. For example, if you are afraid of flying, you can imagine yourself on the plane talking to a fascinating seatmate or reading a racy novel and having a wonderful time. [See chapter on curing phobias, page 158.] If you're frightened about taking a test, you can daydream about something pleasant and peaceful and calm yourself down. By the same token, however, if you allow your daydreams to picture the worst (a plane crash or flunking the test), you could greatly enhance your fears.

• Daydreams can sometimes be a clue to an important problem that is not being resolved or a need not being met. For example, one Madison Avenue advertising executive found himself constantly daydreaming about sailing. He finally decided to invest in a charter yacht and is now happy as a lark running a business in the Caribbean. If you find that daydreams constantly intrude at inappropriate times, it could be a sign that something is wrong in your life and professional guidance may be needed.

For Further Reading

Singer, Jerome, Ph.D., with Ellen Switzer. *Mind Play.* Englewood Cliffs, N.J.: Spectrum Books/Prentice-Hall, 1980.

Hypochondria: Understanding Needed, Not Ridicule

A Los Angeles psychiatrist tells the story, perhaps apocryphal, of the epitaph inscribed on a hypochondriac's gravestone: "See, I told you I was really sick."

Hypochondriacs — people who complain of symptoms for which no physical causes can be found — are believed to number in the several millions in the United States. By one estimate, they account for 20 percent of the nation's medical expenses and as many as half the visits to physicians. Yet they have received little more than derision, scorn, and misunderstanding from the medical profession. Physicians tend to treat them with a patronizing attitude and regard them as costly nuisances who are never satisfied or cured. No sooner is one complaint cleared up than another takes its place.

A Need to Be Sick

As Dr. Robert R. Rynearson, chairman of the Department of Psychiatry at the Scott and White Clinic in Temple, Texas, put it in an interview with *Emergency Medicine* magazine, "The hardcore hypochondriac is someone who needs to be sick, who needs physical symptoms that allow him — or her — to depend on a doctor." Reassuring the hypochondriac that there's nothing physically wrong seems only to exacerbate the disorder and provoke even more demanding complaints.

Sooner or later the doctor is likely to become frustrated, angry, and fed up with the hypochondriacal patient, who then moves on to test another doctor's mettle. En route there may be countless and costly medical tests, examinations, and even operations as each doctor, bent on cure, tries to find an organic cause for the complaints.

Those who live with or are befriended by hypochondriacs may be subjected to a daily litany of woes that they can neither escape nor evaluate. Like the doctor, they may become angry and frustrated and feel helpless because nothing they say seems to make any difference. However, a few who are experts on the subject say that hypochondriacs can be helped if you understand their disorder, appreciate their needs, and perhaps help them find more appropriate ways to express those needs.

According to Robert Meister, author of *Hypochondria* (see "For Further Reading," page 166), doctors would undoubtedly prefer to treat patients they know they can help. "Hypochondriacs have no place to go," he states. "No one takes them seriously. Yet they do suffer, as much as a person with a genuine physical disorder suffers. They're in real pain — only they can't prove it."

Contrary to popular belief, he says, hypochondriacs are not afraid they *might be* sick; rather, they are certain that they *are* sick. He and others note that hypochondriacs use illness to build the self-esteem they lack. They are highly unsure of themselves and have strong dependency needs, usually tied to a parent or parent substitute. They use illness to relate to people, to obtain the security of knowing someone is concerned and will take care of them.

Mr. Meister examined the records of nearly 400 hypochondriacs, talked to more than 300 of them, and interviewed 175 physicians and 63 psychologists and other professionals on the subject. He found that hypochondria can occur at any age. Though it is seen most frequently in adults between the ages of thirty and fifty, children and teenagers may also be afflicted. According to a British study, the problem is as common among men as women, but American physicians say most hypochondriacs are female.

Mr. Meister also discovered that not all hypochondriacs are doctor shoppers. As he pointed out in an article in *Psychology Today,* some, perhaps many, are "closet" hypochondriacs, who confide in only one person and avoid going to doctors. They rely, instead, on a host of self-treatments. He believes that some health-food "nuts," vitamin megadosers, and even jogging fanatics are among the closet hypochondriacs who are obsessively concerned with the well-being of their bodies.

Virtually all of us exhibit a touch of hypochondria from time to time. When tense or depressed or suffering the pangs of a loss, we may develop symptoms and a fear or conviction that we are ill, yet nothing is organically wrong. Rather, the emotional stress we are under shows up in symptoms such as headaches, stomachaches, joint pains, diarrhea, or chest pains. We may report these symptoms to relatives or friends and usually see a doctor about them. This happens less often among people who feel comfortable expressing emotional pain and seeking direct help for it. But for most of us, a physical symptom is far more acceptable and more likely to command the attention and care our psyches really need.

The full-blown hypochondriac has a deeply rooted problem. Typically, hypochondriacs grew up overly dependent on a parent or with a parent who was loving and solicitous only when the child was sick. Also common in the background of hypochondriacs, Mr. Meister found, is an atmosphere of illness: excessive exposure early in life to numerous and persistent complaints; illness or invalidism in the family; personal life-threatening experiences or frequent illnesses; death of a close family member; or strong identification with someone who was often ill or who exaggerated body sensations.

How to Help

Although many psychiatrists believe hypochondriacs are not amenable to treatment, Dr. Gerald C. Crary, professor of emergency medicine and psychiatry at the University of Southern California, says that many are helped by an exploration of the psychological roots of their problem. Some are able to come to grips with the underlying issues and learn to deal with them in healthier ways.

Others may not get over their problem but may learn to control it better. "They don't talk or think about their symptoms so often or so openly, and they learn to get on with life and be more productive," he explained.

In the journal *American Family Physician,* Dr. Norman Altman, a San Diego psychiatrist, says the ordinary physician can help by listening sympathetically, being supportive, and understanding the patient's need for a caring relationship. After an appropriate examination has revealed no physical illness, he recommends that the doctor make sure the patient knows there is nothing dangerous about the condition. However, he says, the doctor should not deny that the patient is sick or say or imply that the "illness" will be cured.

Dr. Altman urges the doctor to show an interest in the patient's life and relationships beyond the medical complaints. Extensive and repeated tests and treatments should be avoided, and a plan should be set up for periodic visits of fifteen to twenty minutes, he recommends.

Dr. Rynearson says it's especially important for the family of a hypochondriac to understand the condition and not to be angry with a doctor for failing to remove the patient's symptoms. He suggests that the family steer the patient to a physician who will deal appropriately with the condition and protect the patient from a constant round of tests, medication, and surgery that other physicians may prescribe "in the name of healing." Rather than a battery of modern therapies, Dr. Rynearson says, "the physician should prescribe *himself* as treatment in whatever ways might be helpful to the patient."

If you are a relative or friend of a hypochondriac, Dr. Crary suggests that you simply listen, nod your head sympathetically, and say, "I understand." Showing concern can be very helpful to these troubled people, he says, but you should avoid assuming responsibility for their problems. If you tire of hearing about them, Dr. Crary recommends that you say in a nonrejecting way, "You've discussed this with me and with your doctor many times, and I'm sorry that you're suffering. Now let's talk about something else."

But Dr. Warren R. Procci, psychiatrist at the University of Southern California, says it's cruel to dismiss a hypochondriac's complaints by saying, "It's all in your head." Pain, he adds, is "no less painful if its cause is imaginary. In fact, hypochondriasis can be more agonizing than diseases with physical causes because the disorder frequently seems hopeless to the victim and commonly disrupts every aspect of the victim's home and work experiences."

166

Furthermore, he warns, "because hypochondriacs have cried wolf so often, they are in constant jeopardy of being ignored when they really need medical attention." Therefore, if a new complaint crops up, a physician should be consulted and the appropriate tests done to determine its cause.

For Further Reading

Ehrlich, Richard. *The Healthy Hypochondriac*. Philadelphia: Saunders Paperback, 1980.
Meister, Robert. *Hypochondria.* New York: Taplinger, 1980.

Holiday Blues: How to Avoid the Doldrums

" 'Tis the season to be jolly," the Christmas carol admonishes us. Yet for millions the winter holiday season, or its aftermath, is the most depressing time of year. Psychiatrists report that they are busiest between Thanksgiving until after the New Year. Patients who have been doing well suddenly take a turn for the worse, and persons previously healthy may find themselves in a deep funk. Traffic accidents increase, and emotional breakdowns peak.

The holidays tend to amplify people's problems and are especially difficult for those who have suffered losses during the year, such as a lost job, ill health, or the death of a close friend or relative. But they may be difficult times even without an obvious cause.

Why It Happens, What to Do

Many reasons have been offered to explain the holiday blues and help people avoid or recover from them. Here are some common precipitants and what to do about them:

Loneliness. The holidays are billed as times when families and friends get together to have a good time. Persons who find themselves alone at holiday time — those who are single, divorced, or widowed, among others — are the most susceptible to depression. Each Christmas carol or holiday greeting becomes a reminder that "everyone is happy but me," and you sink into a pit of self-pity.

Dr. Nicholas Cummings, a California psychologist, recommends resisting all feelings of self-pity. "In the early stages," he says, "you can fight it off." Instead of sitting around feeling sorry for yourself, he suggests, "make it a point to be with people, especially people who enjoy the holidays. Don't wait to be invited. Have people over yourself."

If dinner is beyond you, arrange a potluck party. Or make plans with others to see a show or movie, attend a concert or sports event, visit a gallery or museum. Don't wait until the last minute when everything is likely to be sold out and you're already too depressed to be bothered. Also, plan ahead to do something nice in January to help ward off a post-holiday letdown.

Fatigue. Whether you're staying home for the holidays or going away, there always seems to be more to do than the hours of the day — and often the night — will allow. There's the house to clean, food to cook, decorations and clothing to make or buy, cards to send, gifts to buy and wrap. Stores are open late to permit exhausting shopping expeditions after a full day's work (and usually before eating any dinner).

For those who leave town, there are trip preparations and packing and often long days at the office to get enough work done to permit the time off. The combined stresses of seemingly endless lists of "essential" chores, overbooked days, and inadequate sleep at night can easily precipitate depression, if not set the stage for physical illness.

Exercise, it may surprise you to know, is an excellent antidote to fatigue and depression. Dr. M. Lawrence Thrash, a New York City psychiatrist who requires all his patients to participate in an active physical program, says exercise helps to create a pleasing self-image. "When you like yourself, others tend to like you and want to be with you, and that counters loneliness," he points out. Physical activity helps people organize their lives better so that they have more time to get things done. It also improves sleep and makes you more alert during the day.

Another way to fight holiday fatigue is to divide the preparations and chores among family members so that the full burden of shopping, cleaning, and cooking doesn't fall on one person's shoulders.

Alcohol. Alcohol is a drug, a central nervous system depressant. If you're unhappy to begin with, it will intensify that unhappiness. Holiday cocktail parties at which you try to drown your sorrows only make things worse. Drinking and eating too much also increase fatigue by interfering with restful sleep. If you're feeling blue, stay away from wassail and cocktails, and instead, stick to fruit juices, club soda, mineral water, and unspiked eggnog. Or, Dr. Thrash suggests, "Reach for your running shorts instead of a drink."

Unrealistic expectations. The Christmas spirit is not magical. People who've felt neglected all year often expect that at Christmas their families will make up for it. They almost never do. At holiday celebrations suddenly family members who don't get along all year are supposed to have a wonderful time together. Parents are supposed to stop criticizing; children are not supposed to "act up"; Uncle Joe is supposed to stop being sarcastic and disagreeable. It almost never happens.

You may also expect too much of yourself — the beautifully decorated tree, the perfect dinner, the most appropriately chosen gifts. You drive yourself to exhaustion, trying to make everything perfect, and disappointment is inevitable when the pudding turns out soggy, a toy breaks, the tree lights fail to flicker, or you receive a gift from someone you've crossed off your list. If Christmas dinner is an annual ordeal, why bother? Forget all the invitations and preparations, and have waffles and ice cream or some other homey treat and sing carols with your immediate family.

Gift giving and receiving are common causes of unfulfilled expectations. Many people choose gifts that reflect the giver's, not the receiver's, tastes and needs. Some give what they *want* the receiver to have, not what the receiver would want for himself or herself. Others try to make up for what they lack in feeling by giving a gift that is overly expensive or showy. Even if you can afford it, avoid overspending on gifts.

A homemade gift (food, poem, clothing, or trinket), a gift certificate for a favorite store, or an IOU for a special event might be preferable to a purchase that is likely to disappoint the receiver. For people who simply don't like to receive presents (the "I-don't-know-why-you-bothered" type), forget a gift, and if you must, offer a personal service or make a charitable contribution instead.

Darkness. According to Dr. David V. Forrest, a psychiatrist affiliated with the Columbia-Presbyterian Medical Center, the short days of the winter solstice are an important contributing factor to holiday depression. His patients often complain about the dark and gloomy days of December. With December 21 the shortest day of the year, Dr. Forrest suggests planning a vacation trip to a sunny place, such as a southern beach, or to a ski resort.

A less expensive alternative is to wear light-colored clothing, spend as much time as possible outside during daylight hours, and keep bright lights on indoors, if not in the whole house, then at least in the room in which you spend most of your waking hours. You might consider installing a bright fluorescent light that mimics the spectrum of the sun; it's called Vita-Lite, manufactured by the Duro-Test Corporation, 2321 Kennedy Boulevard, North Bergen, New Jersey 07047. Use it for several hours in the early morning and after sunset. "Bright light has an exhilarating effect," Dr. Forrest notes. "In animals, it stimulates the sex drive."

Guilt. A little self-indulgence at holiday time is natural and desirable. But self-indulgence tends to be guilt-provoking for people who are highly disciplined the rest of the time, and their guilt feeds depression. It's far better to relax your rigid standards and enjoy yourself for a few weeks. Also, don't compound the holiday blues by feeling guilty because you're not as jolly as the carol says you should be. It's normal at holiday time to feel a little sad about the past and the loved ones who can't be with you. Perhaps the best antidote to guilt and depression is to do something nice for someone less fortunate than you.

Hyperactivity: When Children Are Out of Control

Michael is known to his fellow first graders as "the baddest boy in the class." Always talking out of turn, jumping around, disobeying or ignoring the teacher, and picking fights with his classmates, Michael continually disrupts classroom activities. Although of normal intelligence, he fails to keep up with the class.

At home Michael's perpetual motion, bad temper, and unpredictable behavior torture his parents and older sister. The family rarely goes out together because Michael's antics are a constant embarrassment.

Michael has the symptoms of hyperkinesis, or hyperactivity, a poorly understood behavioral syndrome marked by constant, often purposeless, activity, impulsiveness, a short attention span, distractibility, emotional outbursts, and a low tolerance for frustration.

In recent years hyperactivity has been the subject of controversy over its frequency, cause or causes, and proper treatment. The debate has left parents and teachers thoroughly confused about how to recognize and deal with a hyperactive child. Although some say hyperactivity is a wastebasket diagnosis for any child who does not quite conform to society's stereotype of normal childhood behavior, there is little doubt that an identifiable abnormality such as Michael displays actually exists.

For unknown reasons, the hyperactivity syndrome mainly afflicts boys between one and sixteen years old and is usually recognized at about six, when the child enters school. While the symptoms generally subside during adolescence, recent studies of adults who were hyperactive as children suggest that the symptoms may persist in subdued form, sometimes causing psychological difficulties in adult life.

Though hyperkinesis has been variously ascribed to such conditions as minimal brain damage, sensitivity to food additives, low blood sugar, and excessive lead, the real cause is not known, and it is likely that a number of different causes can produce the hyperkinetic syndrome.

Hyperactivity is most commonly treated by stimulant drugs — amphetamines and related substances — which have a paradoxical calming effect on children with "true hyperkinesis." This unusual drug effect suggests that the hyperkinetic child has an abnormal slowness of his brain's "braking" mechanism that is corrected by stimulants.

In 1970 hyperactivity became the focus of public discussion and debate when it was revealed that some public schools were prescribing stimulant drugs to all children deemed "overactive" in class. Many of these children had nothing more serious than the normal exuberance of childhood, had not been examined by an expert, and were not being treated under medical supervision.

Who Is Hyperactive?

Most experts say that true hyperkinesis occurs in only 1 or 2 percent — and certainly no more than 10 percent — of American children. The phenomenon is clearly culturally related since some countries say it does not exist at all and others report an incidence of less than 1 percent.

In making a diagnosis of hyperactivity, experts say these factors should be taken into account:

Attention problems. The child does at least three of the following: often fails to finish things he starts; often doesn't seem to listen; is easily distracted; has difficulty concentrating on schoolwork or other tasks requiring sustained attention; has difficulty sticking to a play activity.

Impulsive behaviors. The child does at least three of the following: often acts before thinking; shifts frequently from one activity to another; has difficulty organizing work; needs close supervision; frequently calls out in class; has difficulty waiting his turn in games or group situations.

Hyperactive behaviors. Child does at least *two* of the following: runs about or climbs on things a lot; has difficulty sitting still or fidgets a great deal; has difficulty staying seated; moves about frequently during sleep; is always "on the go" or acts as if "driven by a motor."

Frequently the hyperkinetic child will have other concurrent difficulties, such as specific learning disabilities, perceptual problems, and emotional disorders, which require special treatment.

Getting Help for Your Child

The American Academy of Pediatrics and others caution that many factors, in addition to true hyperkinesis, can cause hyperactivity, including the child's basic personality, anxiety, depression, inapparent seizures, and the perceptions of the beholder. What a classroom teacher might construe as hyperactivity may be laudable exuberance to parents or an athletic coach. Psychological, psychiatric, and neurological testing of the child should be done before a diagnosis is made and treatment begun.

To find specialists who can do the proper work-up, you or your doctor might call the pediatrics department of the nearest medical school or university hospital, or you can write to the Association for Children with Learning Disabilities, 5225 Grace Street, Pittsburgh, Pennsylvania 15236 (please send a stamped, self-addressed, legal-size envelope).

Drugs, most commonly amphetamine or methylphenidate (Ritalin), are said to alleviate symptoms in about 70 percent of children with true hyperkinesis. Unlike normal people, who become restless, nervous, and overactive from these stimulants, hyperkinetic children are subdued by them. Stimulant drugs, especially amphetamine, diminish weight gain and growth, and experts advise that they be discontinued two years before the child's bones stop growing to allow him to catch up. On the positive side, studies have shown that use of these drugs in treating hyperkinesis does not lead to addiction or abuse of other drugs.

The Feingold Diet

Many parents dislike the idea of giving their children a potent drug day after day and are attracted to seemingly safer therapies, such as the diet devised by the late California allergist, Dr. Benjamin Feingold, who maintained that hyperactivity is caused by foods and medicines that are artificially flavored or colored or that contain aspirinlike (salicylate) compounds. Dr. Feingold, who wrote a book outlining an "elimination" diet to treat hyperactivity, estimated that as many as 25 percent of schoolchildren may be afflicted with this "sensitivity" and its presumed adverse behavioral consequences. He claimed that 50 percent of hyperactive children are greatly improved by his diet, which eliminates foods and drugs with artificial colorings and flavorings and salicylates.

However, a series of independent studies, in which neither parents nor teachers nor independent observers knew which diet the child was on, showed no such dramatic effect of the Feingold diet compared with a diet containing the taboo foods. Some children improved, but others got worse. Rarely did more than a small percentage of children show reduced hyperactivity on the restricted diet. The researchers concluded that further study of the Feingold diet was warranted, but no claims could currently be made about its effectiveness.

Some experts have suggested that the main benefits of the Feingold scheme are the attention it requires of the parents, who may heretofore have had as little to do with their troublesome offspring as possible, plus the fact that the diet necessarily eliminates nearly all junk food. The consequent improvement in the child's nutrition and, perhaps, the concomitant decline in the consumption of sweets may be what actually does the most good.

Other Unproved Theories

Many parents report that concentrated doses of sugar-laden foods and drinks seem to turn their otherwise normal-behaving children into whirling dervishes, and some groups maintain that overconsumption of sugar is at the root of the hyperactivity syndrome. While the latter claim is far from proved, it makes sense in any case to limit your child's sugar consumption, especially if it seems to have adverse behavioral effects.

A team at the Downstate Medical Center in Brooklyn, New York, suggested on the basis of a preliminary study that perhaps half of hyperactive children had excessive amounts of lead in their bodies (shown by elevated levels of lead in the blood and urine), and the removal of the lead with drugs called chelating agents alleviated the hyperactivity in half the cases they studied. Although cautious about making far-reaching claims for their early findings, the researchers urged that lead levels be considered in the evaluation of hyperactive children.

IV.
Sexuality and Reproduction

There is probably no aspect of life that commands more attention, yet is subject to more confusion and anxiety, than our sexuality. Some people worry about when and how and how often to express themselves sexually, while fears of sexual inadequacy and venereal disease deprive millions of the joys of sex. Some are torn between their worries about unwanted pregnancy and their concerns about the safety and effectiveness of the various ways to prevent pregnancies. Still others who would like to have children find that pregnancy or healthy childbirth eludes them.

Although sexuality and reproduction have definitely come out of the closet in recent years, ignorance, myth, and misinformation are still widely prevalent. As a result, many people suffer needlessly and forfeit satisfaction of an appetite that is as basic to our being as eating and sleeping.

Understanding the causes of common sexual and reproductive problems and becoming aware of the sometimes simple solutions to them can often replace sorrow and anxiety with happiness and fulfillment.

Impotence:
How to Avoid and Overcome It

Impotence, the inability to achieve or sustain an erection, is a far more common problem than most men realize. An estimated 10 percent of men are impotent all the time, and as many as 50 percent have potency difficulties some of the time.

Impotence can be one of the most emotionally devastating events in a man's life. The problem may result in severe anxiety, depression, and marital discord and may even lead to suicide. However, though it is a fairly common complaint, impotence is among the most treatable of sexual problems, often through brief therapy.

Erection: A Fragile Response

Potency is the result of a fragile reflex response. An erection results when spaces inside the penis fill with blood as a result of psychic, sensory, and neurologic stimuli. It is an automatic response that cannot be willed. But psychological factors such as fear, guilt, and hostility can inhibit it, as can physical disorders that distort hormone levels or impair the blood supply or the transmission of nerve messages to the penis.

Nearly every man, at one time in his life, finds that his body refuses to cooperate with his emotions. Stress, worry, fatigue, and consumption of alcohol are frequent causes of such "transient" potency problems. They are so common as to be considered within the range of normal sexual functioning.

Unfortunately the first time an erection failure occurs a man may become anxious and begin to question his manhood. In his next sexual encounter his anxiety about what happened the previous time may actually cause a repetition of the difficulty, setting up a vicious cycle of psychogenic — caused-by-the-mind — impotence.

The Causes

Most cases of impotence have psychological roots, but as the following cases illustrate, the causes are varied and complex.

● A thirty-two-year-old sexually inexperienced man married and found he was impotent. Afraid that he could not satisfy his wife, he did not even attempt intercourse. His problem was solved by lengthy discussions with a physician who enhanced the patient's limited sexual knowledge and instilled self-confidence in his sexual ability.

● A fifty-one-year-old man gradually lost his ability to maintain erection, though his sexual desire remained strong. He had had no sexual difficulty in thirty years of marriage. He continued to be happy in his marriage and his job. Medical evaluation showed that his difficulty was a consequence of diabetes, which had damaged his nerves.

• Another man had a blood vessel disease that was apparently contributing to intermittent impotence. However, he became completely impotent after learning that his wife was unfaithful; he also became angry, anxious, and depressed.

When impotence is caused by emotional difficulties within the individual or associated with a particular relationship, the problem usually can be corrected through psychotherapy or sex therapy.

In perhaps a third of cases the cause is organic, or physical — the result of some underlying disease, surgery, the use of certain drugs, including alcohol, or the physical degeneration that comes with old age. In some of these situations, too, impotence can be cured — for example, by stopping the use of the drug. In addition, a significant proportion of impotent men may have correctable hormonal abnormalities, according

MALE GENITAL ANATOMY

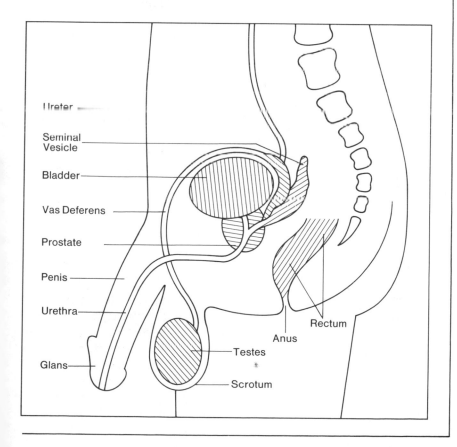

to recent studies at Beth Israel Hospital in Boston.

Even when the cause is organic, there are likely to be complicating psychological difficulties, and they are often the result of the potency problem itself. As Dr. Steven B. Levine, a psychiatrist at Case Western Reserve University in Cleveland, points out, "a mild organic problem may become severe when the man begins to worry." In such cases a combination of treatments may be needed to reduce the difficulty.

Treatment

The treatment of impotence should begin by determining the probable cause. If the man still has sexual desires but is impotent under all circumstances — with all partners and during masturbation, and fails to have erections during sleep or upon awakening — it is likely that the problem has an organic basis. The man should be checked for possible underlying diseases, such as alcoholism, diabetes, heart, lung or kidney disease, previous prostate or urological surgery, or trauma to the spinal cord. Any of these can cause impotence.

Potency-reducing drugs include alcohol, heroin, morphine, injected estrogen, reserpine and related drugs (used to treat high blood pressure), barbiturates, high doses of such tranquilizers as chlorpromazine and other phenothiazines, MAO inhibitors, and — according to some reports — cigarette smoke.

The correctable hormonal problems detected by the Boston studies often involve the body chemicals that serve as triggers for the production and release of testosterone, the male sex hormone, from the testes. Other hormonal derangements can block the response to testosterone. Prior to assuming a man has psychogenic impotence, the researchers urge that all men complaining of impotence be tested for testosterone levels. If an abnormality is found, further study is needed to determine its cause and proper hormonal therapy.

However, the ability of testosterone injections themselves to improve potency, except in rare cases, is a matter of considerable medical controversy. Most experts say the treatment sometimes works because the men *think* it will work and because the injection creates an overall sense of well-being.

Among the psychological causes of impotence are deterioration of the relationship between the man and his partner, an unresponsive or uninterested partner, anxiety, fear, anger, guilt, depression, and sexual misinformation. Doctors and sex therapists have found that simply evaluating the situation helps some couples by reassuring them, correcting misinformation, and removing communication barriers.

Treating psychological impotence focuses on reducing the anxiety that surrounds the couple's sexual interactions. According to sex therapists at the University of California, Los Angeles, "Instead of trying to 'force' an erection (which leads to further failure), the couple must learn to relax and engage in pleasurable activities not dependent on erection, like a sensual massage." The couple may spend a week or more simply caressing, with no attempt at intercourse. With the pressure off, the body is more likely to respond as it should. Therapy, which commonly lasts from two to ten weeks, is successful in about 80 percent of cases, according to the sex therapists Dr. William Masters and Virginia Johnson. Only about 5 percent suffer relapse.

Other Solutions

When impotence, organic or psychological, cannot be reversed through conservative measures, a device can be surgically implanted in the penis to restore potency. These devices have been used in several thousand men, with a success rate of 80 percent in properly selected cases.

One such device is filled with a silicone sponge that gives the penis a permanently erect shape but is flexible enough to be hidden under clothing. The other is a reversible "pump" — silicone tubes are implanted in the penis, and a fluid-containing bulb is placed under the skin of the abdomen or scrotum. The bulb is compressed or released to create or dissipate an erection, as desired.

If it turns out that a man's potency problem is irreversible and he is not a suitable candidate for the penile implant, sex therapy can help him and his partner learn to enjoy their sexuality and reach orgasm without erection and penetration. However, no over-the-counter drug, vitamin, or food can improve potency. According to one New York urologist, "Stories of such improvements with ingestion of items ranging from raw eggs to raw oysters are only old wives' tales."

177

For Further Reading

Brooks, Marvin B. *Lifelong Sexual Vigor: How to Avoid and Overcome Impotence.* New York: Doubleday, 1981.

"Frigidity": When a Woman Is Sexually Unresponsive

The explosion of information about sexuality in the 1970's has prompted many women to question the adequacy of their sexual responses. Women for whom sex has long been an unpleasant or unsatisfying event have come to realize that they need not be doomed to a lifetime devoid of sexual enjoyment or fulfillment.

Thanks largely to the revolution in sex therapy begun by Dr. William Masters and Virginia Johnson in 1970, there are now several effective approaches to treating what has long been mislabeled "frigidity."

A Range of Dysfunctions

The word "frigidity," with its connotation of icy coldness, is a wastebasket term that is incorrectly and indiscriminately used to describe a wide range of female sexual dysfunctions. Rarely a woman may indeed be totally unresponsive sexually, no matter what the circumstances, partner, or techniques used (and in such cases "frigid" may be an apt description). Far more common is the woman who becomes highly excited by sexual stimulation but is unable to reach orgasm.

Some women suffer such painful spasms of the muscles surrounding the vaginal opening that penetration is impossible — a condition called vaginismus. Some find intercourse painful and unpleasant. Others may have lost their orgasmic ability or lost interest in sex altogether, even though it continues to be physiologically satisfying.

"Frigidity" has sometimes been used to describe — again, incorrectly — the woman who can attain orgasm through direct stimulation of the clitoris but not through sexual intercourse. Such women (or their partners) may consider themselves sexually inadequate — Freud and his followers called them immature — but today sex therapists say that orgasm only through direct clitoral stimulation is a normal variant of the female sexual response.

FEMALE GENITAL ANATOMY

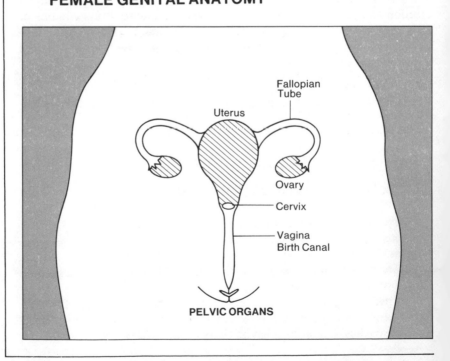

PELVIC ORGANS

According to estimates from several surveys, between one-third and two-thirds of women require direct stimulation of the clitoris to reach orgasm. Dr. Masters and Mrs. Johnson showed that no matter how a woman reaches orgasm, stimulation of the clitoris, either directly or indirectly, is nearly always involved. The clitoris is a woman's most sexually sensitive organ, equivalent to a man's penis.

Dr. Helen Singer Kaplan, Cornell University sex therapist and author of *The New Sex Therapy* (New York: Times Books, 1974) and *The Illustrated Manual of Sex Therapy* (New York: Times Books, 1975), points out that "orgasm is really highly pleasurable no matter how it occurs, provided neither partner considers noncoital orgasm as 'second best.' Secure and loving couples can have gloriously fulfilling sex lives even though the woman requires clitoral stimulation in order to climax."

There are also a fair number of women who are sexually responsive and usually reach orgasm but don't know it. Having read descriptions (most of them written by men) of female orgasms that "start bells ringing" or "make the world stop," they fail to recognize their more subdued orgasmic response for what it is.

A woman who thinks or knows her sexual responses are not what they might be may feel inferior or incomplete and unhappy with her sex

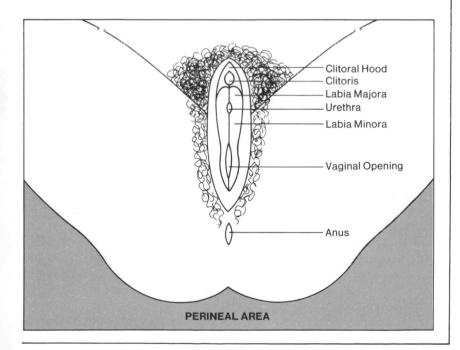

PERINEAL AREA

life. She may blame her partner, or her partner may blame himself for her difficulties, and one or both may go searching for a sexually more satisfying mate. Out of fear of losing or hurting their husbands or lovers, many women regularly fake orgasms, an act that pretty much guarantees that neither partner will ever learn what is needed to bring the woman to orgasm.

The causes of female sexual dysfunctions are as varied as their manifestations. Some women were brought up to think of sex as dirty or forbidden — a man's right, but a woman's duty. They may have heard men portrayed as brutal creatures seeking animalistic satisfactions, whereas women were described as being above such needs. A woman with this background may find it difficult, if not impossible, to overthrow years of aversive conditioning on her wedding night and nights thereafter. The result can be little or no response to sexual stimulation, a relatively rare condition that is difficult to treat and may require prolonged psychotherapy.

Vaginismus, spasm of the vaginal muscles that makes the vagina virtually impenetrable without extraordinary pain, is also a rare condition, most often seen in women who were brought up with very "strict morals." However, sex therapists report that 90 percent or more of women with vaginismus can be "deconditioned" and taught to overcome the spasm with brief therapy.

The loss of orgasmic ability sometimes follows such events as childbirth, some condition that made intercourse painful (such as a vaginal or urinary tract infection), or use of birth control pills. Sometimes — as with psychogenic impotence in men — a woman may begin to worry about her ability to reach orgasm, and this anxiety blocks her orgasmic response.

A woman may lose interest in sex because she has lost interest in her partner or feels anger toward him, or because sex has become so ritualized, predictable, or mechanical that all the excitement is gone. Sometimes the fragile sexual response is disrupted by a partner's habits, actions, words, or sexual techniques.

Treatment

Orgasm, for women as for men, is a natural reflex response, and varying amounts of stimulation may elicit it in different women or in the same woman at different times. Orgasm is also very much in the mind. Guilt, fear, or anger can inhibit it completely, and sexual fantasies can stimulate it. Contrary to popular thinking, neither the onset of menopause nor advancing age spells the end to a woman's sexual responsiveness and orgasmic ability. Although as a woman ages, her response to stimulation is likely to be slower, she can remain orgasmic into her eighties or beyond.

Therapists help couples learn about their bodies (many women as well as men don't know where the clitoris is, for example) and what may enhance or interfere with natural responses. Women with orgasmic difficulties may be taught to masturbate to orgasm, first while alone and then with their partners. Some women can then learn to experience orgasm through intercourse. A vibrator (the electric hand-held massage type, not the widely sold battery-operated phallus-shaped gadget) may be used to stimulate a woman until she acquires orgasmic ability.

In some cases psychotherapy (usually brief) is needed to overcome long-standing inhibitions, in the man as well as the woman. The exploration and correction of a woman's sexual problems may unveil one in her partner, such as premature ejaculation, which also requires therapy.

For Further Assistance

For the most common complaint brought to sex therapists — inability to reach orgasm through intercourse — purely "mechanical" therapy is often effective. Several books have been written by sex therapists to help women acquire orgasmic ability. One of the best of these is *For Yourself* (New York: Doubleday, 1975) by Lonnie Garfield Barbach, a University of California therapist.

Couples in need of sex therapy must beware of the large number of poorly trained individuals who call themselves therapists. To help people find qualified therapists, the American Association of Sex Educators, Counselors and Therapists, Suite 304, 5010 Wisconsin Avenue NW, Washington, D.C. 20016, publishes a national directory. It costs $3. People living in less-populated areas are advised to write to or call the organization (phone 202-686-2523) because the published directory may not cover their area.

Marital Sex: The Many Dimensions of "Normal"

The patterns of "normal" sexual activity among married couples are as varied as the couples themselves.

Example: Mr. and Mrs. S. are in their late thirties and although they share a deep love, affection, respect, and consideration, they have had sexual intercourse fewer than ten times in the more than ten years they have been married, and this is fine with both of them.

Example: Mr. and Mrs. T. had intercourse about ten times a week as newlyweds twenty-five years ago, but the frequency of intercourse is now at a "middle-aged low" of three times a week.

Example: For most of their twenty-five years of marriage, Mr. and Mrs. Y. had sex about once every two weeks, but recently they have experienced a reawakening of sexual interest, and frequency of intercourse has quadrupled.

Example: Mr. and Mrs. B., married nine years, have had a string of serious family problems lately as well as some difficulties between them. Although in the early years of their marriage sex was mutually enjoyed several times a week, they now cannot recall when they last had sex —

"maybe two or three months ago."

Gaining Perspective

Despite such enormous differences, popular wisdom holds that the "normal" married couple has sex twice a week on the average, with the peak in frequency occurring at the beginning of the marriage and declining to almost none after middle age. Many of the millions of couples who do not conform to this "statistical average" — if it is even that — worry that they are somehow abnormal. In other cases married couples experience undesired changes in their sexual patterns but are unaware of the reasons for the change or the fact that often simple home remedies can greatly improve their situation.

Recent studies have shown that while the frequency of intercourse among married couples has generally increased in the last decade, it is common to find couples who share a lot of love but little or no passion or for whom sex has become virtually nonexistent for weeks or months at a time.

A Canadian study among 365 married persons, most below the age of forty and married for an average of eleven years, showed that fully one-third experienced long periods with no sex. For half, the cessation of intercourse lasted more than eight weeks, with the most common reason being marital discord.

It also appears that many happily married couples have what sex therapists consider serious sexual dysfunctions, such as potency problems or inability to reach orgasm. A survey of ninety "normal" married couples by Ellen Frank, a psychologist at the University of Pittsburgh, revealed that although 85 percent described their marriages as "happy" or "very happy," 42 percent of the husbands and 62 percent of the wives complained of having a serious sexual problem.

Dr. David R. Mace, family sociologist at the Bowman Gray School of Medicine in Winston-Salem, North Carolina, and his wife, Vera, who with him founded the Association of Couples for Marriage Enrichment, emphasize the need to put sex in marriage into its proper perspective.

"The idea that it is the joy of sex that sustains a good marriage is putting the cart before the horse," they point out. "It is more appropriate to say that it is the good marriage that sustains the joy of sex" — whether it occurs thrice a week, twice a week, once a week, or once a year. The Maces have estimated that the average married couple spends the hours' equivalent of one weekend a year having sexual intercourse, and therefore, they conclude, it is unrealistic to suggest that sex is the major force sustaining the relationship.

Indeed, among 75,000 women who answered a survey questionnaire prepared by *Redbook* magazine in 1976, sex ranked *after* love, respect, and friendship as the factors the women considered most important to a happy marriage.

Why Sexual Desires Change

Nonetheless, changes that one or both partners find disturbing or baffling often occur in a couple's sexual pattern. Some of these changes reflect the natural ebb and flow of sexual desire through the years. For men, for example, the peak of sexual feelings commonly occurs in early adulthood and gradually declines thereafter, but for women the peak is generally not reached until the thirties and then remains relatively stable into the sixties or beyond. At some point in life a diminished libido in one partner, especially the male, is a common occurrence. However, for both men and women, sexual interest may remain at a relatively high level well into old age.

Other common reasons for changes in sexual desire, many of which are potentially reversible, include the following:

● Adoption of a life-style that leaves little opportunity or mental or physical energy for sex. Dr. John F. Cuber, sociologist at Ohio State University, estimates that fewer than one in five upper-middle-class couples overcomes the pressures and obstacles of their life-style and manages to have an active and satisfying sex life. Too often, he notes, an overworked, harassed, tired husband comes home to a lonely, depressed wife (or a similarly overworked, harassed, tired wife), hardly the setting for scintillating sex.

● Loss of physical attractiveness, such as poor hygiene or excessive weight gain, can turn off the partner's sexual interest.

183

● Changes in self-image as a sexual being as a result of physical or emotional factors. A person who feels inadequate, inferior, or unimportant is likely to experience a decline in sexual interest. But contrary to what many think, the menopause, a hysterectomy, or a prostate operation need not disrupt a person's sexual interest or ability.

● Situational factors, such as a serious problem with a child, loss of a job, financial worries, or major household disruptions. One of the most common of these is birth of the first child. Beset by parental and domestic duties and intrusion of another being, "many couples never fully recover the strong sexual accent which characterized their lives before their first pregnancy," Dr. Cuber notes.

● Sexual dysfunction, such as difficulty in achieving or maintaining an erection, which may discourage a partner from attempting intercourse and lead eventually to suppressed desire. In many cases such problems can be effectively treated by competent sex therapy.

● Deterioration of the marital relationship. If the partner is liked and loved, there is usually more sex. But if one partner feels neglected or there has been a loss of intimacy, or if the relationship is marred by feelings of anger, resentment, frustration, or indifference, sexual desire is likely to diminish. In these cases marriage counseling may improve the entire relationship, including its sexual component.

● Boredom and routine in sexual activity. As Dr. Donald W. Burnap, a psychiatrist in Rapid City, South Dakota, put it, "Year after year a wife may wear the same type of nightgown, and her husband may climb into bed and kiss her in exactly the same way. They may touch each other in the same places for the same length of time. They may say the same things and climax in the same way. They know what to expect. No wonder they lose interest!"

Preserving Passion

Many experts emphasize that the preservation of passion in marriage depends on a couple's having sex when they feel like it, not according to a schedule that satisfies an imagined standard of performance. Quality, they say, is far more important than quantity.

Improving sexual communication is also important. Dr. William Masters and Virginia Johnson, the famed St. Louis sex researchers, report that among married couples there is often a vast communications gap about sexual preferences. For example, their studies showed, genital stimulation by husbands was often too vigorous to be enjoyable or stimulating, but the wives rarely said anything to change it. When the wives did indicate a better way, the husband would often forget or ignore the instructions.

There were also many times when women were made physically uncomfortable by their husbands' manner of touching their breasts, but again nothing was said. When questioned about this, the husbands' unanimous reaction was: "Why didn't she tell me?"

The husbands were no better at communicating with their wives about ways to enhance their own sexual pleasure. Only a few wives said their husbands had suggested specific techniques.

Masters and Johnson also note that many wives assume their husbands are the sex experts and know what pleases their partners. And, the researchers say, if the husband's approach "leaves something to be desired, she simply assumes that he doesn't care."

Other helpful hints for improving marital sex, suggested by Dr. Martin Goldberg, director of marital therapy at the Institute of Pennsylvania Hospital in Philadelphia, include adopting variety in sexual technique (many books that may suggest variations are now readily available), varying the setting for sex, using fantasy, and emphasizing the couple's relationship as man-woman and lovers, rather than as parents.

Many couples find that their sex lives revive dramatically on a vacation — even a weekend away — together, particularly if it is without the children. Free of the day-to-day mental preoccupations, interruptions, and distractions and in a new and different setting, they rediscover the passion within. For some, such a vacation can be the first step toward revitalizing sex back home.

For Further Reading

The following books can help couples discover impediments to their sexual pleas-

184

ure and develop new, more satisfying sexual techniques.

Castleman, Michael. *Sexual Solutions.* New York: Simon & Schuster, 1980.

Comfort, Alex. *The Joy of Sex.* New York: Fireside/Simon & Schuster, 1972.

Masters, William H., and Virginia E. Johnson, with Robert J. Levin. *The Pleasure Bond.* Boston: Little, Brown, 1975.

Sex and Aging: Keeping the Flame Alive

Despite the professed sexual liberalism of the day, when it comes to sex among the elderly, Victorian attitudes persist. Society's disapproval of sexual activity in senescence is reflected in such common expressions as "dirty old man," "old goat," and "lecherous old fool" to describe a man who pursues sexual interests into his twilight years and "robbing the cradle" to describe an older person who selects a much younger mate.

Grown children have difficulty seeing their elderly parents as sexual beings, and many flatly refuse to believe that parental sexuality could persist into the sixties and beyond.

Yet news reports every so often refute the notion that sex precedes the body to the grave. A man in his seventies will be said to have fathered a child. Unmarried couples in retirement communities will be described as "living in sin." Or sexual "hanky-panky" will be revealed among the residents of old-age homes.

Scientific studies of sexual activity have shown that the sexual urge exists for many more elderly people than society realizes or acknowledges. Up to age seventy, one-half to two-thirds of men remain potent and sexually active. Among women, most of whom are without partners by this age, one in three reports an interest in sex, one in four masturbates occasionally, but only one in five actually has a sexual relationship.

For healthy people, regardless of age, sexual interest and activity can continue throughout life. The best predictor of continuing sexual activity into old age is regular expressions of sexuality in preceding years. Even if there is a prolonged interruption in sexual activity, possibly because of illness or death of the spouse, full sexual functioning can often be restored.

In fact, for a number of reasons the "golden years" may well be the Golden Age of Sex for some people. If not for myths and misunderstandings about sex among the aged, many more people than actually do might continue to be sexually active into their seventies, eighties, and beyond.

Sometimes the very professionals who should help to counter misinformation about sex for the elderly instead compound it. A woman in her mid-fifties who asked her gynecologist for help because intercourse had become less satisfying was told, "What do you expect for someone

185

your age?" The same comment was made by a physician to a man in his late sixties who expressed concern about potency problems. More often than not, anticipating disapproval, rebuff, or even ridicule, older patients won't say anything at all to their doctors about their sexual problems and fears.

Effects of Age in Men

In their pioneering studies of the human sexual response, Dr. William Masters and Virginia Johnson determined the normal changes in sexuality with age. If people know what to expect, these researchers have found, their sexual functioning is far less likely to be impaired by the aging process. In men, these are the gradual changes with age that Dr. Masters and Mrs. Johnson and other sex researchers have elucidated:

● The penis takes longer to become erect. Whereas in young men erection may occur in seconds, often at the mere thought of sexual activity, in older men several minutes of direct stimulation, possibly with fondling of their genitals, may be needed to produce erection.

● Longer periods of stimulation are often needed to reach orgasm and ejaculation. For men who in their younger years reached orgasm before their partners did, this delay with age is often welcome. Some wives who never before attained orgasm through intercourse are able to do so now that their aging husbands have better control over ejaculation.

● There is decreased need to reach orgasm at every sexual encounter. Many older men happily participate in sexual intercourse once or twice a week but desire ejaculation perhaps only once every second or third time. The woman who believes that her partner must be "satisfied" every time they have intercourse may actually do them both a disservice. A man who feels pushed to reach orgasm may shy away from sexual activity of any kind. If the man does not ejaculate, he is able to become erect again sooner and can have intercourse more often.

● The volume of the ejaculation and its force are diminished, and the man is likely to lose his erection within moments of orgasm. He is also likely to require a longer time — twelve to twenty-four hours or more — before he can obtain another erection after ejaculation.

A man who notices one or more of these changes and thinks they herald the end of his sexual ability may create a self-fulfilling prophecy. Fear of failure is the greatest inhibitor of potency. According to Dr. Masters and Mrs. Johnson, "Loss of erective prowess is not a natural component of aging." They found that, barring illness or psychological blocks, a man should retain his ability to have erections well into his eighties.

Effects of Age in Women

The changes in a woman's sexuality with age are fewer. Although some women report a decline in sexual interest with age, this may be more psychological than physical. From a physiological standpoint, menopause should not cause a decrease in desire. In fact, for some, libido is enhanced during and after menopause.

Unlike men, women retain indefinitely the potential for reaching orgasm two or three times in quick succession. However, as with men, the buildup to orgasm may take longer. Because of anatomical changes after menopause, it is more likely that discomfort or pain will interfere with a woman's orgastic ability. The fall-off in estrogen production after menopause results in a thinning and flattening of the walls of the vagina. Less lubrication is produced and a longer period of stimulation (foreplay) before intercourse may be needed for the vaginal walls to moisten. The shape of the vagina may change, and its size and elasticity diminish, resulting in increased pressure on the urinary tract. Some women after menopause have painful spasms of the uterus at orgasm. There is also an increased tendency to develop vaginal and urinary infections, which can cause pain during intercourse.

A women's external genital organs also change after menopause. There is less fat and other tissue protecting the clitoral area, and the clitoris — the seat of a woman's sexual response — is more likely to become irritated than aroused by direct stimulation.

Vaginal discomfort after menopause may be relieved by the use of a vaginal lubricant (jelly or cream sold over the counter) or an estrogen cream prescribed by a physician. However, estrogens, both vaginal and oral, must be used with caution, and frequent gynecological checkups are necessary because these hormones may increase the risk of developing uterine cancer. Dr. Masters and Mrs. Johnson found that the best antidote to the effects of aging on the vagina is to maintain an active sex life throughout middle age and beyond.

Countering Myths and Other Impediments

Contrary to common belief, ordinary sexual activity does not endanger an old person's health. Experts say that heart patients who can perform moderate physical activity, such as climbing a flight or two of stairs, can safely have sex. The heart beats faster during a brisk walk or heated argument than during sexual intercourse.

In at least 70 percent of men who have had prostate surgery, potency is retained. Congestion of the prostate commonly results from sexual abstinence and is actually relieved by frequent orgasm. Diabetes can eventually interfere with potency in men and with orgastic ability in women. But impotence in a diabetic who is untreated is usually reversed by medical control of the diabetes. [See chapter on impotence, page 174.]

Various drugs commonly taken by the elderly, including tranquilizers, antidepressants, and certain high blood pressure medications, can impair sexual functioning in men and women. If the drug is necessary, the doctor often can prescribe a substitute medication that does not affect sexual performance.

In their book, *Sex After Sixty* (see "For Further Reading" below), Dr. Robert N. Butler, director of the National Institute on Aging, and Myrna I. Lewis recommend various ways to enhance sexuality in the later years. They suggest that continuing attention be paid to dress and grooming, good hygiene, regular exercise, and proper nutrition. A couple too tired for sex at night might try the morning, when they are relaxed and refreshed. It also helps to avoid eating a big meal or drinking alcoholic beverages before sexual activity.

If an elderly couple encounters a sexual problem, they should not assume it's the inevitable consequence of age. Many problems can be treated; often counseling to erase misconceptions is all that is required to restore full sexual functioning. Even long-standing sexual problems can often be resolved through sex therapy, Dr. Masters and Mrs. Johnson report.

For Further Reading

Butler, Robert N., M.D., and Myrna I. Lewis. *Sex After Sixty.* New York: Harper & Row, 1976.
Starr, Bernard D., and Marcella Bakur Weiner. *The Starr-Weiner Report on Sex and Sexuality in the Mature Years.* New York: Stein and Day, 1981.

Venereal Disease:
A Growing Epidemic

Perhaps the most telling testimony to the sexual freedom of the 1970's was the dramatic rise in the number of Americans afflicted with venereal diseases. Although the reported number of cases of VD seems to have peaked in the last few years and now may be slowly declining, gonorrhea — with an estimated 2.5 million cases a year — remains by far the nation's most common and costly serious communicable disease. And by 1982, genital herpes, an incurable viral disease, had already afflicted an estimated 20 million Americans and was still increasing.

As one VD case worker remarked, "It used to be that love and marriage went together. Now it's love and sex, and in the passion of the moment people don't think about the possibility of receiving an unwanted gift like VD."

Why the Increase?

In addition to the obvious reason of more people's having sexual contact with more than one partner, factors that have contributed to the VD epidemic include the following:

• The declining popularity of the condom and vaginal jellies and foams, which offer some protection (although by no means a guarantee) against the spread of VD. The pill, sterilization, and the IUD, now the most popular contraceptives, have greatly reduced fears of pregnancy but increased the risk of acquiring VD.

● The increasing mobility of Americans, which makes it easy for infected individuals to spread their disease to many others before they themselves even know they're infected. Some 10 to 15 percent of cases are acquired in foreign countries, and many more in cities far from home. In fact, doctors have been alerted to a new syndrome — CB-VD — in which potentially infected pickups made over CB radio are impossible to trace because most use their "handles," or CB nicknames.

● The large percentage of people who are infected with venereal diseases but have no symptoms that they recognize and unwittingly spread the infections to their sexual partners. The majority of women and a smaller percentage of men with gonorrhea may be unaware of their infections until they reach an advanced stage. An increasing proportion of infections are occurring in the throat and rectum, where symptoms may be lacking or confused with other diseases. Even among those who will have recognizable symptoms of venereal disease, the telltale signs may not show up for days or weeks after a person becomes contagious, giving lots of time for spread to others.

● Increased sexual activity among teenagers, who are often ignorant of the signs of VD or too ashamed to seek treatment. However, public health clinics offer free, nonjudgmental therapy, and both clinics and private physicians can treat minors for VD without parental consent. A national toll-free hot line, 800-523-1885, manned by teenagers, can tell anyone where to go for a free VD examination and treatment.

Neither social standing nor intelligence is a barrier to infection. Some of the "nicest people" get VD. In fact, there is no way short of total abstinence to guarantee protection against these diseases. There are no vaccines, and one VD attack does not grant immunity to future infections by the same organism.

Therefore, it behooves every sexually active person to take certain precautions against VD. These include taking more care in choosing sexual partners; using a condom applied before foreplay begins; using a spermicidal vaginal jelly or foam prior to intercourse; urinating and washing the penis with soap and water before and after sexual contact; obtaining frequent tests for syphilis and gonorrhea if you or your partner has other sexual partners; and, if you get a venereal disease, avoiding all sexual contact until the doctor says you are no longer contagious.

The Common Culprits

You should also know enough about venereal infections to prompt you to treat them with the concern they warrant. If you become infected, it is essential that all your sexual contacts be examined and treated as well, whether they have symptoms or not. For despite the euphemistic name derived from Venus, the goddess of love, venereal diseases can have serious consequences. Following is a description of the more serious venereal diseases common in this country.

Gonorrhea. In men, the usual symptoms — severe burning when urinating and a yellowish discharge from the penis — develop within two to ten days of exposure. As many as 80 percent of infected women and 10 to 20 percent of infected men have no noticeable symptoms. Pharyngeal gonorrhea (following oral-genital contact) may produce a scratchy or sore throat, but usually no symptoms at all. Rectal infection is usually symptomless but may produce anal discomfort and discharge.

Contrary to the widespread belief that the causative organism, the bacterium *Neisseria gonorrhoeae*, cannot live apart from moist, warm, mucous membranes, live bacteria have been recovered from contaminated bathroom fixtures fifteen minutes to four hours later.

A certain diagnosis of gonorrhea is made with a culture that takes two days to incubate. However, a physician can often make an accurate presumptive diagnosis on the basis of symptoms and a microscopic examination of the discharge or cervical smear.

Preferred treatment involves an injected double dose of procaine penicillin plus an oral dose of probenicid, which slows the excretion of penicillin. Public heath clinics commonly give ampicillin and probenicid orally, sometimes repeating the treatment eight hours later. In cases of penicillin allergy, tetracycline may be used.

A repeat culture should be taken within one week after treatment. This is especially important now because some gonorrhea organisms have become resistant to penicillin and may require treatment with a different antibiotic. The disappearance of symptoms, however, is not a guarantee of cure.

Untreated gonorrhea can lead to a generalized blood infection that can spread to the heart or nervous system; to swollen, arthritic joints; and — especially in women — to a pelvic infection that can damage the Fallopian tubes and produce sterility. Symptoms of gonorrhea may be absent in up to half the infected sexual partners of women with gonococcal pelvic disease. If a pregnant woman has active gonorrhea when she delivers, the baby may become blinded by the infection.

Syphilis. An estimated 500,000 people are currently in need of treatment for syphilis, but only about a third of them get treated. Caused by the spirochete bacterium *Treponema pallidum*, syphilis occurs in three stages. At first there is an ulcer or sore, usually painless, at the site of infection. In women the sore may occur internally and not be noticed. It appears in ten to ninety days after infection and heals within several weeks with or without treatment. But without proper treatment the disease is not cured.

In the second stage, after three to six weeks, the large numbers of spirochetes that have invaded the bloodstream produce generalized flu-like symptoms and a rash that is easily confused with other disorders.

The rash, too, will heal without treatment, but again the infection is not cured.

In both the first and second stages the victim can easily spread the disease to sexual contacts. In the third stage the victim is no longer contagious, but his or her body remains under relentless attack. Heart disease, blindness, paralysis, brain damage, and death may eventually result in as many as one-third of untreated patients. Syphilis during pregnancy can spread to the fetus and cause severe birth defects.

Syphilis is diagnosed by a blood test. The treatment of choice is an injection of penicillin, sometimes repeated ten to fourteen days later. Erythromycin or tetracycline, although less effective, may be used in cases of penicillin allergy. A blood test should be repeated every three months for two years to be certain of cure.

Genital Herpes. An estimated 20 million Americans harbor genital herpes infections, and more than 1 million new cases occur annually. The virus that causes this venereal infection is a cousin to the cold sore virus. It produces similar painful sores on and around the genital organs. In women the sores may be restricted to the cervix and therefore not noticed, but the discomfort can be considerable.

The sores heal in two to three weeks, after which the person is no longer contagious. But the virus does not go away. It simply goes underground and is likely to recur. Recurrences, however, are usually less painful then and don't last as long as the initial attack.

There is no known cure for a herpes infection, and there are serious disadvantages to most of the specific treatments. The antiviral drug acyclovir, though not a cure for recurrent infections, can relieve symptoms and may prevent recurrence if taken soon enough during the first attack. In addition, the infection can be treated symptomatically: soaking with a salt solution, sitz baths, a pain-killer, soothing ointments, and possibly an antibiotic cream to prevent secondary infections. It is important to avoid touching your eyes while you have an active herpes infection.

If a woman has a herpes infection when she delivers, her baby may become seriously ill and die. Infection of an infant can seem to come out of the blue. A recent study of herpes-afflicted infants showed that 70 percent of their mothers had no symptoms of the virus that lived in their genital tracts. If a woman knows she has had genital herpes sometime in the past, a checkup near term for the presence of active infection followed by delivery by Caesarean section can protect her babies.

Several studies have linked genital herpes infection to the later development of cancer of the cervix. Accordingly any woman who has had herpes should have a regular Pap smear, preferably every six months, for life.

About three-fourths of the recurrences of herpes can be linked to particular triggering factors. A common trigger is trauma to the skin, such as can occur through injury, rubbing, kissing, shaving, sexual intercourse, menstruation, fever, or emotional stress. For genital herpes that is triggered by intercourse, use a lubricant applied just beforehand. If herpes sores flare up with the onset of menstruation, the use of oral contraceptives may help.

For those who want to know more about herpes infections and to keep track of the latest treatment progress, the American Social Health Association has formed a national group, HELP, Box 100, Palo Alto, California 94302. Membership, which includes a quarterly newsletter, access to a telephone hot line and to local chapters, costs $5 a year. *The Herpes Book* by Dr. Richard Hamilton (published in 1981 by J. P. Tarcher, Los Angeles, and distributed by Houghton-Mifflin, Boston) may also be helpful.

Nonspecific urethritis. For every case of gonorrhea, there occurs a case similar in symptoms in men but caused by any of a number of unidentified organisms. These infections can produce urethral burning and discharge in men and, rarely, may result in a tubal infection in women. They are treated with tetracycline taken orally for seven days. Infants born to women with active infections may develop a pneumonialike illness.

There are a host of other usually less serious venereal infections, including trichomonas and candidiasis, common vaginal infections which can be carried with or without symptoms by men. [See chapter on vaginitis, page 536.]

Since a layman cannot differentiate between these various venereal diseases, a medical examination and appropriate tests should be done on anyone with symptoms affecting areas of sexual contact.

For Further Information and Reading

For additional literature on venereal diseases, contact the American Foundation for the Prevention of Venereal Disease, Inc., 335 Broadway, New York, New York 10013. For information about VD clinics, call your local health department.

Corsaro, Maria, and Carole Korzeniowsky. *STD: A Commonsense Guide to Sexually Transmitted Diseases.* New York: Holt, Rinehart & Winston, 1982.

Birth Control: A Cafeteria of Choices

The last two decades have witnessed a revolution in birth control, which has greatly enhanced the ability of sexually active people to prevent unwanted conceptions and helped couples plan desired pregnancies. Today a couple wanting to delay or prevent pregnancy has a cafeteria of methods to choose from. These methods vary in effectiveness, safety, and desirability, determined not just by factors inherent in the methods themselves but also by who is using them. A method that works well for one couple may be totally inappropriate for another. Similarly, a method that is suitable at one time in life may be undesirable during a later stage.

Following is a description of the leading reversible contraceptive techniques — their effectiveness, side effects, and necessary cautions.

PART I: ORAL CONTRACEPTIVES

The history of oral contraceptives has been marred by an intermittent stream of unsettling reports, each describing yet another newly discovered health hazard associated with the pill. For the 8 to 10 million American women taking the pill, and for their families and friends, these reports have created mounting concern about the safety and wisdom of using these synthetic hormones to prevent pregnancy.

Unfortunately the decision about whether to start or continue using the pill is too often made irrationally, without a real understanding of the risks involved and how they may differ for different women. In the wake of new publicity about hazards it is not unusual for many thousands of women to suddenly drop the pill before adopting an alternative contraceptive, thus exposing themselves to the far greater hazards of pregnancy.

Despite the long list of ill effects thus far defined, the pill remains an excellent and safe contraceptive choice for millions of young women. It is the most effective of currently available reversible methods, preventing pregnancy in 97 to 99 percent of consistent users. The pill has to be taken daily. It works by stopping ovulation, the monthly release of an egg from the ovaries. Oral contraceptives contain synthetic versions of one or two female hormones. Hormone doses in the pills now marketed are much lower than when the pill was first introduced two decades ago. Thus, the hazards associated with pill use have also been reduced.

Is the Pill Safe for You?

The trick for potential users is to determine whether the pill may be hazardous for you and, if not, to adopt certain precautions to assure that you continue to use it safely. The serious health problems that have been discussed in relation to the pill include the following:

Circulatory diseases. In a small but significant percentage of women, the pill has caused death and disability from blood clots, stroke, heart attack and other heart diseases, high blood pressure, and hemorrhage under the skull. A British study of 46,000 women revealed that the death rate among pill users was 40 percent higher than among nonusers, with virtually all the excess risk caused by circulatory diseases. However, this same study and others have shown that the risk of such disorders is almost entirely limited to women past the age of thirty-five and to those who smoke cigarettes.

In light of these findings, pill use is considered unadvisable for women past the age of thirty-five, especially if they smoke; for heavy smokers at any age; for those with high blood pressure, a history of clotting disorders, heart disease, or stroke; and possibly also for women who are obese or who have elevated serum cholesterol levels. In addition, women who develop migraine headaches or whose migraines worsen while they are on the pill are advised to discontinue its use because of an increased risk of stroke.

Pregnancy complications. Some women find that after stopping the pill, their normal menstrual cycles do not return immediately. For a woman desiring pregnancy, this could mean a long period of infertility and necessitate the use of drugs to try to stimulate ovulation. The problem is most likely to arise in women whose periods were irregular before they started taking the pill, and infertility specialists advise such women to use other means of contraception.

Since miscarriage occurs more frequently among women who become pregnant in the first month after stopping the pill, it is best to use another contraceptive for a few months before you attempt to conceive. If the pill is inadvertently taken during the early weeks of pregnancy, it may cause a malformation in the fetus, such as a missing limb or a heart defect. Thus, before you start the pill, it is best to check out the possibility that you are already pregnant.

Cancer. Despite fears based on animal studies that the pill may increase a woman's risk of developing cancer, especially breast cancer, nothing definitive has yet shown up in women taking the pill. In fact, the evidence thus far suggests that the pill may help to protect against breast cancer by reducing the incidence of premalignant breast disease.

In the British study of 46,000 women there has been no increased risk of cancer among pill users. Rather, among those on the pill there have been fewer cancer deaths, especially from breast and ovarian cancer. Nonetheless, the pill is not recommended for women who have had cancer, and many doctors advise against using it in women with a family history of breast or genital cancer.

Women who have a cellular abnormality of the cervix (cervical dysplasia) that persists six months or longer after starting the pill may face an increased chance of developing cervical cancer. A Pap smear before a woman starts using the pill and repeat smears at regular intervals (say, every six months) thereafter can detect precancerous changes that warrant stopping the pill.

Liver and gallbladder disease. Benign but potentially life-threatening liver tumors have occurred in perhaps 1,000 American women on the pill. Any woman who develops abdominal swelling, pain, or tenderness while on the pill should be examined promptly by a physician. Pill users are also more likely than nonusers to develop hepatitis (jaundice), and women with a history of liver disease are advised to avoid the pill. Similar advice is given to women with histories of gallbladder disease, since there is twice the normal risk of developing this problem after two or more years on the pill.

Diabetes. The pill may precipitate the onset of diabetes in women predisposed to this disease, especially those who had diabetic changes during a previous pregnancy. The pill should be used with caution in women with stable diabetes, especially since they already face an increased risk of heart disease. If a diabetic takes the pill, periodic blood sugar and glucose tolerance tests are advised.

Psychological effects. Some women seem to become depressed after starting the pill, but in others, depression lifts, suggesting either that individuals react differently or that the reactions are totally unrelated to pill use. Changes in sex drive also vary greatly from woman to woman.

Ideally, before the pill is prescribed, the woman should undergo a thorough medical examination. This should include taking an extensive family and personal medical history to assess susceptibility to diabetes, high blood pressure, obesity, heart disease, stroke, clotting disorders, varicose veins, jaundice, and cancer of the reproductive tract. The physical examination should include a blood pressure check, pelvic and breast exam, and Pap smear, and it should check for obesity and varicose veins. Laboratory tests should examine the urine and blood, including blood fat and cholesterol levels and possibly clotting factors. Women anxious to protect their health should insist on such an exam before taking the pill. In addition, a checkup at least once a year is recommended for all women on the pill, with special exams done more frequently for those thought to face a higher than usual risk of certain complications.

Remember, the pill is a drug, and every drug has unwanted side effects. The most important ones are described in the "Patient Package Insert," a detailed brochure that accompanies pill prescriptions and refills. Every pill user should read it carefully, be alert to early signs of possible dangers, and report them promptly to her physician.

PART II: INTRAUTERINE DEVICES

The first intrauterine devices (IUDs) on record were pebbles inserted into the wombs of camels by Arabs and Turks who wanted to prevent pregnancy in their saddle animals during long treks across the desert. Intrauterine contraception has come a long way since then, though its past is checkered and its present still marked by some important unknowns.

The original reservation about inserting devices into the uterus — the possibility of causing pelvic infection — remains today the most serious drawback of IUDs. Extensive publicity about certain infrequent hazards has frightened many potential users and led to a slight decline in the popularity of IUDs in recent years. Nonetheless, IUDs are a leading form of reversible contraception, second only to the pill in the United

States, where 2 to 3 million women use one or another form of the device.

In general, IUDs are nearly as effective as oral contraceptives in preventing unwanted pregnancy and are safer than the pill in terms of risk to life. Like the pill, the IUD does not interfere with sexual activity and requires no preparation before coitus. Unlike women taking the pill, the IUD user does not have to remember to do something every day. New forms of IUDs introduced in recent years promise improvements in safety and effectiveness as well as increased acceptance by women of all ages and circumstances who want to avoid pregnancy.

The latest IUDs release tiny amounts of hormone or copper to supplement the contraceptive action of a small device that better fits the natural shape of the uterus. These smaller IUDs can more readily be used by women who have never borne children. Most childless women were unable to use the older, larger intrauterine devices, a factor that had limited the popularity of IUDs. The new devices are also associated with fewer bothersome side effects, such as heavy menstrual bleeding and cramping. In the past such problems have compelled many women to give up intrauterine contraception after a few months' trial.

Still, IUDs, in their new or old forms, are not for every woman. Many factors about a woman's life circumstances, attitudes, anatomy, and state of health should be considered before an IUD or any other method of contraception is chosen. If you are considering an IUD, you should know some basic facts about intrauterine contraception to help you separate truth from hearsay. And if you use an IUD, you should know under what circumstances a visit to your physician is advisable.

How They Work

Modern IUDs are constructed from polyethylene, an inert plastic. The older devices, like the Lippes Loop and the Saf-T-Coil, were designed to fill in the entire cavity of the uterus. They stimulate an inflammatory reaction in the uterus, which may lead to destruction of sperm or fertilized egg or prevent a fertilized egg from attaching itself to the wall of the uterus. This in turn prevents pregnancy.

The newer devices — Progestasert, the Cu-7, and the Tatum-T — are designed to fit in the opening of the womb when it is at its smallest. The Cu-7 is shaped like the number 7, and the others are T-shaped. While the device itself helps to reduce pregnancies, its effectiveness is bolstered by one of two substances — copper or progesterone, the hormone of pregnancy. Tiny amounts of these substances are slowly released from the IUD into the uterus, where they exert a localized contraceptive effect. There is no increase in the level of hormone or copper found in the blood, and normal ovulation and menstruation occur. However, the substances eventually get used up, and the devices must be replaced: annually for the hormone-containing Progestasert and every three years for the copper-releasing IUDs.

The ability of IUDs to prevent pregnancy overlaps that of the pill. When used properly, the IUD ranges in effectiveness from 94 to more than 99 percent, with pregnancy rates highest in the first year of use.

Side Effects

The most common problems associated with IUDs are expulsion of the device from the uterus, excessive bleeding during or between menstrual periods, and cramplike discomfort. On the average, about half the women given an IUD stop using it within two years for one of these reasons. The newer devices are less likely to cause these difficulties, and Progestasert — like the pill — actually reduces the amount of menstrual bleeding.

Expulsion of the device can result in an unwanted pregnancy, if the woman doesn't know the IUD is gone and fails to take other precautions. All IUDs have thin tails that hang through the cervix into the vagina, allowing a woman to check periodically to be sure the device is still in place.

A more serious problem involves pelvic infection, which seems to be increased about fourfold among women with IUDs. The risk is highest for women who have never been pregnant and women with multiple sex partners. These infections can damage the reproductive organs and result in infertility.

Another important concern is ectopic pregnancies, or pregnancies that occur outside the womb. Among every 10,000 users of IUDs, a recent study showed, twelve ectopic pregnancies are likely to occur in a year. Ectopic pregnancies can be life-threatening if not treated promptly. It is not known whether IUDs actually increase the number of ectopic pregnancies or whether these devices are merely less effective at preventing pregnancy outside the uterus than inside it. If a uterine pregnancy occurs with an IUD in place, there is an increased danger of infection, miscarriage, and stillbirth. At least twenty deaths have occurred among women who developed IUD-related infections during pregnancy. Therefore, all IUDs are best removed when pregnancy is discovered. Women who use an IUD for several years and then have it removed in order to become pregnant may experience some delay in conception.

On the positive side, IUDs do not disrupt the normal hormone cycle, interfere with ovulation, cause cancer or birth defects, or prompt the formation of blood clots. In the future IUDs may contain chemicals that reduce bleeding and cramping and counter infection.

Who Should Not Use Them

Women with any of the following conditions should not be fitted with an IUD, according to rules set by the Food and Drug Administration: pregnancy or suspected pregnancy; fibroid tumors that distort the uterine cavity; pelvic inflammatory disease (infection) or a history of several such infections; cervical disease or abnormal Pap smears; vaginal bleeding from some unknown cause; previous ectopic pregnancy; serious anemia; leukemia; or continuous treatment with cortisone types of drugs. In addition, copper-containing IUDs should not be used by women with an allergy to copper. These factors rule out about one woman in five as a candidate for an IUD.

Many physicians are reluctant to recommend an IUD for a young woman who has not yet had children and who has more than one sexual partner. Such women are more likely to encounter venereal infections that could make them infertile. At the least, those who want an IUD should be tested for gonorrhea, which in women often produces no symptoms. [See chapter on venereal diseases, page 188.]

If You Use an IUD . . .

Be alert to the signs of infection — fever, pain, or tenderness in the pelvic area, unusually severe cramping, or unusual bleeding — and seek medical help promptly if these symptoms occur. If an infection is discovered, thorough treatment with antibiotics is needed. You should also check the strings of your IUD each month right after your menstrual period; if you cannot locate them or if you miss a period, a call to the doctor is in order.

PART III: BARRIER METHODS

While the modern methods of birth control, like the pill and IUD, have received most of the publicity in recent decades, the old-fashioned barrier methods have been quietly making a comeback. Condoms, diaphragms, and spermicides (contraceptive jellies, creams, and foams) are attracting the attention of growing numbers of sexually active men, women, and teenagers.

Some want to avoid the side effects associated with the newer methods. Others are seeking greater protection against venereal diseases, which are now epidemic among Americans in all socioeconomic groups. Still others have only sporadic need for contraception and therefore less reason to risk the possible hazards and pay the cost of continuous methods. And some who use condoms or spermicides prefer the convenience of a contraceptive that can be obtained without a prescription, medical exam, or doctor's advice.

Yet many people who might benefit from the use of barrier methods are reluctant to do so because of misinformation about their effectiveness and prejudice against their patterns of use. Many doctors have long disparaged these techniques. When quoting statistics to patients, they commonly cite a failure rate of only 1 to 3 percent for pills and IUDs, the rate associated with perfect use of these methods. But for condoms, diaphragms, and foams, patients are likely to be told a failure rate of 20 to 30 percent, which describes their effectiveness when used *im*perfectly.

Studies have shown that couples who do not want to have any more children use all methods of contraception, including barrier methods, more effectively than those who want only to delay the next birth. Unwanted pregnancies are more likely among couples who play Russian roulette with barrier methods, using them only at times of the menstrual cycle when pregnancy is most likely to occur. For greatest protection they should be used all the time, even during a woman's menstrual period.

Known side effects of the barrier methods are generally limited to allergic reactions or irritations caused by the chemicals or rubber. Spermicidal chemicals can be absorbed through the walls of the vagina, though no hazard has been linked to such absorption.

Experts estimate that if the barrier methods were properly presented to people seeking contraceptive advice, about one-third would choose one of these methods. A statistical analysis that took both effectiveness and health effects into account showed that the safest approach to contraception is the use of a barrier method, with early abortion as a backup if the method should fail to prevent pregnancy.

The pros and cons and proper use of the various barrier methods are described below.

Condoms

A penile sheath made of linen and intended to prevent syphilis was first described in 1564. Today condoms help prevent pregnancy as well as venereal disease (hence the common appellation of prophylactics). They remain today the only approved method of contraception used by the male. Largely because of their use by the armed forces, they are unfortunately associated with promiscuity, which is thought to discourage their use by married couples.

Most modern condoms are made from latex rubber, which has the dual advantage of stretchability and strength. A small proportion of more expensive condoms are made from animal membranes, which provide greater sensitivity. Condoms are sold over the counter in drugstores and are often available from vending machines and through mail-order companies. In this country they now come in an assortment of colors, several shapes (including those with a reservoir tip to catch the ejaculate or those preshaped to the contours of the penis), various textures (dots, ribs, and other projections), and with or without lubricants. Under the supervision of the Food and Drug Administration, they are rigorously checked to assure freedom from defects.

The pregnancy rate associated with condom use can be measured in two ways: an overall failure rate of up to 25 percent per year, which includes those who use the condom inconsistently or incorrectly, and a failure rate of only 3 to 5 percent among those who use it properly during every act of coitus. When used in conjunction with a spermicide that is inserted into the vagina, the method is as effective as the pill.

A condom should be rolled onto the full length of the penis when the penis is erect but before entry into the vagina, leaving a half-inch space with no air inside at the tip. The penis should be withdrawn promptly after ejaculation, with the end of the condom held to prevent it from slipping off. Condoms should not be reused. If a condom breaks during use, immediate application of a spermicide into the vagina will help prevent conception.

Diaphragms

These are rubber cups that are coated with a spermicidal jelly or cream and placed in the vagina to cover the cervix, functioning as both a mechanical and a chemical barrier to sperm. Diaphragms come in different sizes and must be fitted by a physician, who provides a prescription for its purchase. The size should be rechecked yearly, and a refitting may be necessary after pregnancy, abortion, or change in weight of ten or more pounds. A diaphragm generally cannot be used by a woman who has a fallen uterus or overly stretched vagina.

The diaphragm can be inserted at any time prior to intercourse, but if more than a few hours elapse or if intercourse is repeated, additional spermicide should be inserted into the vagina. After a diaphragm is inserted, it is essential to check to be sure the soft cap is covering the cervix. The device should be left in place, and no douche should be used for at least six hours after intercourse.

Studies of the effectiveness of diaphragms show a pregnancy rate of 2 to 3 percent among women who use it correctly and consistently. Overall the failure rate is in the range of 5 to 20 percent. A study by Masters and Johnson showed that the diaphragm can sometimes be dislodged during intercourse that involves repeated mountings or in which the woman is on top.

Large-scale studies in the United States and Great Britain suggest that the diaphragm may protect against cancer of the cervix and cervical infections. The spermicide used with the diaphragm may help prevent venereal disease, though not as effectively as the condom.

The cervical cap, which resembles a small diaphragm that fits snugly over the cervix like a thimble, has returned to the contraceptive limelight in the last few years. Its advantages are its small size, its prolonged wearing time, and possibly its effectiveness without a spermicide. However, at the end of 1981 in this country cervical caps were still considered experimental, to be used only by doctors doing research with permission of the Food and Drug Administration. The cap is intended to be worn for prolonged periods — several days or more at a time — and removed only occasionally for cleaning. One experimental device has a one-way valve that permits uterine secretions to escape but keeps sperm out. Some researchers are concerned about the possibility of infection with a device that is worn for a long time.

Spermicides

The insertion into the vagina of various mixtures to prevent conception dates back nearly 4,000 years. The first such barriers used by the Egyptians were made of honey and crocodile dung. The Greeks used oil of cedar, frankincense, and olive oil. Today most commercial preparations rely on one of two spermicidal chemicals, nonoxynol 9 or octoxynol, applied in a cream, jelly, foam, or suppository. Both ingredients were declared safe and effective by an expert advisory panel to the Food and Drug Administration. Recent studies refute charges that vaginal spermicides might cause birth defects when inadvertently used early in pregnancy.

Creams and jellies generally are recommended not for use by themselves, but rather in conjunction with a diaphragm or condom. Foams and suppositories are also more effective when combined with other methods. One large study showed that by themselves, foams, creams, and jellies resulted in 15 pregnancies per 100 women during the first year of use. Another study showed a 31 percent failure rate for contraceptive foams. Proper and consistent use results in a failure rate of less than 5 percent.

While foams, creams, and jellies are effective spermicides as soon as they are inserted, foaming tablets and suppositories require a waiting period before intercourse of five to fifteen minutes to allow them to dissolve and disperse. One study showed that Encare suppositories, which were heavily and erroneously promoted as "99 percent effective" among teenagers and college students, failed to dissolve within fifteen minutes in 9 of 20 users. Users of foaming tablets and suppositories are advised not to get up and walk about after inserting the contraceptive to assure that they will disperse in front of the cervix.

Spermicides should be applied within about twenty minutes of intercourse and additional applications are necessary each time intercourse is repeated. The products are considered effective for only one hour. Douching should not be done for at least eight hours after the last intercourse.

Laboratory tests have shown that spermicides can inhibit growth of the microorganisms that cause the venereal diseases, gonorrhea, syphilis, and herpes infection, as well as the vaginitis organisms trichomonas and candida. A study of regular users of contraceptive foam showed they had fewer cases of gonorrhea than nonusers. Disease protection requires consistent use of the spermicide at every sexual contact.

Sterilization: The Permanent Contraceptive

Each year more than 1 million American couples find permanent freedom from pills, IUDs, diaphragms, condoms, foam, and the fear of unwanted pregnancies because either husband or wife undergoes a simple operation that ends their fertility. Surgical sterilization today is the leading method of birth control among couples who've been married ten or more years or when the wife is over thirty, and it ranks second only to the pill among younger couples.

Sterilization comes closer than any other method of birth control to reducing the chances of an unwanted pregnancy (it is about 100 times more effective than the pill, the next most effective method), and so far as is known, the health risks of sterilization are one-time risks faced at the time the procedure is done. The pill and IUD, on the other hand, present a continuing risk for as long as they are used. [See chapter on birth control, page 192.]

The important thing to remember about sterilization is that it is a permanent method of fertility control, useful for couples or individuals who are certain they will never want another pregnancy. Although operations to reverse sterilization are under study, their results are currently too uncertain to count on.

If you are considering sterilization, first think through possible situations that might change your decision to have no more children. How would you feel if one or more of your children died, if you were divorced and did not retain custody of your children, if your spouse died, if you remarried someone who might want to have children with you, if you had nothing to fill your life after your children grew up and moved away? You should not expect sterilization to solve emotional, marital, or sexual problems that are unrelated to a fear of unwanted pregnancy.

PART I: FEMALE STERILIZATION

Approximately half of the more than 13 million Americans who were sterilized as of 1982 are women. The female operation, commonly referred to as tying the tubes, is now somewhat more popular than the male operation (vasectomy) largely because new techniques have greatly simplified the procedure and put it more nearly on a par with vasectomy in terms of the cost, safety, and time involved. Short of hysterectomy, female sterilization is the most effective contraceptive.

In recent years a number of women have publicly described the simplicity and positive aftereffects of their own "Band-Aid" or "belly-button" sterilization operations, reports which undoubtedly encouraged others to follow suit.

Female sterilization involves tying, cutting, or otherwise sealing the

Fallopian tubes, which each month carry an egg from the ovaries to the uterus. Fertilization of the egg by the male sperm takes place in the tubes. The operation makes it impossible for the sperm to reach the egg, thereby permanently barring fertility. However, the surgery does not affect the woman's menstrual cycle, change the normal production of sex hormones, or interfere with sexual expression or desire. Studies of hundreds of women who have been sterilized have shown that sexual satisfaction and activity improve in about one-quarter to one-half, remain unchanged in half or more, and deteriorate in at most a few percent.

In the past for a woman to be sterilized meant a major abdominal operation, several days in the hospital, and weeks of recovery. But new techniques developed over the last decade or two (with further improvements continually being made) have transformed female sterilization into relatively minor surgery that can be done under local anesthesia on an outpatient basis, leaving little or no visible scar and requiring only a brief recovery period.

Also changed is the old "rule of parity" that established how many children a woman must have had before sterilization would be permitted. Now, throughout the country, a woman may be sterilized regardless of the size of her family.

The Various Methods

Although female sterilization operations are now much safer than in the past, they still involve anesthesia, surgery, and risk of complications, including, very rarely, death. The various techniques of female sterilization vary in effectiveness and in the likelihood of complications. The procedures most commonly performed today include the following:

Laparotomy. This is the traditional sterilization operation, which involves a large abdominal incision, followed usually by tying and cutting the tubes. It requires about a five-day hospital stay and weeks of recovery. It leaves a lasting scar. Although laparotomy is the most effective approach to sterilization, it has largely been replaced by the safer, quicker, and less traumatic procedures described below.

Laparoscopy. This approach, commonly called belly-button surgery, can be done on an outpatient basis or at most with a night or two in the hospital. It takes fifteen to twenty minutes to complete, but the physician must be highly skilled in the technique. Laparoscopy involves the use of a lighted instrument that gives the doctor a view of the tubes through a half-inch incision made in the lower rim of the navel (which leaves no apparent scar).

First the abdomen is inflated with carbon dioxide gas to allow an unobstructed view and to reduce the chance of injuring other organs. Then the laparoscope is inserted. The doctor may use an operating laparoscope, through which the tubes can be blocked, or a surgical tool can be inserted through a second tiny incision made just above the pubic hairline.

Most commonly in laparoscopic sterilization, the tubes are sealed by being burned electrically, a procedure called cautery or fulguration. The resulting damage to the tubes is extensive, and the chances of reversing the operation are very slim. There is also a risk of burns to nearby organs. Burning of the tubes is more effective if it is combined with cutting out a segment of each tube and sealing the ends.

Instead of burning the tubes, some doctors now obstruct them with clips or bands of silicone to block egg transport. These techniques are considered more readily reversible than burning or cutting, although they have not been fully tested for reversibility in women. The silicone band is a more effective contraceptive than either the tantalum or the spring-loaded clip. The tantalum clip has reported failure rates as high as 11 percent. Other techniques, such as injecting various chemicals into the tubes or inserting plugs of Silastic or other materials, are still experimental.

Although laparoscopy is an extremely safe operation, complications occur in about 5 percent of patients. Most are short-lived, but 1 percent of patients develop serious complications, and 2 in 10,000 die as a result of the procedure. Following the operation, about one-third of patients return to normal activities within a day, another third rest for a day or two, and the remaining third need several days to recover.

Minilaparotomy. In this procedure an incision about one inch long is made just above the pubic hairline, and by manipulation of the uterus through the vagina, the tubes are brought into direct view. Any method of sealing them can be used, but most often they are tied and cut. The operation can be performed by a skilled physician in ten to thirty minutes, usually under local anesthesia, and the patient can go home the same day unless complications develop. Recovery time is comparable to that of laparoscopy.

The rate of complications is also similar to that associated with laparoscopy, but as doctors become more familiar with the technique, the complication rate is falling. Although full evaluation of the method's effectiveness is not yet possible, it appears to be similar to the traditional laparotomy: 4 pregnancies per 1,000 women per year.

Other methods. Less frequently used methods of female sterilization include approaching the tubes through the vagina or through the uterus, which involves no visible incision but is somewhat more hazardous and less effective than other methods. Some women resort to hysterectomy (removal of the uterus) to become sterile. However, hysterectomy is by far the most dangerous method and should not be used as a method of sterilization unless there are also other medically urgent reasons for removing the uterus. Fifteen percent of women having hysterectomies suffer serious complications, ten times more than with tubal sterilization.

[See chapter on hysterectomy, page 232.]

As for the long-term effects of female sterilization, there have been several reports from England stating that years after sterilization, some women develop very heavy and painful menstrual periods that may necessitate a hysterectomy. However, further research is needed to clarify the accuracy and significance of these reports.

The costs of female sterilization operations generally range from $150 to $1,000. Medicaid and about two-thirds of Blue Cross-Blue Shield plans cover part or all of the costs. It's wise to check your policy beforehand. Two states, New Mexico and Virginia, require the husband's consent to the procedure. In Medicaid-funded sterilization operations, a thirty-day waiting period between the request for the procedure and its execution is required.

Reversing female sterilization is a difficult and not highly successful operation. A few doctors who use microsurgical techniques are reporting better results, but on the average no more than 25 percent of women who have their tubes reconnected conceive.

PART II: VASECTOMY

"It was the only sensible thing to do," said a Middlewestern father of four children, only one of them planned. "I just couldn't see my wife staying on the pill for another ten to fifteen years. Her spirits lifted as soon as I decided to have the operation."

He was speaking of his decision to have a vasectomy, the operation that ends a man's ability to father children. As of 1982 more than 7 million American men had voluntarily and permanently ended their fertility through vasectomy. Each year half a million American men join their ranks.

However, a number of "scare" reports describing real and hypothetical hazards of vasectomy undoubtedly have discouraged others from seeking the operation. In addition, many men — and some women, too — harbor unrealistic beliefs and fears about the consequences of vasectomy.

The usual reaction to vasectomy is nothing short of enthusiastic. "At last, we're completely free to make love, without first having to insert, push, pull, or swallow anything," a mother of three who is in her mid-twenties reported. "For the first time since our marriage, we're totally unworried," said a father of four children, all of them born within three and a half years, despite contraception. "Our sex life has never been better."

The Operation

The operation itself is usually a fifteen- or twenty-minute procedure done under a local anesthetic, either in a doctor's office or in a clinic. Through two small incisions on either side of the scrotum, the doctor lifts up the tubes, called the vas deferens, which normally carry sperm from the testicles into the urethra for ejaculation. Each tube is cut to block the flow of sperm. Sperm continue to be formed, but cannot be ejaculated. Instead, the sperm are broken down and absorbed into body tissues. Some surgeons prefer to seal the vasa electrically rather than cut them.

Sterilization operations, which are covered by most insurance plans, usually cost $150 to $250 when performed by private physicians, $75 to $150 in clinics. Many clinics have a sliding scale so that the indigent pay little or nothing. Medicaid covers the cost for men over twenty-one. Two states, New Mexico and Virginia, still require the wife's consent.

Following a vasectomy, there's likely to be some discomfort, pain, and swelling, usually relieved by ice packs, that lasts for a few days to a week. Usually no more than an over-the-counter pain-killer is needed. The scrotum may appear temporarily discolored and bruised.

In a small percentage of cases there occur more serious but treatable complications, including formation of a blood clot in the scrotum (which usually disappears without treatment), infection, and inflammatory reactions. Experts say that there have been no deaths associated with vasectomy in this country.

The operation is commonly done on a Friday afternoon, and by Monday most men are able to go back to work. Some go to work the day after surgery. Doctors usually advise their patients to wear athletic supporters and avoid heavy labor for a week to ten days after the surgery. Sexual activity can usually be resumed comfortably in five days to a week, but it is essential that some other form of contraception be used for the first six to twelve weeks after a vasectomy, until two consecutive samples of semen show no sperm.

Except for female sterilization, vasectomy is the most effective method of contraception. The pregnancy rate among wives of vasectomized men is only about 2 per 1,000 women a year; the pill has an annual failure rate ten times greater.

The main reasons for failure are resumption of sexual intercourse without adequate protection before all sperm that were in storage before the vasectomy have been ejaculated; the presence (rare) of a third vas that the doctor failed to detect; cutting of the wrong tube, leaving behind an intact vas; and, most commonly, regrowth of the vas to permit ejaculation of sperm. To help prevent contraceptive failure caused by regrowth, some doctors recommend that the semen be rechecked six months after surgery.

Safety
No serious long-term consequences of vasectomy have yet been uncovered, despite the millions of operations that have been done. How-

ever, there have as yet been no careful studies following large numbers of vasectomized men for many years, so it's not possible to say with certainty that vasectomy is not related to an increased risk of developing some serious health problem years later.

Most concerns center on the fact that one-half to two-thirds of the men develop antibodies that inactivate sperm following vasectomy. (Such antibodies also develop in a significant proportion of men who have *not* had vasectomies.) Thus far these antibodies have not been shown to have any health effect in men other than to reduce the chances of restoring fertility should a vasectomized man change his mind.

A study of monkeys fed a high-cholesterol diet showed that those that had also undergone vasectomies were more likely to develop cholesterol-clogged arteries. It is not known whether men experience a similar effect. In two studies of men who had suffered heart attacks, no link to prior vasectomy was found. But it would be wise for all men — vasectomized or not   to adopt a heart-saving diet low in cholesterol and saturated fats. [See chapter on fats and cholesterol, page 14.]

As for hormonal effects, if anything, vasectomy seems to increase the amount of male sex hormones produced, but not above the normal range. Also, the sterilization operation does not cause sexual or emotional problems in men who did not have them to begin with and who were properly counseled prior to the operation. Vasectomy does not impair virility or libido, nor does it cause impotence or inability to ejaculate. The absence of sperm has no noticeable effect on the volume of the ejaculate, most of which consists of seminal fluid.

Studies of thousands of vasectomized men and their wives have revealed an overwhelmingly positive response to the procedure. Well over 90 percent of the men who have vasectomies say they would make the same decision now, and they would readily recommend the operation to others. However, adverse psychosexual effects can occur after vasectomy if the men undergoing it are carelessly selected.

Who Should Not Get a Vasectomy

Experts regard the following characteristics as indications that a man may not be suitable for a vasectomy:

• If one partner has doubts about the operation, either about the decision to have no more children or about the aftereffects of surgery.

• If the man is young (early twenties) and has only one child or no children, or if he is unmarried.

• If the couple has sexual problems that are unrelated to their fertility.

• If the marriage is shaky or the couple thinks vasectomy will improve a poor marital adjustment.

• If the man expects the surgery to do more than just make him sterile, perhaps to make him young again or cure a sexual problem.

- If the man is a macho type whose sense of masculinity is closely tied to his fertility.
- If the man has problems with potency, homosexual tendencies, or doubts about his masculinity.
- If the man is mentally or emotionally incompetent to give proper informed consent to the surgery.
- If the man has a serious neurosis or is receiving psychotherapy that could result in a change in marital status.
- If either of the couple believes that the operation is easily reversed should they change their minds.

Possibilities of Reversal

While anyone who has a vasectomy must regard it as a permanent decision, there have recently been considerable improvements in techniques for restoring fertility. These involve reconnecting the vasa, using an operating microscope, a technique in which relatively few urologists have been trained. In selected cases, up to 90 percent of men undergoing microsurgical vasovasotomy (reconnecting the vasa) subsequently ejaculate sperm and three-fourths are able to impregnate their wives.

Older techniques of vasovasotomy, which most doctors still use, result in a pregnancy rate of only about 25 percent. All types of vasectomy reversals involve major surgery, necessitating two or more days in the hospital.

Neither the new nor the old reversal operations are likely to work if the vasectomy was performed many years earlier, if a large piece of each vas was removed, or if there was extensive damage to the vasa. Even under the best of circumstances, in the individual case, there is no guarantee that a reversal operation will work. Vasectomy today must still be considered a permanent procedure for men who are certain that they don't want to father any more children.

The Association for Voluntary Sterilization also advises men not to count on sperm banks for fertility insurance since there is no guarantee that a particular man's sperm will remain healthy and viable after it has been frozen for years.

For Further Assistance

To help men and women find doctors experienced in the techniques of vasectomy, vasovasotomy, and female sterilization, the Association for Voluntary Sterilization, 708 Third Avenue, New York, New York 10017, maintains a roster of qualified physicians and clinics throughout the country. The association can also provide further information about the procedures.

Infertility:
New Hope for Childless Couples

At a time when better birth control, legal abortion, rising costs, and population consciousness have made it possible and desirable for millions of American couples to control precisely their family size, a growing proportion of couples are finding themselves faced with the opposite problem: difficulty having the children they want. Infertility was never a problem discussed openly, and it can be even more embarrassing these days when the societal emphasis is on declining birthrates.

Causes

For a variety of reasons more and more couples today are seeking medical help to have children. There has been an increase in the direct and indirect causes of infertility, which traditionally afflicted about one couple in six. A major factor has been the growing tendency to marry later or at least to delay childbearing, often into the thirties.

Fertility in both men and women declines with age. A woman reaches her peak fertility at age eighteen or nineteen with little change into the mid-twenties. Then fertility begins a slow decline to age thirty-five, a sharper one to age forty-nine, and a precipitous drop as the woman nears menopause. A man's fertility decline is neither as rapid nor as definite, since there is no clear-cut end to it, but a man of fifty is likely to be less fertile than he was at twenty-five or thirty.

The epidemic rise in venereal diseases, particularly gonorrhea, among all social classes and age-groups is contributing importantly to the increase in both male and female infertility. Gonorrhea that is not promptly and thoroughly treated can permanently damage the tubes that carry eggs and sperm. Women are especially at risk of suffering irreversible fertility damage because three out of four women with gonorrhea don't even know they have it. [See chapter on venereal diseases, page 188.]

Ironically, the pill and the IUD, popular methods of preventing unwanted births, can sometimes stand in the way of wanted births later on. [See chapter on birth control, page 192.] Some women, upon stopping the pill, find that their periods don't return or come very irregularly, indicating a disruption of normal ovulation. Most of these women, it turns out, had irregular menstrual cycles to begin with, and the cycle irregularity apparently was further aggravated by the pill. Such women are advised to avoid taking the pill if they expect to want children later. Even a woman who had a normal menstrual cycle before starting the pill might be wise to stop the pill for a month every two years to see if she ovulates and menstruates normally.

The IUD increases a woman's chances of suffering a pelvic infection that may damage the tubes, and infertility experts recommend that women who have a history of pelvic infection should avoid using the IUD if they value their future fertility. To reduce the chances of tubal damage, all pelvic infections should be promptly treated with antibiotics.

Abortion, too, may result in later infertility, although the chances of this happening following a legal abortion are far less than when pregnancies were terminated in back alleys. Between 1 and 5 percent of women develop infections following abortion, some of which may damage the tubes. Multiple abortions or ones done late in the first three months of pregnancy may weaken the cervix (the mouth of the womb) and result in miscarriages of future pregnancies.

A precipitous decline in healthy infants available for adoption has also prompted more couples to seek the aid of infertility specialists. Many couples who might otherwise have adopted a baby after several years of trying to conceive today must pursue other routes if they desire a family.

Treatments

Many infertile couples have been encouraged to seek help as a result of the tremendous and well-publicized progress made during the last decade or so in treating infertility problems. Couples who in the past would have been told, "It's hopeless," or, "Nothing wrong can be found" (yet their infertility persisted), now can have their fertility problem correctly diagnosed and successfully treated by appropriate specialists. More than half of couples with infertility problems can now be helped to achieve pregnancy and childbirth. Drugs to stimulate ovulation, surgery under magnification to repair a woman's damaged tubes and reconnect the sperm ducts of men who had vasectomies (see chapter on sterilization, page 202), and an operation to correct a vein disorder that can impair sperm production are among the recently developed techniques to restore fertility.

Although many people think of infertility as a "woman's problem," in approximately 40 percent of cases a problem in the husband is the main or a contributing cause. A couple's fertility is really a combination of the fertility of the individuals. Thus, Dr. Richard Amelar, a New York specialist in male infertility, points out, "A superfertile woman often can make up for a subfertile man," a compensation which tends to be lost as the woman ages and her own fertility drops off.

Therefore, when the reasons for a couple's inability to conceive are explored, it is crucial to examine the husband as well as the wife. In fact, since a semen analysis is relatively simple and inexpensive, compared to the tests done to assess a woman's fertility, it is advisable to have it done within the first weeks of an infertility work-up. The semen analysis must be done by a laboratory that specializes in the procedure, and two or three analyses should be done before a final pronouncement is made on a man's fertility status, Dr. Amelar advises.

An obstetrician-gynecologist or a urologist who specializes in the treatment of infertility is your best source of referral to a competent lab and your best bet for an accurate diagnosis and proper treatment of an infertility problem.

For Further Reading and Assistnce

If you need help in locating an infertility specialist, write to the American Fertility Society, 1608 Thirteen Avenue South, Birmingham, Alabama 35205 (phone: 205-933-7222), which lists its members by geographical area; please enclose a stamped, self-addressed envelope. You might also check to see if there is an infertility clinic at the medical center or Planned Parenthood clinic nearest you.

Books that can provide further information on infertility problems and their treatment include:

Decker, Dr. Albert, and Suzanne Loebl. *Why Can't We Have A Baby?* New York: Dial Press, 1978.

Harrison, Mary. *Infertility: A Couple's Guide to Causes & Treatments.* Boston: Houghton Mifflin, 1977.

Kaufman, Dr. Sherwin A. *You Can Have a Baby.* Nashville: Thomas Nelson, 1978.

Menning, Barbara Eck. *Infertility, a Guide for the Childless Couple.* Englewood Cliffs, N.J.: Prentice Hall, 1977. Ms. Menning is the founder and director of Resolve, Inc., a mutual support organization for infertile people, with headquarters at P.O. Box 474, Belmont, Mass. 02178.

Stangel, Dr. John J. *Fertility and Conception: An Essential Guide for Childless Couples.* New York: Plume/New American Library, 1979.

211

Prenatal Health: How a Mother Affects Her Unborn Child

It is nothing short of a miracle that my twins were born healthy and normally formed. In fact, it is a miracle they were born at all, considering the hazards they faced at the start of gestation. During the crucial first three months of fetal life, when limbs and organs form, my unborn children were bombarded by infectious organisms and a half dozen different drugs, all of which could have severely damaged or even destroyed them.

The week after I conceived, even before I knew I was pregnant, I came down with a severe case of Hong Kong flu, which I self-treated with aspirin and cough medicine when I could keep them down. The flu yielded to double pneumonia, treated by a physician with antibiotics and a stronger cough medicine. I coughed so hard that I cracked a rib, but the pregnancy continued. Bronchitis and sinusitis followed, and it was three months before I felt healthy enough again to start worrying about the fetal effects of all I had been through. To boot, toward the end of my pregnancy two X rays had to be taken of my abdominal area.

The Vulnerable Fetus

The prenatal period is the most vulnerable time of a child's life. Though it was once thought that the fetus was well protected from external harm, in recent decades hundreds of substances, organisms, and circumstances have been shown to have a malignant effect on fetal development and survival.

Despite widespread publicity about the fetal harm done by such things as thalidomide, rubella infection, cigarette smoking, and alcohol, many pregnant women continue to expose their unborn children to needless hazards. It is now known that fetal vulnerability changes during the course of pregnancy; a substance harmless during the early months may become harmful later on, or vice versa. Furthermore, questions have been raised about the prenatal hazards of sexual intercourse, previously thought to be safe.

About 20 percent of birth defects are caused by environmental factors, such as drugs, viruses, and vitamin deficiencies and excesses. Another 60 percent result from the interaction of some environmental factor and a genetic predisposition. An unknown but presumably large proportion of spontaneous abortions and stillbirths are also attributable to the harmful effects of prenatal exposure to some noxious agent or condition.

Thus, it is important for every woman — whether already pregnant or contemplating pregnancy — to know the potential hazards and how to protect against them. The single most important form of protection is to go to a good doctor (preferably an obstetrician) or maternity clinic as soon as pregnancy is suspected. Early prenatal care, and continued care throughout pregnancy, reduce the risk of stillbirth and death of the newborn by 75 percent. It is also important for the pregnant woman to eat a well-balanced diet, gaining, on average, 25 pounds in the course of pregnancy (somewhat less if she was obese to start with and more if she was very thin). Continuation of prepregnancy exercise habits, including jogging, is not known to have any harmful effect on the fetus or the woman. However, pregnant women are cautioned against deep scuba diving and prolonged sauna bathing since both may harm the fetus.

Hazards to Beware

Other factors to consider include the following:

Drugs. The tragic harm caused by the sleeping potion thalidomide when administered during pregnancy apparently has had little effect on the drug-taking habits of most pregnant women. A study in 1973 showed that 82 percent of women had taken prescription drugs during their pregnancy, with an average of four drugs prescribed per woman. A study five years later that included over-the-counter medications showed that all the women had taken two or more drugs, with the average exposure being eleven drugs per woman.

Virtually all drugs can cross the placenta and reach the fetus.

Eighty percent of drugs currently on the market have never been tested for safety during pregnancy. The list of drugs that are known to be potentially harmful to the fetus includes aspirin (near the end of pregnancy acetaminophen is a safer choice); the antibiotics tetracycline, streptomycin, and sulfa drugs (penicillin, ampicillin, and cephalosporins are safer); antithyroid drugs; the anti-inflammatory drugs indomethacin and naproxen; the anticonvulsant Dilantin; the anticoagulant warfarin; the high blood pressure drugs thiazide diuretics and reserpine; iodine (including that used in vaginal douches); excessive amounts of the essential nutrients vitamins C, D, and K, calcium, and copper; sex hormones (including oral contraceptives); and the tranquilizer Librium.

The rule of thumb during pregnancy is to take no medication — not even an antacid, antiemetic, or a laxative — unless it is essential to your health and prescribed for you by a physician who knows you are or might be pregnant.

Alcohol. Women who drink heavily during pregnancy face a high risk of bearing a child with a syndrome of defects, including abnormal facial features, heart defects, growth retardation, and mental and motor deficiencies. It is now known that more moderate drinking is also harmful. Women who drink one to two ounces of absolute alcohol (the equivalent of two to four cocktails, beers, or glasses of wine) a day have nearly a 10 percent risk of bearing a child with some features of fetal alcohol syndrome, and those who drink this amount twice a week face an increased risk of spontaneous abortion. A single drink toward the end of pregnancy can temporarily abolish fetal "breathing" motions.

Since it is not yet known what, if any, amount of alcohol might be safe, experts now recommend that pregnant women keep their drinking to a bare minimum or abstain completely.

Caffeine. Miscellaneous reports of increased rates of spontaneous abortion and birth defects among coffee drinkers and a variety of animal tests have prompted the federal Food and Drug Administration to recommend that women stop or reduce their consumption of coffee, tea, and other caffeine-containing products during pregnancy.

Tobacco. Cigarette smoking during pregnancy interferes with the blood and oxygen supply to an unborn child, resulting in an increased risk of spontaneous abortion, stillbirth, prematurity, reduced birth weight, pregnancy complications, death of the newborn, crib death, cleft lip and cleft palate, strabismus (eye that turns in or out), and hernias, as well as long-term adverse effects on growth and development. Children of smoking mothers score lower on tests of neurological, psychological, and intellectual ability and are more likely to be irritable and hyperactive than those of nonsmokers.

Infections. The list of infections that can harm the fetus if they occur during pregnancy includes rubella (once called German measles), regular measles, mumps, herpes simplex virus, syphilis, gonorrhea, viral hepatitis (in the second half of pregnancy), cytomegalovirus, toxoplasmosis, and influenza. With few exceptions, a woman should not be immunized with live virus vaccines during pregnancy. Flu vaccine is recommended only for pregnant women with serious underlying diseases. If avoidable, travel to foreign countries where shots are required against such infections as yellow fever, cholera, typhoid, etc., is not recommended.

To protect against toxoplasmosis (spread through raw meat and cat feces), pregnant women are urged to eat only thoroughly cooked meats, wash hands after handling raw meat, and avoid handling cat litter boxes and anything that may be contaminated with cat feces. An experimental vaccine is under study against cytomegalovirus, which can impair brain development even if the newborn has no obvious symptoms of infection.

A recent study of nearly 27,000 pregnancies revealed a link between potentially harmful infections of the amniotic fluid (in which the fetus floats) and sexual intercourse occurring within the month before delivery. These infections sometimes result in stillbirth and neonatal death. Aside from abstinence during pregnancy, a possible preventive might be use of a condom and careful cleansing of the genital area of both partners prior to intercourse.

Radiation. Though prenatal exposure to X rays in dosages up to 10,000 mrad (well above the amount used in ordinary diagnostic X rays) apparently does not cause birth defects, higher doses can, and there is conflicting evidence that the risk of childhood leukemia may be increased at far lower dosages.

Several protective measures are recommended: (1) nonemergency X ray examinations of a woman's abdominal and pelvic area should be done within ten days of her last menstrual period and, if she is pregnant, postponed until after pregnancy; (2) when feasible, ultrasound, which involves no radiation and has as yet no known harmful fetal effects, should be used instead of X rays during pregnancy (although even ultrasound should be kept to a minimum); (3) during all nonabdominal X rays, the woman's abdominal and pelvic area should be protected with a lead apron; (4) all nondental X ray examinations should be done by a fully qualified radiologist, and (5) a woman should complete X ray examinations of her teeth and gums prior to becoming pregnant.

The risks of ordinary radiation exposure are not sufficient to justify an abortion should an X ray have to be taken during pregnancy. Nor is it wise for a pregnant woman to refuse an essential X ray examination.

For Further Reading

Gots, Ronald E., M.D., and Barbara A. Gots, M.D. *Caring for Your Unborn Child.* New York: Bantam, 1979.

Norwood, Christopher. *At Highest Risk.* New York: McGraw-Hill, 1980, and Middlesex, England: Penguin, 1981.

214

Amniocentesis:
The Miracle of Prenatal Diagnosis

Thanks to a revolutionary technique called amniocentesis, through which doctors can assess the health of an unborn child, countless couples who would not otherwise have dared to risk a pregnancy have had one or more healthy children. Many others have been spared the tragic birth of a child with a life-limiting disorder. For still others, planned abortion was averted when prenatal diagnosis revealed that the fetus would not have the expected abnormality.

Amniocentesis allows doctors to examine the cells of a young fetus to see if it might be afflicted with any of a variety of serious genetic disorders. When prenatal diagnosis reveals a defect, as happens in about 5 percent of cases, the pregnancy can be terminated and the couple can try again to have a healthy baby.

A Chicago woman whose two sisters were mentally retarded had refused to have a baby out of fear that the disorder ran in her family. Medical studies, indeed, showed that the retardation was caused by an abnormal chromosome — a strand of genes in the women's cells — and that each of the woman's children would have a fifty-fifty chance of inheriting the abnormality.

Since it would be possible through amniocentesis to tell whether the fetus carried the abnormality, the woman decided to become pregnant. Examination of fetal cells removed during the sixteenth week of pregnancy showed that the child would have the defective chromosome. The woman had an abortion and tried again. During the second pregnancy amniocentesis indicated that this time the fetus had been spared the defect, and five months later the birth of a healthy boy confirmed the happy diagnosis.

The Procedure

Amniocentesis involves inserting a needle — resembling a large hypodermic — through the abdomen into the womb during the fourth month of pregnancy and extracting a small amount of the amniotic fluid that surrounds the fetus. A local anesthetic is used. The test is nearly always completed without overnight hospitalization.

To make sure that the needle will not puncture the placenta or the fetus, an examination by ultrasound is carried out first to locate the fluid-filled portion of the womb. The ultrasound examination can also reveal a multiple pregnancy and alert the doctor to the need to test for the normality of two or more fetuses.

The extracted fluid contains cells shed by the fetus. These cells are then grown in the laboratory and analyzed for the number and shape of the fetal chromosomes or for a crucial enzyme or a metabolic product that would indicate the presence or absence of the disorder in question. Doctors cannot determine through amniocentesis that the fetus is completely healthy and normally formed, only whether a particular disorder is present. It is not feasible to check a sample of amniotic fluid cells for all those defects that can be diagnosed prenatally.

What It Detects

Currently nearly 200 different genetic disorders can be diagnosed through amniocentesis, including some of the most common and more serious: all the major chromosomal abnormalities, scores of biochemical disorders in which body chemicals that are missing or that accumulate in excess impair the baby's development, and structural defects of the brain and spinal column.

Since it is also possible to determine the sex of the unborn child through amniocentesis, at least thirty genetic diseases that are passed on only to sons can be prevented by selectively aborting male fetuses. (However, experts say the procedure is not so safe that it should be used merely to satisfy parental curiosity or to select a boy or girl.) Still experimental are prenatal treatments — instead of abortion — to prevent abnormal development of a fetus found to be afflicted with a genetic disorder.

More than half the women who undergo amniocentesis today are age thirty-five or older. They have it done not because they fear a genetically transmitted disease but because older mothers — and possibly older fathers as well — run a greatly increased risk of producing a child with an abnormal number of chromosomes. The most common of these chromosomal abnormalities results in a disorder called Down's syndrome (formerly referred to as mongolism), producing mental retardation and, usually, early death.

Among women in their early twenties Down's syndrome occurs once in about 2,500 births. However, the risk increases dramatically after thirty-five, rising to 1 in 250 among women thirty-five to thirty-nine, 1 in 100 among women forty to forty-four, and 1 in 46 among women forty-five and older. Women over thirty-five have only 10 percent of the babies born in this country, but they have half of those born with Down's syndrome.

Amniocentesis is now generally recommended for any woman who becomes pregnant after age thirty-five, unless she would not have an abortion even if an abnormality were found. Today more and more women are having children late in life — they may have married late, or preferred to establish a career first, or reversed an earlier decision to remain childless — and amniocentesis for reasons of age is becoming increasingly popular.

Nonetheless, the National Foundation–March of Dimes estimates that only a small proportion of the pregnant women who could benefit from amniocentesis undergo it. In addition to those over thirty-five, such women would include those who have already given birth to children with inherited defects diagnosable through amniocentesis and those who are known to carry the genes for such defects and could pass them on to their offspring.

Specialists at several medical centers are now working to perfect a technique through which samples of fetal blood or other fetal tissues can be obtained and analyzed for any of several severe disorders, such as sickle-cell anemia. A number of pregnancies have been correctly diagnosed so far, but generally speaking, the procedure is still considered too hazardous and uncertain for common use.

The Safety Question

As for amniocentesis itself, a study conducted by the National Institute of Child Health and Human Development among 2,032 pregnant women from July 1971 through June 1973 showed that the procedure "is highly accurate and safe" and "does not significantly increase the risk of fetal loss or injury." Nor is the mother harmed. Diagnosis of the presence or absence of the fetal defect in question was accurate in 99.4 percent of cases. Fewer than 4 percent of the 1,040 women in the study who underwent amniocentesis had elective abortions.

Despite this record of safety and accuracy, some doctors discourage their patients from undergoing the test, warning them of possible fetal harm or miscarriage. One thirty-seven-year-old Minnesota woman, told

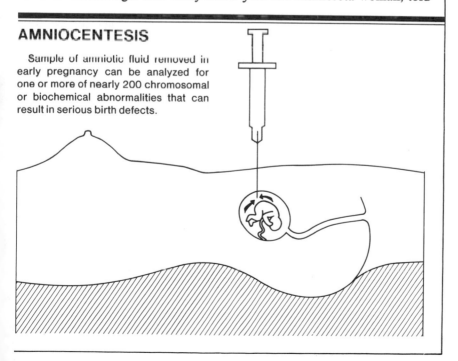

AMNIOCENTESIS

Sample of amniotic fluid removed in early pregnancy can be analyzed for one or more of nearly 200 chromosomal or biochemical abnormalities that can result in serious birth defects.

by her doctor that amniocentesis was too dangerous, is now very bitter about his advice. Her child was born with Down's syndrome and is severely retarded.

The usual fee for amniocentesis is about $400. Medicaid covers it, and some insurance plans reimburse for part or all of the costs.

For Further Information

For accuracy and safety, it is critically important that amniocentesis be done by hospital-based experts, with the cells analyzed by experienced laboratories. The National Foundation, P.O. Box 2000, White Plains, New York 10612, and the National Genetics Foundation, 250 West Fifty-seventh Street, New York, New York 10019, can help you and your doctor find qualified sources of genetic counseling and amniocentesis. In some areas local or state health departments provide free or low-cost services.

Miscarriage: Myth and Reality

Miscarriage, a far more common and more emotionally devastating event than most people realize, is riddled with myths and misapprehensions that often lead to profound guilt, deep grief, fear of subsequent pregnancies, and, sometimes, irreparable damage to the marital relationship.

"The miscarriage was all my fault. My mother warned me against moving the furniture."

"If only I hadn't reached up into the closet to get down that suitcase."

"We should never have gone on that long bike ride."

"I know this happened because I had an abortion before I was married."

"We made love last night. I'm sure that's why I lost the baby."

"I felt that God was punishing me — that because I didn't want this pregnancy, here I was miscarrying."

All these statements, taken from interviews with women who had miscarriages, are based on mistaken beliefs. It is nearly impossible to disrupt a normal, healthy pregnancy through physical exertion or trauma, as many women who have attempted self-abortion have discovered. In a majority of cases, detailed studies have shown, miscarried fetuses are genetically or anatomically abnormal and unable to survive. However, couples suffering miscarriages are rarely told this and commonly attribute their misfortune to a host of events that can be guilt-provoking and life-disrupting.

A Common Event

Numerous surveys have shown, furthermore, that 15 to 20 percent of known pregnancies end in spontaneous abortion, the medical term for miscarriage. In addition, a much higher percentage of very early conceptions — before a diagnosis of pregnancy is made — are spontaneously aborted.

The risk that a miscarriage will occur in the first three months of pregnancy increases with advancing age of the woman, roughly doubling from the twenties to the early thirties, and then doubling again from the early to the late thirties. With more women today postponing childbearing until their thirties — and then wanting a child as soon as they've decided they are ready for motherhood — miscarriage is likely to become more common and more poignant an experience, according to Pamela Daniels and Kathy Weingarten, Wellesley College researchers and authors of *Sooner or Later: The Timing of Parenthood in Adult Lives* (New York: W. W. Norton, 1982).

Despite the frequency of miscarriage and the severe emotional trauma it can cause, it remains an almost taboo subject. Even after the event there is often a breakdown in communications between doctor and patient that leaves couples with festering emotional wounds. The proper time and place for discussing why a miscarriage occurred and what it might mean for future pregnancies are at a woman's follow-up visit to her physician.

Dr. Rhonda Klorman, a clinical psychologist at the University of Rochester who had a miscarriage herself, urges that husbands be included in the discussion. "Too often the husband is forgotten, though it's just as much his loss as his wife's," she explained. She told of a man who became impotent during his wife's second pregnancy because she lost the first baby soon after sexual intercourse; no one had corrected his mistaken belief that sexual intercourse caused the miscarriage.

Causes and Treatments

According to Dr. Richard Schwarz, chairman of obstetrics and gynecology at the Downstate Medical Center in Brooklyn, New York, the fetus in 60 percent of spontaneously aborted pregnancies is either anatomically or genetically abnormal. Long-standing beliefs that physical or emotional trauma or hormonal irregularities are common causes of miscarriage have been disproved; only occasionally are hormonal imbalance, infection, or immunological factors involved. There is no solid evidence that particular vitamins or minerals make a difference.

"Miscarriage is a natural-selection process in most cases, not someone's fault," Dr. Schwarz said. "A healthy pregnancy continues whether you hang curtains or stay in bed."

This is particularly true of miscarriages during the first three months of pregnancy, which represent the overwhelming majority. Later, however, miscarriage is more likely to result from anatomical abnormalities in the mother, such as a cervix that cannot withstand the pressure of the expanding uterus. This problem, called incompetent cervix, can usually be treated by stitching to prevent it from opening prematurely in subsequent pregnancies. If uterine fibroids are a problem, they can be removed surgically.

When no other basis can be found for repeated miscarriages, an immunological abnormality is the likely cause, according to Dr. Ross E. Rocklin and colleagues in Boston. In eight patients studied, all lacked antibodies known as blocking factor, which apparently protects the fetus from being rejected as foreign tissue. It may eventually be possible to supply the missing antibodies.

If a woman has had one or more miscarriages, there is a 25 to 40 percent chance that she will have another, a probability not much greater than the 20 percent she faced before her first pregnancy. Dr. Joe Leigh Simpson, obstetrician at the Northwestern University Medical Center, maintains that after two miscarriages a full medical work-up is in order. For repeated first-trimester miscarriages the work-up should include chromosome studies of husband and wife, a thyroid function test, and a biopsy of the endometrium (lining of the uterus) to check for hormonal deficiencies. Repeated miscarriages later in pregnancy warrant a careful examination, by X ray and other methods, of the uterus and cervix.

Both Dr. Schwarz and Dr. Simpson emphasize that there is no justification for giving hormones to a woman who is threatening to abort — for example, bleeding slightly or having uterine cramps — in the absence of clear-cut evidence of hormonal insufficiency. There is considerable fear that hormone treatment could cause birth defects and, possibly, cancer in fetuses that survive.

Dr. Simpson, noting that a patient threatening to abort is usually told to go home, get into bed, and relax, said: "In reality, for first-trimester abortion, I don't think it matters one way or another. It just gives the doctor something to say and gives the woman the feeling she's done what she could."

Even this advice can backfire, Dr. Klorman maintains, since "the woman is often not told of the low probability that it will make any difference. Can she get out of bed to go to the bathroom? When the miscarriage finally does occur, the woman may blame herself for getting up to get a book!" Furthermore, Dr. Simpson said, "Chances are you're aborting because nature wants you to. It doesn't make sense to try to stop that."

The situation is different for threatened abortion later in pregnancy. Then bed rest and the use of drugs that relax an "irritable" uterus may indeed help to save an otherwise healthy fetus.

The Emotional Aftermath

Although some couples recover quickly after a miscarriage, it provokes in others a deep, prolonged mourning reaction and fear that they will never be able to have a child. Some arm themselves against repeated disappointment by "ignoring" the next pregnancy — delaying a pregnancy test and a visit to a doctor — because they fear another miscarriage. Dr. Klorman recalled that in her second pregnancy she kept herself from getting excited about it for a long time and then became deeply depressed when she reached the same stage at which she had had the miscarriage. Now, after the birth of a healthy child, she said, "The pain abates, but you never really forget."

For Further Reading

Borg, Susan, and Judith Lasker. *When Pregnancy Fails: Families Coping with Miscarriage, Stillbirth, and Infant Death.* Boston: Beacon Press, 1981.

Friedman, Dr. Romo, and Bonnie Dauber Gradstein. *Surviving Pregnancy Loss.* Boston: Little Brown, 1982.

Pizer, Hank, and Christine O'Brien Palinski. *Coping with a Miscarriage.* New York: Dial Press, 1980.

Caesarean Births: Medical Progress or Regression?

At a time when more and more women are insisting on "natural" childbirth, an increasing proportion of babies are being delivered by what most women consider the least natural way of all — Caesarean section. Nationally one in five births is now by Caesarean — four times the rate in 1970 — and in some hospitals as many as 40 percent of babies are born via a surgical incision through the mother's abdomen instead of vaginally after passage through the birth canal.

221

Some view this trend with alarm and charge that many of the operations are unnecessary. Others regard it as a progressive move in obstetrics that is helping to bring forth living, healthy babies in situations that might otherwise be tragic. Recent surveys suggest that both views are correct, depending on the circumstances.

For the parents a Caesarean delivery is often a traumatic experience for which they are totally unprepared. The fathers may feel left out and helpless; the mothers may be overwhelmed with disappointment and taken aback by the pain and temporary incapacitation that follow all major surgery. Since the large majority of Caesareans are last-minute operations, decided upon after labor has begun, it behooves every pregnant woman to know something about the operation and its aftermath. At least one study showed that couples who were knowledgeable about Caesareans, who understood the reasons for them and knew what to expect, experienced less postpartum emotional trauma as a result.

There are now increasing numbers of prenatal classes for couples who are anticipating a Caesarean delivery as well as postnatal support groups for women who are trying to adjust to a Caesarean birth. More and more Caesareans are being done under local anesthesia, and some hospitals now allow fathers to remain with their wives during a Caesarean delivery, a move that seems to make the entire experience less trying for both.

Why the Increase in Surgical Deliveries?

Whereas in the past obstetricians concerned themselves mainly with the mother and delivery, today they are much more interested in the quality of the product they deliver. This new focus on the welfare of the baby is the main reason for the recent upsurge in Caesarean births. Until recently Caesareans were considered operations of last resort, to be done only after extended efforts to deliver the baby vaginally had failed. However, now that all surgery, including Caesarean section, is much safer thanks to improvements in anesthesia, obstetricians are departing from the "heroic" measures of the past which too often resulted in the delivery of a brain-damaged or stillborn baby.

Rather than risk injuring the baby through the use of forceps or by turning the baby around in the womb, doctors today are more inclined to operate when an easy vaginal delivery is not forthcoming. Thus, most breech or transverse babies — those that are not lying head down in the womb — are today delivered by Caesarean.

At the same time new equipment has enabled doctors to monitor the effects of labor on the unborn baby. They can detect when a fetus is in distress and predict which babies may be harmed if a vaginal delivery is allowed to proceed. Unfortunately, however, electronic fetal monitoring came into widespread use before doctors fully appreciated the significance of the abnormalities it can detect, and many babies today who would have had no problem with a vaginal delivery are being delivered surgically.

Other reasons for performing Caesareans include the following:

- The failure of labor to progress satisfactorily perhaps because of a too-tight fit through the birth canal.
- A delivery complication, such as the appearance of the placenta or umbilical cord before the baby's head, which could result in a loss of oxygen to the baby.
- A complication in the mother, such as diabetes or severe high blood pressure, which could endanger her health and possibly that of her baby if she had a natural delivery.
- A previous birth by Caesarean, which in rare circumstances can lead to rupture of the uterus if a subsequent pregnancy goes to term and the woman goes into labor.
- The threat of malpractice suits, which prompts some physicians to operate when there is the slightest doubt that a healthy baby would result from a vaginal delivery. In an informal survey of fifty leading obstetrical experts in 1975, nearly all mentioned the threat of malpractice as a reason for the recent growth in the Caesarean birthrate.

The Risks of Caesareans

Although much safer than in the past, Caesareans still entail some risks to the mother and to the baby as well. The death rate among Caesarean mothers today is one-tenth what it was in the 1940's, but a Caesarean is still two to four times more hazardous than a vaginal delivery. Major complications, which in one recent study occurred in 6 percent of cases, include hemorrhage, serious infections, blood clots, and injury to the bladder or intestines. Approximately a third of Caesarean mothers suffer some complications as a result of the surgery.

The major risk to the baby born by Caesarean is premature delivery. This can happen when the Caesarean is scheduled in advance, usually because the woman had a previous Caesarean, and an incorrect estimate is made of her due date. To guard against delivering a premature baby, who may suffer from life-threatening lung disease, doctors in many hospitals first test for the maturity of the baby's lungs by taking a sample of the amniotic fluid and determining the so-called L/S ratio, which measures the relative amount of two chemicals produced by the lungs.

In other cases the doctor may allow labor to begin before operating, thus allowing nature to reveal when the baby is ready to be born. Some doctors, in fact, are letting women with previous Caesareans attempt subsequent vaginal delivery (unless the same condition that necessitated the first Caesarean section is present again); half or more of the women who try it are able to deliver vaginally without strain to mother or child, two studies showed.

Except in the case of an ultraemergency, Caesareans today are often done under a local anesthetic (far less hazardous than general anesthesia) that numbs the pelvic region but leaves the woman awake. While she cannot see the actual surgery, she can hear everything that is going on and can be handed her baby right after it is born. The type of incision has also changed, with most women now getting what is called the bikini cut — crosswise just above the vaginal hairline — which is much less destructive to abdominal muscles and which permits the scar to be covered by a skimpy bathing suit and greatly reduces the risk of uterine rupture if the woman delivers vaginally in subsequent pregnancies.

Following a Caesarean, the woman is given pain-relieving drugs as needed and is fed intravenously until her intestinal tract overcomes the temporary paralysis that often follows abdominal surgery. The average hospital stay in uncomplicated cases is four to eight days. However, full recovery to normal energy levels can take six weeks or longer.

The emotional complications of a Caesarean sometimes last for years. It is not uncommon for women to feel depressed and inadequate for not delivering vaginally as well as cheated out of a natural birth experience. Caesarean fathers may have similar feelings, especially if they prepared for natural childbirth and wound up being banned from the operating room. Breast-feeding, which Caesarean mothers can do as well as others, often helps to counter the mother's negative feelings, but there is little to relieve the father's disappointment.

If you are pregnant, be sure to ask your physician about Caesareans and about the hospital's policies governing anesthesia and father participation, if these are a concern to you.

For Further Information

Caesarean support groups, nearly 100 of which now exist around the country, can help many couples. To find out about such groups and about prenatal classes that discuss Caesareans, contact the Lamaze or other childbirth preparation course in your area or write to one of the following groups:

Caesarean Birth Association, 133-29 122nd Street, South Ozone Park, New York 11420; C-SEC, 181 High Street, North Billerica, Massachusetts 01862; Maryland Caesarean Section Association, Inc., 2403 Shellydale Drive, Baltimore, Maryland 21208; or International Childbirth Educational Association, P.O. Box 20852, Milwaukee, Wisconsin 53220.

The following books may also prove helpful:

Donovan, Bonnie. *The Caesarean Birth Experience.* Boston: Beacon Press, 1977.

Hausknecht, Dr. Richard, and Joan Rattner Heilman. *Having a Cesarean Baby: The Mother's Complete Guide for a Happy and Safe Cesarean Experience.* New York: E.P. Dutton, 1978.

Mitchell, Kathleen, and Marty Nason. *Caesarean Birth: A Couples' Guide for Decision and Preparation.* San Francisco: Harbor/Putnam, 1981.

Wilson, Christine Coleman, and Wendy Roe Hovey. *Caesarean Childbirth: A Handbook for Parents.* New York: Dolphin/Doubleday, 1980.

Menstruation: Problems and Solutions

In the first century A.D. the Roman naturalist Pliny described menstruating women as capable of turning milk and wine sour, ruining crops, killing bees, rusting iron, and driving dogs mad. In Leviticus the menstruating woman is proclaimed "unclean" (spiritually dangerous), and anyone who touches her or anything she touches also becomes unclean. Even into the twentieth century, say three women (Janice Delaney et al.) who wrote *The Curse, a Cultural History of Menstruation* (New York: New American Library, 1977), beliefs that menstruating women were tainted persisted: A permanent wave during the menses would not take, plants would wither and die, meat would spoil, butter would not churn, and bread would not rise. No normal bodily function has been the subject of as much myth, superstition, shame, pain, confusion, and concern as the monthly shedding of the uterine lining by women of childbearing age.

Rarely are the menses thought of positively as the periodic reaffirmation of womanliness and health. When pregnancy is unwanted, a delay of a few days in the start of menses is the cause of great anxiety. When pregnancy is wanted, the arrival of menses heralds disappointment and depression.

When I was in high school in the 1950's, girls who were menstruating were said to be "unwell" and were excused from participation in gym class. Many stayed home altogether and spent a day or two in bed with a heating pad. A decade later the physical and emotional upheaval that commonly precedes the menses was said by some public figures to make women inferior and incapable of assuming demanding jobs, such as the presidency, which required mental and physical stability seven days a week.

Only recently have many such old wives' tales been exposed for what they are. Exercise has been shown to be beneficial to menstruating women. An American Olympic swimmer broke a world record and won three gold medals during the height of her period. Although about 70 percent of women experience one or more premenstrual symptoms, it is the rare woman who is physically or emotionally unable to carry out her normal activities during that time.

Although for centuries women were told to "grin and bear" their monthly miseries and suffer in silence, recent studies show that most menstrual problems have a physical basis. The vast majority are caused by cyclical changes in the secretion of hormones and other body chemicals and the effects of these substances on various tissues. Further, the new research demonstrates, women who are seriously bothered or incapacitated by these changes can usually be helped significantly by one or more simple treatments. For most women it is no longer necessary to suffer in silence or to suffer at all.

The Menstrual Cycle

The menses are the culmination of the menstrual cycle, which commonly ranges from twenty to thirty-six days and averages twenty-eight days. Counting as day one the first day of menstrual bleeding, in the average cycle the period lasts about five days. During the next week an egg is prepared for release from a follicle in one ovary, and the lining of the uterus (endometrium) is built up by estrogen produced by the maturing follicle.

About two weeks into the cycle (days twelve to sixteen), ovulation (release of the egg) occurs, and the ruptured follicle produces estrogen and progesterone to develop further the uterine lining in anticipation of having to nurture a fertilized egg. After about twelve days the follicle stops producing hormones, with the amount dwindling toward the end of this time. If the egg has not been fertilized, the hormone levels drop and buildup of the uterine lining ceases. The lining is then shed to produce the menstrual flow a few days later, and the cycle begins anew.

In the average American female, menarche — the first menses — starts between the ages of twelve and thirteen (which represents the end, not the beginning, of puberty) and lasts until age forty-nine, when ovulation ceases and the menopause begins. Thus, the average woman is fertile for about three and a half decades — nearly half her life.

Menarche may be delayed until age fifteen or sixteen, but beyond that (or if other signs of puberty are not present) the girl should be checked to determine if there is a cause, which is sometimes correctable. Similarly, if the menses stop unaccountably much before the age of forty or when childbearing is still desired, an examination may reveal a treatable cause (such as cystic ovaries), and fertility can be restored.

Sometimes prolonged use of oral contraceptives or a crash diet can cause the periods to stop temporarily. Women who exercise very vigorously and whose bodies have little fat (like long-distance runners and ballet dancers) may also fail to menstruate. Drugs can frequently stimulate ovulation and the return of menses in such women, but sometimes reduced exercise and weight gain are needed to restore a natural cycle. If bleeding resumes during menopause a year or more after it has stopped completely, a prompt checkup is necessary, since uterine cancer may be the cause.

It is the rare woman who is "regular" from month to month. Many factors, including emotional stress, can delay the menses or shorten the cycle. If the woman does not ovulate one month, her cycle will probably be irregular, and she may skip a period entirely. Other causes of irregularity include jet lag, the use of tranquilizers containing chlorpromazine or meprobamate, and chronic iron deficiency.

As a woman approaches menopause, her periods generally become scantier, shorter, and farther apart (but occasionally heavier, longer, and more frequent). A woman who uses oral contraceptives can safely "induce" irregularity (delay her period for a couple of days or cause it to start sooner) on special occasions by taking a few extra or fewer pills that month.

Premenstrual Tension Syndrome

Premenstrual symptoms are thought to be largely the result of the cutoff of progesterone, the reputed hormone of tranquillity. Symptoms may include breast swelling and tenderness, pelvic bloating, weight gain (three to six pounds), backache, headache, complexion problems, constipation, fatigue, insomnia, irritability, anxiety, emotional outbursts, and crying spells. The symptoms vary from woman to woman and even differ in the same woman during different cycles.

A recent study suggested that women's perceptions of their premenstrual symptoms can be influenced to some extent by their "knowledge" of where they are in their menstrual cycles. But there can be no denying that for most women the symptoms are real and physiologically based, not "in their heads." Various studies have shown that during the premenstrual and menstrual period women are more likely to commit crimes and suicide and to be admitted to mental hospitals and treated for accidental injuries.

Other women, just before the menses, experience bursts of energy and ambition as well as an increase in sexual desire (probably the result of pelvic congestion). For some, the menstrual period is the best time of month — the one time they are sure they are not pregnant and in all probability cannot become pregnant involuntarily.

Many of the discomforting premenstrual symptoms — the emotional as well as the physical ones — are related to water retention. Accordingly they are best prevented by following a diet high in protein and low in salt, alcohol, and carbohydrates (which hold water in the body) and possibly by taking a diuretic for a week before the period. The over-the-counter menstrual drugs are diuretics, such as caffeine and ammonium chloride, sometimes with aspirin. Stronger diuretics can be prescribed by a physician. Dr. Penny W. Budoff, a family practitioner associated with the State University of New York at Stony Brook and author of *No More Menstrual Cramps and Other Good News* (see "For Further Reading," page 228), recommends Dyrenium (triamterene) instead of the more powerful diuretics that are normally used to lower blood pressure.

Sometimes treatment with progesterone for about ten days brings relief of symptoms. It also helps to get regular exercise and adequate sleep and to limit your consumption of alcohol. Several studies have shown that cutting out coffee (with or without caffeine), tea, chocolate, and colas can prevent breast swelling and soreness.

Valium may be prescribed for a few days before menstruation for women with anxiety attacks. The drug Parlodel, which works on brain chemicals, has been reported to help some women with premenstrual mood changes.

Perhaps the most important step is awareness on the part of the woman and her family that premenstrual symptoms are real and less devastating if others are tolerant and supportive. It helps a great deal if the woman keeps a calendar of her menstrual cycle, alerts her family to the approach of difficult days, and plans her schedule to reduce stress. This is the time for daddy to keep the children out of mother's hair and to walk away from arguments.

Dysmenorrhea

Although most women feel some discomfort during the first day or two of menstrual bleeding, others can hardly walk for the pain. Other symptoms may include spasms of laborlike pains in the lower abdomen, backache, pain in the inner thighs, diarrhea, nausea and vomiting, dizziness, headache, hot flushes, and chills. These distressing symptoms associated with the start of menstrual bleeding can result from a number of physical factors, such as endometriosis (an abnormal growth of uterine tissue), pelvic infection, uterine fibroids, or the use of an intrauterine device. All women with dysmenorrhea should first be checked for such possible causes.

Menstrual cramps usually abate after the start of flow. Aspirin (with or without codeine) can relieve pain, and aspirin's anticoagulant properties may help prevent painful clots in the menstrual flow. Exercise is an excellent preventive, since it helps to ease the flow and relieve congestion and constipation as well as rid the body of excess water.

Recent evidence has shown that dysmenorrhea most likely results from natural hormonelike chemicals called prostaglandins, which are released in the uterus in large amounts at the time of menstruation. Women with dysmenorrhea tend to produce excessive amounts of prostaglandins. These substances stimulate contractions of the uterus and gastrointestinal tract and can cause sudden dilation of blood vessels, effects that account for most of the symptoms of dysmenorrhea.

The majority of women with dysmenorrhea can obtain dramatic relief from drugs that counter the production and action of prostaglandins. Aspirin, a mild prostaglandin inhibitor, helps those with mild cramps; it works best if taken in advance of symptoms. Several prescription drugs are now available, including Motrin (ibuprofen), Anaprox (naproxen sodium), and Ponstel (mefenamic acid). These do not have to be taken until the first sign of menstrual bleeding and only for the duration of symptoms. Side effects are few (they may include constipation, nausea, itching, or dizziness), but the drugs should not be used by women with asthma or ulcers. Some women benefit from taking oral contraceptives, which also inhibit prostaglandins and produce a lighter and less painful period, but they are not recommended unless also needed for birth control.

Bad cramps are most common among adolescents and young women. They generally subside after the first pregnancy, when the cervical opening stretches. Sometimes severe cramps in young women result from an abnormally positioned uterus. Sometimes psychological factors, such as fear or feelings of disgust, are the cause.

Later in life severe cramps and very heavy or persistent bleeding may result from fibroids (benign uterine tumors found in one out of five women past the age of thirty-five) or endometriosis (abnormal growth of uterine tissue), which may require surgery if hormone treatments bring inadequate relief.

Bleeding between periods (other than staining mid-cycle at the time of ovulation) should be checked out medically. It is normal and not a cause for concern if you only occasionally have a heavy period or pass small clots. But women with regularly heavy or prolonged periods (whether natural or caused by an IUD) should have a blood test since they may need an iron supplement to prevent iron deficiency.

For Further Reading

Budoff, Penny W. *No More Menstrual Cramps and Other Good News*. New York and Middlesex, England: Penguin, 1981.

228

Schrotenboer, Kathryn, M.D., and Genell J. Subak-Sharpe. *Freedom from Menstrual Cramps.* New York: Pocket Books, 1981.

The Menopause: A Normal Change

Much of the misery commonly associated with menopause is an outgrowth of society's negative image of this natural, inevitable time in a woman's life.

"The popular stereotype of the menopausal woman has been primarily negative: she is exhausted, irritable, unsexy, hard to live with, irrationally depressed, unwillingly suffering a 'change' that marks the end of her active (re)productive life," notes the Boston Women's Health Book Collective, the authors of *Our Bodies, Ourselves* (New York: Simon & Schuster, 1976). Such misconceptions can easily become self-fulfilling prophecies and turn what might otherwise be a smooth adjustment into a tumultuous upheaval.

If you think cessation of menstruation means a loss of femininity or the end of sex, in all probability it will (though it shouldn't, since sexual response is determined more by psychological than physical factors). If you think it marks the beginning of rapid physical deterioration, you may be more likely to "let yourself go" and become fat and flabby or dress unattractively (although good eating and exercise habits and attention to your appearance can help to keep you looking younger than your years). If you expect your creativity to suffer or your energy to flag, you may then stagnate (though many women have made their greatest contributions after age fifty).

"Menopause is a normal change, not a tragedy, not an immense challenge, not a bad joke — just a change," states the introduction to *The Menopause Book* (see "For Further Reading," page 232). How well informed you are about menopause will largely determine how well you handle it and its aftermath.

Menopause means the permanent end of menstruation. It is the final result of a gradual decline (starting at age twenty-five) in the function of the ovaries. During a woman's reproductive years the ovaries produce the female sex hormones, estrogens, and each month release an egg for possible fertilization. As a woman approaches menopause, her menstrual periods tend to become irregular and scant, until they stop altogether. In some women menstruation ceases abruptly.

After a year of no periods a woman is said to have gone through menopause. In American women this typically occurs between the ages

229

of forty-eight and fifty-two, although some women naturally enter menopause in their late thirties to mid-forties and others undergo an early surgical menopause following the removal of their ovaries. A hysterectomy that removes the uterus but not the ovaries will, of course, bring an end to monthly uterine bleeding and fertility, but it will not precipitate menopause since the ovaries continue to produce hormones and eggs.

Until menopause is complete, it is unsafe to discontinue contraception, because you may continue to ovulate erratically for a while even if your periods seem to have stopped.

Discomforting Effects

After menopause small amounts of estrogens may still be produced by the ovaries as well as by the adrenal glands. In most women, however, the hormonal level is not great enough to prevent totally the two symptoms unequivocally linked to the hormonal shifts during menopause: hot flushes and thinning and drying of the vaginal walls. There is currently no way to predict how severe menopausal symptoms are likely to be in a particular woman, though 75 percent report some degree of discomfort.

Hot flushes — feelings of extreme heat usually confined to the upper part of the body and often accompanied by drenching sweats — can be a cause of extreme discomfort, embarrassment, and sleep disruption. They are caused by an instability in the blood vessels that results from biochemical shifts in the brain.

Hot flushes gradually diminish in frequency and usually disappear entirely within a year or two. Treatment with estrogen drugs is highly effective, though their use can increase a woman's risk of developing uterine cancer. Recent studies have indicated that another hormone, progesterone, and a drug called clonidine also can relieve hot flushes.

The loss of vaginal lubrication and elasticity, which can result in painful intercourse and urinary tract irritation, is also alleviated by estrogen therapy, perhaps applied as a vaginal cream. However, a safer approach is to use a water-soluble lubricant, such as K-Y jelly or Ortho personal lubricant, since vaginal estrogen creams are absorbed into the body and may be no safer than the hormone taken orally.

Because of its potential hazards, estrogen therapy, if it must be used, should be limited to as brief a period as necessary, and the woman should be examined first to detect possible precancerous changes in the uterus, perhaps with repeat examinations annually. A woman considering estrogen replacement therapy should realize that it is no fountain of youth and does not retard visible signs of aging. Estrogen can help to ward off bone loss (see chapter on osteoporosis, page 610) and the fractures that may result from weakened bones. However, continued physical activity (which helps to keep your bones strong) and treatment with calcium and an activated form of vitamin D are safer and may be as effective as estrogen therapy.

The Myth of Lost Sexuality

Aside from possible physical discomfort, however, there is nothing about menopause per se that should disrupt a woman's sexual desire or activity since estrogen, the ovaries, and the uterus have no direct effect on libido. Sex researchers have found that the best way to prevent a loss of sexual capability with age is to continue to be sexually active throughout the menopausal period and beyond. [See chapter on sex and aging, page 185.]

"A woman's sex life during and after menopause is very much influenced by her sexual patterns premenopausally," notes Dr. Sherwin A. Kaufman, a New York gynecologist and author of *Sexual Sabotage* (New York: Macmillan, 1981). "Basically well-adjusted couples are likely to enjoy sexual relations well beyond 'change of life.' "

Sex researchers Bernard D. Starr and Marcella Bakur Weiner, authors of *The Starr-Weiner Report on Sex and Sexuality in the Mature Years* (New York: Stein and Day, 1981), note that sexual intercourse may occur less often as a woman gets older, but the quality of the experience does not necessarily diminish, and for some it actually improves.

For those who find intercourse painful, Dr. Kaufman suggests oral-genital contact and manual stimulation as alternative routes to sexual pleasure. However, he adds, if a menopausal woman thinks she is losing her main purpose in life, "the result is often depression, with loss of sexual interest and activity" caused by the depression.

The Myth of Mental Depression

As for the purported link between menopause and serious depression (so-called involutional melancholia), recent psychiatric studies have shown that hospitalizations for depression and suicides occur no more often during this time of life than at any other. A study by Dr. Myrna M. Weissman of the Yale University School of Medicine found no differences in depressive symptoms, severity, or precipitating life stresses among women younger than forty-five, those between ages forty-five and fifty-five, and those fifty-six and older.

Other emotional disturbances supposedly associated with menopause have not been subjected to rigorous study. Most of the reports of menopause-related emotional instability stem from the files of psychotherapists, who would naturally see only people with problems. There is no scientific evidence to support the notion that many menopausal women become anxious over the loss of their reproductive capabilities. If some do, at least an equal number are elated because they no longer have to worry about an unwanted pregnancy or be bothered by monthly menstrual bleeding. One study of 100 women showed that those with previous psychological problems, such as low self-esteem and little satisfaction from life, were most likely to have difficulties with menopause. Similarly, middle- and upper-class women — who have more options open to them

— have fewer problems adjusting to menopause, studies have shown.

Dr. Sophie Freud Loewenstein, a Boston psychiatrist who is Sigmund Freud's granddaughter, believes that middle age is easier for women who eat well, exercise, go easy on cigarettes and alcohol, and are committed to causes, studies, or careers. She quotes the late anthropologist Margaret Mead, who said, "The most creative force in the world is a menopausal woman with zest."

For Further Reading

Cherry, Dr. Sheldon H. *The Menopause Myth.* New York: Ballantine, 1976.
Gray, Madeline. *The Changing Years: The Menopause Without Fear.* New York: Doubleday, 1981.
Rose, Louisa, ed. *The Menopause Book.* New York: Hawthorn Books, 1977.

Hysterectomy: Cause of Controversy and Concern

In both myth and medicine the womb, when not engaged in childbearing, has been seen as the source of many female woes, ranging from emotional disorders to cancer. Thus, it is hardly surprising that the advent of relatively safe surgical and anesthetic techniques in the mid-twentieth century brought with it an explosion in the incidence of hysterectomy — surgical removal of the uterus, or womb, usually after a woman has completed childbearing.

If the current rate continues, more than half the women in this country will undergo hysterectomies by the age of sixty-five.

In the 1970's hysterectomy, as the leading operation performed in the United States, nearly always by male surgeons, became a cause célèbre among feminists, health care economists, and consumer groups, who viewed much of the surgery as a means of lining the doctor's pocket rather than protecting the patient's health.

Various studies have shown that the hysterectomy rate varies widely: It is twice as high in the South as in the Northeast; it is higher if doctors are paid a fee for doing the operation than if surgery is done under a prepaid health plan; it is higher if only one doctor decides on surgery than if a consultant's opinion must also be sought. Studies of this kind have suggested that about a third of hysterectomies are "unnecessary" and involve the removal of a healthy uterus for reasons that are hard to justify.

Amid such controversy a woman whose uterus is being considered for removal may rightly wonder whether the operation is really needed. A woman's thinking is likely to be further confused by a host of prevalent myths (for example, that hysterectomy causes mental illness or ends a woman's sex life) and over-the-back-fence horror tales of the experiences of neighbors and friends. Thus, while some women undergo needless surgery, others may avoid a hysterectomy that is clearly to their benefit.

Since the vast majority of hysterectomies are elective (nonemergency) operations, the prospective patient usually has an opportunity to weigh the advantages and disadvantages of surgery and make a decision based on the reasons for surgery and what it entails, the circumstances of her life, and the dictates of her body.

What Is a Hysterectomy?

Much misunderstanding surrounds the nature of the operation, what tissues are removed, and with what effect. Hysterectomy — including those called total or complete — involves removal of the uterus and cervix (the portion of the uterus that extends into the vaginal cavity). If the operation is done on a woman who is still menstruating, her periods will stop and she will be unable to conceive and bear a child. But her ovaries will continue to produce hormones until menopause, which may occur a few years earlier than it would have had the uterus not been removed.

Sometimes the ovaries and Fallopian tubes are removed along with the uterus. The operation is then called hysterectomy with salpingo-oophorectomy. In a premenopausal woman it results in surgical menopause: Both her periods and her ovarian hormone production cease abruptly. The woman is usually given hormone treatments to alleviate the symptoms of menopause.

Depending on the condition being treated, the operation may be done from inside the vagina (leaving no visible scar) or through an abdominal incision, usually a horizontal cut made just above the pubic hairline. The abdominal approach enables the doctor to examine carefully the health of nearby organs and is the method used when the uterus is greatly enlarged or cancer is involved.

As with all surgery, hysterectomy has hazards. The death rate is between one and two per 1,000 patients, and as many as half of patients experience one or another operative complication, among them reaction to the anesthesia; hemorrhage requiring a blood transfusion; abdominal or urinary tract infection; abdominal adhesions; injury to the bladder, rectum, or pelvic blood vessels; and life-threatening blood clots.

The surgery commonly involves a week to ten days in the hospital and another three to five weeks of recovery at home before a woman can fully resume her usual activities. However, strenuous activity is usually curtailed for several months, and some women experience prolonged fatigue and loss of energy for up to a year after surgery.

When Should It Be Done?

Doctors agree that hysterectomy is needed for the following conditions: cancer or precancer of the uterus, tubes, or ovary; incapacitating, irreversible damage from infection (pelvic inflammatory disease); large benign tumors (fibroids) that cause pressure or bleed excessively; uterine bleeding that does not respond to D and C (dilatation and curettage) or hormone therapy; severe endometriosis (misplaced growth of uterine tissue); a uterus severely damaged by childbirth or abortion; and prolapse of the uterus, in which it drops into or through the vagina and causes pain or pressure.

There is a gray zone in which medical opinions differ. This usually involves a woman near or past menopause who has extreme abnormal bleeding or pain but no apparent uterine abnormality. Some regard hysterectomy as the preferred alternative to frequent examinations, repeated D and C, or prolonged hormone treatments.

Finally, there is an area of great conflict: removal of an otherwise normal uterus as a means of contraception or to prevent the later development of medical problems, including cancer. Tubal ligation and other methods of female sterilization are far safer than hysterectomy, although in many Roman Catholic hospitals hysterectomy is done to skirt the church's prohibition of voluntary sterilization.

Most experts say the surgery cannot be justified as a cancer preventive except possibly in women past childbearing who are known to face a high risk of developing uterine cancer. In a woman past forty or forty-five who is undergoing an abdominal hysterectomy for other reasons, the doctor may also recommend removal of the ovaries, since 1 percent of women over forty develop ovarian cancer, a disease that is hard to detect and cure.

Long-term Consequences

Controversy has raged for years over the emotional effects of hysterectomy, with some experts claiming that more than a third of women suffer prolonged depression and others maintaining that 90 percent are happier after the procedure. To a large extent, a woman's reaction may be influenced by her expectations as well as by her emotional health and life circumstances prior to surgery. If a hysterectomy is done on a woman who would have liked to become pregnant, depression is a natural reaction. Similarly, if a woman inappropriately expects a hysterectomy to solve marital conflicts, she's likely to be disappointed.

One study showed that two-thirds of postoperative depressions occurred in women who had had emotional problems prior to surgery. The hysterectomy triggered a recurrence, but so might any other traumatic event in the woman's life. And a woman who incorrectly equates her womb with femininity or sexual responsiveness (or whose spouse holds to such notions) is likely to react badly to a hysterectomy.

When a hysterectomy is done to get rid of life-inhibiting symptoms, such as painful intercourse, frequent and potentially embarrassing bleeding, or loss of bladder control from a prolapsed uterus, the woman is likely to feel much better afterward. Emotional considerations aside, a hysterectomy should not impair a woman's enjoyment of or response to sexual activity, although the quality of sexual response may change in those women for whom cervical and uterine movement enhances the intensity of orgasm.

In one widely quoted study by Dr. D. H. Richards of Oxford, England, 36 percent of 200 women who had a hysterectomy were treated for postoperative depression, and among premenopausal hysterectomy patients, 55 percent required such treatment. Dr. Richards subsequently described a posthysterectomy syndrome of depression, headache, dizziness, insomnia, and extreme tiredness occurring in up to 70 percent of patients.

However, in another study, Dr. Bruce C. Richards, a Colorado physician, asked 340 women, most of whom had a hysterectomy for "quality-of-life" considerations, how they felt afterward. The questionnaire was returned by 80 percent, with the following results: 91 percent were pleased they had had the surgery; 85 percent would encourage a friend to have it; 78 percent said they felt better (less inconvenience, more energy, better sex life, less pain); and only 4 percent felt worse (weight gain, worse sex life, depression). Of course, it is not known whether the 20 percent of patients who failed to send back the questionnaire would have had similar responses.

In January 1981, a British research team described sixty premenopausal patients who were tested before and up to three years after their surgery. No evidence was found of depression or sexual difficulties related to the hysterectomy. In fact, in comparison to their problems before surgery, most showed "improved mood and vigor" and no change in sexual activity. The few who experienced postoperative depression had been depressed prior to surgery.

For Further Reading

Giustini, F.G., M.D., and F.J. Keefer, M.D. *Understanding Hysterectomy: A Woman's Guide.* New York: Walker, 1979.
Jameson, DeeDee, and Roberta Schwalb. *Every Woman's Guide to Hysterectomy.* Englewood Cliffs, N.J.: Prentice-Hall, 1978.

235

Prostate Problems: Combatting Fears of Lost Potency

As the age structure of the population tips increasingly toward the twilight years, we are likely to hear more and more complaints about the prostate, the part of the male genital anatomy that supplies a third of the fluid portion of the ejaculate. Normally an obscure, chestnut-sized organ, the prostate has a propensity for enlarging, perhaps to the size of an orange, when a man is past the age of fifty.

In the process the enlarging prostate can interfere with urinary and sexual functions and cause painful and embarrassing — although reversible — symptoms. Contrary to widespread belief, treatment of most prostate problems does not destroy sexual potency. In fact, potency may be restored by treating patients whose prostatic disease caused painful or weak erections.

In addition to this annoying but otherwise benign overgrowth, the prostate is subject to infections, both acute and chronic, and to cancer. The prostate can be the source of recurrent urinary tract infections in men, and cancer of the prostate is the third most common cancer killer of American men and the leading cause of cancer deaths among men aged seventy or beyond. Paradoxically, up to 20 percent of elderly men seem to harbor a microscopic cancer of the prostate that for unknown reasons remains dormant indefinitely.

The Gland: Its Functions and Problems

The prostate is situated just below the bladder and surrounds the beginning of the urethra, the eight-or-so-inch tube that carries urine from the bladder to outside a man's body. (Women have a series of glands and ducts along their much shorter urethras; these glands are considered the evolutionary vestiges of the prostate.) Although it is an internal organ, the prostate can be examined by a physician who inserts a gloved finger into the rectum. The doctor can thus detect enlargement of the gland; soft, infected tissue; or hard, potentially cancerous nodules.

The full role of the prostate may not yet be known, but without this organ a man produces no apparent ejaculate and is in effect sterile. Normally sperm produced in the testicles and nourished by the sugars of the seminal vesicles pass by the prostate, where liquid containing enzymes and other essential components are added to the semen.

Although present from fetal life, the prostate does not become active until puberty. Prostatic fluid is produced and released in response to sexual stimulation. Repeated or prolonged sexual stimulation without ejaculation or abrupt changes in sexual frequency can sometimes result in painful prostatic congestion.

Young men are rarely bothered by prostate problems. When problems do occur, they usually take the form of acute infections, or bacterial prostatitis, most often caused by a common intestinal bacterium or a venereally transmitted organism, such as the gonorrhea bacterium. The afflicted individual is likely to experience painful urination, perhaps with pus or blood in the urine, an urgent and frequent need to urinate, high fever, chills, and pain in the lower back or perineal region (between the scrotum and rectum).

Acute bacterial prostatitis is usually treated with appropriate antibiotics, bed rest, pain-killers, and lots of fluid. In venereal infections, both sexual partners must be treated simultaneously. [See chapter on venereal diseases, page 188.]

Chronic bacterial prostatitis may produce few, if any, symptoms much of the time but can cause recurrent painful flare-ups. Pain in the lower back and perineal region, painful urination, and urgent need to urinate are typical symptoms. Long-term treatment with antibiotics, including a new drug called trimethoprim-sulfamethoxazole, or TMP-SMZ, can usually suppress symptoms of chronic bacterial prostatitis.

More common than bacterial infection of the prostate is chronic inflammation that has no apparent causative organism. Hot sitz baths, anti-inflammatory drugs, ejaculation with regular frequency, and sometimes massage of the prostate by a physician through the rectum can help relieve the congestion.

Treating Prostatic Enlargement

By far the most frequent prostatic ailment is benign prostatic hypertrophy, a noncancerous enlargement of the prostate gland. Approximately half of men past the age of fifty develop some symptoms of this overgrowth of tissue, which can cause such difficulties as a frequent and urgent need to urinate, especially at night, slowness of the urinary stream, difficulty starting urination, dribbling of urine, incomplete emptying of the bladder (which can set the stage for a bladder infection), or pain with erection or orgasm. Prior to the age of eighty, the symptoms become severe enough in about 10 percent of men to warrant surgical correction.

Sometimes the operation is done under anesthesia through the urethra and is called transurethral resection. This type of surgery does not impair sexual potency. However, if the prostate is greatly enlarged, a more extensive operation that approaches the prostate through the abdomen may be necessary; it also does not usually result in impotence. But if the operation is done through the perineal region, impotence is a likely consequence because nerves and muscles that are involved in penile erection are severed in the course of this surgery.

Only a physician can tell the difference between benign and cancerous enlargement of the prostate. To the patient the symptoms are likely to be identical. Early, curable prostate cancer, in fact, generally produces few, if any, symptoms. Therefore, from the age of about forty, every man should have an annual digital rectal examination to check for prostate enlargement. Currently only 10 percent of prostate cancers are discovered before the disease has spread beyond this organ; once such spread has occurred, there can no longer be an assurance of cure. There is now available a blood test for a substance called acid phosphatase that may be able to detect prostatic cancer before it has spread. Some experts recommend that it be part of the routine checkup for adult males, though others say its value has not yet been proved.

If an elderly man is found to have a dormant prostate cancer, the surgeon is likely to leave it alone, although frequent checkups are necessary. Treatment of a prostate cancer that is not dormant usually involves extensive surgery that in most cases leaves the man impotent. Increasingly now, intensive radiation therapy is being used in place of surgery to treat cancer, without compromising chances for cure. Radiation treatments also result in impotence in about a third of patients. In more advanced cases spread of the cancer can often be controlled for years by removal of the man's natural source of male sex hormone, the testicles, and by treating him with the synthetic female hormone diethylstilbestrol.

Through regular examinations and prompt treatment of any cancers discovered, the ten-year cure rate of prostate cancer can approach 100 percent, a study at the University of Minnesota showed. A Columbia University study indicated that the wives of men with prostate cancer face a higher than usual risk of developing cancers of the breast and genital organs, and therefore, such women should have frequent checkups for these diseases.

V.
Abused
Substances

Many of the substances we enjoy as part of everyday life are really powerful drugs that influence mood, mental capacity, and physical functions. They are also subject to abuse, injuring our health in the process. Heavy smokers or coffee drinkers may not think of themselves as drug addicts, but in fact, that is just what they are. Caffeine, for example, is a stimulant, and many coffee and tea drinkers become dependent on the lift it gives them. But large amounts of caffeine can cause anxiety, nervousness, and insomnia. Alcohol is a central nervous system depressant that can disrupt mental and motor skills as well as injure internal organs, if consumed to excess. Most herbal teas contain drugs, some of which can inflict serious health damage. Even ordinary food, though drug-free in and of itself, can sometimes be abused by those who can't control its consumption.

Yet many of these substances can be enjoyed in limited amounts without hazard *if* they are used properly. Alcohol, for example, may help to prevent heart attacks if consumed moderately. A singular exception is tobacco, which is harmful in any amount; here abstinence should be your goal.

Understanding the sources and effects of commonly used recreational drugs can help you limit your exposure to protect your well-being without diminishing your pleasure.

Effects of Alcohol:
The Good and the Bad

If there ever was a Janus-faced phenomenon, it's alcohol. It eases tension and smooths social interactions, but it blurs judgment and muddles reason. It's a nutrient that supplies 10 to 20 percent of the calories consumed by American adults, but it's also an antinutrient that jeopardizes the body's supply of essential vitamins and minerals. It heightens the desire for sexual activity at the same time that it hampers sexual performance. Alcohol is a well-known killer — by way of heart and liver disease, cancer, and accidents — but it's also a potential extender of life.

This last statement may shock you. Americans have become so inured to the idea that anything enjoyable must be bad for them that a statement linking alcohol to improved health is likely to be regarded with suspicion, if not downright disbelief. In fact, the best available evidence indicates that those who imbibe with moderation live longer, on the average, than abstainers or very light drinkers. Moderate drinkers also live longer than heavy drinkers and former drinkers, many of whom undoubtedly gave up alcohol because of an existing health problem.

For most healthy people there is apparently some level at which the benefits of alcohol outweigh its risks. That level is roughly one to two drinks a day — a drink meaning approximately one shot (one and a half ounces) of distilled spirits, or twelve ounces of beer, or five ounces of table wine. Certainly, recovered alcoholics should not take this observation to be an invitation to resume drinking, but for those who do not suffer from alcohol addiction a drink or two a day might help to keep the doctor away.

The Benefits . . . and the Risks

The heart. This most vital organ seems to be the main beneficiary of moderate doses of alcohol. The nationally funded Honolulu Heart Study and studies by researchers in Yugoslavia and at the Kaiser-Permanente Medical Center in Oakland, California, have indicated that nondrinkers and light drinkers are more likely to suffer heart attacks than those who consume one or more drinks a day. Researchers at the University of Minnesota and the federally financed heart study at Framingham, Massachusetts, have shown that persons who drink moderately have higher levels of high-density lipoproteins, which are blood proteins that apparently protect against coronary heart disease. [See chapter on fats and cholesterol, page 14.] Certainly alcohol in small doses has a relaxing effect — which is why most people drink — and perhaps it best helps the heart by relieving stress.

Even here alcohol has a Jekyll-Hyde personality. It can damage heart muscle cells, reduce the heart's ability to pump blood, and raise the blood level of triglycerides, fatty substances that promote clogging of the arteries. Among heavy drinkers, high blood pressure, a type of heart disease known as cardiomyopathy, and abnormal heart rhythms are common, and many heavy drinkers succumb to cardiovascular disorders at relatively early ages. Cardiologists usually caution heart patients to limit their alcohol intake to the equivalent of one shot of whiskey a day, and patients with severe heart damage or congestive heart failure are advised to abstain completely.

Cancer. Alcohol-related cancer risks are faced primarily by those who drink more than moderate amounts, especially if they also smoke cigarettes. Alcohol seems to promote the growth of cancers that are caused by other factors. Cancers of the mouth and throat are two to six times more common among heavy drinkers than among nondrinkers, and the combination of heavy drinking and heavy smoking raises the risk fifteen times.

EFFECTS OF ALCOHOL

Amount of Distilled Spirits Consumed In 2 hours (ounces)	Alcohol in Blood (percent)	Typical Effects
3	0.05	Loosening of judgment, thought, and restraint Release of tension; carefree sensation
4½	0.08	Tensions and inhibitions of everyday life lessened
6	0.10	Voluntary motor action affected; hand and arm movements, walk and speech clumsy
10	0.20	Severe impairment, staggering, loud, incoherent, emotionally unstable, very drunk 100 times greater traffic risk
14	0.30	Deeper areas of brain affected. Parts affecting stimulus response and understanding confused, stuporous
18	0.40	Asleep, difficult to arouse, incapable of voluntary action, equivalent of surgical anesthesia
22	0.50	Coma, anesthesia of centers controlling breathing and heartbeat. Death.

Note: Adapted from information furnished by the National Clearing House for Alcohol Information.
Source: "Why Drinking Can Be Good for You," by Morris Chafetz, M.D.; Stein and Day, 1976.

Similar links exist between heavy drinking and smoking and cancers of the larynx (voice box) and esophagus. Among moderate smokers, those who drink heavily face a twenty-five times greater risk of developing cancer of the esophagus than do nondrinkers.

Liver cancer is also a common problem among alcoholics who develop cirrhosis, a degeneration of the liver caused primarily by prolonged heavy drinking.

One study has found a strong relationship between deaths from rectal cancer and the amount of beer consumed in various states and countries. Beer and scotch whiskey, both of which are made from malt, have been found to contain a very potent cancer-causing substance, N-nitrosodimethylamine, or NDMA. As one of a family of carcinogens called nitrosamines, NDMA has caused cancer in nearly every laboratory animal tested so far. Manufacturers are under government orders to reduce the amount of this chemical in their beverages.

The liver. As the only organ in the body capable of metabolizing alcohol, the liver is also the main target for alcohol damage. This organ is forced to use alcohol as an energy source in preference to its usual reliance on fatty acids. Through a variety of mechanisms, fatty acids then accumulate in the liver, causing fatty liver, a condition that can be cured by abstinence. A liver injured by alcohol may be unable to detoxify fully the poisons and carcinogens that find their way into the body.

Drinking bouts can precipitate alcoholic hepatitis, an inflammation of the liver, and prolonged excessive drinking can result in potentially fatal cirrhosis. [See chapter on liver diseases, page 664.]

Accidents. Alcohol is the nation's single most important cause of traffic accidents and fatalities. Excessive drinking is a factor in nearly half of the traffic deaths. It plays a role in many home accidents as well.

Although very small amounts of alcohol can improve skilled performance, higher levels interfere with reflex responses, slow reaction time, and impair judgment. Alcohol can also disturb visual ability by slowing recovery from glare and making it hard to identify and track moving objects.

Birth defects. Excessive amounts of alcohol consumed during pregnancy can produce a group of birth defects called fetal alcohol syndrome, which involves growth deficiency, developmental delays, small head, facial abnormalities, and abnormal fine motor function. The advice to pregnant women varies. Some recommend that they limit themselves to at most two drinks a day; others say that since the safe level is not known, pregnant women should abstain completely, especially during the crucial first three months.

Other health effects.

• It causes the liver to break down *testosterone*, the male sex hormone, impairing potency at the same time that another hormone, called LH, heightens desire. Prolonged heavy drinking can result in chronically low testosterone levels, causing shrinking of the testicles and growth of the breasts in men.

• Alcohol increases the need for the *B vitamins*, niacin and thiamin, which are used in the metabolism of alcohol, and may interfere with the absorption and storage of others, especially folacin. Because alcohol is a diuretic, it may result in shortages of water-soluble *minerals* (magnesium, potassium, and zinc) that are lost through urination. These deficiencies can occur even if the drinker consumes an otherwise nutritionally adequate diet.

• Alcohol, except perhaps in very small amounts, is a poor sleeping potion. Like sleeping pills, it interferes with REM, or dream, sleep and can actually make *insomnia* worse. It can also intensify *depression* and should not be used to help lift yourself out of a bad mood. [See chapters on insomnia, page 557, and depression, page 146.]

• Although it doesn't cause *gout*, alcohol can precipitate a gout attack if large amounts are consumed at one time. This results from an accumulation of uric acid in the blood, which is cured by abstinence. [See chapter on gout, page 608.]

• Large doses of alcohol can cause *impaired immunological responses*, increasing a person's susceptibility to bacterial infections and possibly also to cancer.

The answer to alcohol's split personality, as with most of life's other pleasures, seems to lie in moderation. While small amounts may improve your life, large doses can kill you.

Safe Drinking:
Using Alcohol for Pleasure

Alcohol, the nation's favorite mood-altering drug, is supposed to make people feel warm and friendly — to ease social interactions, loosen tongues and spirits, and warm body and soul. Little wonder, then, that so many consider it an ideal — perhaps even an essential — accompaniment to holiday and other celebrations as well as ordinary social gatherings or at the end of a long, hard day.

Unfortunately alcohol also has a dark side. [See chapter on effects of alcohol, page 240.] Nearly half the nation's traffic fatalities and more than half of home accidents can be partly or entirely blamed on misuse of "demon rum." Many people occasionally overindulge in alcoholic drinks and in the process embarrass themselves and their companions, perhaps endanger their lives, and nearly always pay a painful price the next day.

Happily there are ways to use alcohol so that you can derive all the benefits and incur few, if any, of the risks. All it takes is to understand some basic facts about different kinds of drinks and how the body handles alcohol and to adopt sensible drinking habits.

What and How You Drink

According to Dr. Morris Chafetz, former director of the National Institute on Alcohol Abuse and Alcoholism, the most important fact to remember is that alcohol's effects can be controlled only on the way in. After the drug has been consumed, only time can mitigate the consequences.

The effects of alcoholic beverages depend largely on how much pure alcohol is consumed over what period of time. The less concentrated the drink and the more slowly it's consumed, the less high you're likely to become. If you guzzle beer or gulp wine, you can get drunker than if you sipped a concentrated "hard" drink.

Twelve ounces of beer or six ounces of wine contain about the same amount of alcohol as a jigger (ounce and a half) of 80-proof liquor. Six ounces of a fortified dessert wine (such as vermouth, sherry, or port) contain nearly double the amount of alcohol in a jigger of 80-proof liquor. The alcohol in wine and beer is not weaker than that in hard liquor — it's only less concentrated. Your body can handle it better than liquor only if you consume it slowly.

244

Whatever its source, alcohol does not need to be digested. About 20 percent of it is absorbed directly from the stomach into the blood, which carries it to the brain. (The remaining 80 percent is absorbed more slowly through the intestine.) Once absorbed, alcohol will affect the brain until it's metabolized. The average person metabolizes the alcohol in a jigger of hard liquor, a medium-size glass of wine, or twelve ounces of beer in sixty to ninety minutes.

Controlling the Impact of Alcohol

There are several good ways to slow the absorption or reduce the concentration and resulting impact of alcoholic drinks.

• First eat something, preferably bulky foods and foods high in protein or fat; then wait fifteen minutes before drinking. Such foods line the stomach and sponge up the alcohol, slowing its absorption.

• Dilute your drinks with lots of ice and water to lower the concentration of alcohol. But avoid carbonated mixes, which speed the absorption of alcohol because the gas creates pressure that pushes the liquid through the stomach wall. Wine and beer are absorbed less rapidly than hard liquor because they contain nonalcoholic substances that slow absorption.

• Drink in a relaxed, comfortable setting. If you're emotionally upset, under stress, or tired, you're likely to get a stronger impact from a given amount of alcohol. Dr. Chafetz comments: "If I had to come up with an unhealthy drinking situation, it would be the American cocktail party. Standing around uncomfortably in a crush of people, most of whom we don't know, makes us want to gulp that first drink."

• Your expectations also influence your reactions: If you expect to get drunk, you're likely to feel intoxicated on less alcohol than if you plan to keep a fairly tight rein on yourself.

• Be aware of your capacity. Don't try to keep up with your drinking companions or prove how well you hold your liquor. A given amount of alcohol will affect small people more intensely than heavier people and, generally, women more than men. Among women, alcohol's effects are more intense just before the menstrual period. If you don't want to drink or you feel you've had enough, keep your glass filled with something nonalcoholic and no one will know or bother you to "have another."

• Avoid mixing drugs with drinks. The effect of many drugs, including narcotics, tranquilizers, antidepressants, and antihistamines, are enhanced by alcohol. Alcohol may also interact with certain antibiotics, antihypertensive drugs, and anticonvulsants. If you are taking medication and you want to drink, be sure to ask your doctor or pharmacist if it's safe to mix the drug with alcohol.

How to Protect Your Guests

Party givers can do a great deal to help their guests drink to joy rather than excess.

• Always serve snacks with drinks. Meat or cheese with crackers or bread, or cheese or cream dips with raw vegetables are best, according to the Rutgers Center of Alcohol Studies. But avoid salty snacks because they increase thirst and will encourage imbibers to drink faster.

• Pour your guests' drinks yourself, and measure them with a jigger. Don't be generous to a fault by serving too-stiff drinks. Remember, you're doling out a drug.

• Don't hasten to refill every glass the moment it falls below the halfway mark. Most people can pace themselves to consume alcohol at the rate they can handle, as long as they're not pushed to do it faster.

• Keep the bar in a separate room to discourage self-service and too-fast refills, but keep a tub of ice handy for guests to help themselves.

• Always have nonalcoholic beverages available, and offer them when you take drink orders.

• Never serve "one for the road." Rather, you should stop serving drinks at least an hour before you expect the party to end and serve coffee and cake or some other food instead. These won't do anything to sober up your guests, but they will give people time to metabolize what they've already consumed.

• It's generally safe to drive after one or two drinks consumed over a period of an hour or two. But driving can be extremely dangerous after three drinks of hard liquor, five eight-ounce glasses of beer, or four six-ounce glasses of wine. If a guest appears intoxicated when he's ready to leave your party, do everything possible to discourage him from driving. Call a cab, ask someone else to give the guest a lift, take his car keys, have him spend the night if necessary, but keep him from getting behind the wheel of a motorized vehicle.

Hangovers: Coping with the Aftermath

Generally speaking, sobering up is a list of things that won't work. There's no way to speed the rate at which alcohol is metabolized or burned up by your body. Walking around the block doesn't help because muscles can't use alcohol for energy. Drinking black coffee may turn a sleepy drunk into a wide-awake drunk, but it won't sober him up. Nor will taking a cold shower or breathing pure oxygen. Only time will do the trick. Generally it takes as many hours to sober up as the number of drinks consumed.

Time is also the only real cure for that bilious feeling that afflicts so many the morning after the night before — time and rest and aspirin if your stomach can take it. For, in the view of some experts, the single most common cause of hangover is fatigue. Alcohol anesthetizes portions of the brain that send out early warning signals that we have stayed up long enough and really should go home and go to bed. Even without alcohol, people sometimes get hangover symptoms — headache, shakiness, etc. — when they've pushed themselves too far, says Dr. Chafetz.

246

Accordingly, hangover remedies like coffee (a stimulant) and walking are like whipping a tired horse, forcing more activity on a body clamoring for rest. A "hair of the dog" — that is, more alcohol — is also counterproductive. It will probably relieve temporarily the discomfort of a hangover, but once again the body's fatigue sensors will be dulled and the needed rest postponed, only delaying — not avoiding — the moment of reckoning.

Of course, alcohol itself plays a direct and crucial role in hangovers. Alcohol dulls the brain mechanisms that regulate body chemistry, disrupting the normal balance of water and salts. While the alcohol level in the blood rises, much water is lost from body tissues, possibly causing the thirst of a hangover. Alcohol also causes blood vessels to dilate, and hangover headache is believed to result from the swelling of cranial arteries. Alcohol irritates the mucous membranes that line the gastrointestinal tract, undoubtedly causing the heartburn, nausea, and vomiting common to overindulgers. To minimize this effect, you should eat a decent amount of food — especially a fatty protein food like cheese or meat — *before* drinking.

The amount and kind of alcohol consumed, the rate at which it is drunk, and the mixers used can also influence hangover symptoms. The more diluted your drinks and the more slowly they are consumed, the less likely you'll suffer a hangover.

The different alcoholic beverages also contain varying amounts of substances known as congeners. These are toxic chemicals present in amounts of less than 1 percent that result from fermentation and maturation of the liquor. Alcohol is rapidly eliminated by the body, but congeners are not, and thus they may be around the next day to contribute to hangover symptoms.

Congeners are substances that add flavor to liquor. The main one — fusel oil — is mostly removed during distillation and sold for paint solvent. Vodka and gin have a very low congener content; blended scotch has four times more than gin; and brandy, rum, and pure malt scotch have six times more. Bourbon contains the most — eight times more than gin and thirty times more than vodka. In one experiment, researchers produced hangovers by giving congeners in water — with no alcohol. In another, a high-congener drink (a laboratory-made superbourbon) produced more and longer-lasting hangover symptoms than either vodka or regular bourbon. You might be able to mitigate the effects of congeners by consuming some activated charcoal (it can be purchased in drug stores in tablet or granular form) before, during, or after you have indulged. Chew one tablet for each ounce of liquor consumed.

Despite the attendant miseries, many Americans seem to take pride in their hangovers, regarding them perhaps as proof of their big night — the more miserable in the morning, the more fun they must have had the night before. Quite the contrary, says Dr. Chafetz. "A person is more likely to get a hangover after drinking in a situation where he is tense or emotionally distressed."

In fact, guilt, fear, and anxiety about drinking can predispose a person to hangover. When research subjects were given huge amounts of alcohol in a relaxed permissive setting, no one got a hangover. In another study those who most disapproved of drinking (but did it anyway) got the worst hangovers. The moral is to drink without remorse and only when you feel relaxed and happy and not tired.

Although there is a direct relationship between the amount of alcohol consumed and the likelihood of hangover, there are also some people who seem able to drink a lot and still feel fine the next morning, whereas others get hung over from very small amounts of alcohol. Undoubtedly some people have an unusual sensitivity to alcohol or to various congeners, and some people have guilt-induced hangovers — they think they deserve one after their indulgence, so they get one.

There are at least as many myths about preventing hangovers as about curing them. But in fact, it does little good (except inasmuch as you *think* it will do good) to take various combinations of vitamins or over-the-counter medicines, to sober up or eat before going to bed, or to drink lots of water before the alcohol.

The only surefire preventive is to avoid alcohol altogether or consume it with great circumspection. In view of the agonies of some hangovers, it's a wonder they are so rapidly forgotten when the next opportunity arises to drink to excess.

For Further Reading

Chafetz, Morris, M.D. *How Drinking Can Be Good For You.* New York: Stein & Day, 1978.
Outerbridge, David E. *The Hangover Handbook.* New York: Harmony Books, 1981.

Problem Drinking: Recognizing the Signs

Probably no other progressive and potentially fatal disease is more often denied than alcoholism. Even members of the alcoholic's family, who may suffer as much as the victim, often fail to recognize or refuse to acknowledge the existence of alcohol abuse by their relative.

The longer an alcohol problem is denied, the more damage it does to body, mind, and family, social, and occupational circumstances. Yet denial is so common as to be almost an inherent characteristic of the disease.

As David C. Hancock, president of Lynnville, Inc., an alcoholism treatment center in Jordan, Minnesota, puts it, "Unfortunately part of the nature of alcoholism is its tendency to deceive and delude its victim so that he cannot recognize that he is sick. He can no longer look at himself and his behavior objectively. Alcohol has diminished his capacity for accurate self-evaluation and self-judgment."

Many myths and misunderstandings about the earmarks of alcohol abuse and its victims contribute to this deception. On the other hand, sometimes people worry needlessly about the seriousness of alcohol consumption by loved ones who are regular drinkers but not alcoholics and not likely ever to become alcoholics.

What to Look For

Loss of control. The alcoholic cannot consistently predict the duration of any particular drinking occasion or the amount of alcohol that will be consumed. In other words, a social drinker can decide whether to drink at a certain time and whether to continue drinking after the first few drinks. The alcoholic's drinking behavior tends to be compulsive, often continues to the point of drunkenness, and the uncontrolled episodes usually become increasingly frequent. It is not the amount of alcohol consumed but rather the effect on the person that determines alcohol addiction. Depression that precedes or follows a drinking bout is a serious warning sign of alcoholism.

Chronic abuse. While a social drinker may on rare occasion drink more than he or she intended and become inebriated, for the alcoholic,

248

such behavior repeats itself often. Though drinking to the point of intoxication may be interspersed with periods (days, weeks, months, even years) of abstinence, uncontrolled drinking can recur at any time and often does.

Injurious consequences. Alcohol abusers often don't realize it, but their uncontrolled drinking inevitably takes its toll on their health, sleep patterns, and ability to function socially and/or occupationally. These effects tend to worsen as abusive drinking continues.

Development of tolerance. With repeated excessive drinking, the brain adapts to high concentrations of alcohol in the blood, so that more and more alcohol is needed to produce obvious intoxication.

Physical dependency. Body tissues become accustomed to being bathed in alcohol, and withdrawal symptoms (such as the shakes) result when alcohol consumption is stopped or greatly reduced.

Symptoms of Alcohol Abuse

Dr. Morris Chafetz, former director of the National Institute of Alcohol Abuse and Alcoholism, cites the following people as showing symptoms of an alcohol problem:
- Anyone who has been drunk four times a year.
- Anyone who drinks in order to work.
- Anyone who goes to work intoxicated.
- Anyone who is intoxicated and drives a car.
- Anyone who sustains bodily injury requiring medical attention as the consequence of drinking.
- Anyone who comes in conflict with legal authority as a consequence of drinking.
- Anyone who, under the influence of alcohol, does something he would not otherwise do.

Who Becomes a Problem Drinker?

Alcoholism usually develops over a period of years in a person who starts out as a normal social drinker seeking to enhance pleasure. For some people, however, alcohol provides more than just ordinary good feelings and relaxation, and it is these people who are at greatest risk of developing an addiction, many experts believe.

Dick Selvig, a recovered alcoholic who has been involved in the treatment of more than 20,000 alcoholics in the Midwest, says future alcoholics commonly experience euphoria and a greatly inflated sense of well-being from their early contacts with alcohol. The drinker is headed for trouble when alcohol becomes a route to fulfillment, used to produce feelings of superiority, self-confidence, ego strength, happiness, romance, aggressiveness, or any feelings not natural to the drinker's personality, says Mr. Selvig, who is the author, with Dan Riley, of *High & Dry* (see "For Further Reading," page 251).

According to Mr. Selvig and Mr. Riley, "A typical telltale sign of alcoholism is the person who, ordinarily quiet, becomes loud; the person who ordinarily is reticent who becomes aggressive; the person who ordinarily is neat becomes untidy. The person who changes after his alcohol drinking is probably an alcoholic or on his way to becoming diseased."

Dr. Chafetz says someone with an alcohol problem uses the drug in order to function — to ease the way, obliterate pain, blur perceptions, dissolve inhibitions, tolerate their circumstances.

Unfortunately, Mr. Selvig notes, the very people best able to recognize such signs don't and often don't want to because they are more comfortable with the alcoholic than with the real person. "All too often the change in personality is so welcomed by friends and family that no one even wants to believe it is caused by alcohol," he adds. This is particularly true when the alcohol abuser is a teenager who previously has been shy, withdrawn, and socially isolated but who seems to "blossom" under the influence of alcohol.

But the good feelings induced by alcohol are sought more and more often and become progressively elusive as alcohol abuse worsens. For alcohol is a depressant and soon leaves its abusers feeling worse than they did to begin with. They continue to drink in hopes of recapturing the initial euphoria or blotting out the current pain.

Don't Be Fooled By Rationalizations

In an illuminating pamphlet called *I Can't Be an Alcoholic Because ...* (available from Lynnville Treatment Center, Jordan, Minnesota 55352), David Hancock counters some of the more popular rationalizations:

... "I'm not a skid row bum." Anyone can be an alcoholic — doctor, housewife, student, executive, car mechanic, factory worker, professional athlete. Only 3 to 8 percent of the nation's 10 million alcohol abusers are falling-down-drunk skid row bums.

... "I never drink before 5 P.M." It is not *when* a person drinks, but whether the amount can be controlled. Nor does an alcoholic have to get drunk every time he or she drinks.

... "I never drink anything but beer." The consumption of alcohol to the point of abuse, not its form, determines alcohol addiction. A person can become an alcoholic even if nothing stronger than beer, wine, or cough medicine is drunk.

... "I drink only on weekends." Many alcoholics can go a long time without taking a single drink but are unable to control their drinking when they do drink.

... "I am too young." Neither a person's age nor the number of years he or she has been drinking determines alcoholism. Twelve-year-olds have been known to become dependent on alcohol within a matter of months.

... "I can quit at any time." It matters not how many days an alcoholic can abstain from alcohol. More important is how the person feels during periods of abstinence — happy, calm, relaxed, and even-tempered or nervous, tense, easily frustrated, irritable, resentful, anxious, or lonely? Alcoholics Anonymous refers to the latter set of reactions as a "dry drunk" that sooner or later leads to a resumption of drinking.

For Further Information and Treatment

If you or someone in your family has a drinking problem, the following organizations should be able to direct you to an appropriate treatment facility.

● The National Council on Alcoholism: local affiliates or the national office at 733 Third Avenue, New York, New York 10017.

● Alcoholics Anonymous: local branches or the national office at P.O. Box 459, Grand Central Station, New York, New York 10017. In addition to AA groups for alcoholics, there is Al-Anon, an organization for relatives and friends of alcoholics, and Alateen, for young people concerned about alcoholism in the family.

The National Clearinghouse for Alcohol Information (lists treatment resources by community throughout the country), P.O. Box 2345, Rockville, Maryland 20852.

Guidance may also be obtained from local mental health associations, family service agencies, local health and social services departments, United Way, or your local community council.

For Further Reading

Langone, John, and Dolores deNobrega Langone. *Women Who Drink.* Reading, Mass.: Addison-Wesley, 1980.
Milam, James R., and Katherine Ketcham. *Under the Influence.* Seattle: Madrona, 1981.
Selvig, Dick, and Dan Riley. *High & Dry.* Blue Earth, Minn.: Piper Publishing, 1980.

Cigarette Smoking: How Lethal Is the Habit?

"Smoking-related diseases are such important causes of disability and premature death in developed countries that the control of cigarette smoking could do more to improve health and prolong life in these countries than any single action in the whole field of preventive medicine."

— *The World Health Organization*

You've heard it before. More than 30 million Americans have taken it to heart and quit smoking. But 55 million continue to puff away on those little white "cancer sticks," perhaps closing their minds to the grim facts about cigarettes and/or fearing the emotional and physical agonies of giving them up.

Indeed, three out of four American smokers *say* they want to quit, and 60 percent claim to have taken at least one serious stab at it. Their failure in the long run is testimony to the strength of the habit and the likelihood that for many hard-core smokers cigarettes are an addiction similar to alcoholism and heroin abuse.

While quitting smoking can be difficult, it is by no means impossible. Many voluntary health organizations and proprietary clinics run stop-smoking programs that have helped large numbers of would-be quitters who could not succeed on their own. [See box in chapter on quitting smoking, page 256.]

Confronting the evidence indicting cigarettes — and learning the health value of being an ex-smoker — can be an important first step toward successful quitting. Fortified with the facts, you are likely to have an easier time giving up smoking. Here is a summary of the reasons, many of them described in an excellent eighty-one-page booklet, "Dangers of Smoking, Benefits of Quitting," prepared by the American Cancer Society, why you should not smoke.

Your Personal Risks

Smoking cigarettes is likely to shorten your life. The damage is

WHY YOU SHOULD QUIT SMOKING

Risks of Smoking	Benefits of Quitting
Shortened life expectancy Risk proportional to amount smoked. A twenty-five-year-old who smokes two packs a day can expect to live 8.3 years less than nonsmoking contemporary.	After ten to fifteen years, ex-smoker's risk approaches that of those who never smoked.
Lung cancer Cigarettes are major cause in both men and women. Overall, smokers' risk is ten times higher than nonsmokers.	After ten to fifteen years, risk approaches that of those who never smoked.
Larynx cancer Smoking increases risk by 2.9 to 17.7 fold that of nonsmokers.	Gradual reduction in risk, reaching normal after ten years.
Mouth cancer Smokers have three to ten times as many oral cancers as nonsmokers. Alcohol may act as synergist, enhancing effect of smoking.	Reducing or eliminating smoking/ drinking lowers risk in first few years. Risk drops to level of nonsmokers in ten to fifteen years.
Cancer of esophagus Smoking increases risk of fatal cancer two to nine times. Alcohol acts as a synergist.	Since risk is proportional to dose, reducing or eliminating smoking/ drinking should lower risk.
Cancer of bladder Smokers have seven to ten times greater risk. Synergistic with certain occupational exposures.	Risk decreases gradually to that of nonsmokers over seven years.

dose-related, with the number of years of reduced life expectancy proportional to the amount you smoke and the length of time you've been a smoker. Smoking directly causes or contributes to the three main causes of premature deaths among Americans: heart disease, cancer, and accidents.

Cigarettes are responsible for about one-quarter of heart attack deaths. Along with high blood pressure and high cholesterol, smoking is a main factor in premature death and chronic disability caused by coronary heart disease. The carbon monoxide in cigarette smoke may replace oxygen in as many as 12 percent of a smoker's red blood cells. Thus, it interferes with oxygen delivery to the heart as well as to other muscles and the brain.

Twenty percent of cancer cases are directly caused by smoking, and

Risks of Smoking	Benefits of Quitting
Cancer of pancreas Risk of fatal cancer is two to five times higher than for nonsmokers.	Since risk seems related to dose, stopping smoking should reduce it.
Coronary heart disease Smoking a major factor, causing 120,000 excess heart deaths each year.	Risk decreases sharply after one year. After ten years, risk is same as for those who never smoked.
Bronchitis and emphysema Smokers face four to twenty-five times greater risk of death; lung damage even in young smokers.	Cough and sputum disappear within few weeks. Lung function may improve; deterioration slowed.
Stillbirth and low birth weight Smoking mothers have more stillbirths and babies both at below normal weight, with greater vulnerability to disease and death.	If mother stopped smoking before the fourth month of pregnancy, risk to fetus is eliminated.
Peptic ulcer Smokers get more ulcers and are more likely to die from them; cure more difficult in smokers.	Ex-smokers get ulcers, too, but they heal faster and more completely than in smokers.
Drug and test effects Smoking changes pharmacological effects of many medicines; changes results of diagnostic tests and increases risk of blood clots from oral contraceptives.	Most blood factors raised by smoking return to normal after quitting. Nonsmokers on birth control pill have much lower risks of hazardous clots and heart attacks.

a third of all cancer deaths are caused at least in part by smoking, sometimes in concert with occupational exposure to noxious substances like asbestos, uranium, and dyes. Cigarette smoke contains a number of known cancer-causing agents, including radioactive elements. In fact, a major portion of a smoker's total radiation exposure comes from cigarettes, which may result in forty times the recommended maximum annual exposure to radiation. For those who smoke, cigarettes are also the main source of the potent carcinogens nitrosamines.

Smoking is responsible for three-fourths of cases of the nation's leading cancer killer, lung cancer, which is fatal to 90 percent of its victims. As females of all ages have taken up smoking with a vengeance, their once-low risk of lung cancer has risen dramatically, and this disease may soon surpass breast cancer as the leading cancer killer of American women. Other cancers to which smoking makes an important contribution are the nearly always fatal cancers of the esophagus and pancreas as well as the disabling and sometimes fatal cancers of the larynx, mouth, and bladder.

Smoking even for a short while impairs the functions of the respiratory system. Coughing and spitting are common afflictions of smokers. They suffer from reduced lung capacity, which means they get short-winded more quickly than nonsmokers. Smokers are also less able to keep their lungs clear of infectious organisms and harmful debris. Cigarettes account for about 70 percent of the cases of life-limiting chronic bronchitis and emphysema.

Smoking has also been linked to peptic ulcers, earlier onset of menopause, excessive wrinkling of the skin, hearing loss in older men, sleep problems, impaired athletic performance, excessive numbers of red blood cells, and malignant (life-threatening) hypertension. Furthermore, smoking adversely affects the action of several important drugs, including pain-killers and tranquilizers.

Risks to Others

The unborn child is probably the most vulnerable of passive smokers. Smoking during pregnancy reduces the oxygen supply to the fetus and increases the risk of stillbirth, low birth weight, and death shortly after birth. It may also impair the physical and social development of surviving offspring. The children of smoking parents have poorer lung function and a higher incidence of wheezing and respiratory infections, including life-threatening pneumonia.

A large Japanese study showed that the nonsmoking wives of smoking men were four times more likely than those married to non-smokers to develop lung cancer. A Greek study showed similar results. Although a long-term study of 1 million people conducted by the American Cancer Society found no such effect, the data from this study cannot directly address this question.

Other risks of passive smoking are firmly established. In addition to general discomfort and allergic reactions caused by the smoke of others, significantly reduced lung function has been shown to occur in people who work near smokers. Nonsmokers inhaling the air in a smoke-filled room can develop high levels of carbon monoxide in their blood, which can interfere with heart function and cause angina pains. [See chapter on passive smoking, page 361.]

Apart from health considerations, but no less important, smoking also causes more fatal fires than any other source of combustion, resulting in an estimated 2,500 deaths a year. Annually at least 25,000 people are injured and $313 million in property lost as a result of smoking-caused fires.

Benefits of Quitting

Although many smokers justify the continuation of their habit by thinking that it's too late to quit because the damage has already been done, the facts show otherwise. In ten to fifteen years after stopping smoking, your risk of dying prematurely comes close to that of people who have never smoked. Although those who stop smoking before the age of forty benefit the most, at any point that you give up smoking, your risk of smoking-caused death and disability declines. Contrary to what some believe, so-called stress-related deaths do not increase among former smokers.

The risk of suffering a heart attack among men under sixty-five is reduced by 25 percent if they stop smoking. The risk starts dropping within a year after quitting and after ten years reaches the level of those who never smoked. Similarly, lung cancer risk approaches that of the never-smoker ten to fifteen years after quitting. The chances of developing other smoking-related cancers similarly decline when the smoker quits.

In addition, there are immediate benefits of quitting — namely, a decline in the oxygen-robbing carbon monoxide in your blood, improved sleep, disappearance of smoking-caused headaches and stomachaches, enhanced stamina, keener sense of taste and smell and, after a few weeks or months, disappearance of smoker's cough and sputum.

Switching to a low-tar, low-nicotine brand of cigarettes has nowhere near the benefits of quitting, although some reduction in the risk of developing lung cancer and heart disease does occur. For most of the disorders listed in the accompanying chart, however, no benefit has been identified as associated with low-tar, low-nicotine brands.

Quitting Smoking: You Can Do It If You Really Try

If you would like to be among those who have rid themselves of the expense, smell, bad breath, stained fingers, nagging cough, and serious health hazards of smoking, here are some tips based on the experiences of successful quitters and the formats of effective stop-smoking programs.

Cigarette smoking is a habit, a learned behavior that — like other behaviors — can be unlearned, or a new behavior can be learned in its place. No matter how strong this habit or how frequently it is reinforced, anyone who wants to quit badly enough can. The secret is in the wanting. Quitting smoking is a personal decision that no one else can make for you.

Ingredients for Successful Quitting

Motivation. If you find strong, important, personal reasons for wanting to give up cigarettes, they will help to reinforce your decision to quit when the going gets rough.

Insight. If you understand what cigarettes do for you, you can find substitutes and learn to do without them. Since different people smoke for different reasons, what works for one would-be quitter may not work for another.

Attitude. Viewing quitting as a plus, as attaining a new sense of self-control and esteem, will make it a lot easier than if you think you are giving something up.

Practice. After years of "practicing" smoking, you must now be willing to practice *not* smoking.

Dr. Daniel Horn, former director of the defunct National Clearinghouse for Smoking and Health at the Centers for Disease Control in Atlanta, has devised a self-test that can help you gain insight into your attitudes and knowledge about smoking and quitting, what kind of support you will get in trying to quit, what smoking does for you, and how you use the different cigarettes you smoke during the day. Single copies of the *Smokers Self-Testing Kit* (for adults) and the *Teenage Cigarette Smoking Self-Test* can be obtained free from the Office of Smoking and Health, 1-58 Park Building, 5600 Fishers Lane, Rockville, Maryland 20856.

Why People Smoke

To optimize your chances for success, your approach to quitting should be tailored to the reasons you smoke. Psychological studies have defined six roles that cigarettes can play in people's lives.

Stimulation: to help you get going and focus on what you are doing. Stimulation smokers tend to smoke heavily in the morning, sometimes having their first cigarette of the day the moment they get up. As a substitute for cigarettes, they might try such stimulants as a cool shower, brisk walk, deep breathing, or an exercise routine.

Handling: to glean the satisfactions of manipulating an object and to have something to do with your hands and mouth. Such smokers enjoy the process of taking out a cigarette, lighting up, feeling it in their mouths, watching the smoke, and toying with the ashes and butt. Substitutes such as doodling with a pen or pencil may help. Many such smokers switch to pipes, which involve a lot more handling but fewer health risks than cigarettes.

Pleasurable relaxation: to add to already good feelings and help you relax. Pleasure-seeking smokers tend to light up after meals or making love or finishing a task. They usually find it easy to quit, sometimes by substituting other pleasurable but less hazardous activities.

A DO-IT-YOURSELF PLAN

The stop-smoking plan that is the basis for a number of successful clinics and programs can also be used by individuals on their own. Although designed as a four-week program, it can be condensed into two weeks or less:

First week. List the reasons you want to quit, emphasizing the positive effects, and read the list daily. Complete the self-test. Wrap your cigarette pack with paper and rubber bands. Each time you smoke, write down the time of day, what you are doing, how you are feeling, and how important that cigarette is to you (on a scale of one to five, with one being the most important and five the least). Then rewrap the pack.

Second week. Keep reading your list of reasons and adding to it if possible. Keep wrapping your pack and recording your smoking. Don't carry matches or a lighter, and keep your cigarettes some distance away (not on you or within arm's reach). Each day try to smoke fewer cigarettes than you did the day before, systematically eliminating those that are least or most important, whichever way works best. Decide every morning how many cigarettes you can get by on that day, and see how close you come.

Third week. Continue with the second week's instructions. In addition, don't buy a new pack until you finish the last one, and never buy a carton. Change brands twice during the week, each time choosing a brand lower in tar and nicotine. Select a time period that is likely to be easy, and try not smoking for forty-eight hours. If you succeed, try another forty-eight.

Fourth week. Continue the above. Increase your physical activity. Try to avoid the situations you most closely associate with cigarettes (for example, get up immediately after meals and do something that makes smoking difficult). Find a temporary but harmless cigarette substitute — gum, celery or carrot sticks, toothpicks. Whenever you feel the urge to smoke, try a deep-breathing exercise: With your body limp, inhale slowly and deeply, hold your breath and count to five, then exhale slowly. Have a plan of action for when temptation comes that would make it difficult or impossible for you to smoke, such as knitting, typing, or jogging (but stay out of the refrigerator and pantry).

Many smokers find that they have to quit several times before they succeed permanently at being a former smoker. So if you fail the first time or even the second or third, don't get discouraged or give up. Simply try again . . . and again . . . because in the end, if you really want to, you'll make it.

Crutch, or tension reduction: to relieve bad feelings, such as tension, anxiety, anger, disappointment, fear, or depression. Such smokers are more likely to light up when things go wrong or the pressure builds up. They must try to face difficult situations without smoking, a task that often turns out to be much easier than anticipated.

Psychological addiction: to fulfill a perceived "craving" for cigarettes, which begins to grow the moment the last cigarette is stubbed out. Addicted smokers usually have to quit "cold turkey" — they can't cut down slowly since each cigarette simply reinforces the addiction. Although they find it difficult to quit, they are often more successsful at staying nonsmokers because they don't ever want to go through the agony again.

Habit: as an almost automatic response, with little or no thought involved. Habit smokers often light up a new cigarette while the previous unfinished one is still burning in the ashtray. Habit smokers have a much easier time quitting than most others. They have to make smoking a conscious behavior (such as by wrapping up each pack or not carrying cigarettes or matches) and ask themselves each time, "Do I really want this cigarette?"

Each smoker, then, must find his or her own route to quitting, and countless gadgets and schemes have been devised to help. For those who can't do it alone, there are thousands of clinics where the support of a leader (often a former smoker) and a group of fellow sufferers can be bought.

Aids to Quitting Cigarettes

The old saw that it is easy to quit smoking — as Mark Twain said, "I ought to know because I've done it a thousand times" — is all too familiar to millions of smokers who would like to be free of their habit. Numerous strategies have been devised to help enlarge the ranks of former smokers, ranging from special chewing gums and countdown filters to hypnosis and group therapy.

Some say successful quitting is reinforced by having to pay a large sum to do it; others prefer to go it alone and use their cigarette money for a special reward. One fact is clear: Different strategies work for different smokers. The trick is to find the one that best suits your needs and personality.

The following are among the better programs available:

Freedom from Smoking, a twenty-day, do-it-yourself program devised by the American Lung Association and distributed by local chapters. The two manuals *Freedom from Smoking in 20 Days* and *A Lifetime of Freedom from Smoking* are available for a suggested $5 donation. Contact your local chapter of the Lung Association, or write to national headquarters: American Lung Association, 1740 Broadway, New York, New York 10019.

Stop Smoking System, a five-day multifaceted program sponsored by the American Health Foundation at a cost to individuals of about $100 to $120. For information about the program and sessions that may be held in your area, contact the foundation offices, at 320 East Forty-second Street, New York, New York 10017, or at 3000 Town Center, Suite 2900, Southfield, Michigan 48075.

Quit Smoking Clinics, sponsored by local chapters of the American Cancer Society. The course is run over a period of several weeks. Many are given for no fee. Do-it-yourself "Quitters' Aides" also are available from local chapters. For information contact your nearest cancer society chapter or American Cancer Society national headquarters, 777 Third Avenue, New York, New York 10017, 212-371-2900.

SmokEnders, an eight-week course that costs several hundred dollars, held periodically throughout the country. For information about courses in your area, check your local phone book or contact the national office of SmokEnders, 37 North Third Street, Easton, Pennsylvania 18047, 215-250-0700.

A major deterrent to many would-be quitters, especially women, is the prospect of weight gain when cigarettes are no longer available to satisfy oral cravings. Two books may help you avoid substituting unwanted pounds for unwanted cigarettes: *Stop Smoking Lose Weight*, by Neil Solomon, M.D. (New York: Putnam, 1981), and *The Stop Smoking Diet*, by Jane Ogle (New York: Evans, 1981).

Marijuana:
More Hazardous Than Most Realize

Millions of marijuana-smoking young Americans, jaded by alarmist, politically motivated but poorly documented reports of marijuana's alleged risks, are convinced that it is a safe drug, especially when compared to alcohol.

However, with so many people smoking an increasingly potent marijuana at ever younger ages, scientists are gathering impressive, though still inconclusive, evidence indicating that the nation's third leading recreational drug (alcohol is number one; cigarettes are number two) is indeed hazardous to health. In fact, some leading drug experts who once dismissed marijuana as a drug of minor consequence now express serious concern about the possible risks and patterns of use, particularly among teenagers.

Among those who now take a dim view of marijuana are Dr. Sidney Cohen, a drug expert at the University of California at Los Angeles, who once described marijuana as "a trivial weed," and Dr. Robert L. Dupont, former director of the National Institute on Drug Abuse, who once favored decriminalizing personal possession of marijuana. According to these and other experts, it is no longer possible to say that marijuana is an innocuous drug with few, if any, health effects aside from intoxication. Although the evidence for immediate effects on the brain is the most convincing, a number of recent studies show damaging effects that suggest long-term health hazards involving many different body functions. These include the heart, lungs, and reproductive organs.

The problem with accurately defining the hazards of marijuana is that the way in which it is used by Americans has not yet been subjected to long-term study. Decades of experience with marijuana in other countries is not necessarily relevant here, where a stronger form of the drug is used primarily by people in their formative years and where patterns of inhalation are likely to differ.

It may be twenty years or more before the necessary studies can be conducted among Americans. Therefore, it is especially important to heed the early warnings signs of the delayed effects of smoking marijuana. Remember that it took half a century of heavy cigarette smoking by millions of Americans before the health risks of tobacco were widely recognized. By then so many had become so hooked on the "innocuous weed" that today, twenty-five years after the first major report on the health hazards of cigarettes, more than 50 million Americans still smoke cigarettes, and smoking remains the nation's leading preventable cause of illness and premature death.

The Reasons for Concern

Patterns of use. Some 43 million Americans have tried marijuana, and a national survey in 1977 showed that 16 million were current users. They included 4 percent of twelve-year-olds, 15 percent of fourteen-year-olds, and 31 percent of eighteen- to twenty-one-year-olds. More than 4 million youngsters aged twelve to seventeen were using marijuana in 1977, and 1 in 9 high school seniors used marijuana daily. The survey showed that the proportion of youngsters who had begun using marijuana before the ninth grade had nearly doubled since 1972.

Two-thirds of young adults say they use marijuana, but most older adults who use it tend to smoke it only occasionally. There is relatively little concern about occasional use by adults, except for pregnant women and individuals with heart disease, lung disease, or emotional disorders.

Potency. Drug experts are disturbed about the rapidly increasing potency of the marijuana generally available to Americans. In 1975 the average sample of confiscated marijuana contained 0.4 percent of the mind-altering chemical THC (tetrahydrocannabinol). By 1979, because of improved cultivation practices, the average was 4 percent of the active drug — a tenfold increase in potency — and concentrations of 5 percent were not uncommon. One cultivated form increasingly available in this country contains 7 percent THC.

This is especially worrisome because unlike alcohol, which is soluble in water and rapidly washed out of the body, THC and related cannabinoids in marijuana are fat-soluble and can remain and accumulate in the body for a week or longer after marijuana is smoked.

Brain effects. Immediate effects on the brain are the least controversial and best defined of marijuana's hazards. Like alcohol, marijuana is intoxicating. A marijuana high interferes with memory, learning, speech, reading comprehension, arithmetic problem solving, and the ability to think. Driving skills are impaired, as is general intellectual performance. Long-term intellectual effects are not known.

Some researchers have described what they called amotivational syndrome among young marijuana smokers, who, with frequent use of the drug, tend to lose interest in school, friends, and sexual intercourse. However, it is not known whether marijuana use is a direct cause or merely one symptom of a general underlying problem. Persistent brain abnormalities and changes in emotion and behavior have been demonstrated in monkeys given large doses of marijuana.

Also like alcohol, marijuana interferes with psychomotor functions such as reaction time, coordination, visual perception, and other skills important for driving and operating machinery safely. Actual tests of marijuana-intoxicated drivers have clearly shown that their driving is impaired, yet they tend to think they are driving better than usual. In several surveys 60 to 80 percent of marijuana users said they sometimes drive while high.

Marijuana is not physically addicting, but people can become psychologically hooked on the drug. Marijuana may aggravate existing emotional problems. The most common adverse emotional effect is an acute panic reaction, in which the user may become terrified and paranoid and require hospital treatment. In 1978 some 10,000 people were treated in hospital emergency rooms for adverse marijuana reactions.

Lung damage. Marijuana cigarettes are unfiltered, and smokers tend to inhale deeply, exposing sensitive lung tissue to potent, irritating chemicals. One study among marijuana smokers showed that five marijuana cigarettes a week were more damaging to the lungs than six packs of cigarettes smoked over the same period. Marijuana smoking irritates the air passages and diminishes the amount of air the lungs can hold and exhale, the studies show. Like tobacco, marijuana smoke impairs lung defenses against infections and foreign inhaled matter. In animal studies it has caused extensive lung inflammation. Bronchitis and emphysema may occur in people who smoke marijuana regularly.

Marijuana smoke contains 150 chemicals in addition to THC, and the effects of most of these are not known. One ingredient is benzopyrene, a known cancer-causing agent that is 70 percent more abundant in marijuana smoke than in tobacco smoke. There is also more tar in marijuana than in high-tar cigarettes. When painted on the skin of mice, marijuana tar can produce tumors. However, there is as yet no good evidence of any cancer-causing effects in people. If there is a carcinogenic effect akin to that of tobacco, it is not likely to become apparent for another two decades.

Heart effects. Marijuana has an even greater effect on heart function than tobacco. It can raise the heart rate by as much as 50 percent. This is of no known consequence to young healthy people. But in those with poor heart function, this effect can be dangerous and may also produce chest pains (angina). Heart patients would be well advised to steer clear of marijuana.

Hormone and reproductive effects. Several, but not all, studies have shown that marijuana smoking can lower the level of the male sex hormone, testosterone, in the blood, though it usually remains within the range of normal. Sperm abnormalities, including reduced numbers of sperm and abnormal sperm movement and shapes, have also been found in relation to marijuana use.

In females, preliminary studies suggest an adverse effect on the menstrual cycle in 40 percent of the women who smoke marijuana at least four times a week. The result may be infertility. In animal studies the levels of growth hormone and the female sex hormones, estrogen and progesterone, have been reduced by marijuana.

262

Marijuana can cross the placenta and reach the developing fetus. Miscarriage is more common among users. Pregnant monkeys given THC were far more likely to suffer abortions or deliver dead babies.

Studies by Dr. Gabriel G. Nahas of Columbia University showed an effect of marijuana on the hypothalamus, the body's master gland that directs the functions of other hormone-producing glands.

Immune impairment. Evidence from both animal and human studies have suggested damage to basic body defenses against disease. However, it is not known whether marijuana smokers are any more likely to get sick than other people of similar life circumstances. As the National Institute on Drug Abuse concluded in a recent report to Congress on marijuana: "It is very difficult to anticipate the problems which will arise in a given society in advance. Thus, any attempt to compare the health impact of marijuana with that of alcohol and tobacco at *current* levels of use is certain to minimize the hazards of marijuana."

For Further Information

"Marijuana and Health," 1980 report to Congress prepared by the National Institute on Drug Abuse, DHEW Publication No. (ADM) 80-945; available from the institute, P.O. Box 2305, Rockville, Maryland 20852. The institute also has available a ten-page fact sheet, "Marijuana: What It Is and What It Does," which contains the highlights in lay language of the 1980 report.

"For Parents Only: What Kids Think About Marijuana," a free-loan film plus two booklets, "For Parents Only: What You Need to Know About Marijuana" and "For Kids Only: What You Should Know About Marijuana," all prepared by the National Institute on Drug Abuse. The film and booklets are available to organizations without cost from Modern Talking Picture Service, 5000 Park Street North, St. Petersburg, Florida 33709. Single copies of the booklets are available free from the institute (see address above).

Marijuana Today, by George K. Russell, distributed by The Myrin Institute for Adult Education, 521 Park Avenue, New York, New York 10021.

"Twelve Things You Should Know About Marijuana," *Consumers' Research* magazine (April 1980). Reprints available ($1 per single copy) from Consumers' Research, Washington, New Jersey 07882.

Marijuana and Health, by a committee of Institute of Medicine, National Academy of Sciences (1982). Copies are available for $11.25 each from the National Academy Press, 2101 Constitution Avenue, NW, Washington, D.C. 20418.

Caffeine:
The National Pick-Me-Up

"Light, no sugar" ... "Regular" ... "Black." ... Few who have grown up in the eastern part of this country need to be told that these orders refer to the all-American drink, coffee. More than half the world's coffee beans are brewed in the United States. The average adult American consumes sixteen pounds, or approximately 800 cups, each year of this brown, nonnutritive liquid extracted from the beans of *Coffea arabica* and related species.

Whether they drink it light or dark, sweet or bitter, hot or iced, with caffeine or without, one cup a day or ten, many people are confused about the effects — good and bad — of coffee and its constituents and where else these ingredients may be obtained.

Recent warnings about the possible health hazards of caffeine and coffee have forced some to think seriously about the role coffee plays in their lives and whether they could — or would want to — give it up or at least reduce their consumption of it.

Its Benefits

The most important ingredient in coffee — and the one primarily responsible for its continuing popularity — is caffeine, a drug that powerfully stimulates the central nervous system and gives that familiar coffee lift. Caffeine clears away mental cobwebs, relieves drowsiness, masks fatigue, and creates a general sense of well-being. Its sleep-inhibiting properties led, according to legend, to coffee's discovery some thousand years ago by Arabian shepherds who watched their charges gambol about all night after eating the berries of the coffee plant.

Caffeine in small doses helps produce a clearer train of thought, a keener appreciation of sensory stimuli, and a swifter reaction time. Its pick-me-up properties largely account for the popularity of cola drinks, twenty ounces of which have roughly the same amount of caffeine as a six-ounce cup of brewed coffee.

Since children are more sensitive to the stimulant effects of caffeine

263

than adults, some doctors discourage youngsters from drinking colas (regular and diet) and other caffeine-containing soft drinks (Mello Yello, Mountain Dew, Dr Pepper, Mr. Pibb are among those with caffeine) as well as cocoa (depending on the source of the chocolate, cocoa can have up to half the caffeine in a cup of coffee). In addition to stimulating the brain, caffeine stimulates the kidneys to produce more urine.

Caffeine's virtues have prompted many drug manufacturers to include it in medications designed to relieve pain, premenstrual tension, and cold symptoms (caffeine counters the drowsiness produced by antihistamines in cold remedies). Caffeine is also the active ingredient in over-the-counter drugs to help people stay awake. In fact, the dose of caffeine in a single stimulant tablet is no greater than that in a cup of brewed coffee, but the unaware consumer may pay a lot more for caffeine in the drug than in the drink.

Caffeine, which constricts cerebral blood vessels, is used to treat migraine types of headaches and to counter the effects of drugs that depress the central nervous system. It has shown some promise as a treatment for hyperactivity in children (in whom it has a calming effect) and as a means of stimulating breathing in premature babies who tend to stop breathing during sleep.

Its Risks

At the same time, however, caffeine may have untoward effects. It can interfere with fine muscular coordination and, possibly, accuracy of timing. Large doses of caffeine — the result, say, of drinking several cups of coffee at one time or ten or more cups in the course of a day — can cause irregular or rapid heart beats; insomnia; upset stomach; increased breathing rates, blood pressure, and body temperature; nervousness; and irritability. Caffeine "addicts" have sometimes been mistakenly diagnosed as suffering from anxiety attacks and treated incorrectly with tranquilizers instead of having the cause of their difficulty eliminated. Caffeine-induced anxiety reactions can happen with as few as three cups a day in sensitive individuals, but the more caffeine you consume, the greater the likelihood of this effect.

Sometimes caffeine has paradoxical effects. In some people it may cause a headache; in others it may relieve one. In some it raises the amount of sugar in the blood; in others it lowers it and may consequently stimulate hunger pangs or, rarely, a hypoglycemic reaction — a dizzy, weak, nauseated, headachy, irritable feeling.

The effects of caffeine show up within thirty to sixty minutes of its ingestion and last several hours. Half the amount consumed is gone from the body within three and a half hours. The source of caffeine does not seem to make much difference in how rapidly it is absorbed into the blood, how high a level is reached, and how long it stays around.

Many people incorrectly believe that while coffee in the evening will keep them awake, tea won't. A typical cup of tea does have less caffeine than coffee — between half and three-quarters the amount, depending on the kind and strength of tea used and how long it steeps. One careful study showed that on an empty stomach, the caffeine in tea is absorbed as readily as that in coffee, and when the same doses of caffeine are given as tea or coffee, the same levels of caffeine are reached in the blood. Instant coffee has less caffeine than brewed coffee, but usually more than tea.

Coffee and tea — even decaffeinated and acid-neutralized coffee — stimulate the release of acids in the stomach and therefore are ill-advised for ulcer patients. Patients with high blood pressure or fever may also be told to avoid caffeine since it raises both body temperature and

CAFFEINE CONTENT OF COMMON PRODUCTS

Product		Amount of Caffeine in mg
		Per Serving
Foods and	Brewed coffee, 6-oz cup	100–150 mg
Beverages	Instant coffee, 6-oz cup	86–99 mg
	Decaffeinated coffee, 6-oz cup	2–4 mg
	Tea, 6-oz cup	60–75 mg
	Cocoa, 6-oz cup	5–10 mg
	Colas and Dr Pepper, 12-oz	32–65 mg
	Milk chocolate, 1 oz	6 mg
	Bittersweet chocolate, 1 oz	20 mg
	Baking chocolate, 1 oz	35 mg
		Per Tablet
Prescription Drugs	Cafergot and Migralam	100 mg
	Migral	50 mg
	Fiorinal, Esgic, and Apectol	40 mg
	Darvon Compound and Soma Compound	32 mg
		Per Tablet
Over-the-Counter	Vivarin	200 mg
Drugs	NoDoz	100 mg
	PreMens	66 mg
	Excedrin	65 mg
	A.P.C.'s, Anacin, Cope, Vanquish, Goody's headache powders, Empirin Compound, Midol, Easy-Mens, Sinapils	32 mg
	Triaminicin and Coryban-D	30 mg
	Dristan	16 mg
	Neo-Synephrine Compounds, Cenegisic	15 mg

blood pressure. Although one major study indicated that coffee drinkers face an increased risk of heart attack, three subsequent studies that took other factors — including cigarette smoking — into account found no such relationship.

However, pregnant women have been cautioned by the federal Food and Drug Administration to avoid all caffeine-containing foods and drugs, after studies indicated that caffeine can increase the risk of stillbirth, miscarriage, and malformations of the fetus. Although this relationship has not yet been proved, caffeine-containing substances should be used sparingly, if used at all, during pregnancy, the agency said.

An initial suggestion that coffee consumption may increase the risk of bladder cancer has not stood the test of further research. A Harvard Medical School study suggesting that coffee drinking significantly increases the risk of pancreatic cancer has not been confirmed by other studies, although further research is needed to determine if and how coffee and this cancer may be related.

In laboratory studies, caffeine can cause cancerlike changes in cells at doses twenty to forty times higher than the highest level ever measured in a habitual coffee drinker. At lower doses caffeine seems to inhibit the cancer-inducing effects of other chemicals and thus may be protective. However, British studies suggested that another substance in coffee, chlorogenic acid, may enhance the formation of cancer-causing nitrosamines in the stomach.

Caffeine and its chemical relatives, the methyl xanthines, have been linked in several studies to the painful swellings of fibrocystic breast disease. This benign condition is associated with an increased risk of developing breast cancer. Doctors who have studied the matter report that the disease subsides in most women who stop consuming all sources of methyl xanthines — including coffee, decaf, tea, chocolate, colas, and other caffeine-containing soft drinks.

How to Cut Down on Coffee

Heavy coffee drinkers who decide to break their addiction to caffeine should avoid abrupt withdrawal. Dr. Morris A. Shorofsky of Beth Israel Hospital in New York City reports that sudden withdrawal can cause headache, nausea and vomiting, mental depression, drowsiness, and a disinclination to work. The symptoms, which begin twelve to sixteen hours after the last dose of caffeine, can be relieved by caffeine.

The best way to withdraw from caffeine, Dr. Shorofsky advises, is slowly, weaning yourself a cup or two at a time over a period of a week or more.

You can also reduce your caffeine consumption by brewing your coffee from a mixture of regular and decaffeinated coffees. Or substitute a grain-based beverage, such as Postum or Cafix, for some or all of your cups of coffee. But beware an uneducated foray into the field of herbal teas; some present even greater hazards than ever associated with coffee or caffeine.

While such dramatic ill effects as these are not very common, increasing numbers of cases of herbal toxicity have come to the attention of health professionals in recent years. Those cases that are recognized medically are believed to represent the tip of the iceberg. It is not known, for example, how many people risk their health by abandoning prescribed medications in favor of herbal remedies or who use herbal preparations that interfere with the effectiveness of needed drugs. Some chemicals in herbal teas can cause such abnormal effects as increased blood pressure or lowered blood sugar. Tannin-rich teas, which include a number of herb teas, may be linked to an increased risk of developing cancer of the esophagus.

Foods or Drugs?

Although they are sold as foods and thus not subject to federal drug regulations, "herbal teas are drugs, not foods," says Dr. Ara Der Marderosian, professor of pharmacognosy at the Philadelphia College of Pharmacy and Science. "They are crude complexes containing many impurities and active components with a variety of possible undesirable effects. Some are actually too dangerous to be used at all."

Dr. Der Marderosian points out that because the active constituents are generally present in very low concentrations, moderate consumption of herbal teas rarely presents a problem for the healthy. But, he continues, the concentration of active ingredients can vary widely, depending on the growing conditions of the plant, the parts of the plant used, and the way the tea is brewed.

In addition, some people think that if something is good for you in small amounts, more is better, and as a result, they may consume enough of the active herbal ingredients to produce a toxic effect. "These are not substances to be used frivolously," Dr. Der Marderosian warns.

Dr. Der Marderosian should know. Pharmacognosy, his specialty, is the science of drugs of natural origin. At one time all drugs came from natural products, for the most part plants. Even now 47 percent of prescription drugs sold contain active ingredients extracted from plants. Among them are the heart drug digitalis; reserpine, a tranquilizer and blood pressure-lowering agent from snakeroot; quinine, an antimalarial drug from the bark of the cinchona shrub; atropine, a powerful alkaloid with many effects extracted from deadly nightshade (belladonna); ephedrine, a nasal decongestant and central nervous system stimulant from the shrub ephedra; colchicine, a drug to treat gout, its source meadow saffron; ipecac, from the root of a South American plant, used today to induce vomiting and to treat amebic dysentery; and kainic acid, from red seaweed, used by the Japanese to treat intestinal parasites. Fewer than half the plant compounds of possible pharmacological value have been identified, and even fewer have been tested for effectiveness. Nonetheless, the herbal folklore is replete with reputed remedies.

Herbal Teas:
Source of Potent Drugs

Herbal preparations, used for 5,000 years as medicines and tonics and still the mainstay of folk remedies throughout the world, are enjoying a surging revival in the United States. Many people, disillusioned with or distrustful of modern medicine, have turned to them in an attempt to cure whatever ails them or to "preserve" their health. Others, concerned about the possibly harmful effects of coffee and ordinary tea, have switched to supposedly healthier or safer herbal teas, dozens of which are now widely sold in health food and other stores. These amateur "naturopaths," unaware that herbal teas may contain any number of potent chemicals that can disrupt the normal function of body and mind, are often unprepared for the consequences of their innocent foray into the plant kingdom.

Example: An elderly couple from Chehalis, Washington, had been to a health spa that recommended comfrey tea as an herbal remedy for their arthritis. The wife picked what she thought was comfrey and prepared tea, which the couple drank with lunch. Within an hour they were overcome with nausea, vomiting, and dizziness. The husband discovered that what his wife had picked was not comfrey but a very similar-looking plant called foxglove, the source of the toxic heart drug digitalis. By the time the ambulance arrived his wife was dead and his own heart rhythm was so unstable that hospital treatment could not save him.

Example: Three young women with an interest in health foods bought senna tea as an herbal substitute for ordinary tea and coffee. They suffered such severe diarrhea after drinking just one or two cups that they required emergency medical treatment. They hadn't realized that senna tea, a strong laxative, is a common folk remedy for constipation.

Example: A thirty-year-old man who avoided alcohol, cigarettes, coffee, and other psychoactive drugs began taking daily capsules of Gotu Kola after reading an ad describing the herbal preparation as a general tonic and a "brain food" helpful in treating mental and nervous disorders, memory problems, and ulcers. After three weeks he became chronically nervous and unable to sleep. The preparation was found to consist of ground kola nuts, containing pharmacological doses of caffeine.

Risks Outweigh Benefits

Although the packages and advertisements for herbal teas and capsules cannot legally make claims for their health value (that would subject them to the drug laws of the Food and Drug Administration), often on shelves right next to these herbal products are stacks of books, pamphlets, magazines, and charts describing the supposed health benefits of herbs. Herbs of one sort or another are said in this literature to be capable of curing everything from acne, alcoholism, and allergies to hemorrhoids, miscarriage, and ulcers, all supposedly without any adverse side effects.

It is true that many plants contain substances that can, in sufficient quantity, alleviate some of these conditions. It is also true, however, that these substances are really drugs, not foods, and that all drugs can have dangerous side effects.

Because herbal compounds sometimes counter the effects of drugs prescribed by doctors, Dr. Alvin B. Segelman, pharmacognosist at Rutgers University, advises people who are taking prescription drugs to avoid herbal teas. People with chronic ailments should tell their physicians of any use of herbal preparations.

Those who try to treat themselves herbally, Dr. Der Marderosian says, may make a number of unwarranted and possibly dangerous assumptions: that they know what's wrong, that they know the strength and composition of the herbal preparation, and that there are no side effects from herbs. Four persons developed life-threatening infections and one died after self-treatment with Chinese herbal medicines to relieve arthritis and back pains. The herbal medicines were laced with potent pain-killing and anti-inflammatory drugs that can destroy infection-fighting white blood cells.

"People don't realize that herbal preparations were once available only in pharmacies," Dr. Der Marderosian said. "They were used as drugs and the druggist would tell the purchaser how to prepare them to get the desired effect. Now it's very difficult to get reliable information about the effects of herbs. The literature in health food stores may be peppered with a little truth, but on the whole it is very dubious. To really know what's in herbal teas and what is safe, you have to take a specialized course like pharmacognosy or study a textbook on the subject."

Cautions Worth Heeding

A number of field guides to edible wild plants are available, but Dr. Der Marderosian cautions: "No one should pick and eat wild plants without having first taken a course or read an authoritative book *and* gone out with a knowledgeable collector." Dr. Segelman advises consulting first with your community pharmacist about the safe use of herbal medicines.

Some medicinal teas are too dangerous to be on the shelves of any food store, according to Dr. Der Marderosian. Among them are mistletoe, a "calmative" containing toxic proteins that can produce anemia and hemorrhage in the liver and intestines; shave grass (horsetail or equisetum, a diuretic and dyspepsia agent), which has toxins that can produce severe neurological reactions; and sassafras tea (made from sassafras root bark), which contains safrole, an established cause of cancer and a potent inhibitor of certain liver enzymes.

Other herbal preparations can have severe and terrifying effects on the mind. Some contain psychoactive compounds, including stimulants, hallucinogens, narcotics, sedatives, and euphoriants. A thirty-seven-year-old woman who drank nutmeg tea became incoherent, giddy, flushed and dizzy and had frightening hallucinations. A young man who drank a tea made from jimsonweed suffered hallucinations and became totally disoriented, wandering in the woods barefoot, cutting his feet badly, and lighting fires to scare off the "voodoo people."

Dr. Ronald K. Siegel, pharmacologist at the University of California at Los Angeles School of Medicine, who reported these two cases of herbal intoxication and five others, cautioned doctors to ask their patients about the use of herbal preparations whenever investigating the origin of any medical complaint.

How Dangerous are Herbal Teas?

The Medical Letter, an independent drug-advisory newsletter for physicians, has cited the following hazards associated with popular herbal teas:

● **Cathartics.** Teas that can cause severe diarrhea include those made from senna leaves, flowers, and bark; buckthorn bark; dock roots; or aloe leaves.

● **Allergens.** Teas from camomile, goldenrod, marigold, and yarrow can cause severe allergic reactions, even fatal shock, in persons sensitive to ragweed, asters, chrysanthemums, and related plants. St.-John's-wort tea can cause delayed allergic reactions and sun sensitivity.

● **Carcinogens.** Cancer-causing substances are present in tea made from sassafras. Tannins in ordinary tea and peppermint tea may increase the risk of cancer of the esophagus and stomach. If tannin-containing teas are consumed, add milk to bind up the tannins.

● **Diuretics.** Chemicals that cause the body to lose large amounts of water through increased urination are found in teas from buchu, quack grass, and dandelion. Their effects, however, are no worse than those from the caffeine in ordinary tea and coffee.

● **Poisons.** Toxins that could cause fatal reactions are found in Indian tobacco, shave grass, and mistletoe leaves, none of which should ever be used to make tea. Toxins that affect the nervous system, sometimes causing hallucinations among other frightening effects, are found in catnip, juniper, hydrangea, jimsonweed, lobelia, nutmeg, and worm-wood.

Compulsive Overeating: A Hidden Epidemic

Most people now recognize alcoholism as a sickness warranting sympathy and treatment, but compulsive overeating is still widely regarded as a character defect or moral weakness that victims could overcome through willpower if they wanted to. But the stories told by compulsive overeaters present a very different picture, one strikingly similar to that of a compulsive drinker or gambler or drug addict.

It is a picture of profound unhappiness, loneliness, shame, and loss of control to an inner demon that cries out, "Eat, eat," even when the rational self says, "Stop that. What are you doing to yourself?" To the victims of compulsive overeating, it is an illness that most are unable to cure or control on their own. As Laura R. confessed to a meeting of Overeaters Anonymous, "My daughter was going to spend Christmas with her grandmother, and she baked some cookies to bring along. While she was at school, I ate all the cookies."

Compulsive overeating is a life-disrupting addiction to food that can lead to severe obesity and profound unhappiness. But not all compulsive eaters are fat. Some are normal-weight individuals, and others are dangerously thin anorexics, who alternate eating binges with punishing purges or starvation diets.

According to Dr. Marcia Millman, a sociologist at the University of California at Santa Cruz and the author of *Such a Pretty Face: Being Fat in America* (see "For Further Reading, page 274), "Compulsive eating is like all other compulsions. The eating gives you a temporary sense of control over whatever is making you anxious. But it's not a permanent solution because it doesn't get at the source of the anxiety. Your 'hunger' is never satisfied. That's why the behavior becomes compulsive."

In *The Overeaters* (see "For Further Reading," page 274), Dr. Jonathan Kurland Wise, a Boston endocrinologist, and Susan Kierr Wise, a dance therapist, describe a variety of emotional clusters that trigger some to overeat, including a dependence on food for warmth, comfort, and safety; a fear that expressing anger will lead to uncontrolled rage; a fear of independence, and confused or ambivalent feelings about sexuality. A common pattern expressed by compulsive overeaters is their need to be perfect, to be totally in control of life, and to be all things to all people. Dr. Millman suggests that no one can maintain such perfect control.

Compulsive overeaters use food to help them face life. An Overeaters Anonymous pamphlet says, "Every emotion from agony to ecstasy is met by fleeing to the 'comfort' and oblivion of food." OA members report that when they abstain from compulsive eating, they are besieged with the painful feelings that food used to mask.

Dr. Millman notes that the vast majority of OA members are women, and although no survey has been done to determine if there are many hidden food addicts among men, she believes men are more likely to lapse into other types of compulsions, such as compulsive overwork, to cover up their anxieties.

Like abstaining members of AA, compulsive overeaters in OA don't ever consider themselves cured, only recovered. They try to refrain from compulsive eating one day at a time and try to keep coming back to OA meetings to maintain their abstinence and help others achieve it. As with alcoholism, relapse is common. But with time, many victims find that the old addictive eating patterns have been sufficiently suppressed to prevent minor slipups from turning into major blowouts.

Because OA groups are anonymous and no records are kept, it is not possible to say how successful they are in helping people to control their abnormal eating, lose unwanted pounds, and maintain normal weights. Nor is it known what proportion of compulsive overeaters might benefit from the OA approach. Individual and group psychotherapy has been used successfully in many cases to treat victims of what psychologists and psychiatrists call the binge-purge syndrome, in which frenetic episodes of gorging are interspersed with drastic purges, such as self-induced vomiting, abuse of laxatives and diuretics, or abnormal amounts of vigorous exercise.

OA is not considered a "cure" for obesity. But, Dr. Millman says, "often those who stay [in OA] feel their eating has come under control and also feel they have undergone a profound personal transformation." Many members tell of dramatic success through OA after years of failure with every other kind of weight-loss program.

Grace, for example, weighed 290 pounds in May 1977, when she came to her first OA meeting. She had been fat, very fat, all her life and paid the usual social debts of no dates, no clothes that fit, no participation in school sports. But she was highly successful in other areas: a leader in church groups, dependable team assistant, superb baby sitter, and valedictorian of her college class.

Grace told an OA meeting in Brooklyn, New York, "I did many of those things so that people would love me. I wasn't good enough to be loved just for me. But no matter what I did, I felt a gnawing emptiness inside, an 'I-got-to-have-more, something's-missing' feeling." She attempted to fill that emptiness with food, but though eating provided a temporary distraction, the old hollow feeling eventually returned, crying out to be fed again.

Today it is hard to recognize Grace in her "fat pictures." In less than three years she has lost 130 pounds and is still going down, slowly, purposefully, by relentless adherence to the OA program and by treating abstinence from compulsive eating as the single most important thing in her life. Grace says she has also learned how to deal more directly with her feelings, how to express anger, resentment, and disagreement, instead of trying in vain to bury them with food. "I'm learning that they're just feelings, not facts, and I'm not a bad person for having them," she said.

The OA program that helped Grace achieve her present state is neither a diet plan nor a psychotherapy clinic. It is, rather, a fellowship that provides unconditional love, acceptance, understanding, empathy, and support. Many who join discover for the first time that they are not alone in their bizarre eating habits, their self-hate and self-pity, and the difficulties they have accepting events that are beyond their control.

The OA program seeks to give members choices other than food for coping with their lives. As members of Alcoholics Anonymous do with alcohol, members of OA are first asked to admit that they are powerless over food and that the problem has made their lives unmanageable. Then they are supposed to ask a higher power (God, for those who believe) to help with their recovery. Abstaining OA members serve as sponsors for others. Individuals are advised to write down a daily food plan and read it to their sponsors and to telephone their sponsors whenever they feel threatened by the desire to eat compulsively.

At meetings members learn to start confronting their feelings and dealing with them constructively instead of burying them in food. Some members supplement this with psychotherapy. Some have dual or multiple addictions and join other anonymous groups as well.

The OA program, now more than twenty years old and 4,000 groups strong, is a free, independent, self-help program that offers no professional counseling. It involves no special diet, though it suggests food plans and guidelines for achieving and maintaining abstinence. Many members, for example, find it necessary to abstain from refined carbohydrates and sugars, which trigger in them cravings to eat compulsively. Participants are encouraged to consult a physician before starting on their chosen eating plan.

Those interested in attending a meeting of Overeaters Anonymous can find the group listed in the telephone directory of many cities. Or write to Overeaters Anonymous, World Service Office, 2190 190th Street, Torrance, California 90504, for local meeting information. If you find that the group you are considering insists on a rigid adherence to a particular diet plan (even though your own may be adequate), or if group loyalty is encouraged at the expense of professional psychological counseling, seek out a different group. There is little point in substituting one compulsion for another.

For Further Reading

Greene, Herbert, and Carolyn Jones. *Diary of a Food Addict*. New York: Grosset & Dunlap, 1974.

Millman, Marcia. *Such a Pretty Face: Being Fat in America.* New York: W.W. Norton, 1980.

R., Karen. *That First Bite: Journal of a Compulsive Overeater.* New York: Pomerica Press, 1979.

Wise, Jonathan Kurland, and Susan Kierr Wise. *The Overeaters.* New York: Human Sciences Press, 1979.

VI.
Dental
Health

Teeth are easy to neglect. You probably don't think of them as vital parts of your anatomy — that is, not until they hurt or fall out. Then they start costing, not just in dollars but also in lost time and pleasure and possibly impaired appearance and compromised nutrition. Yet nearly all dental misery can be prevented. Your teeth can and should last you a lifetime, pretty much intact.

Most people brush their teeth every day, but many have never learned the right way to brush and floss to dislodge the bacteria that corrode gums and tooth enamel. Only half the population now benefits from the decay-inhibiting properties of fluorides.

Some people equate good dental care with getting cavities filled, but they neglect the gums and bones that hold teeth firmly in the mouth. Often the result is expensive, extended periodontal treatments or teeth lost to periodontal disease.

Confusion about the nature and cost of proper dental care abounds, and some people fall prey to shoddy dentistry that ends up costing them greatly in both health and dollars. Care that might have been considered adequate two decades ago may no longer be so in light of new, improved techniques.

How to Get Good Dental Care

Other than wisdom teeth, I have lost one permanent tooth, and I have shoddy dentistry and myself to blame for it.

I was camping in the wilderness out West when the tooth began to throb so badly that I had to keep aspirin and a canteen next to my sleeping bag for when the pain awakened me during the night. The California dentist I finally saw shook his head in dismay: The tooth had decayed so extensively beneath a crown that it could not be saved.

The crown had been made some years earlier by a neighborhood dentist who functioned more like a short-order cook than a careful health professional. He "worked" at least three patients at a time, frenetically flitting from one treatment room to another, doing a little bit on one patient, then another, while a full waiting room kept on the pressure for speed. It was hardly the setting for careful dentistry. But it was close to home, swift, the fees were moderate, and the dentist kept up a friendly chatter that took your mind off the inevitable discomfort.

The price I paid for this convenience — besides the pain, a fixed bridge with two crowns to support it, requiring many weeks of treatment and hundreds of dollars — was hardly worth it.

Even more than with medicine, consumers of dental care are hard put to evaluate the competence of the practitioner. A medical patient who does not get well or suffers frequent recurrences or mishaps from treatment may get suspicious about a doctor. But the hallmarks of careless dentistry are rarely obvious to the patient, at least not immediately. Complicating the matter is the fact that many people expect their teeth to rot or fall out as they get older, so they fail to relate this occurrence to the poor quality of previous care.

All too often the choice of dentist is based on criteria that may actually be counter to proper dentistry: that the work is painless, fast, inexpensive, and that few, if any, demands are placed on the patient.

By contrast, good dentistry is often time-consuming, sometimes uncomfortable, and it always requires the patient to continue care at home to prevent future decay and tooth loss. Furthermore, good dental care is often expensive.

Beware Dental Bargains

In dentistry perhaps more than in any other health area, you usually get what you pay for. The dollars you save today often end up costing you a lot more down the road. If a dentist does a quick inexpensive filling but fails to clean out all decay and properly prepare the tooth first, the tooth will continue to deteriorate and eventually may require a crown or root canal work.

Various cost-saving measures, including dental insurance and high-volume dental centers, have become widespread in recent years. But while they make dental care available to more people, the quality of that care sometimes leaves something to be desired.

For example, department store dentistry (so-called because the centers are often housed in department stores or shopping centers) advertises lower fees and faster care than is usually available from private practitioners in the area. Bulk equipment purchases and shared overhead costs help to keep prices down. But attention to detail is often sacrificed in these centers, where the quality of practitioners varies widely and profits are determined primarily by how many patients are treated each day.

As Dr. Howard B. Marshall, a New York City dentist, puts it, "Dentistry is an art as well as a science. Art requires tremendous attention to detail. One cannot mass-produce art." Dr. Marvin J. Schissel, another New York dentist, is more pointed in his criticism: "If the big clinics find that taking the time to do good dentistry results in lower profits, then good dentistry will go by the wayside."

A reporter from *Dental Economics* magazine had his teeth cleaned at such a center: $12 for a six-minute process. Later the same day he visited his own dentist, who told him his teeth needed cleaning. The hygienist then spent half an hour scraping tartar from his teeth.

There may also be hidden costs at such centers since the advertised price for a crown may cover just that, with extra charges for the examination and temporary crown. Before beginning treatment, be sure to ask what the advertised charges cover and what other costs might be involved in your care.

This is not to say that all dental centers do careless work. Those that employ experienced, well-trained dentists who take their time, use quality materials, and are truthful about costs can be excellent. But you will pay for what you get, though the cost should still be lower than that which an individual dentist would charge.

The care obtained under some dental insurance programs may also fall short of the best. Two basic kinds of programs exist: those that rely on a closed panel of dentists to do all the work covered by insurance and those that reimburse for part or all of the costs of work done by independent dentists. Closed panels restrict patient choice; dentists who participate in them agree to accept a set fee, which may prompt them to shortchange services in order to make a profit when too many patients require extensive work.

Most insurance plans permit patients to choose their own dentist but may require submission of a pretreatment plan for review by the program's own consultants, who may suggest alternative treatment that costs less. The alternative may or may not be in the patient's best interests. In many programs the patient is free to accept the more expensive treatment so long as he or she pays the difference in cost. Before you start treatment, find out exactly what your insurance covers.

If private dental care is more than you can afford and you are not eligible for dental insurance (most programs are negotiated by employers or unions), you can often obtain quality care at a hospital-based dental clinic or at a student clinic at a dental school. It will probably take more of your time, however. Medicaid coverage is also available for medically indigent persons.

How to Evaluate a Dentist

How do you know that the care any dentist proposes is appropriate? How, in fact, can you tell whether a particular dentist is giving you thorough treatment that will help you keep your own teeth for life? Here are some guidelines to use in evaluating a dentist.

The examination. The first time you see a dentist, a thorough examination should be done. According to Dr. Marshall, this should include the following: a visual examination of the soft tissues of your mouth (cheeks, tongue, throat, etc., as well as gums) and your teeth, bite, and how your chewing muscles and joints work; a periodontal examination in which a probe is used to measure the depth of pockets that may have formed between your gums and teeth (indicating periodontal disease); and a dental examination that includes a full set of X rays, unless you have a recent complete set taken by your previous dentist. [See chapter on X ray examinations, page 445.]

The treatment plan. Following a complete examination, the dentist should discuss what treatment you need and why, about how long it will take, what it will cost, and what alternative treatments might be available

HOW TO FIND A GOOD DENTIST

One of the best methods is to contact the Academy of General Dentistry, 211 East Chicago Avenue, Chicago, Illinois 60611 (312-440-4300), and ask for a list of members who practice in your neighborhood. The academy requires its members to take carefully supervised continuing education courses.

Call a nearby dental school and ask for the names of faculty members who have private practices. Or speak to a faculty member and ask for a recommendation.

Contact a periodontist in town, and ask for the names of the best dentists in the community. Periodontists usually know because they see the fallout of inadequate dental care and can evaluate the quality of restorative work (fillings, crowns, and bridges).

Ask your family physician or the local pharmacist for the name of the dentist he or she uses. Or check with the dental clinic at a nearby hospital.

Ask friends, relatives, or co-workers whose opinions you have reason to trust for the names of the dentists they use. Quiz them about the dentists' practices and the reasons they are satisfied with the dental care they get.

if the "ideal" plan costs more than you can afford. If the dentist doesn't mention fees, ask. The plan should emphasize trying to save teeth, rather than extracting them. Though saving teeth may cost more initially, you will save dollars and time in the long run.

If extensive work is needed, or if the proposed treatment involves the extraction of teeth, obtain a second opinion from another dentist before you proceed. If your dentist is confident of the plan recommended, he or she should welcome a second opinion.

If you have serious gum disease (for example, if any pockets measure six millimeters or more), you should be referred to a periodontist for treatment unless your dentist has such specialty training. [See chapter on periodontal disease, page 290.] Periodontal disease, which is the major cause of tooth loss in adults, is preventable and readily treated in the early stages. Yet dentists often ignore periodontal disease because they fear that referral will cause them to "lose" their patients.

Emphasis on prevention. Decay and loss of teeth are not inevitable, but saving them is largely up to you, not your dentist. [See chapters on preventing decay, page 281, and fluorides, page 284.] Any good dentist will stress the importance of a proper diet and daily home care — proper brushing and flossing — as well as periodic cleanings by the dentist or

HOW TO TAKE CARE OF YOUR TEETH

The goal of home care is to cleanse your teeth both of food debris and of deposits of destructive, acid-producing bacteria, called plaque, that live on tooth surfaces and just beneath the gum line. Here are some tips on tooth and gum care from the American Dental Association.

Brushing

Replace your brush often. A worn-out toothbrush will not clean teeth properly.

Change the position of the toothbrush frequently. The toothbrush will clean only one or two teeth at a time.

Brush gently and with very short strokes, but use enough pressure so that you feel the bristles against the gum. Remember, only the tips of the bristles clean; don't squash them.

While it's better to brush several times a day, be sure to brush and floss thoroughly at least once every day to help prevent plaque damage.

Toothpaste

Some fluoride toothpastes prevent 25 to 30 percent of the decay a child might otherwise develop. However, not all fluoride toothpastes are effective. The seal of the American Dental Association Council on Dental Therapeutics is carried on the cartons or tubes of those that have been proved helpful.

Mouthwashes

A mouthwash can temporarily freshen your breath or sweeten your mouth, but it does not remove plaque and cannot prevent decay or gum disease. However, mouthwashes that contain fluoride do help protect the teeth against decay.

Do not rely on mouthwashes for a prolonged period to relieve pain or other symptoms of disease. Bad breath may be a sign of poor oral health or other bodily disorders.

dental hygienist (the frequency, which may vary from once every two or three months to once a year, depends on how rapidly tartar accumulates on your teeth).

How you are treated. The dentist should explain what is going to be done and what discomfort you might feel. Painless dentistry might also be that which fails to dig deep enough to remove all sources of decay and infection. On the other hand, thanks to a variety of anesthetic techniques, severe or prolonged pain should be avoidable in nearly all patients.

Treatment should never be rushed, nor should the dentist flit back and forth from one patient to another. If the work cannot be completed in the appointed time, you should be asked to return for another appointment. Crowded waiting rooms and constantly having to wait hours beyond your appointment time are signs of a disorganized dentist, not nec-

HOW TO BRUSH AND FLOSS

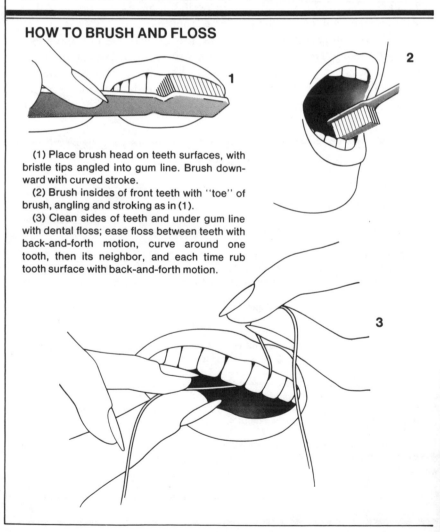

(1) Place brush head on teeth surfaces, with bristle tips angled into gum line. Brush downward with curved stroke.

(2) Brush insides of front teeth with "toe" of brush, angling and stroking as in (1).

(3) Clean sides of teeth and under gum line with dental floss; ease floss between teeth with back-and-forth motion, curve around one tooth, then its neighbor, and each time rub tooth surface with back-and-forth motion.

essarily a good one who is in great demand.

The late results. If in the months or years following treatment, you continue to develop a lot of cavities, if fillings keep falling out, gums bleed often, or teeth loosen, find another dentist.

For Further Reading

Marshall, Howard B., D.D.S. *How to Save Your Teeth.* New York: Everest House, 1980.
Schissel, Marvin J., D.D.S. *Dentistry and Its Victims.* New York: St. Martin's Press, 1980.

Preventing Tooth Decay: Look Ma, No Cavities!

It may surprise many parents to know that nearly all tooth decay is preventable. Teeth that are properly cared for can — and should — last a lifetime, and many fewer children than now do should have to spend dozens of hours in a dentist's office. Even orthodontic work can often be avoided through preventive measures.

What keeps these possibilities from becoming realities are countless misconceptions and fatalistic attitudes about teeth and their proper care, combined with the low priority some parents place on childhood tooth care. In addition, many parents are unaware of the latest developments for protecting children's teeth from decay and misalignment.

Misunderstandings that jeopardize the sanctity of children's teeth surround such factors as the proper time to start worrying about them, the importance of baby teeth, the benefits of fluorides, the role of heredity, the influence of diet and eating patterns, and the effects of various mouth habits, such as thumb-sucking.

Here are some facts to help set the dental record straight and let you, as parents, in on the secrets of saving your children's teeth.

Prenatal Care

By the third month of gestation, baby teeth have already begun to form under the fetal gums. Heredity actually has very little to do with decay resistance; environment is nearly all. Dr. Stephen J. Moss, head of children's dentistry at the New York University College of Dentistry, points out that the ability of teeth to resist decay depends largely on how well mineralized they are when formed.

Good nutrition during pregnancy is obviously important overall, but unless the mother is severely undernourished, her unborn baby will derive from her blood all the minerals needed to form healthy teeth. If the mother's diet is deficient in calcium and phosphorus, some will be removed from her bones to meet the baby's needs. Though very little fluoride, essential to the formation of decay-resistant teeth, crosses the pla-

281

centa, a few studies have suggested that prenatal fluoride supplements may help to protect the baby's teeth. [See chapter on fluorides, page 285.]

Infections or fever during pregnancy can interfere with tooth mineralization in the baby and result in decay-prone primary teeth. In such cases, devoted care to the child's teeth after birth is even more crucial. The same is true if the baby is ill during the first year of life.

Infancy

A baby's primary teeth are already fully formed at birth, and the permanent teeth begin forming immediately after birth. They are best protected by fluorides obtained from drinking water, from infant formula, or as a liquid dietary supplement (sold by prescription). Breast milk has very little fluoride, so an additional source of fluoride might be advisable for a baby who is fed only mother's milk. A daily bottle of fluoridated drinking water is probably the best source. If your water is not fluoridated, consult your pediatrician and dentist about fluoride supplements; some experts recommend waiting until the baby is six months old before giving fluoride supplements to prevent an overdose that could cause white spots on the child's teeth.

But don't wait until the baby has a mouthful of teeth before you think about keeping them clean. Start long before the first tooth comes through to remove deposits of decay-causing bacteria from the baby's mouth. Dr. Moss suggests holding a gauze pad between thumb and forefinger and vigorously wiping the gum pads (the ridge where the teeth will come through) twice a day. The same cleaning routine can be used to protect the baby's first teeth.

As soon as babies can grasp solid food (even before any teeth emerge), Dr. Moss recommends that they be given foods to chew, such as slices of apple or pear or pieces of toast. Good chewing habits help prevent decay and malpositioning of the teeth.

Perhaps the most common cause of rampant decay of the primary teeth is a habit totally within parental control: giving the baby a bottle of milk or juice to go to sleep with. The result — widespread decay of the upper front teeth — usually doesn't show up until the child is three or four. It is caused by the pooling of sugar-containing fluids around the teeth; mouth bacteria then use the sugars to produce decay-causing acids. The same thing can happen if a baby is allowed to linger too long at the breast. If the baby is given a bottle at bedtime, it should contain plain water. Otherwise, feed the baby and take the bottle away before bedtime.

The effects on teeth formation of sucking on a pacifier are no different from those caused by a thumb. In either case, if the habit is given up by the age of six, it will not push the teeth out of position. A pacifier, however, may be easier for a child to relinquish because it can be conveniently "lost" at age four or five.

The Baby Teeth

The baby, or primary, teeth usually start coming through the gums at around seven months of age. By eighteen months most babies have about twelve teeth, and by age two or three all twenty primary teeth should be through. If a child has not already been to a dentist, this is the time to go.

The primary teeth do more than allow the child to chew food. They pave the way for the permanent teeth that follow. Unrepaired decay in a primary tooth can lead to decay of the permanent tooth that will replace it. It can also cause the teeth to move too close together, diminishing available space for the permanent teeth. Premature loss of primary teeth can also result in malpositioning of the permanent teeth and improper development of the jaw and facial bones.

Fluorides, diet, and oral hygiene are the main factors that affect the health of the primary (and the permanent) teeth. Although a child should start using a toothbrush as early as possible to establish the habit, until a child is about eight years old, parents should assume responsibility for daily tooth cleaning. Younger children usually lack the dexterity to do a thorough job themselves. By holding the child's head in your lap, you can clean all the teeth, cheek side and tongue side. Use a soft brush and small amount of fluoridated toothpaste on your child's teeth twice a day: after breakfast and before bed. After the molars come in, daily use of dental floss to clean debris from between them is recommended. An electric toothbrush is OK and may encourage young children to brush their own teeth and help them do a good brushing job by themselves.

The benefits of fluoride are additive. Along with fluorides in drinking water (which can reduce decay by two-thirds) or as diet supplements, a child's teeth should be brushed with a fluoride-containing toothpaste. Twice a year, or more often if the teeth are especially prone to decay, the dentist can apply a fluoride gel. Additional benefit can be derived from home use of a fluoride-containing mouthwash. [See chapter on fluorides, page 285.]

Plastic sealants can be applied to the biting surfaces of the permanent molars to protect them from decay caused by food that lodges in crevices. Consult your dentist about this measure, which can reduce decay in coated teeth by two-thirds.

The Role of Sweets

Everyone "knows" that sugar is bad for teeth. Sugar is the food decay-causing bacteria use to produce acid that eats away tooth enamel. What everyone doesn't know is that rather than the total amount of sugar consumed, it is the frequency and consistency of the sweets eaten that make the difference to teeth. Sweets consumed as part of meals contribute little to tooth decay. But sweet snacks, especially sticky foods like caramels, dried fruits, cookies, and pastries, wreak havoc with teeth.

Honey, which adheres to teeth, is worse for them than refined sugar.

Sweet drinks are not a problem unless, like colas, they contain acids and are consumed several times a day. Sucking on lemons can also destroy the protective tooth enamel. A child who craves sweets might be given an occasional chocolate bar since chocolate has been shown to have some decay-inhibiting properties.

Studies of sugar-coated breakfast cereals (though they are hardly the best from a nutritional standpoint) show they cause no more decay than unsweetened cereals if they are eaten with milk as part of a meal. Regardless of what food is eaten, it is best to brush — or at least rinse the mouth with plain water — after every meal and snack.

For Further Reading

Cranin, A. Norman, D.D.S. *The Modern Guide to Family Dental Health.* New York: Stein and Day, 1971.

Moss, Stephen J., D.D.S. *Your Child's Teeth.* Boston: Houghton Mifflin, 1977.

Fluorides: Dental Bargain of the Century

Dental decay is the nation's most prevalent disease, afflicting 98 percent of Americans and costing more than $8 billion a year in dental bills and 100 million hours of lost labor. That doesn't even count the estimated one billion decayed teeth in American mouths that have not been treated. Dental decay often leads to loss of teeth and the need for dentures, which may interfere with good nutrition. Besides, nothing hurts quite like a toothache.

Dentists have known for more than a quarter of a century that up to two-thirds of tooth decay can be prevented by a simple, safe, inexpensive public health measure: the addition of tiny amounts of fluoride to the water supply. For every dollar invested in fluoridation, approximately $50 is saved.

Yet today, thirty-five years after the first American community — Grand Rapids, Michigan — had its water fluoridated, only half the nation's population is receiving such benefits. The main impediment to wider use of fluoridation has been a campaign by small but vociferous groups that maintain that fluoride causes a host of disorders, including birth defects, heart and kidney disease, allergies, and cancer. Careful, extensive research — including major studies sponsored by the federal government — has shown these claims to be false and misleading.

The studies on which the claims of hazard are based have been reviewed by the American Medical Association, the National Cancer Institute, the National Heart, Lung and Blood Institute, the American Academy of Allergy, and the United States Public Health Service, among others, and found to be inadequate to prove the conclusions drawn. Yet they have led many communities, including Los Angeles, to vote down fluoridation or to abandon it after years of effective use.

The Benefits of Fluoride

Fluoride is considered an essential nutrient. [See chapter on micronutrients, page 42.] It protects the teeth by forming crystals of the mineral hydroxyapatite in the tooth enamel. These crystals resist the action of decay-causing acids produced by bacteria that live on tooth surfaces. Fluoride also inhibits the ability of these bacteria to become attached to teeth and to produce acid. Although fluorides are most effective if consumed from birth onward, allowing them to become part of the teeth as they form, they also help to reduce tooth decay in adults.

Bones may also benefit from fluoridated water. Adults who live in communities where the water is naturally high in fluorides have been found to have fewer problems with osteoporosis, the bone loss of aging that causes shortening of the spinal column and costly, painful, life-limiting fractures. Fluoride combines with calcium in bones to form a mineral, fluorapatite, that slows the loss of calcium and the softening of bones with age. [See chapter on osteoporosis, page 610.]

The benefits of fluoridation to teeth have been clearly demonstrated in numerous studies involving whole communities. In some studies dental disease in communities with fluoridated water was compared with that in neighboring communities that lacked fluorides. In others, communities were compared before and after fluoridation. The benefits include the following:

285

* A reduction of up to 65 percent in the number of dental cavities in school-age children who consume fluoridated water from birth and an increased resistance to decay that continues throughout life.
* A decrease of about 75 percent in the loss of first permanent molars in children from twelve to fourteen years old.
* A sixfold increase in the number of children who reach their teens with no cavities.
* A decrease of at least 30 percent in the number of adults who need dentures.

Perhaps the most dramatic demonstration of fluoride's dental benefits took place in the town of Antigo, Wisconsin, which first added fluoride to the city water supply in 1949. The activities of an antifluoridation group brought fluoridation to a halt in 1960. The proportion of kindergarten children free of cavities decreased, from 39 percent in 1960 to 18 percent by 1966, and the number of decayed, filled, or missing teeth in second graders increased more than 200 percent in the same period. In 1965 Antigo — unwilling any longer to sacrifice its dental health to a politically motivated minority — voted to resume fluoridation.

Safety is Well Established

As for fluoride's purported health hazards, at the levels used in water fluoridation (an average of one part fluoride per million parts of water), they are simply nonexistent, according to the American Dental Association and the national Centers for Disease Control. To obtain a lethal dose of fluoride, 2,500 quarts of water would have to be consumed at one time, the dental association says. The water would kill you first. Studies of whole communities of children who grew up with fluoridated water showed no harm to growth, hormones, sexual development, blood, bones, skin, kidneys, or any other organ system or aspect of development.

Supposed links to heart disease and the birth of babies with Down's syndrome (a genetic abnormality formerly called mongolism) were based on wholly inadequate studies that failed to take into account the myriad other factors, such as age and residence, that influence the rates of these disorders, Dr. Ernest Newbrun, a San Francisco dental researcher, has pointed out. Nor is there any effect on the kidneys, liver, blood, maternal milk supply, or hormone-producing glands, the dental association says.

The most terrifying of the charges against fluoridation involves cancer. These charges are invoked by such antifluoridation groups as the National Health Federation when fluoridation is put to a community vote. Regardless of how the matter has been looked at by researchers, no relationship could be found between cancer and consumption of fluoridated water.

In studies by the National Cancer Institute, when such factors as age, sex, and residence were taken into account, cancer death rates were no greater in fluoridated communities than in those without fluoride in the water. Similarly, comparisons of cancer rates before and after fluoridation showed no relationship.

The only known adverse effect of fluoride — a mottling, or discoloration, of teeth and bones — occurs only among people whose water is naturally heavily fluoridated (about eight times the dose used in artificially fluoridated water supplies). No such noticeable effect occurs from drinking artificially fluoridated water.

The benefits of fluoridation can be supplemented by periodic fluoride treatments, including the regular use of a fluoridated toothpaste with the American Dental Association endorsement and periodic application of fluoride paste or solution by the dentist. Adults as well as children can benefit from such fluorides, studies have shown.

Millions Miss Fluoride's Benefits

About 10 million Americans live in communities where the water is naturally fluoridated to a level of one part per million or more. For another 98 million, fluoride is added to the community water supply to approximately that level. (The actual amount varies from 0.7 to 1.2 parts per million, depending on the climate and the amount of water residents can be expected to consume.)

There are state laws requiring fluoridation in Connecticut, Delaware, Georgia, Illinois, Michigan, Minnesota, Nebraska, Ohio, and South Dakota. But for most areas of the country, fluoridation is decided by municipal ballot, and in 1982, 75 million Americans served by public water supplies were still not receiving fluoridated water. In addition, about a quarter of Americans — those who use well water — cannot benefit from community-wide fluoridation, although in some cases well water is naturally fluoridated.

If your water is not fluoridated, your children can still benefit from fluorides through tablets (or drops for infants) or vitamin-fluoride combinations available on prescription from a dentist or physician. Be sure the brand you buy is not prepared in a sugar base lest you partly defeat the purpose. Choose one with a base, such as sorbitol, that does not promote tooth decay.

Orthodontics:
Straight Teeth for Children and Adults

When you go to the dentist, you're usually told to "open wide." But in a proper dental exam you should also be told to "close" so that the dentist can see how your teeth come together.

Misaligned, crooked, protruding, or overcrowded teeth can interfere with the proper development of body and mind. They can make chewing difficult, and because they are difficult to clean, they increase the risk of tooth decay, periodontal disease, and tooth loss. Crooked teeth can also thwart the development of a healthy self-image and sociable personality. Many adults with dental malocclusion, as these problems are called, report that they were teased as children (Bucky is a popular nickname for those with a pronounced overbite) and have always felt self-conscious and reluctant to smile.

A national health survey recently showed that only 46 percent of youngsters aged six through eleven have a normal bite or only slight abnormalities in how their teeth are formed and come together. However, 25 percent have definite malocclusion (literally, "bad bite") and could benefit from orthodontic treatment, and 29 percent have more severe problems for which treatment is considered "highly desirable" or "mandatory."

Although most people think that malocclusion is primarily inherited and little can be done to prevent it, in fact, the emphasis today is on heading off orthodontic problems before they develop. In most cases, if a child is properly examined and followed from about the age of five, costly orthodontic work can be avoided and those cases that require treatment will be far simpler to correct. Today at least 15 percent of orthodontic patients are adults who are having their teeth straightened to improve their looks or prevent tooth loss from periodontal disease that is fostered by malocclusion.

Treating Malocclusions

For children and adults with pronounced malocclusion, there are now a wide variety of orthodontic devices in addition to the "mouthful of metal" associated with traditional orthodontics. The best device to use in a particular case is determined by the severity of the malocclusion and the tolerance of the patient.

Some devices are removable, some are worn part time outside the mouth (such as external headgear), and others are permanently attached to the teeth for the duration of treatment (usually two or three years). Permanent braces can be constructed out of plastic that blends into the color of the teeth, though these may not be strong enough for some cases. Facial bones, as well as teeth, can be realigned to improve both appearance and bite.

The principle behind orthodontic treatment is that pressure placed on teeth causes the bones that support them to resorb on one side and increase on the other, thus repositioning the tooth by changing the shape of the bony socket in which it sits. In a child whose bones are softer and still growing, the process of reshaping the bone through pressure is faster than in an adult. Direct pressure on facial bones can have a similar effect. The amount and direction of the pressure determine the shape the bone will assume.

Genetic factors, such as an inherited disharmony in the size, shape, or position of the jaws, do play a role in malocclusion. But according to Dr. George Silling, orthodontist at the New York University College of Dentistry, environment is more important. A tooth cutting through the gum doesn't "know" where to go. Rather, it chooses the path of least resistance. The American Academy of Pedodontics (children's dentistry) estimates that 50 to 85 percent of orthodontics can be avoided if the problems are caught early enough.

Breaking Bad Mouth Habits

Among environmental forces that can influence which path a tooth follows are bad mouth habits such as thumb- and finger-sucking past the age of six, lip-sucking, cheek-biting, nail-biting, mouth breathing, thrusting the tongue against the front teeth when swallowing, and resting the face against a fist. A pacifier is no better for tooth development than a thumb. However, the pacifier habit is more easily broken because of peer pressure and the fact that unlike a thumb, the pacifier can be conveniently lost.

To break a bad mouth habit, Dr. Harvey Miller of New York Hospital says, the child first has to be made conscious of it, encouraged to cooperate by being told about its effects, and then trained to change it. A cooperative child, even one as young as three or four, can be helped by habit "reminders" — a Band-Aid on the thumb that is sucked, a greasy salve on the lip that is sucked, or a removable mouth appliance that holds the tongue back or makes the habit difficult to pursue — and by simply being reminded in a nonemotional way every time you notice the habit being practiced. In a child who is willing, a thumb-sucking habit can be broken in about ten days, Dr. Miller reports.

Take Care of Baby Teeth

Decay, premature loss, or delayed loss of primary (baby) teeth also can interfere with proper alignment of the permanent teeth. Saving $20 by not repairing a cavity in a primary tooth because it will be lost in a year or two anyway can lead to $2,000 worth of orthodontic treatment later. The premature loss of a front primary tooth usually causes no problem. But if a molar is lost too soon, the surrounding teeth shift and the space into which the permanent tooth must later emerge may close up. This shift can be prevented by the use of a small metal device called a space maintainer; in fact, lost space can be regained with a similar device wedged between the teeth.

On the other hand, if a primary tooth has not fallen out by the time the permanent tooth is ready to come in, the latter could be forced into an abnormal position. In such cases the dentist should pull the primary tooth to clear the way for the permanent one.

The full set of permanent teeth is already formed in the gums by the age of five and can be seen with an X ray. A plaster model can be made of the child's mouth, and in many cases the dentist can predict whether there will be room for all the teeth as they emerge. Sometimes, through a series of well-timed extractions of primary teeth, room can be made for teeth that would otherwise have come in overcrowded and crooked. Eventually one or more permanent teeth may have to be extracted, but the ones that remain will be straight and come together normally.

Containing the Costs

Many people are deterred by the cost of orthodontic treatment. The price can vary greatly depending on the region of the country and the extent and length of therapy. Two factors can help defer costs: orthodontic insurance, purchased through your health plan or insurance company, and the fact that payments to the orthodontist can be spread out over the entire treatment period. Patients without insurance can expect to pay about $100 a month for orthodontic treatment, not counting the costs of tooth extractions, Dr. Silling estimates.

Dr. Stephen Goodman, a New York periodontal specialist, emphasizes that it's unwise to "rush" orthodontic treatment to save money or bother. "The pressure on the teeth should be slow and gradual," he explains. "If the stresses are too great, you can end up with loose teeth." By the same token, orthodontic treatment that lasts for many years and involves extensive movement of the teeth can also loosen teeth, Dr. Goodman notes. In cases requiring extensive readjustment, other approaches besides traditional orthodontics may be needed.

Periodontal Disease: Preventing Tooth Loss

Vincent has bad breath that no mouthwash can erase. June's gums often bleed when she brushes her teeth. Robert's front teeth have begun to spread out, and the spaces between them get wider and wider.

All three have periodontal disease, a problem that could ultimately lead to loss of all their teeth. For more than 20 million Americans, this has already happened. But it doesn't have to happen to Vincent, June, or Robert — or to you.

Dentures are not an inevitable consequence of old age. Your teeth can and should last you a lifetime, whether that be twenty-five, fifty-five, or a hundred five years. Periodontal disease, the most common cause of tooth loss, is almost entirely preventable if you spend ten to fifteen minutes a day cleaning your teeth and visit your dentist twice a year for a professional cleaning.

The alternative to prevention is false teeth or painful, lengthy, costly treatment in an attempt to save the teeth, which is not always successful. As an added benefit, preventing periodontal disease is likely to reduce greatly your problems with tooth decay.

By the age of fifteen, four out of five Americans have the beginnings of periodontal (literally "around the tooth") disease, which can insidiously destroy the supporting structures of their teeth the way termites chew up the foundations of a house. Since in the earlier, reversible stages, the disease is nearly always painless, most people have no inkling of the relentless destruction that may be taking place in their mouths. But nearly all adults and most children can safely assume they have it.

Dental experts have found that those who understand the origins and progression of periodontal disease and its consequences and are taught how to clean their teeth properly are most likely to make good oral hygiene a part of their daily routine. Therefore, it pays for you to read on.

Periodontal disease is primarily the result of the destructive action of bacteria that set up housekeeping in your mouth. These bacteria take advantage of any opportunity to settle down and establish organized colonies. Their favorite habitats are protected areas along the margins where your gums meet your teeth, between your teeth, and in crevices caused by a lost tooth, ill-fitting bridgework, dentures, or worn-down fillings. The bacterial colonies reside in a gummy film called plaque that sticks to the teeth. Unless plaque is removed once every twenty-four to thirty-six hours, it can harden into tartar, or calculus, and become a persistent source of irritation to the gum and underlying bone.

Plaque bacteria produce toxins that damage the gums, causing them to become inflamed and swollen and to pull away from the teeth. Pockets of pus and cell debris may form between the teeth under the gum line, allowing the bacteria and their toxins to move down along the roots of the teeth to the bone that supports them. Eventually the bone retreats, the fibers that hold the teeth to it are gradually eaten away by bacterial action, and the teeth loosen and fall out.

How to Remove Plaque

Plaque is soft and is easily scrubbed off the outer surfaces of your teeth by a soft-bristled toothbrush. But the real problem lies in the plaque that forms between the teeth and just under the gumline. This can't be removed by ordinary brushing. A special brushing technique and daily flossing are necessary to dislodge this otherwise inaccessible plaque. [See chapter on good dental care, page 276.]

Most people use the wrong technique to brush their teeth and spend too little time at it. Your dentist should demonstrate the correct way to brush and floss and review the procedure with you periodically. According to the American Dental Association, to brush properly, use a soft, multitufted brush with rounded-end bristles and a flat brushing surface. The head should be small enough to reach all sides of all your teeth (use a child's brush if necessary).

Holding the brush sideways against your teeth with the bristles at a forty-five-degree angle facing into the gum, wiggle it with very short, almost circular strokes (don't scrub) so that the bristles get in just under the gum to loosen the plaque. Move to the next group of teeth, and repeat, doing both the cheek and the tongue sides of all your teeth.

For the tongue side of the front teeth, hold the brush the long way and use the wiggling strokes. Clean the chewing surfaces with short back and forth scrubbing strokes. Then brush your tongue to remove plaque and reduce problems of bad breath. Since these brushing techniques may not be suitable for everyone, check with your dentist first.

An electric toothbrush can also be used effectively, especially by persons with limited dexterity, such as small children, the handicapped, or the elderly. Avoid highly abrasive toothpastes or powders. Although a mildly abrasive dentifrice can help you clean your teeth, no toothpaste can prevent periodontal disease. Mouthwashes provide only temporary sweetening of the breath. They cannot remove plaque or halt the progression of periodontal disease.

Oral irrigating devices, such as a Water Pik, can supplement but not substitute for the cleansing action of a toothbrush. They are especially useful for people with bridgework or braces on their teeth. Gum stimulators (pointed rubber tips at the end of a toothbrush or handle) can help you massage gum tissue and are especially useful for those with bridgework or large spaces between their teeth.

Dental floss, preferably the unwaxed kind since it is more abrasive, is needed to clean between the teeth. Take an eighteen-inch piece of floss and wrap the ends around your middle fingers, holding a section of about one and a half inches between the thumbs and forefingers of each hand.

With a gentle sawing motion, ease the floss down between the teeth (avoid cutting into the gum). Curve the floss into a C shape around the tooth, and slide it into the space between the gum and the tooth until you feel resistance. Move the floss up and down, scraping against the side of the tooth. Then curve it around the neighboring tooth and repeat. Ease the floss back out through the teeth and move to the next pair of teeth; repeat until all your teeth have been flossed. After flossing, rinse your mouth thoroughly to wash out loosened bacteria.

At first this process will seem extremely awkward and may take you fifteen or twenty minutes to complete. But with practice you should soon be able to do a thorough job in just three to ten minutes. Parents can and should floss their children's teeth, but by age eight or nine most children can do an adequate job themselves.

To help you know whether you've done a thorough job, use a "disclosing" solution or tablet containing a vegetable dye that stains plaque. These can be purchased at pharmacies and are best used after brushing but before flossing. At first use the disclosing agent every day, but as you become more proficient at plaque removal, a spot check once or twice a week is enough.

These dyes also stain the tongue and lips for a few hours, so you may prefer to use them before bed. Put Vaseline on your lips to help prevent staining. Or you may want to use a fluorescent dye that doesn't show in ordinary light; this, however, necessitates the purchase of a special light to show up the stained plaque.

Factors That Promote Gum Disease

Many factors influence the production of plaque and the susceptibility of your gums to its destructive effects. Diet is one. Fibrous foods like raw carrots and celery, lettuce and apples have a natural cleansing action, but soft, gummy foods like white bread cling to the teeth and provide nourishment for plaque bacteria. These bacteria use sucrose (sugar) in the diet to manufacture a substance called dextran that helps them cling to the teeth, so frequent consumption of sugary foods fosters plaque formation. If you eat sweets, it's better to consume them all at one time, preferably before you give your mouth its daily thorough cleaning. But remember that plaque will form even if you eat nothing at all, so there is no substitute for daily plaque removal.

A serious deficiency of vitamin C can promote gum deterioration. However, nearly all Americans with gum disease already consume adequate amounts of vitamin C, so taking extra vitamin C does not help to prevent periodontal disease. Don't be misled by unproved nostrums such as special diets, bone meal preparations, or exotic mouth rinses.

Saliva has a natural cleansing action, and the constituents, consistency, and amount of your saliva affect plaque formation. While awake, you swallow perhaps 2,000 times a day, constantly washing away mouth bacteria. But during sleep you may swallow only 20 times a night. Therefore, just before bed is the best time to remove the bacteria from your teeth. While sleeping, some people breathe through their mouths, further reducing the cleansing by saliva. Emotional stress is known to thicken saliva, maybe one reason why stress increases susceptibility to periodontal disease.

Certain conditions, such as pregnancy, diabetes, and thyroid disease, also foster periodontal disease, as do some drugs, including the oral contraceptives and Dilantin, an antiseizure medication. Other factors include poorly positioned or crowded teeth, excessive pressure on parts of the teeth when chewing, bad oral habits such as teeth grinding and lip biting, smoking, and improper use of toothpicks (don't stick them into your gums — if your gums itch, that's a clue to gum disease that should be treated promptly by the dentist, not scratched with toothpicks).

When to See a Dentist

If your gums bleed when you brush or floss, that is probably a sign that you have the beginning stage of periodontal disease — gingivitis — and should visit your dentist promptly for a professional cleaning and periodontal examination. Other early symptoms of periodontal disease may include soft, tender, reddened, or swollen gums; persistent bad breath; gums that recede from the teeth; a feeling of pressure between the teeth after eating, and an itchy feeling in the gums. Other symptoms of more advanced periodontal disease may include loose teeth, a change in your bite or the fit of dentures, and the formation of spaces between your teeth. Make sure your dentist uses a probe to measure the depth of the space between your gums and teeth and check for pockets of periodontal disease. An X ray will show if there has been any bone loss.

No matter how good a job of plaque removal you may do, a semiannual visit to your dentist is necessary to remove the tartar (hardened plaque) that forms despite your efforts. Tartar cannot be removed by flossing; it must be scraped off by a dentist or dental hygienist with special tools. If plaque forms very readily in your mouth, more frequent professional cleanings — say, once every three months — are advisable.

Treating Periodontal Disease

The treatment of periodontal disease and who does it depend on how advanced the disease has become. For the early reversible stage called gingivitis, your regular dentist can remove the tartar from the crowns and roots of your teeth by scaling and root planing. Scraping the gums may be necessary to remove infected gum tissue.

More advanced disease is best treated by a periodontist. Gum surgery may be done to remove shallow pockets around the teeth. Very advanced disease may require reshaping and grafting of bone and gum transplants. Treatment may also involve grinding or capping teeth to correct abnormal pressure points or the use of splints and other appliances to control harmful mouth habits and reduce movement of loose teeth.

Recent studies at the National Institute of Dental Research suggest benefits from an alternative approach that involves daily treatment with a solution of salt, baking soda, and hydrogen peroxide and the use of an electric toothbrush and pulsed-water irrigator, supplemented by frequent professional cleanings and antibiotic treatments when needed. A number of dentists claim to have used this therapy successfully, but further research is required to confirm its effectiveness and long-term safety.

Depending on the extent of your problem, periodontal treatment can take six to eight months or longer and cost several thousand dollars. The more advanced the disease, the more painful, time-consuming, and costly the therapy. Therefore, it's important to start treatment at the first sign of periodontal disease.

HOW A TOOTH DECAYS

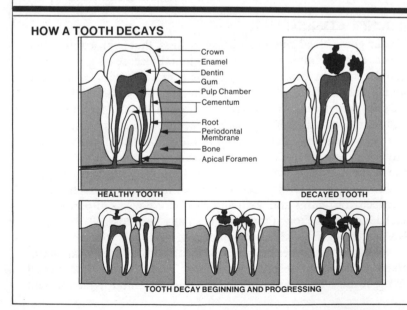

Crown
Enamel
Dentin
Gum
Pulp Chamber
Cementum

Root
Periodontal Membrane
Bone
Apical Foramen

HEALTHY TOOTH

DECAYED TOOTH

TOOTH DECAY BEGINNING AND PROGRESSING

Preventive care is especially important after periodontal treatment because the disease is likely to recur among those who have already had it. Periodontal disease is a disease of neglect, and of all the human chronic health problems, it's the one you can do the most to prevent.

Dentures:
How to Avoid Difficulties

Although often comically treated in movie cartoons, dentures are serious matters to the more than 50 million Americans who wear them and the 30 million who don't but should. By the age of fifty, two in five Americans have already lost their teeth, and by age sixty-five, half are toothless.

Without teeth for chewing, a person's menu is limited to soft, easily mashed foods, and good nutrition may be compromised. Speech is also likely to be distorted, and facial structure can change dramatically, resulting in a sunken look around the mouth. The psychosocial consequences are harder to measure, but being toothless is hardly conducive to a positive self-image and easy social acceptance.

Even those who have dentures may not be deriving the maximum benefit from their false teeth — and may even be doing themselves harm — because of a poor initial fit or failure to get periodic professional adjustments. If dentures that don't fit properly are worn over a long period, destruction of underlying bone and serious mouth irritations, possibly leading to oral cancer, may result, not to mention difficulties in chewing and speaking if the dentures are loose or uncomfortable.

Getting Dentures that Fit

Although they may seem like simple mechanical gadgets, dentures are actually highly sophisticated devices that must be individually tailored to each patient. Before you are fitted with either a partial or a complete denture, your mouth should be thoroughly examined by a dentist, both visually and with X rays. Future difficulties with dentures can result from a failure to detect such problems as cysts, tumors, inflammation, bone loss, teeth that never erupted, tooth roots that are lodged in the jaw, and distorted positions of the jaw.

Your dentist may also be able to save some of your teeth, which could serve as an anchor for a partial denture and result in a more secure fit. When a full denture (upper, lower, or both) is needed, the muscles of the cheeks and the tongue must be relied upon to keep it in place. Thus, even if you've lost most of your teeth, it's to your advantage to take good care of the few that remain.

Careful measurements and impressions must be made to assure a good-fitting denture. The mouth is extremely sensitive to even tiny differences in size — a one-millimeter protrusion can feel like a large mound. An ill-fitting denture may put undue tension on the muscles of the jaw, irritate the sensitive tissues of the gums and cheeks and cause loss of underlying bone as well as fail to provide good chewing action.

Fitting of dentures immediately after tooth extractions can spare you a lot of embarrassment and avoid the development of bad mouth habits, but it means more visits to the dentist, more refittings, and greater expense than if you had waited until your gums healed completely. The decision to get immediate dentures is best made after a thorough discussion with the dentist of their advantages and disadvantages. Sometimes dentists use modules in which the artificial teeth are already in place in a preformed denture and the base is then fitted to the patient's mouth. Though fast, such dentures may not fit as well as those prepared from individual teeth and adjusted to the patient's natural bite.

Another recent development involves the growing use of dental implants — pieces (usually metal) implanted into the bone of the jaw into which false teeth can be anchored. For years implants were nothing but trouble for many of the thousands of patients who tried them, resulting in their removal within months, serious bone loss, and irreversible damage. However, recent experience indicates that today in 65 to 90 percent of patients who are properly selected, implants can be expected to last at least five years and the risk of complications is low.

Implants are recommended for use only in older adults who are unable to use conventional dentures, who are otherwise in good health, and who have good supporting bone in the jaw. If you are considering implants, make sure the oral surgeon and prosthodontist are experienced in their use and are using a device that has been cleared by the federal Food and Drug Administration. If an experimental device is being considered, ask how it has worked out to date.

Adapting to Dentures

Getting used to new dentures can seem as challenging as learning to live without teeth. If you have been without a complete set of teeth for a while, you may have to learn a new way to speak and eat. Your dentist should accompany new dentures with counseling to help you adjust both physically and emotionally.

Dr. Richard A. Abrams, head of the Division of Community Dentistry at Marquette University, points out that "the patient's attitude is the most critical thing in wearing dentures. Patients have to realize that dentures are not real teeth and never will be like real teeth. They've got to work at it, practice."

Most problems are temporary; sensations of bulk, gagging, and crowding disappear with time. At first it's best to select soft foods, take small bites, and chew slowly. Gradually introduce firmer foods, but avoid those that are sticky or very hard until you are well adapted to your dentures. Reading aloud can help improve speech with dentures. Speak more slowly if you find that your dentures click as you talk.

How to Care for Your Dentures

You should take as good care of your dentures and your mouth as you should of teeth. Dentures should be cleaned daily with special brushes and dentrifices (but not ordinary toothpastes) and placed in water (never hot) or a cleansing solution if they are out of your mouth for any length of time. This will help prevent bad breath and staining of the dentures. Your mouth should be rinsed each morning, after every meal, and before bed to clean out harmful bacteria and food particles.

At least once a year you should return to your dentist for an examination and refitting, if needed. Do not try to reline dentures yourself; a small error in fit can be compounded into a major problem. Sometimes, if major changes occur in your jawbones, a new denture may have to be made.

Be Wary of Denture Clinics

You may have heard of denture clinics in which a dental technician, rather than a dentist, does the fitting and preparation of the dentures. These technicians, called denturists, have been working legally in Canada for more than twenty years but are permitted to operate (usually under the supervision of a dentist) only in four states — Maine, Colorado, Arizona, and Oregon. They offer dentures at perhaps half the usual price and thus appeal to people living on fixed incomes. In fact, in some areas senior citizens' groups have been fighting to legalize denturists.

If you are considering a denturist, you should be aware of the possible risks involved. In most states denturists are not licensed, nor are they trained to detect diseases that may show up in or around the mouth. They may also be unable to diagnose conditions that could adversely affect a proper denture fit. If you are thoroughly examined by a dentist beforehand, these risks can be minimized. But make sure the denturist has completed a training program in prosthodontics.

VII.
Eyes, Ears, Nose, and Throat

The upper respiratory tract is probably the cause of more distress than any other system of the body. Perhaps because your eyes, ears, nose, and throat have such intimate contact with the outside environment, they are subject to abnormalities that at the least are annoying and at the worst compromise your ability to function.

The problems are also extremely common. Few children grow up without suffering from one or more ear infections. Sinus trouble is practically epidemic, at least if you believe the ads for decongestants. If you are lucky enough to escape visual defects during your youth, chances are you'll succumb to the need for corrective lenses after mid-life. Nearly everyone has had to contend with snoring at one time or another.

Yet much of the misery associated with EENT (eyes, ears, nose, and throat) can be avoided or alleviated, once you understand the problems and how to prevent or treat them.

Sinusitis:
A Problem Everywhere

Sinuses — we all have them, and given our druthers, many of us would gladly send them to Arizona . . . without us. Each year more than 20 million Americans are plagued by inflamed and painful sinuses, and for some the problem is persistent or recurrent. Frustrated patients who have exhausted the standard repertoire of therapies and are still complaining may be advised by their equally frustrated physicians to move. But where?

Sinusitis, it turns out, is a nationwide complaint. People in the Northeast and Northwest say they get it because it's cold and damp; in the Middle West, because it's cold and dry; in the Southeast, because it's hot and damp; and in the Southwest, because it's hot and dry. There are, however, ways to head off and relieve sinus inflammation short of packing up for parts unknown in the vain hope that the weather will be kinder to those holes in your head.

Sinus means "cavity," and sinuses — hollow air spaces or recesses in the bones — can be found in many parts of the body. The ones that concern most people, however, are the sinuses that surround their noses. The true function of the paranasal sinuses, as they are called, is unknown. It has been suggested that they add resonance to the voice and lighten the weight of the skull. There are four important groups of paranasal sinuses: the frontal sinuses, just above the nose behind the eyebrows; the maxillary sinuses, behind each cheekbone; the sphenoid sinuses behind the nose; and the honeycomblike ethmoid sinuses behind each side of the bridge of the nose.

Why Sinuses Cause Trouble

Each sinus is lined with a mucous membrane and is connected to the nasal cavity by a passageway the width of pencil lead. Herein lies the problem. Whenever this narrow passage becomes obstructed and the sinuses are unable to drain freely and exchange air with the nose, they can become inflamed and painful. Air and secretions trapped in an obstructed sinus can cause pain, as can the vacuum that results when air in the sinus is absorbed into the bloodstream and no fresh air can enter through the nose. Accumulated fluids can become a breeding ground for bacteria, with a sinus infection the result.

It takes very little to block sinus drainage. The most common cause is a cold or other respiratory illness that is associated with swollen mucous membranes and thickened nasal secretions. The "cold" that lingers for weeks and is accompanied by copious thick yellow or greenish nasal discharge is, in fact, a sinus infection. Allergies, a deviated septum (the bony partition in the nose), polyps (benign growths) in the nose, or enlarged and inflamed adenoids can also interfere with sinus drainage and set the stage for sinusitis.

A second major cause of sinusitis is the forced entry of bacteria or other infectious organisms into the sinus cavities. This can happen when infected secretions are carried into the sinuses by forceful blowing of the nose, by increasing air pressure (as during a descent in an airplane), or by water that enters the nose during swimming or diving. An abscessed or badly decayed tooth in the upper jaw can also spread infection into the sinuses.

The hallmark of sinusitis is a headache or pain in the face, usually on only one side of the head (the side of the involved sinus). Pain is likely to be most intense ("splitting") when the frontal sinuses behind the eyebrows are involved. The ethmoid sinuses cause discomfort between the nose and eye beside the bridge of the nose. The lids and tissues surrounding the eye may swell. The maxillary sinuses may be associated with pain in the upper jaw, aches in the teeth, and tenderness in the cheeks. The sphenoid sinuses, less commonly involved in sinusitis, can produce an earache, neck pain, and aching at the top of the head.

Generally sinus headache is most severe in the late morning. Bending over forward tends to make the pain worse, as does jolting, jarring, or tapping the tender area with a finger. The nostril on the painful side of the head (or both nostrils) tends to be blocked.

People commonly mistake tension headaches for "sinus trouble." Unlike sinus headaches, tension headaches are usually relieved by lying

THE FACIAL SINUSES

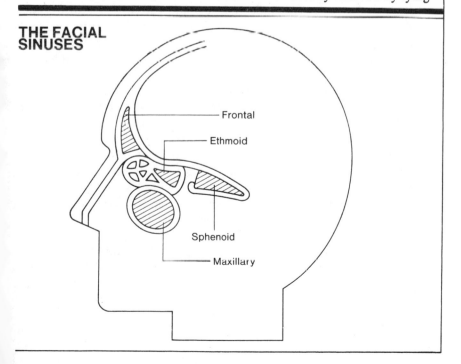

Frontal

Ethmoid

Sphenoid

Maxillary

down and generally are not associated with stuffed nostrils. Since the majority of headaches are not caused by sinus disease and other types of headache can resemble sinus pain, X rays are often necessary to diagnose sinusitis, particularly in its chronic form. In addition to pain, sinusitis may be accompanied by malaise, swelling, postnasal drip, bad breath, and fever.

Sinus attacks come in two forms: acute, which generally lasts a week to ten days, and chronic, which can persist for months, with continual discomfort or periodic flare-ups. Chronic sinus inflammation can flare up with the slightest obstruction, such as that caused by smoking or inhaling someone else's smoke, exposure to an allergen, eating spicy foods, drinking alcohol, or being exposed to chilly, damp weather.

Although most cases of sinusitis are brief and mild, repeated acute attacks can lead to a permanent thickening of the membranes in the sinuses and result in a chronic problem. Complications of sinusitis are rare, but when they do occur, they can be very serious. Untreated, sinus infection may lead to an ear infection, bronchitis, or pneumonia. More serious complications include osteomyelitis (a bone infection) and infection of the eye cavity, the meninges (lining of the skull), or the brain.

How to Prevent Sinusitis

302

The first line of defense in preventing sinusitis, as with all other infectious illnesses, is to be sure to get enough rest, eat well-balanced meals, and exercise regularly. Many joggers report that running helps their sinuses to drain. A similar effect would accompany vigorous exercise of any sort. When your home is heated, especially if the system is forced-air heat, the use of a humidifier may help to prevent drying of mucus and blockage of sinus drainage. [But first, see chapter on humidifiers, page 372.]

If you smoke, stop. Tobacco smoke paralyzes the cilia (hairs) in the nasal passages that help clear out debris and invading organisms. [See chapter on quitting smoking, page 256.] If you have allergies, try to identify and avoid the provoking substances. Air conditioners may help remove dust and pollen from the air. [See chapter on hay fever, page 542.] Swimming in chlorinated water can also precipitate sinusitis by irritating the membranes that line the nose and sinuses. Use goggles and nose plugs to prevent chlorinated water from entering your nasal passages and sinuses. When blowing your nose, blow gently, blow both nostrils simultaneously, and don't pinch your nose.

To keep nasal passages open when you have a cold, use decongestant nose drops or spray (such as ¼ percent phenylephrine), but be sure to follow directions on the label, and limit their use to once every three or four hours (some recommend that they be used only twice a day) for no more than three days. Such medication should not be used by people with high blood pressure or heartbeat irregularities without a doctor's advice. A decongestant spray and sometimes an oral decongestant as well are helpful before you descend in an airplane. Antihistamines can reduce nasal swelling and congestion in people with allergies.

Treating Sinus Problems

Treatment of sinusitis is designed to restore normal drainage of the nasal passages, to relieve pain, and to reduce inflammation. Many people are helped by inhaling steam or using hot, wet compresses over the sinuses and nostrils. Some find that alternating hot packs and cold packs brings the greatest relief. Aspirin often reduces the pain of sinusitis, and an oral decongestant and decongestant nose drops or sprays may relieve congestion.

If you have chills or fever and a thick, yellow nasal secretion along with sinus discomfort, you probably have a bacterial infection. If the infection is severe, antibiotics may be needed. If possible, the doctor should culture the causative organism before prescribing an antibiotic. Penicillin — or its substitute, erythromycin, for those allergic to penicillin — can kill the bacteria that most commonly cause sinusitis. Antibiotics are prescribed for seven to ten days in acute cases and four to six weeks or longer for chronic forms.

In severe cases, a physician who specializes in the ear, nose, and throat (otolaryngologist) may have to drain the sinuses physically, either by suctioning or by washing out the accumulated pus and mucus. Chronic cases may require surgery to scrape out the thickened linings of the sinuses or to remove polyps.

Snoring: Always Bothersome, Sometimes Serious

The bedroom is filled with snorts and chortles. A woman is perched, lamp in hand, ready to strike the somnolent source of the distressing sounds — her husband. This and similar scenes are common in comedies and in cartoons.

Though often a subject of derision and humor, sonorous breathing during sleep, better known as snoring, is really no laughing matter. It's certainly no joke to those who have to listen to it and sometimes not to the creator of the grunts, rumbles, whistles, rasps, and hisses. In addition to its sleep-disrupting effects on spouses, roommates, and neighbors, snoring, particularly the persistent, loud kind, can be a signal of a serious health problem.

Hundreds of "remedies" — including such bizarre contraptions as snore alarms, harnesses that prevent turning over, straps that hold the mouth shut — have been devised or suggested. Most afford little or no relief, and some can jeopardize the health and life of the sleeper by preventing breathing through the mouth. Sometimes, however, simple, practical measures can eliminate or reduce the frequency of snoring. In other cases medical or surgical treatment can correct the problem.

Snoring is the audible symptom of a blocked airway during sleep. The noise is caused by a vibration in the soft palate as the lungs pull hard to take in the diverted or weakened current of incoming air. The blockage may result from any number of circumstances, and these offer clues to alleviating the problem. Obesity, nasal deformities, and enlarged tonsils and adenoids may create structural obstacles to air. Nasal allergies, heavy smoking, gluttonous bedtime eating, and heavy consumption of alcohol and food can swell nasal passages and similarly block the free flow of air. Snoring is also more likely to occur among people who sleep on their backs; the tongue falls back toward the throat and partly closes the airway.

Sleep Apnea and Other Hazards

Most of the time snoring is intermittent and innocuous, except for its disrupting effects on the sleep of others. But some people snore all night, indicating a possible shortage of oxygen for a significant portion of a person's life. In turn, recent studies suggest, this may lead to daytime fatigue and eventually may precipitate high blood pressure and other disorders of the cardiovascular and nervous systems.

In a few cases heavy snoring is a sign of a potentially life-threatening problem: sleep apnea, in which breathing stops for seconds or even minutes at a time and finally resumes with raucous snorting and tossing about. The pattern may be repeated hundreds of times all night long. The resulting chronic oxygen shortage may lead to abnormal heart rhythms, high blood pressure, and heart strain.

Sleep apnea affects the obese almost exclusively. Nine of every ten victims are male. Anyone with such snoring patterns who is excessively sleepy during the day (possibly dozing off while driving, while reading, or even while talking) or who has signs of memory loss or intellectual deficiencies would be wise to undergo a thorough medical examination and have his or her sleep patterns evaluated in a sleep laboratory.

The apnea is often corrected by weight loss. Sometimes surgical relief of a blockage in the nose or upper throat is helpful. Other cases may be helped by antidepressant drugs or nasal tubes, but some victims require a tracheotomy (a surgically created breathing hole cut through the windpipe) to eliminate the risk of fatal complications.

Causes and Treatment

About one in every eight people snores — more men than women. Snoring is common among children under the age of ten, usually because of enlarged tonsils and adenoids or nasal allergies. It becomes less common during adolescence and young adulthood, only to increase again after the age of thirty. (Animals, especially such blunt-faced dogs as boxers and Boston terriers, also snore.)

For all the people it afflicts, snoring has not attracted much research attention. There are fewer than 100 papers in the medical literature that discuss it at all, and only a handful reflect good research. "Treating snoring as a joke discourages research and perpetuates our ignorance," says Dr. Charles Pollak of the sleep clinic at the Montefiore Medical Center in the Bronx, New York.

One who has studied snoring, Dr. Kenneth Hinderer, an ear, nose, and throat specialist at the University of Pittsburgh, points out that people normally breathe through their noses while sleeping, but if the nose doesn't bring in enough air, mouth breathing is used to supplement it. Snoring may result (though some people manage to snore with their mouths closed). He goes on to note that devices that attempt to eliminate snoring by keeping the mouth closed can interfere with an adequate oxygen supply to the body and brain.

Dr. Hinderer has found that there is a natural nasal sleep cycle that can be interrupted by nasal deformities or injuries. Normally, he explains, you would go to sleep on your side and the nasal passage on top would open while the bottom passage slowly swells and closes. After a while you turn over, and the nostril now on top opens while the bottom one closes. This helps assure normal, quiet breathing all night. However, if some abnormality or nasal congestion prevents the opening of the upper nostril, the cycle is interrupted and mouth-breathing or other snore-promoting sleep positions may result.

Nasal congestion may be relieved by eliminating allergens in the bedroom (dust, down pillows or quilts, nonfoam mattresses), taking antihistamines or decongestants, stopping smoking, avoiding excessive consumption of food and alcohol in the evening, and reducing salt intake.

Surgery may be needed to correct certain structural defects, such as deviated septum. But Dr. Hinderer suggests first trying to equalize the pressure in the nostrils by rolling up a tiny ball of tissue (from a piece about the size of a postage stamp) and placing it inside the pocket in the forward part of the tip of the nose. If the pocket is bigger on one side than the other, he suggests a slightly larger ball of tissue on that side. This, Dr. Hinderer says, helps to open the nostrils and change the direction of the air current through the nose, so that the air will no longer cause a vibration of the soft palate, or snoring.

The breathing blockage may also result from excess fatty tissues in obese people or from flabby muscles in the back of the mouth — for example, when dentures fit improperly or are removed at night. Some find that sleeping with their dentures in place eliminates snoring, and weight loss usually does. If chronically enlarged tonsils are the cause of breathing difficulties, a tonsillectomy is likely to help.

Finally, there are numerous tricks to maintain a snore-inhibiting sleeping position, such as stacking up pillows or a head rest so that the sleeper is more upright. Sleeping in a cervical collar (the type used to treat a neck sprain) will keep the chin elevated and often prevent snoring, according to one expert. Some have tried sewing a marble or rubber ball into the back of the pajama top, which prompts a quick return to one's side. But avoid barricades that prevent the sleeper from turning over from side to side, since Dr. Hinderer's studies indicate that this may make matters worse.

Tonsils and Adenoids: When to Operate

Just a few decades ago community newspapers proudly printed portraits of entire families who were about to enter the local hospital to have their tonsils removed. Often it was only one child who really "needed" the operation, but while the doctor was at it, parents asked that those pesky tissues be removed from everyone in the family.

The picture today is vastly different. Although tonsillectomy was the nation's leading operation as recently as 1971, it has declined dramatically since and now ranks third — below hernia repair and hysterectomy, according to the National Center for Health Statistics.

Still, it remains by far the most common major operation among children under fifteen, and many specialists believe that the great majority of the 600,000 or so tonsillectomies done annually are unnecessary operations, subjecting thousands of children to surgical risks for little or no demonstrable benefit. Although tonsillectomies have been done for thousands of years — at least since 600 B.C. and perhaps as long ago as 3000 B.C. — their true value is only now being examined.

What Are the Tonsils?

Tonsils are patches of lymph tissue — a part of the body's immunological system — that are attached to the sides of the throat just behind the teeth. Companion tissues, the adenoids, are located at the top of the throat where the nasal passages end and the Eustachian tubes that go to the middle ear begin.

Tonsils enlarge in early childhood, usually reach their maximum size between the ages of three and six years, and then shrink. Adenoids also shrink, but often not until puberty. As a child gets older, the frequency of infections of all kinds decreases, and most children outgrow any possible need for a tonsillectomy by the age of eight.

Contrary to what many people think, tonsils (and presumably adenoids) are not useless tissues. They have definite immunological activity and may help defend against a variety of infections, ranging from colds to polio. However, whether there are important disadvantages to being without tonsils and adenoids is still unknown. One report, by the New York State Health Department, that tonsillectomy may increase the risk of Hodgkin's disease, a cancer of the lymph system, has not been borne out by later research.

When To Remove Them

Whatever their function, experts now agree, tonsils are not to be removed just because they're there. Tonsillectomy is an operation, and all operations entail some risk, both from the anesthesia and from the surgery itself. Bleeding after surgery is the most common complication. It is estimated that between 1 in 10,000 and 1 in 100,000 patients dies as a result of tonsillectomy. Psychological harm may also result if the child's hospital experience is not handled sensitively. Aside from the possible risks, removal of the tonsils does not guarantee an end to throat infections.

There is only one undisputed reason for removing tonsils: if they are so enlarged that they interfere with breathing or swallowing. Except for this uncommon situation, there is a wide range of medical opinion. Some doctors suggest removing the tonsils if a child suffers two or three sore throats during one year; others say tonsillectomy is no cure for sore throats, so no amount of illness is justification for the surgery.

Parents who seek several opinions are likely to get just that — opinions, often radically different, that have limited foundation in fact.

A major study at Children's Hospital in Pittsburgh is using as its criteria for surgery one of the following situations: seven or more sore throats in one year, or five sore throats in each of two consecutive years, or three sore throats in each of three consecutive years. Furthermore, the sore throat episodes have to be documented as medically significant by a doctor's examination.

An earlier phase of the study, being conducted by Dr. Jack L. Paradise and his colleagues, showed that parental memory of the frequency of sore throats may sometimes be in error and that children sometimes complain of a sore throat when no infection is present. In fact, only one in five children initially thought to meet the criteria for surgery were shown to actually have had as many throat infections as believed.

Although the study is not yet complete, Dr. Paradise says the results so far suggest that children who meet the criteria for surgery and undergo a tonsillectomy thereafter suffer few throat infections, whereas children who do not have the surgery are more likely to have further sore throats. However, about half of those *not* operated on do nearly as well as those who have the operation. So far, Dr. Paradise says, there's no way to predict who will and who will not continue to have sore throats if no surgery is done.

Thus, the Pittsburgh pediatrician has tentatively concluded on the basis of this preliminary evidence that "tonsillectomy is not a useless operation from the standpoint of preventing throat infections among children who suffer a lot of medically documented infections. But the degree of benefit is variable. Some who are not operated on do just as well as those who have the surgery."

However, Dr. Paradise points out, the majority of tonsillectomies are done for far less stringent criteria than those used in his study, and the benefit to such children is highly questionable. Even those who meet the Pittsburgh criteria for surgery should not automatically be pushed into a tonsillectomy, he maintains.

"You have to deal with each child individually and consider such matters as whether the repeated infections are hurting the child educationally and whether the family has geographical and economical access to medical care," Dr. Paradise says. "Tonsillectomy is a useful operation that should be reserved for a highly select group of children, and even then done only for certain reasons." His rule of thumb: "When in doubt, don't operate. There's no harm in waiting awhile to see what happens."

Other claimed benefits of tonsillectomy — such as dramatic increase in appetite and growth — are, for the most part, apocryphal, possibly true for only a tiny fraction of patients who were sick so much of the time that they ate poorly, experts say.

Sometimes adults who suffer repeated infections have their tonsils removed. At Yale University, where about 20 percent of the tonsillectomies involve adults, the operation is done because the tissue has become chronically infected, and instead of functioning as a barrier to infection, serves as a source of repeated throat infections. More than seven such infections a year is the Yale criterion for removing an adult's tonsils.

The operation is more painful in adults than in children. Children usually go home the day after surgery and return to school in a week, but adults may be hospitalized for several days and spend about two weeks recovering from the operation.

Should the Adenoids Go, Too?

Traditionally, when tonsils are removed, adenoids are taken out along with them, giving the surgery the common name of T and A. This practice, too, has been called into question in recent years.

In the Pittsburgh study, adenoids are removed along with tonsils only when they interfere with breathing or speech or if the child suffers from chronic or recurrent middle ear infections that impair hearing or cause other serious ear problems. [See chapter on middle ear problems, page 312.] Adenoids may also be removed by themselves (an adenoidectomy) for these reasons.

Dr. Paradise says it's too soon to know what benefit adenoidectomy might have for ear infections, but it is clearly useful for those with long-standing obstruction of the nasal passages if the cause of the obstruction is enlarged adenoids and not something else, such as allergy.

If either tonsillectomy or adenoidectomy is done, the procedure is best performed by a board-certified ear, nose, and throat specialist.

Hearing Loss: Often Missed and Mistreated

Hearing loss is the most common chronic disability in the United States. A national survey completed in 1971 showed that 14.5 million Americans have a hearing loss that interferes with their ability to understand conversations and to function socially and vocationally. Nearly 2 million cannot hear or understand speech and are classified as deaf. The survey showed that 1.3 percent of children under seventeen and at least 40 percent of adults over sixty-five had hearing disabilities.

Despite its commonness, hearing loss is frequently mistreated. A recent survey showed that 70 percent of people who buy hearing aids do so without the benefit of a professional examination by an independent medical specialist (an otologist or otolaryngologist) or by an audiologist (a certified hearing specialist). Many of these people have hearing problems that could be corrected through medical or surgical treatment, making an aid totally unnecessary. Others could expect little help from a hearing aid unless it was individually prescribed to suit their particular problem and then followed by a rehabilitation program. Still others simply do not need a hearing aid or could not benefit from one under any circumstances.

All told, about 40 percent of the hearing aids purchased without a professional examination — at an average cost of $300 to $400 (the markup is commonly 300 percent) — are inappropriate or unnecessary, according to the American Speech and Hearing Association.

Causes of Hearing Loss

A child's hearing may be damaged by overgrown adenoids that block the Eustachian tube; chronic infections and fluid in the middle ear; allergies; a bone abnormality called otosclerosis that interferes with the movement of bones in the inner ear; or simply an accumulation of wax. These difficulties cause a *conductive* hearing loss — a disruption in the transfer of sound waves from the external ear to the inner ear. Nearly all conductive losses can be corrected through surgery or medical treatment, and normal hearing restored or the condition stabilized. [See chapter on middle ear problems, page 312.]

The other type of hearing loss — *sensorineural* — may result from damage to the sensitive hair cells of the inner ear that receive sound waves or from interference with the transmission of the sound-induced nerve impulses to the brain via the auditory nerve. A professionally selected hearing aid can be of enormous benefit when a sensorineural hearing loss interferes with a person's ability to communicate.

Some people are born with sensorineural hearing loss as a result of certain genetic diseases, prenatal exposure to a viral infection (such as rubella) or to a drug that damages hearing, a birth injury, or inadequate oxygen at birth. Although most such defects are permanent, properly fitted hearing aids and speech and language therapy can help many children to learn to speak and understand spoken language.

More commonly, sensorineural hearing loss is caused by prolonged exposure to excessive noise, by deterioration of nerves and blood vessels through aging, by viral and bacterial infections, by drugs that damage hearing (including high doses of aspirin, certain antibiotics, and some diuretics used to treat high blood pressure), and occasionally by a tumor on the auditory nerve. [See chapter on tinnitus, page 316.]

"Noise probably accounts for more hearing loss than all other factors combined," according to Dr. Maurice H. Miller, professor of audiology at New York University and chief of audiology at Lenox Hill Hospital. "Forty million people work in an environment noisy enough to damage their hearing after prolonged exposure."

Even though the federal noise limit of 90 decibels set in 1970 will protect the hearing of most workers, many industries still do not meet that limit and don't protect workers exposed to louder noises. Significant sources of noise in the home include vacuum cleaners, air conditioners, hair dryers, garbage disposals, and electric blenders. Snowmobiles, rock-and-roll music, and the steady roar of traffic can damage hearing; the noise in some subway cars can reach a potentially hazardous 118 decibels. [See chapter on noise, page 364.]

Prevention and Early Detection

Since serious hearing damage by noise cannot be reversed, prevention through noise control or wearing muffs to protect hearing is by far the best medicine, Dr. Miller emphasizes. Other preventive measures include prompt treatment of all ear infections, avoiding airplane flights when you have a cold, not using instruments — including cotton swabs — to remove ear wax (wax in the ears should be left there or removed by an otologist if it interferes with hearing), and changing drugs or adjusting dosages to prevent hearing damage.

Adults are advised to have a hearing test as part of their regular physical examinations. Such tests are especially important for people who work in noisy environments, those who are over age sixty-five, and those who regularly take drugs that could damage hearing. Professional audiologic examinations should also be conducted during the first two months of life on infants who weighed less than three and a half pounds at birth as well as on those who had high bilirubin levels, suffered prenatal viral infections, have a family history of childhood hearing impairment, or have birth defects involving the ear, nose, or throat.

The early stages of hearing loss may be hard to detect and easy to deny. Any of the following should warrant an examination by an otologist and/or an audiologist:

• Inability to hear the ticking of a watch.

• Ringing in the ears (if this happens while you are taking a drug, inform your physician immediately).

• A need to strain to hear what is being said or to have people repeat themselves.

• Giving inappropriate answers to questions.

• Difficulty hearing if you are not in the front rows of a theater or near the loudspeaker in a movie.

• Difficulty distinguishing between words like "fit," "sit," "kit," and "hit."

• Difficulty hearing on the telephone or identifying the source of a voice in a group.

• Finding yourself increasingly left out of conversations.

Getting Proper Treatment

"People wait an average of about five years before they do something about a hearing problem," Dr. Miller says. "They first blame factors outside themselves for their hearing difficulty — they say, 'People don't talk clearly,' or, 'There's too much noise to hear.' Then, when they finally decide to do something, they do the wrong thing by going directly to a vendor to get a hearing aid."

The examination for hearing loss should be done by a qualified professional who has no ties to the sale or rental of hearing aids, and no aid should be fitted without such an examination. A few states — New York, California, and Michigan among them — have laws requiring a professional exam before you buy an aid, and the federal Food and Drug Administration prohibits sales of hearing aids without a prior medical examination. A hearing evaluation by a professional can distinguish between a correctable conductive loss and sensorineural loss.

If an aid is deemed appropriate, audiological training and adjustment are needed if the costly device is not to end up permanently stored in a bureau drawer. People fitted with hearing aids must be taught how to be good listeners and how to clarify distortions in hearing introduced by the aid. They need assistance in re-entering the world of sound.

How to Find Professional Help

Your family doctor may recommend a hearing specialist, or you can call your county medical society or nearby medical school or get in touch with your local crippled children's program. The American Speech-Language-Hearing Association, 10801 Rockville Pike, Rockville, Maryland, 20852, can provide a list of certified audiologists or centers that perform complete audiological examinations in your area.

For Further Reading

Rosenthal, Richard. *The Hearing Loss Handbook.* New York: St. Martin's Press, 1975.

Middle Ear Problems: Prevention and Treatment

Erik had the sniffles, hardly unusual for a four-year-old. But as the day wore on, he became cranky and feverish. He awoke from a nap holding his head and crying with the stabbing pain of an ear infection.

Every winter, the peak season for upper respiratory infections, millions of young Americans suffer the agonies of ear infections. For some it's a problem that recurs perhaps four or five times a season. In addition to the discomfort, fever, and malaise, many suffer hearing loss that can seriously interfere with learning and getting along with others.

Ear infections nearly always result from infections of the nose and throat that work their way through the Eustachian tubes, the air channels that run from the middle ear and serve as an outlet for secretions and an equalizer of air pressure on either side of the eardrum. Middle ear infections may develop as complications of colds, sore throats, or viral or bacterial diseases like measles, mumps, scarlet fever, and flu.

Children are more prone to ear infections than adults because the straight, horizontal Eustachian tubes of children more readily carry infectious organisms into the middle ear than the curved, tilted tubes of adults. However, adults as well as children may develop an inflammation of the middle ear in response to changes in air pressure, such as during airplane flights.

Most ear infections are readily cured by treatment with antibiotics and decongestants, but failure to treat them adequately can sometimes lead to such serious consequences as mastoiditis or permanent hearing loss. The most common forms of middle ear problems are painful enough to force the patient to seek medical treatment. Sometimes, however, the symptoms are less obvious or practically nonexistent, and the victim suffers chronic, undetected hearing loss. A child with this problem is likely to have difficulty learning and hearing instructions and may be labeled stupid or disobedient.

The more common types of middle ear problems, their symptoms, treatment and, in some cases, methods of prevention, include the following:

Acute Otitis Media (Ear Infection)

A stabbing earache, a feeling of fullness in the ear, impaired hearing, and sometimes fever and ringing in the ear are the hallmarks of this disorder, the most common type of middle ear inflammation. The problem may occur in one ear or both ears simultaneously, nearly always in conjunction with another infection. Sometimes, enlarged adenoids block the opening of the Eustachian tubes and increase susceptibility to otitis media; in such cases, an adenoidectomy may be necessary to prevent recurrent infections. [See chapter on tonsils and adenoids, page 306.]

It's wise to avoid swimming — and especially diving — when you have an infection in the nose, sinuses, or throat because water that enters through the nose may force germs into the middle ear. Ear plugs are no help since the infection enters from the inside, not the outer ear.

The pain of acute otitis can be relieved by aspirin and heat, such as provided by a hot-water bottle. The infection should be treated with an antibiotic (such as penicillin, ampicillin, or erythromycin) or sulfa drugs, with the medication continued for five or more days after the infection has apparently cleared. This usually means about ten days to two weeks of therapy. In an increasing number of cases the infecting organism is resistant to ampicillin, and a broader-spectrum antibiotic like cefaclor is

313

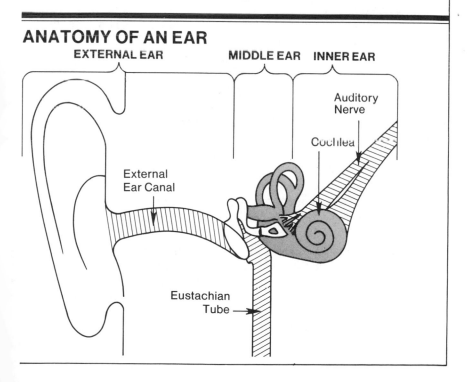

ANATOMY OF AN EAR

EXTERNAL EAR   MIDDLE EAR   INNER EAR

Auditory
Nerve

Cochlea

External
Ear Canal

Eustachian
Tube

needed to prevent recurrences. Antihistamines or decongestants may also be prescribed to clear the middle ear and Eustachian tube of congestion by mucus and fluid that can impair hearing and act as a breeding ground for a recurrent infection.

Sometimes in an acute ear infection the eardrum ruptures and blood-tinged fluid drains out. This relieves the pressure on the drum and the intense earache, but drug therapy is still needed to eradicate the infection. The drum will nearly always heal, but because repeated ruptures may result in a chronic infection with potentially serious consequences, it's important to get prompt treatment of ear infections before the drum ruptures.

Untreated, acute otitis could develop into mastoiditis, an inflammation of the bone in the ear which may require surgery and can result in permanent hearing loss. Other complications of untreated ear infections include meningitis and brain abscess.

Chronic Otitis Media

This problem often occurs as the aftermath to acute otitis or repeated upper respiratory infections that involve the Eustachian tubes. Or it may result from enlarged adenoids or the effects of pressure changes. Pain may be present at first, but then it disappears. However, the feeling of fullness and hearing loss persists. The patient may complain of a sensation of "water in the ear." Ringing in the ear and dizziness are also common symptoms.

Sometimes the loss of hearing is so gradual that neither patient nor family is aware of the problem. If the patient is a child, the insidious hearing loss can lead to serious learning difficulties, as well as to irritability and other behavior problems. Failure to recognize and treat chronic otitis can also result in serious physical consequences, including mastoiditis.

In recent years there has been a tremendous increase in the number of children diagnosed as having a chronic middle ear problem called *serous otitis media*. There is no pain or discharge from the ear, and the eardrum may look normal to the doctor; but sterile fluid has collected behind the drum, where it impairs hearing and provides an ideal growth medium for the next infectious organism that happens along. The condition may develop following treatment for acute otitis or as a consequence of allergies.

If hearing is affected and decongestants cannot clear up the accumulated fluid, or if the fluid is gummy, a simple operation, in which tubes are placed through a tiny opening in the drum, can correct the problem and produce dramatic changes in the child's behavior. The tubes are kept in place for six weeks to several months and usually come out by themselves. The operation is best done by an otolaryngologist.

Anyone who has had numerous ear infections or who is diagnosed as having serious otitis media should have a professional hearing examination by an audiologist, with periodic follow-up examinations if the problem persists.

Aerotitis (from Changing Air Pressure)

Closing of the ear during airplane flights or other high-altitude activities is a common experience. Usually during the descent many people experience pain or a sense of fullness and deafness that may then last for hours or days. Sometimes the pain is excruciating and a hemorrhage occurs inside the middle ear.

The problem results from a failure of the Eustachian tube to equalize the pressure on either side of the eardrum. Pressure in the middle ear becomes negative relative to the outside air, causing sterile fluid to exude into the middle ear, as it does in serous otitis media. It is most likely to happen if the tubes are already swollen, perhaps as the result of a cold or an allergy. Consumption of alcoholic beverages before or during the flight can make the problem worse because alcohol causes swelling of the mucous membranes.

To avoid aerotitis, it's best to stay out of airplanes if you have an upper respiratory infection, including "a little cold," or an allergy that has congested your nasal passages or sinuses. In addition, you might avoid alcoholic beverages before or during the flight. Babies should be seated upright during the descent to minimize Eustachian tube closure. Yawning, swallowing, chewing gum, sucking on mints, and using a nasal decongestant spray (administered before the descent begins — within two hours of the plane's anticipated landing) can help to keep the Eustachian tubes open. Try not to sleep during the descent because you may not swallow often enough to keep up with the pressure changes.

For more stubborn problems, a decongestant tablet may be taken once or twice on the day of the flight, including one tablet within four hours of the plane's scheduled arrival time. An excellent medication for this purpose — Sudafed   can be purchased without a doctor's prescription, but it should not be used by persons with high blood pressure or excessive nervousness. If you are suffering from allergies, be sure to take your antihistamine tablets at the beginning of the flight.

If your ears fail to pop and you feel increasing pressure as the plane descends, you might try to unblock your ears in this way: Pinch your nostrils shut, take a mouthful of air, and using your cheek and throat muscles, force the air into the back of your nose as if you were trying to blow your fingers off your nostrils. You should hear a loud pop as your ears unblock, but you may have to repeat the procedure several times during the descent. *Be sure not to use pressure from your chest or abdomen when trying to clear your ears.*

If aerotitis does not clear up by itself within a few hours after landing, it should be treated with decongestants administered by a physician.

Tinnitus:
When the Noise Is Internal

Ringing, roaring, buzzing, hissing, chirping, whining, or whistling noises in the ear or head: Nearly everyone hears such sounds now and again, perhaps when he or she has been exposed to a loud noise or has a cold or sinus congestion. But an estimated 37 million Americans hear them in one or more forms all the time.

To some they are intolerably loud, as loud as a subway car roaring into the station or a jet plane taking off. But even at much lower volumes they can interfere with work, sleep, personal relationships, and the ordinary pleasures of life. Sounds that some people tolerate well, others find maddening. Sometimes they drive people to drink, drugs, or even suicide.

The problem is called tinnitus (pronounced tinn-EYE-tus by the American Tinnitus Association), and until recently most sufferers were told, "There's not much we can do. You'll just have to learn to live with it." But the outlook today for many victims is far brighter. Though no cure is known for the majority of cases, several new techniques that can bring significant relief and sometimes the temporary disappearance of the life-disrupting symptom are now available.

Causes

Persistent internally generated head sounds can have many causes, and some have long been amenable to medical or surgical treatment that may provide a permanent cure. Obstructing ear wax, tumors of the auditory nerve, middle ear infection, otosclerosis (a bone disease in the middle ear), and other ear disorders are among the potentially correctable causes of tinnitus.

In addition, certain drugs — including aspirin, several antibiotics in the "mycin" family, certain drugs used to treat high blood pressure, indomethacin, quinine medications, and some tranquilizers — may cause ringing in the ears that is sometimes reversible. Inform your physician immediately if you develop ringing in your ears while taking any drug. Allergies, especially a food allergy, may also cause tinnitus as well as hearing loss.

Thus, it is critically important for all persons afflicted with tinnitus to have a thorough medical and audiological examination to determine if there is an underlying correctable cause before pursuing some of the newer treatments that offer relief but not cure. The examination should be done by an otolaryngologist (a physician who is a specialist in the ear, nose, and throat) and by a certified audiologist (a hearing specialist). It should include an ear, nose, and throat examination; a complete audiology test; X rays of the internal auditory canal; and a balance test called electronystagmography.

The majority of cases of tinnitus are not yet curable. Most are caused by prolonged exposure to noise, usually at work. The noise damages the sound-sensitive hair cells of the cochlea in the inner ear. Persons with cochlear damage often also suffer hearing loss. [See chapters on noise, page 364, and hearing loss, page 309.] Dr. Maurice H. Miller, professor of audiology at New York University and chief of audiology at Lenox Hill Hospital, warns that a person with tinnitus who has been exposed to noise should not automatically be assumed to have a noise-induced problem. A treatable disease or tumor may be the real culprit.

Other causes of tinnitus include deterioration of the cochlea or other parts of the ear with age, Menière's disease, cardiovascular disease, head injury, and acoustic trauma — exposure to a sudden extremely loud noise.

Treatment

Some victims with mildly disturbing tinnitus find that they can treat themselves by playing background music, tuning the radio to the noise between FM stations or playing a recording of "white noise" (like ocean waves) to block out the noise in their own heads. For others, however, these are not adequate solutions. Those who also have hearing loss often find that use of a hearing aid reduces or eliminates their awareness of the tinnitus by focusing their attention on outside sounds.

The most exciting recent advance has been the development of a device that resembles a hearing aid, called a tinnitus masker; it produces a noise to cover up the tinnitus. According to various estimates, between 30 and 70 percent of tinnitus patients find relief by using the masker either intermittently or continuously. Dr. Jack Vernon, a professor of otolaryngology at the University of Oregon Health Sciences Center, who was instrumental in the development of the masker, reports that studies of 160 patients who have used the device for up to two years showed no adverse effect on speech discrimination or on the severity of the tinnitus itself.

In fact, Dr. Vernon told an international conference on tinnitus, many patients using the masker reported a reduction in the intensity of their tinnitus, and in a few the internal noise disappeared entirely after a while. Some patients found that they could use the masker in cycles; after they had used it for several hours, days, or weeks, their tinnitus disappeared for an equal or greater amount of time and then gradually returned to its former volume.

In explaining how the masker works, Dr. Vernon said that people ordinarily learn to ignore many external sounds, such as ventilator noise, traffic sounds, or office racket, but "internal sounds such as tinnitus cannot be easily ignored." When the external noise from the masker covers the tinnitus, patients learn to ignore the masker noise and automatically ignore the tinnitus at the same time, Dr. Vernon believes.

The masker, which has been developed in various forms to cover noises of different frequencies, has not yet been subjected to carefully controlled tests. It is possible — indeed likely — that some patients helped by it are responding to the power of suggestion (placebo effect) rather than to the instrument itself.

There is also available a combination hearing aid and tinnitus masker that is helpful to some patients with hearing loss for whom a hearing aid alone is not enough. The masker alone costs about $300, not including the cost of fitting and testing.

Another new approach involves biofeedback, a method that enables people to exercise conscious control over ordinarily automatic body processes. In a dozen or more sessions, which may vary in length from twenty minutes to an hour each, the patient learns to recognize cues of circumstances that may provoke the tinnitus and to apply specific relaxation techniques to avert it.

Biofeedback is said to be especially useful for tinnitus patients whose symptoms are aggravated by anxiety or tension, but not for those suffering from serious depression or psychosis. Thus far biofeedback has been used primarily in patients for whom other methods of treatment have failed. In one study forty of fifty-one patients reported significant improvement through biofeedback. All patients in the study were able to stop taking the sedatives they were using to help them cope with their problem. The improvement seems to last for a year or longer.

In addition to these approaches, treatment with various drugs has proved helpful to individual patients, but on the average, drug therapy has proved to be disappointing, Dr. Miller reports.

For Further Information and Assistance

For information about tinnitus, write to the American Tinnitus Association, P.O. Box 5, Portland, Oregon 97207. For a proper examination, ask your physician or local medical society to refer you to an otolaryngologist who has an interest in problems of the auditory system. The name of a qualified audiologist can be obtained from the American Speech-Language-Hearing Association, 10801 Rockville Pike, Rockville, Maryland 20852.

Vision Problems: Nearly Universal

A Gallup poll in the mid-seventies showed that Americans fear loss of vision more than any other medical mishap, an understandable concern considering that four-fifths of what we know is said to be learned through the use of our eyes.

Yet few are alert to the early warning signs of correctable visual difficulties. Especially in children, problems too often go undetected until serious consequences or permanent damage result. Adults as well as children may suffer needlessly for years with a visual defect that could be readily corrected. In addition, many people have serious misconceptions about eye care — about what hurts vision, what may help it, who should check vision, what tests should be done and how often.

In some cases simple home tests can alert you to a problem involving your own or your child's vision that requires prompt professional attention. And since the eye is like a window to the rest of the body, a professional exam can often reveal early signs of other serious disorders, such as high blood pressure, atherosclerosis, or diabetes.

How the Eye Works

The eye resembles a highly compact television camera. The conjunctiva, a protective membrane over the white of the eye, is attached to a transparent circle in the center of the eye called the cornea. Behind the cornea is the iris, the colored portion of the eye, and between the two is a watery fluid. In the center of the iris is a hole called the pupil, which, like the aperture of a camera, can expand and contract to let in more or less light.

Behind the iris is the lens of the eye, a curved, transparent disk that can be made more or less rounded by contraction or relaxation of the eye muscles. The center of the eye is filled with a clear jellylike fluid — the vitreous humor — and along the back of the eye lies a light-sensitive net-

319

HOW THE EYE FOCUSES

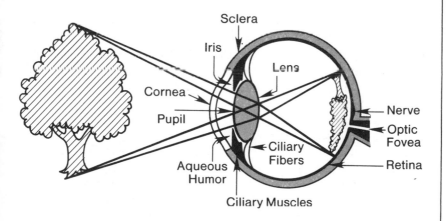

Sclera
Iris
Lens
Cornea
Pupil
Nerve
Optic
Fovea
Ciliary
Fibers
Aqueous
Humor
Retina
Ciliary Muscles

work of nerves called the retina.

When an image enters the eye, the rays of light are refracted, or bent, as they pass through the cornea and lens. In normal vision the refracted rays from all images, near and far, converge, or meet, on the retina. The information gathered on the retina is converted to electrical impulses and carried by the optic nerve to the brain, which interprets what the eye "sees."

Common Vision Defects

The most common abnormalities of the eye are called refractive errors. Because of an abnormal curvature of the lens or because the distance between the cornea and the retina is too long or too short, the rays may converge either in front of or (theoretically) behind the retina. This results in a blurred image of near or far objects.

Nearsightedness. In nearsightedness, or myopia, nearby objects can be focused on the retina, but the image of distant objects focuses in front of the retina, causing blurred vision. The myopic person tends to squint to bring distant objects into focus.

Farsightedness. In farsightedness, or hyperopia, people can adjust their eyes to see distant objects clearly, but they may develop eyestrain when trying to see things nearby. The constant adaptation needed to do close work can tire the eye muscles and cause headaches. Small print may occasionally blur, or things appear momentarily out of focus when the farsighted person looks up from close work.

Astigmatism. In people with an astigmatism, vision is partially blurred because of irregularities in the curvature of the cornea, causing haphazard focusing on the retina of both near and far images. In addition to suffering from headaches and eyestrain, someone with an astigmatism may squint, frown when reading, or twist his or her body to position the eyes in order to see more clearly.

Nearly all these abnormalities can be readily corrected by properly prescribed eyeglasses or contact lenses. The value of eye exercises to correct refractive errors is questionable, but exercises may help to strengthen weak eye muscles.

Presbyopia. For most people the lens prescription they receive at age twenty will serve them well for twenty to thirty years. But then, during their forties, a noticeable change takes place: It becomes increasingly difficult to focus on close objects. This is a normal part of aging, a result of wear and tear on the muscles that adjust the lens as well as a loss of elasticity in the lens itself. This condition, called presbyopia, necessitates corrective lenses for close work. Those already needing correction for distance vision may require bifocals or even trifocals to see clearly near and far.

Cataracts and glaucoma. Older people are also more likely to develop cataracts, a clouding of the lens that, if not corrected surgically, can lead to blindness, and glaucoma, an increased pressure within the eye that can also produce blindness if not treated daily with medication. [See chapters on glaucoma, page 325, and cataracts, page 328.]

Strabismus and amblyopia. In youngsters the most threatening visual difficulties are conditions called strabismus and amblyopia. In strabismus, crossed or drifting eyes don't focus together on the same object. In order to see clearly, the child "rejects" the image registered by one eye and gradually this eye falls into disuse. This is amblyopia, or lazy eye, which may also result from an astigmatism or refractive error in one eye. If not corrected before the age of six, strabismus or amblyopia can lead to permanent loss of vision in one eye. A slightly crossed or drifting eye is just as serious as one that is very obviously out of line. [See chapter on amblyopia, page 323.]

Detecting Vision Problems

Children should be examined by an ophthalmologist (a medical doctor who specializes in eye care) long before they reach school age, preferably before the age of three, and again when they enter school. If an abnormality is found, annual checkups may be needed since the eyes can change dramatically as the child grows. A myopic adolescent may require a new prescription for corrective lenses as often as every six months.

One in four school-age children has an eye problem. Undetected, the problem can impair the child's learning ability, personality, and adjustment in school. According to the National Society for the Prevention of Blindness, a professional exam is in order if your child rubs his eyes excessively; shuts or covers one eye; has difficulty doing close work; often blinks, squints, or frowns; is unduly sensitive to lights; or has inflamed, watery, itchy, or burning eyes.

The society provides a free home eye test for preschoolers to help alert parents to the need for a professional checkup. The test, in English or Spanish, can be obtained by writing to the society at P.O. Box 426, New York, New York 10019.

Young adults (approximately aged twenty to forty) require less frequent eye exams. Contrary to popular belief, your eyeglass prescription need not be checked annually. A checkup is needed only if some change has occurred. Be alert to signs like the need to thrust your head backward or forward to look at distant objects, tilting your head to one side, avoidance of close work, placing your head abnormally close to what you are reading, or blurring of vision.

You can also test yourself by comparing your vision with that of your relatives, by covering one eye and then the other to see if there is a noticeable difference in what you see with each eye, or by looking straight ahead at an object in a room first with one eye and then with the

other and noticing how much you can see on either side of the object —
your peripheral vision.

The Professional Eye Exam

Ideally professional eye examinations are best done by *ophthal-mologists,* who are qualified to diagnose and treat eye diseases as well as difficulties in visual acuity. An *optometrist,* a graduate of a school of optometry, not a medical school, is an expert in diagnosing and treating refractive errors of the eye. Optometrists are also trained to detect signs of eye disease, but patients must be referred to a physician — an ophthalmologist or other appropriate specialist — for a definitive diagnosis and for therapy.

Eye care should never be provided by an *optician,* who is a specialist in grinding and dispensing lenses according to the prescription written by an optometrist or ophthalmologist.

A proper routine eye checkup should consist of both a vision exam and a medical exam. First, the ophthalmologist or optometrist will examine the eyes externally, testing such things as their ability to focus on an object that is moved closer toward a point between the eyes, the size of the pupils and their reaction to light, the movements of the eyes up and down and side to side, and the distance between the pupils while the patient looks at near or distant objects. The specialist will also examine the external eye tissues for signs of inflammation or injury.

Then the examiner will look inside the eye from the outside, using a special lighted instrument called a ophthalmoscope and checking for signs of blood vessel damage, blank spots, and detachment of the retina from its moorings. Using targets and moving objects, the examiner can detect a loss of peripheral vision. Color vision can be tested through the use of special cards with colored numbers on a different colored background. Tonometry, a test of internal eye pressure, should be done at all ages to check for signs of glaucoma.

The refractive state of the eyes can be tested both by instruments that automatically measure refraction and by the examiner's asking the person how well he or she sees when different lenses are placed in front of the eyes.

For Further Reading

Eden, John, M.D. *The Eye Book.* New York: Penguin Books, 1978.
Esterman, Ben, M.D. *The Eye Book.* Arlington, Va.: Great Ocean Publishers, 1977.

Amblyopia:
Common Threat to Young Eyes

No one ever suspected that Richard might have something wrong with his eyes. He learned to read before the age of four and raced through book after book. He had no trouble in school. But he never could learn how to catch a ball, or how to hit one for that matter.

It wasn't until fifth grade, when a team of eye doctors came to his town to examine schoolchildren, that Richard's problem was detected. He could see pretty well with his right eye, but the visual acuity in his left eye was very poor. Early in childhood, before he entered the first grade, his brain "learned" to block out the fuzzy image from his poor eye and to rely solely on the good eye. As a result, he never developed normal binocular vision, the ability to use both eyes together, which is important in judging distances or determining the location of a moving object, such as a ball.

Richard had developed amblyopia, or lazy eye. The eye may gradually stop functioning because the image it receives is blocked out by the brain. Richard could still see with his left eye, although poorly, and his vision was greatly improved by strong prescription lenses. But it was too late for his brain to learn to fuse the images from both eyes. To this day he has difficulty estimating such things as how far away an oncoming car or highway exit may be, and he has never learned to catch or hit a ball.

Amblyopia affects one in twenty-five preschool children, and if the cause is not corrected before the age of six or seven, the child will never develop the ability to use both eyes together. Amblyopia is the most frequent serious visual disorder in young children, and it is one that is likely to go undetected and uncorrected until it is too late to restore full vision in the weaker eye. But if a proper eye examination is done before the age of three and any abnormality found is corrected soon after, the brain will still have time to acquire normal two-eyed vision.

Causes

A significant disparity in visual acuity in the two eyes, such as far-sightedness or astigmatism in one eye but not the other, may result in the weaker eye's falling into disuse. Or amblyopia may result from a crossed eye or walleye or an eye that drifts. In this condition, called strabismus, or squint, there is an imbalance in the six muscles that hold the eye straight, causing it to turn in or out, up or down, without the other eye.

Sometimes the eye will drift only when the child looks in a particular direction or from a certain position, or the eyes may alternately turn in or out. Although vision may be normal in both eyes, strabismus causes the brain to receive a double image because each eye gets a different view. Since the brain cannot fuse the two different images, it blocks out the one that is less true. That eye falls into disuse, and eventually it becomes functionally blind.

Heed the Warning Signs

Michael was six months old when his mother first noticed that his left eye was slightly crossed, but the pediatrician told her not to worry, he'd "outgrow" it. Well, Michael didn't outgrow it, and now, as he enters the second grade, he has lost full use of his "slightly crossed" eye forever. The eye can still be straightened to improve his appearance, but he can never have normal binocular vision.

Many people, doctors included, assume that most children will outgrow crossed eyes, particularly if the condition is not extreme. In fact, many infants' eyes seem crossed because the eye muscles are still weak at birth or because the skin at the corners of the eyes covers so much of the white. If a child's eyes still seem crossed at six months of age, you can assume he won't outgrow it and should be treated by an ophthalmologist, the sooner the better.

A child's eyes may not noticeably cross or drift at all, and he could still have a serious problem in need of correction to prevent amblyopia. The muscle imbalance may be so slight that it can be detected only through an eye doctor's special tests. Therefore, every child should be examined by an ophthalmologist by the age of three.

Warning signs of a possible amblyopic problem include frequent rubbing of the eyes, frowning or blinking, tilting the head or thrusting it forward to look at something, shutting or covering one eye, stumbling over small objects, and, like Richard, difficulty with games that require good distance or binocular vision. Any child with such symptoms should get a thorough eye examination as soon as possible.

Remember, children with amblyopia have no way of knowing they are not seeing as they should because they have no basis for comparison, and there may be nothing about the outward appearance of the eyes to suggest trouble.

Amblyopia is more common among children born prematurely and those with a family history of amblyopia, nearsightedness, or astigmatism.

Treatment

Treatment of an amblyopic condition usually does not require surgery. If the cause is a refractive error, such as Richard had, prescription lenses can correct it and prevent deterioration of normal vision. For an eye with a muscular weakness, temporary patching of the stronger eye or the use of eye drops that force the child to exercise the muscles may help to strengthen it. Special eye exercises may be part of the treatment, but exercises alone are not likely to correct the problem in a young child.

In other cases surgery may be necessary to correct a muscle imbalance. The operation is safe as operations go and does not involve entering the eyeball since the muscles are outside it. Nonetheless, considerable skill is required, and the surgery should be done only by an experienced ophthalmologist.

For best results, an amblyopic problem should be corrected before the age of four. From ages four to seven the percentage of those who improve following treatment declines. For children not treated early, a type of exercise called pleoptics can be used at age seven or eight to help improve vision.

Glaucoma:
Common Threat to Adult Eyes

Marian had been a safe, accident-free driver for thirty of her fifty-three years and was baffled at how she could have failed to see that car coming from the left. As she started through the intersection, the car appeared "as if out of nowhere" and hit her car broadside. Marian was lucky to escape with cuts and bruises and a broken arm.

As it turned out, Marian had a vision problem, one she shares with some 2 million Americans. The problem is glaucoma, the second leading cause of new cases of blindness in this country. Like Marian, half of the victims of glaucoma don't know they have it and suffer irreversible visual impairment as a result, even though there are simple ways to detect it and halt the damage. Although glaucoma is currently incurable, the permanent visual damage it inflicts can be prevented.

Glaucoma usually starts by destroying sight in the outer edges of the visual field, creating increasingly narrow tunnel vision. With her peripheral, or side, vision impaired, Marian missed seeing the car approaching on her far left.

How Glaucoma Causes Blindness

Glaucoma is the result of abnormally high pressure within the eyeball caused by a buildup of aqueous humor, the circulating fluid within the eye that washes over the lens. Normally this fluid is constantly formed and drained out of the eye through a channel called the canal of Schlemm. But in glaucoma normal drainage is blocked.

The resulting pressure in the eyeball squeezes the blood vessels that nourish the retina and optic nerve. The blood supply is consequently reduced, and some of the visual nerve cells and fibers die, producing permanent visual loss. As glaucoma progresses, more and more nerve cells are damaged, and the "tunnel" of vision becomes narrower and narrower, culminating eventually in total blindness.

While blindness ranks second only to cancer as the "most feared" physical affliction, only 49 percent of adults interviewed in a Gallup poll knew about glaucoma, the cause of one out of seven new cases of blindness.

The National Society for the Prevention of Blindness, which sponsors a nationwide campaign to detect early cases of glaucoma, calls the disease the "sneak thief of sight" because many victims have no symptoms until they have lost much of their peripheral vision. Only rarely do patients with the common type of glaucoma experience such symptoms as pain, redness, blurring of vision, or seeing rainbow-colored halos around lights.

More than 80 percent of glaucoma cases occur insidiously over a period of months or years. They are called chronic, open-angle glaucoma. Most of the remaining cases — acute, closed-angle glaucoma — begin suddenly, causing symptoms such as pain, blurring, redness, or halos that prompt the patient to see a doctor. If not treated immediately, acute glaucoma can permanently damage vision in as little as twenty-four hours.

Who Gets It?

The risk of developing chronic or acute glaucoma increases with age. The national society estimates on the basis of health surveys that 1 in 50 Americans over the age of thirty-five and 3 out of 100 over age sixty-five have glaucoma.

Much rarer — constituting about 1 or 2 percent of cases — is congenital glaucoma, in which a defect in fetal development interferes with drainage in the eyeball. According to Dr. Steven Podos, chairman of ophthalmology at Mount Sinai Medical Center in New York, an infant with glaucoma has readily recognizable symptoms, including an aversion to light, an enlarged cornea, a lot of tearing, and an enlarged, cloudy-looking eye. Prompt surgery can preserve the infant's vision.

While the cause or causes of most cases of glaucoma are unknown, cortisone drugs taken orally or put into the eye can precipitate it in certain people, and drugs that control high blood pressure may increase the susceptibility of the eye to the damaging effects of increased eyeball pressure. People with diabetes or a family history of glaucoma face a higher than usual risk of developing the eye disease themselves. When glaucoma runs in the family, there is a tendency for people to develop it at a younger age than their parents or grandparents did.

Detection and Treatment

The best defense against glaucoma is an eye examination at least once every two years (more often for those at high risk). Increased pressure in the eye is detected by an examination with a tonometer. With the kinds of tonometers most commonly used in doctors' offices, the eye is first anesthetized and the instrument is placed against the open eye for a few moments.

Several measurements of eyeball pressure should be made at different times before the examiner concludes that a person has abnormal (or normal) pressure since pressure can be influenced by such factors as time of day, season, consumption of caffeine-containing beverages (which tend to raise pressure) or alcohol (which lowers it) and lead to an erroneous conclusion.

A new instrument — the noncontact tonometer, which measures eye pressure with a jet of air and requires no anesthesic — is now being used in glaucoma screening programs. Glaucoma can be detected by an ophthalmologist (a medical doctor) or an optometrist (a vision specialist), but treatment must be prescribed and monitored by an ophthalmologist.

A survey released by the American Optometric Association in the mid-1970's indicated that 45 percent of the adults interviewed did not know the difference between optometrists and ophthalmologists, and nearly one-fifth of those interviewed did not even know which kind of eye specialist they were going to for eye care. Since glaucoma is a disease and only medical doctors are adequately trained and licensed to treat it, it is critically important for all glaucoma patients to be examined and treated by an ophthalmologist or other medical doctor, not by an optometrist.

Treatment is aimed at reducing the pressure in the eyeball, either by drugs or by surgery. The vast majority of cases of chronic glaucoma can be controlled by one of several drugs that either improve drainage or reduce the formation of fluid in the eye.

Glaucoma drugs must be used as eye drops three or four times a day to keep down the pressure. A new approach in which a tiny sustained-release device containing a week's supply of drug is placed under the eyelid is helpful for those who are unable to put drops in several times a day, but it costs five or six times more than the drops. Marijuana has been found to reduce pressure in the eye, and drug researchers are trying to isolate the responsible factor so that a useful glaucoma drug that is free of effects on the brain can be devised.

For fewer than 10 percent of cases in which visual damage cannot be halted by drugs, surgery is necessary to make a new opening in the eye by which the fluid can escape.

Not all cases of increased pressure in the eye need to be treated. Most ophthalmologists treat only those cases in which there are signs of beginning damage to vision (determined by tests of the visual field) or to vital parts of the eye (determined by an ophthalmoscopic examination). People without signs of damage may simply be monitored by frequent eye exams and treated only if and when damage begins to appear.

Once treatment is begun, it must be continued as prescribed. Many patients fail to follow their doctor's instructions and suffer visual damage as a result.

For Free Tests and Information

Chapters in twenty-three states of the National Society for the Prevention of Blindness conduct free glaucoma screening programs. Check your phone book under "name of state" Society . . . etc.

The society's national office provides free pamphlets for glaucoma patients and the general public, obtainable by writing to the society at 79 Madison Avenue, New York, New York 10016.

Cataracts: When Vision Clouds

Nearly half a million Americans will have "clouds" removed from their eyes this year, the first step toward restoring sight lost because of cataracts. At the same time, however, more than 5,000 people will become needlessly blind because they are ignorant of or irrationally fear the operation that can help them to see again. Better than 95 percent of patients who undergo cataract surgery see better as a result, and the surgery is among the safest of operations.

Example: A pilot for a major airline was removed from flight duty at age forty-one because cataracts had seriously reduced his visual clarity. The cataracts were removed surgically, and his own defective lenses were replaced by implanted artificial lenses. Now he's back working as a top-grade pilot.

Example: A seven-year-old boy accidentally pushed a fork into his baby brother's eye, and a cataract developed in the injured lens. The cataract was removed, and the baby was fitted with a contact lens, which he, at age three, is now able to insert and remove himself.

What Is a Cataract?

A cataract is an opacity, or clouding up, of the normally transparent lens of the eye. The lens, a tiny oval capsule about an eighth of an inch thick and convex on both sides, fits behind the pupil and the iris, the colored part of the eye. Its job is to focus light rays so that they converge on the light-sensitive cells of the retina. Muscle fibers attached to the lens contract or relax, enabling the lens to flatten so that distant objects are in focus or to fatten (become more rounded) so that near objects can be seen clearly.

Cataracts are the result of a chemical change in the protein of the lens which converts the lens from transparent to opaque, thus interfering with the passage of light rays. A cataract usually starts as a very small spot in the center or near the side of the lens. At first there may be no noticeable effect on vision. As the cataract enlarges, clouding of vision becomes apparent. As one victim described it, "It's as if there were a veil in front of your eye that you always had to look through." Gradually more veils are added and vision becomes cloudier and cloudier.

In addition to fuzzy or blurred vision, which may prompt people with cataracts to seek brighter and brighter light for reading or to hold things very close to their eyes, symptoms of cataracts include occasional double vision and difficulty with night driving because light from oncoming headlights is scattered by the cloudy lens. As a cataract develops, frequent changes of eyeglass prescriptions may be necessary, but after a while new glasses no longer help.

Cataracts may form in only one eye or in both eyes at the same time. They may grow very slowly and never develop to the point where surgery is needed. Or they may enlarge rapidly. If there are cataracts in both eyes, they may not grow at the same rate.

Causes

The most common cause of cataracts is simply degeneration associated with age — so-called senile cataract. Of the more than 3 million Americans who have cataracts, three-fourths are sixty-five years of age or older. Only 1 victim in 5 is between ages forty-five and sixty-five.

Other causes of degenerative cataracts include exposure to X rays, microwaves, and infrared radiation; an injury in which the eye is penetrated; an illness such as diabetes associated with high blood sugar levels; an inflammation of the eye called uveitis; and certain drugs and chemicals taken orally or by injection, including cortisone and its derivatives, a cholesterol-lowering agent called MER-29 (no longer marketed), and a now-banned food chemical, dinitrophenol.

Some cataracts are developmental, rather than degenerative. These may be congenital (present at birth) cataracts that are caused by some noxious prenatal influence, or they may develop shortly after birth, possibly the result of a genetic disorder.

If the mother has rubella (German measles) early in pregnancy, her baby may be born with cataracts. Infants afflicted with the hereditary metabolic disease galactosemia will develop cataracts shortly after birth. Both these types of developmental cataract can be prevented, the first by giving a woman rubella vaccine or actually having rubella before pregnancy, the second by placing the newborn infant on a special diet that lacks galactose, a sugar found in milk.

The Treatment Is Surgery

No drug, diet, or exercise can prevent or dissolve cataracts. Surgery is the only effective treatment, and it is best done by an ophthalmologist who has a lot of experience with cataract surgery or has been trained in microsurgical techniques. The operation should be done when the cataract has reached the point where it interferes with a person's normal life.

There is no need to wait until the cataract is "ripe" and vision is totally obscured.

There are a number of different ways to remove a cataract. The entire lens and its capsule may be removed (intracapsular extraction), a method usually done for senile cataracts. Or a large portion of the lens and capsule is removed, but part of the capsule left intact (extracapsular extraction). In children the soft lens may be aspirated through a hollow needle.

A cold probe may be used to freeze the cataract, which then sticks to the probe, making it easy to remove. Another method, called phakoemulsification, uses ultrasound to break up the cataract, the pieces of which are then sucked out through a hollow needle. Although initially hailed as a breakthrough, this method has since been shown to give no better results than older techniques. Some ophthalmologists have been trained to operate through a special microscope, which enables greater precision and the use of finer needles, minimizing the trauma and complications of surgery.

Local or general anesthesia may be used. With local anesthetics, surgery can be done safely on elderly and chronically ill people. The operation usually takes less than an hour. If both eyes need surgery, only one eye is operated on at a time; the second is best done months later to reduce the risk that a complicating infection would spread from one eye to the other.

A number of physicians do not even keep their patients in the hospital overnight; others require only an overnight stay. However, although usually unnecessary, it is still common practice among ophthalmologists to keep cataract patients hospitalized for several days to a week. Ask your doctor about his or her practice regarding hospitalization before you decide who should do the operation. [See chapter on outpatient surgery, page 455.]

Convalescence is also much simpler than in the past. No longer must patients lie heavily bandaged and perfectly still, with their heads immobilized for days by sandbags. Most patients can return to normal activities within a few days, as soon as their visual abilities allow them to. If the surgery is properly executed, and the wound correctly sutured, there should be no need to restrict activities significantly for many weeks after surgery.

Restoring Vision After Surgery

Surgery is only half the story. To restore vision, a new lens must be used to replace the one that was removed. In the past cataract patients were obliged to wear thick glasses — "Coke bottle" lenses — which so magnified the image in the operated eye that the brain could not integrate the images from both eyes. (This is not a problem if both eyes are operated on.) The glasses also restrict undistorted vision to straight ahead, requiring the wearer to turn his head to see clearly to the side of him.

Now there are other choices. One is a lens that is implanted permanently in the eye at the time the cataract is removed. Since experience with this intraocular lens varies greatly from doctor to doctor, it's important that such an implant be done only by one who is specially trained in the procedure. The results with this type of lens are particularly good for the elderly.

Most patients, however, are fitted with an external lens — a hard or soft contact lens. These do not grossly magnify the image, allowing the brain to see with both eyes at once. Peripheral (side) vision is also normal. But the wearer must be able to insert and remove contact lenses daily and to keep them clean. [See chapter on contact lenses, page 332.]

The particular choice of lens type should depend on the patient's needs, abilities, and wishes. Often, however, it is determined by the doctor's expertise and experience. Before surgery ask the doctor what type of lens correction works best in his or her hands. If you are not satisfied with the method to be used, consult another ophthalmologist.

Following cataract surgery, protection from intense sunlight may be needed to prevent serious eye problems. Dr. Jerald Tennant of the Dallas Eye Institute recommends the use of "UV400" lenses, made by the Optical Radiation Corp. of Azusa, California.

For Further Reading

Single copies of a booklet, ''Cataract: NEI Focus on Research,'' are available free from the Office of Information, National Eye Institute, National Institutes of Health, Bethesda, Maryland 20014.

Contact Lenses: Revolution in Vision Correction

President Reagan, tennis pro Eddie Dibbs, and actress Carol Channing are among more than 14 million Americans who have turned to contact lenses to improve their vision without obscuring their visage with a second pair of "eyes." Contact lenses are a particular boon to cataract patients, self-conscious adolescents, and those who are bothered by fogging of eyeglasses or who need good peripheral vision to do their jobs.

As with most other "miracles" of medicine, contact lenses are a mixed blessing. While they grant freedom from the annoyances and limitations of spectacles and in many cases provide superior vision, contact lenses can, if misfitted or mishandled, threaten the very thing they are meant to help — your eyesight.

There is now a confusing array of choices available to the prospective contact lens wearer — hard, soft, and gas-permeable, either as a single or as a bifocal, or a clear or tinted lens that is removed daily or worn for several weeks at a time. The type your best friend wears may be ill-suited to you, and vice versa. Furthermore, contact lenses are not for everyone.

Lenses require an investment of time and money and daily care that often make them far more complicated to use than eyeglasses. Persons lacking commitment to their use are poor candidates for contact lenses. Too often improperly chosen and/or poorly fitted lenses end up buried in a bureau drawer, a wasted investment of several hundred dollars.

How to Get Them

If you are considering contact lenses, it is critically important to secure the services of a highly trained professional who will take the proper time and care in introducing you to contacts. Your eyes are far too precious to trust to an assembly-line fitting or a supermarket-style selection of contact lenses, as currently offered at some heavily advertised contact lens "centers" throughout the country. Though these clinics may be quick and easy and seem to offer lenses at bargain-basement prices, there are usually hidden costs — to your pocketbook and possibly to your visual health as well.

You would be far better off investing more time and money to get thorough care and careful follow-up from a private or hospital-based ophthalmologist or optometrist who specializes in the prescription of contact lenses. Depending on the type of lens and the specialist who treats you, contact lenses — complete with exam and after-fitting checkups — can cost anywhere from $200 to $500. It's a good idea to discuss the fee beforehand and find out what it covers. Lens insurance is extra, and when the deductible is taken into account, you may find that it does not pay, except perhaps for a new lens wearer.

Lenses should be fitted only after a complete checkup has assured that you have no health problem or abnormality that would make contact lenses inappropriate or hazardous. The exam should include a general medical history that explores, among other things, your allergies, the drugs you take, visual complaints, and related symptoms like headaches.

Contact lenses may be inappropriate for people with allergies that cause severe eye irritation; workers who are exposed to dust and chemical vapors; or people with overactive thyroids, dry eyes, uncontrolled diabetes, or arthritis involving the hands. In addition, women who are pregnant or taking birth control pills and persons taking diuretics, antihistamines, or decongestants, all of which can produce dryness in the eyes, may have difficulty wearing lenses.

The eye exam itself should involve a test of your visual acuity and refractive properties of your eyes using a retinoscope; the use of a slit lamp to check the health of the external eye; an ophthalmoscopic examination of the interior of the eye; tests for eye coordination; and tonometry to check eye pressure.

Proper fitting is the key to success in wearing lenses. Though they may feel uncomfortable or odd at first, lenses should never cause actual pain and you should not have to suffer to "break in" new lenses.

Often lenses can be fitted immediately from stock sizes in inventory, perhaps with minor adjustments to suit your eyes. Other times made-to-order lenses must be prescribed. New lenses should be rechecked after one or two weeks and again a month later to be sure that they are not damaging your eyes. Repeat exams once every six to twelve months are essential.

Kinds of Lenses

All contact lenses are made of one or another kind of plastic. All fit on the cornea, the see-through covering over the colored part of the eye. The lenses are shaped to correct anatomical distortions that cause near or far vision to blur. Like glasses, they focus the image of objects on the retina, allowing visual information to be transmitted to the brain. Unlike glasses, lenses can interfere with the oxygen supply to the cornea, which has no blood supply and depends on exposure to the oxygen in air and tears. This is why most lenses must be removed each day.

The major types of lenses available, and their relative advantages and disadvantages, are these:

Hard lenses. As the first lenses available, these are still worn by more people than any other type, although in recent years soft lenses have become a two-to-one favorite among new lens wearers. Hard lenses generally provide superior visual correction and are the only type appropriate for persons with a severe astigmatism or an irregular corneal surface. [See chapter on vision problems, page 318.]

Hard lenses are the least expensive and most durable of contact lenses. They also require minimal care — daily removal and a simple cleaning. They can be polished to remove scratches and reground to adjust to small changes in your eyes, helping you to avoid the expense of a completely new pair.

However, hard lenses require getting used to — a weeks-long breaking-in period that gradually extends the hours they are worn to a maximum of fourteen to eighteen hours at a time. They cannot be worn occasionally, such as while performing, participating in athletics, or out for the evening. If you stop wearing them for a few days, you must repeat the gradual break-in. Rushing the adjustment can lead to serious and painful inflammation. After removing hard lenses and putting on glasses, you may experience visual blurring that lasts for several minutes or longer.

Hard lenses can be tinted or made as bifocal lenses (the thicker half of the lens needed for reading is heavier and automatically moves to the bottom after the lens is inserted in the eye). Bifocal lenses are more expensive and more complicated to fit.

Gas-permeable lenses. These are more expensive hard lenses that let through some oxygen and carbon dioxide, enabling the cornea to "breathe." Most people find them more comfortable and easier to adapt to than ordinary hard lenses. They are often recommended for people who need the visual correction offered by hard lenses but who cannot tolerate the conventional hard lens.

Soft lenses. These lenses, made of a water-absorbing plastic, fit flush against the cornea, assuming whatever shape it has. (Thus, they are inappropriate for people with irregular corneas, though newer lenses are being developed to overcome this limitation.) They are more comfortable than hard lenses and require little adjustment; within just a few days they can be worn for a full day. Unlike hard lenses, they can be used intermittently. Athletes prefer them because they are also less likely than hard lenses to pop out of the eye and are better at keeping out dust and soot.

However, soft lenses have several disadvantages: They cost considerably more initially and in their routine care; they are more likely to rip and become clouded (and thus need more frequent replacement, probably every two years); and they require meticulous daily cleaning either through boiling or with a chemical solution. Failure to follow the recommended cleaning procedure can lead to serious eye infections and permanent clouding of the lenses.

Because they dry out easily, soft lenses may cause difficulties for people with dry eyes or if they are worn while under a hair dryer, in an overheated room or vehicle, in a high wind, or in a very dry climate.

Extended-wear (up to two weeks at a time) soft lenses are now available. These would be especially useful for persons with arthritis or other handicaps that make daily insertion and removal of lenses difficult. There now are also bifocal and tinted soft lenses.

Helpful Hints for Contact Lens Wearers

Little things can markedly influence your success in wearing contact lenses. Experts recommend the following precautions:

● Wait about twenty to thirty minutes after waking up to insert your lenses. This will give sleep-swollen corneas a chance to return to normal.

● Don't swim with lenses in, especially not soft lenses, which can absorb chemicals from water. Similarly, remove soft lenses in the presence of irritating vapors.

● Unless you have been fitted with extended-wear lenses, never go to sleep with your lenses in. Sleeping with lenses interferes with circulation of fluid in your eyes, depriving the cornea of needed oxygen. However, a short nap with lenses in place is not harmful.

● If you do a lot of driving, carry an extra pair of lenses with you in tant decline in the consumption of sweets may be what actually does the most good.

Other Unproved Theories

Many parents report that concentrated doses of sugar-laden foods and drinks seem to turn their otherwise normal-behaving children into whirling dervishes, and some groups maintain that overconsumption of sugar is at the root of the hyperactivity syndrome. While the latter claim is far from proved, it makes sense in any case to limit your child's sugar consumption, especially if it seems to have adverse behavioral effects.

A team at the Downstate Medical Center in Brooklyn, New York, suggested on the basis of a preliminary study that perhaps half of hyperactive children had excessive amounts of lead in their bodies (shown by elevated levels of lead in the blood and urine), and the removal of the lead with drugs called chelating agents alleviated the hyperactivity in half the cases they studied. Although cautious about making far-reaching claims for their early findings, the researchers urged that lead levels be considered in the evaluation of hyperactive children.

case a lens gets lost en route.

● If you have a chronic illness that may cause you to lose consciousness, such as epilepsy or diabetes, note on an identification bracelet that you wear lenses.

● If you play racket sports or ball games, be sure to wear safety glasses over your lenses.

● Women should insert their lenses prior to putting on face or eye makeup. Water-soluble eye makeup is best for lens wearers.

● Use aerosol deodorants and hair sprays before you put your lenses in. Better yet, avoid using sprays.

● Wash your hands before putting in lenses so as not to introduce irritating substances into your eyes. Never touch the inner surface of the lens that rests against the cornea.

● See an ophthalmologist (medical doctor who specializes in eye care) promptly if you develop a persistent irritation, redness, pain, blurred vision, or any other eye abnormality.

For Further Reading

Morrison, Robert J., D.O. The Contact Lens Book. New York: Cornerstone Library, 1978.

VIII.
Environmental
Health
Effects

The emphasis these days is definitely on getting out. Sun, wind, rain, snow, cold — nothing is supposed to stop the intrepid twentieth-century wanderer bent on fresh air and exercise. No sun is too hot, no sea too deep, no mountain too high.

Yet too often you pay an unexpected price for your excursions into the elements: sunburn, frostbite, altitude sickness. Even the ordinary person who rarely ventures far from home is sometimes discomforted by confrontations with the mean side of Mother Nature as well as with environmental hazards inside the home and workplace, such as cigarette smoke and other air pollutants.

The air you breathe, the water you drink, the sounds you hear, the sun that warms your body and soul — all can be hazards to your health. If you appreciate the risks and take the proper precautions, you will greatly minimize the damage they can do.

Your Drinking Water: How Safe Is It?

For many decades Americans have taken the healthfulness of their water supply for granted. Most people still do. After all, you rarely, if ever, hear these days of outbreaks of typhoid, cholera, dysentery, and other waterborne diseases common before the advent of chlorinated community water supplies and restrictions on the placement of wells and cesspools.

But sales of bottled water have zoomed in recent years as millions of Americans have become concerned about their health and the safety of the colorless liquid that comes out of their taps. Others have purchased filtering devices to purify their home water supplies. Studies suggest that this concern may be justified but that the alternatives people choose are often no better than the tap water they spurn. Stronger community-based action may be needed to clean up our water.

Not only do infectious diseases transmitted through tap water still occur — afflicting at least 10,000 Americans a year (and probably many more since most cases of illnesses like intestinal "flu" are not recognized as attributable to water) — but a far more serious threat may exist. Studies have shown that the nation's 50,000 water supplies are liberally laced with potentially harmful substances — including asbestos, pesticides, heavy metals like lead and cadmium, arsenic, nitrates, sodium, viruses, and organic chemicals that are known to cause cancer.

Ironically, the very process by which we cleanse our water of infectious organisms — chlorination — is responsible for creating cancer-causing substances, or carcinogens, from otherwise innocent chemicals in water. The chlorine can combine with other pollutants in water to form such carcinogens as chloroform, carbon tetrachloride, and bis-chloroethane and other chemicals called trihalomethanes.

Contamination with Carcinogens

In the mid-1970's the Environmental Protection Agency (EPA), the federal unit responsible for the purity of our water, made two surveys of municipal water supplies around the country and found chlorinated organic chemicals in significant amounts virtually everywhere.

To date more than 300 different organic chemicals have been identified in American drinking water; most have not yet been tested for their ability to cause cancer. Even though these chemicals may be present in only minuscule amounts, the average person consumes one and a half or more quarts of water every day for life. Chronic exposure to small amounts of carcinogens can add up to a significant hazard.

Indeed, in at least fifteen studies carried out so far a real hazard has been suggested. In New Orleans, where the Mississippi drains agricultural chemicals into the water supply and where the hazard of chlorinated carcinogens was first noted, cancers of the kidney, bladder, and urinary tract are more common than in most other American cities.

A study of eighty-eight counties in Ohio showed that death rates for cancer of the stomach and bladder were more common in counties served by surface water supplies (from rivers and lakes) than in counties with ground water (from wells). The EPA surveys revealed that the concentration of organic chemicals was considerably higher in surface water supplies. Another nationwide study showed a relationship between the levels of trihalomethanes in the drinking water and deaths from cancers of the bladder, brain, kidney, and lymph glands.

While none of the studies so far proves that a waterborne cancer hazard exists, they all suggest there's cause for concern. The hazard can be greatly reduced by filtering the water through activated carbon granules prior to chlorination. However, only a few water systems currently do this and then only to remove foul odors and tastes. Another approach involves the use of ozone instead of chlorine to purify the water.

Other Bad Actors in Water

Other substances in water that are worrisome include the following:

Nitrates. These chemicals, present in both surface and well water from agricultural runoff and seepage from septic tanks, are a direct hazard to infants, causing methemoglobinemia, or blue-baby syndrome. In people of all ages, nitrates may contribute to the formation of potent carcinogens called nitrosamines in the digestive tract. Nitrates can be removed from the water supply by treatment through an ion exchanger.

Sodium. The Environmental Defense Fund, which has petitioned the EPA for stronger water safety rules, notes that water supplies may contain up to 500 parts of sodium per million parts of water. In some sections of the country, such as the Northeast and Middle West, the problem is seasonal, the result of runoff from highways that have been salted in winter. In others the water is naturally high in sodium.

This may be no problem for most people, but for the 20 percent who are predisposed to high blood pressure and the 60 million Americans who already have this disease, the high sodium content of drinking water could be a hazard. [See chapters on salt, page 66, and high blood pressure, page 631.] While sodium is hard to remove from water, the fund suggests that the sodium content be monitored regularly and the public be warned when high levels occur in the water supply.

Heavy metals. In communities where the water is soft — that is corrosive because it contains relatively few dissolved minerals and salts — toxic metals from water pipes may leach into the tap water. For reasons not yet known, studies have shown that in soft-water areas the death rates from cardiovascular diseases are considerably higher than they are in areas where the water is hard. This may result from higher levels of cadmium (leached from galvanized pipes) and sodium in soft water. Some communities, like Boston, where many houses have lead pipes, now harden the water supply by adding lime and carbonates to reduce its corrosive action.

Asbestos. Asbestos fibers enter the water supply primarily through erosion of asbestos-containing rocks and asbestos cement water pipes and runoff from sanded roads. Several years ago, people who drank water from Lake Superior were shown to be consuming large amounts of asbestos fibers dumped in the lake by a mining company. Although the hazards of asbestos in water are not known, asbestos workers exposed to the persistent fibers of this mineral have high rates of cancers of the lung and gastrointestinal tract and an otherwise rare fatal cancer called mesothelioma. Asbestos levels in water can be reduced by hardening the water to make it less corrosive, and the fibers can be removed by conventional filtration techniques.

The Bottled Alternative?

Bottled water is not your only — or even necessarily the best — alternative. Aside from being costly, bottled water may be no better than that which comes out of your tap. Some is just processed tap water to which minerals, with or without carbonation, have been added.

Dr. Robert Harris, water specialist at the Environmental Defense Fund, suggests that before you make a major investment in bottled water, check with the manufacturer about its source, the type of processing, and results of tests of its contents and purity. Most nationally sold brands are probably free of organic carcinogens. However, an EPA survey showed that many bottling plants had sanitary deficiencies, and some bottled water was contaminated with intestinal bacteria.

In general, Dr. Harris suggests you choose natural spring water derived from a spring located in a nonindustrial area. The addition of minerals or carbonation by the processor does not compromise the safety of the water. However, carbonation can be a problem for persons with hiatus hernia or other digestive disorders. Also beware of bottled waters to which sodium-containing chemicals are added (read the label).

How to Make Your Water Fit to Drink

As for home water purifiers, the EPA has tested the effectiveness of thirty filter systems. The results ranged from "totally useless" for a $12 model that fits on your faucet to "as effective as filtration at a water treatment plant" for a $300 unit that's attached to your main water source. The main problem, however, is that even the expensive units permit the growth of bacteria on the intake side of the unit; the bacteria can then contaminate the water that comes out of your tap. Home filter units can magnify the bacterial content of tap water by tens of thousands of times, although the Consumer Product Safety Commission says no illnesses have been linked to the use of such filters.

The Environmental Defense Fund suggests an inexpensive and safer homemade alternative: Put a coffee filter paper in a large funnel. Wash enough granular activated carbon (it can be purchased in one-pound bags from Walnut Acres, Penns Creek, Pennsylvania 17862) to fill one-quarter of the funnel. (To wash carbon, put it in a jar, fill it with water, cover, and shake. Let the carbon settle, and pour off the water at the top. Repeat until the water you pour off is clear.) Now set the funnel in a large clean jar, add the washed carbon, and slowly pour your tap water through the funnel. Change the carbon every three weeks or after twenty gallons of water have been filtered through it. Store the filtered water in the refrigerator.

For further purification, you might boil your tap water gently for fifteen or twenty minutes to evaporate many of the carcinogens. After you have boiled the water, bottle and store it, closed, in the refrigerator.

Certainly any water that appears turbid (cloudy, indicating possible contamination by sewage, not the aeration effect that clears within a minute) or any water taken from an unpurified and untested source (such as a stream) should be boiled for at least ten minutes if you have no choice but to use it. An alternative is to add liquid chlorine laundry bleach or tincture of iodine. Use two drops of bleach per quart of clear water or four drops per quart of cloudy water. Mix thoroughly, and let stand for thirty minutes. You should detect a slight chlorine odor. If not, repeat the treatment, and let the water stand for an additional fifteen minutes. For iodine, use five drops per quart of clear water, ten per quart of cloudy water, mix it, and let it stand for thirty minutes.

If your water is soft, first thing in the morning or after hours of not using it, let the cold water run for a few minutes before you draw it for drinking or cooking. Don't use hot water from the tap for these purposes since it's likely to have a higher metal content. If your water is hard, soften only the hot water, since softening adds sodium to the water.

Turning On the Regulatory Pressure

For citizens interested in knowing what's in their water and doing something to improve it, the Consumers Union recommends that they organize a community group and start by familiarizing themselves with the facts about drinking water. A useful pamphlet for individuals or groups — "Safe Drinking Water for All: What You Can Do" — may be obtained for 25 cents from the League of Women Voters Education Fund, 1730 M Street NW, Washington, D.C. 20036. Citizens' groups might also find useful the *Manual for Evaluating Public Drinking Water Supplies*; single copies are available free from the Water Supply Division, Environmental Protection Agency, Washington, D.C. 20460.

Then get in touch with the local water superintendent, and ask for the results of water-sampling tests and sanitary surveys. *Consumer Re-*

ports suggests that if you get no cooperation, you should inform the local media — they may want to find out what the water officials are trying to hide. Compare the test results with the Public Health Service standards in the EPA manual. Was the water tested at the tap as well as in the plant? If the federal standards are being met, broach the matter of further purification or alternative methods of purification. Many improvements can be made for just pennies a day per family that may save you thousands in future health care costs.

Heat Disorders:
When the Body Gets Too Hot

"Mad dogs and Englishmen go out in the mid-day sun" — and so do a good many Americans who are unaware of the hazards or who refuse to be stymied by the weather. As a result, every summer millions of Americans suffer heat-caused disorders, ranging in seriousness from mild heat fatigue and temporarily incapacitating heat cramps to imminently fatal heat stroke. During an ordinary American summer some 175 Americans die from an overdose of heat and sun, and in some years heat waves have claimed more than 1,000 lives.

While hot weather is especially taxing for people with chronic illnesses, such as heart or lung disease, it can also endanger the lives of perfectly healthy people. Witness the young athletes who die from heat stroke during late-summer football practice.

The body temperature of warm-blooded animals is regulated by a tiny control center in the brain called the hypothalamus. When a person's blood rises above 98.6 degrees Fahrenheit, the hypothalamus sends chemical messages that prompt the heart to pump more blood and dilate the blood vessels, especially the tiny capillaries in the upper layers of the skin. More blood flows through these surface vessels so that excess heat will drain off into the cooler atmosphere by heat conduction. At the same time water diffuses through the pores of the skin (called insensible perspiration because the water evaporates before you see it and the skin remains dry).

If this is not adequate to cool the blood, the hypothalamus signals the sweat glands to pour out larger amounts of water and heat in what is called sensible perspiration, or sweating. When perspiration evaporates, heat energy is needed to change the liquid to vapor. This heat comes from your skin; that is why sweating helps to cool your body.

All this works reasonably well as long as the air temperature is considerably below normal skin temperature (which is several degrees lower than body temperature) and the humidity is not so high that your sweat cannot evaporate rapidly. When the temperature of the air is near normal body temperature, there is no conductive cooling of the blood as it circulates through the skin. And when the relative humidity rises above 60 percent, even sweating becomes a poor cooling device; at 75 percent humidity it ceases being effective.

Even on a not too hot, fairly dry day, it is possible to induce heat illness by overworking your muscles and overheating your body, thereby overtaxing the cooling mechanism. Profuse sweating and perspiration may result in a large loss of body salts, disrupting the body's electrolyte balance and precipitating heat illness.

Sunburn impairs the body's ability to get rid of excess heat, and coating your body with a greasy suntan lotion or sunburn spray makes matters worse. People with heart disease have a particular problem in hot weather because the heart must work harder to get rid of excess body heat.

Recognizing and Treating Heat Problems

Here's how to recognize the various heat disorders, in order of their severity, and what to do about them:

Heat fatigue, or asthenia (weakness). The symptoms of this disorder include fatigue, headache, mental and physical inefficiency, poor appetite, heavy sweating, high pulse rate, and shallow breathing. These result from exposure to excessively hot, humid conditions. The sufferer should rest in a cool, dry place; drink plenty of fluids; and, if not counter to doctor's orders, consume extra salt, but not as tablets (try one teaspoon of salt in a quart of lemonade, or drink a commercial salt-balanced drink, such as Gatorade or Take Five).

Heat cramps. The most likely victim of these sudden incapacitating pains in the abdomen or extremities is someone in good physical condition who overexerts himself or herself during a heat wave. The cramps are caused by excessive sweating and loss of salts from the blood and tissues. They are best treated by drinking a salty liquid — up to four doses of one-half teaspoon of salt dissolved in half a glass of water, drunk fifteen minutes apart. Firm pressure on the cramped muscles and warm wet towels may also give relief, but the victim should not try to knead or work out the cramp. A twenty-four-hour rest before resuming normal activity is advised.

Heat exhaustion. This is usually caused by a prolonged hot spell, overexposure to heat and humidity, and overexertion. It is important to be able to distinguish between heat exhaustion and the far more serious heat stroke. In heat exhaustion the victim sweats profusely, feels weak and dizzy, and may faint or vomit. The skin is pale and feels cold and clammy, and body temperature is normal or below.

The victim should lie down in a cool spot. Remove his or her clothing, and sponge the body with cool water. After a rest, if the victim is not vomiting, give him or her a salty liquid to drink. Although the victim may feel better quite rapidly, he or she should take it very easy and use extra salt for several days. If the victim is elderly, has a chronic disease, or cannot retain salty liquids, it is best to get him or her to a hospital.

Heat stroke. This life-threatening condition can result from extreme overexertion or from circulatory impairment caused by illness, old age, or drugs. In contrast with heat exhaustion, the victim of heat stroke will stop sweating, he or she will feel very feverish, body temperature will soar (often rising to 106 or higher), the pulse will pound, and he or she may become unconscious. The skin at first appears flushed, then may become ashen or purple.

Minutes count in this syndrome in which the body's thermoregulatory system has completely shut down. Body temperature must be reduced as rapidly as possible. Call an ambulance. Then remove the victim's clothing, and plunge the person into a tub of cold water (don't add ice), or sponge with cold water or alcohol and massage the arms and legs with ice cubes. When the victim's body temperature has dropped to below 102, cover him or her to prevent chilling. Victims of heat stroke should be hospitalized for several days.

Preventing Heat Problems

To avoid hot-weather problems, the following safety measures have been recommended by the American Medical Association, the American Heart Association, *Patient Care* magazine, and others:

● Stay cool. Spend as much time as possible in air-conditioned areas. If necessary, go to a movie or shop in a cool store for a few hours. But stay out of the sun. If the weatherman says it's 85 degrees, it's likely to be 95 on the tennis court or in your backyard. Take lukewarm, not cold, showers or baths.

● Avoid strenuous outdoor activity during midday. When you exercise, rest in the shade for five to ten minutes every half hour, and drink lots of water. If you drink more than three quarts of water, extra salt is needed, perhaps in the form of cold bouillon or salted lemonade. It is a myth that drinking cool liquids while exercising will cause stomachaches.

● Eat lightly — lots of fruits, vegetables, cold salads, cottage cheese, but little meat or fish and no heavy meals. You may salt your food liberally, but don't take salt tablets unless your doctor prescribes them. Drink water often even if you're not thirsty. Avoid alcoholic beverages — they produce heat in the body and interfere with the heat control mechanism.

● Wear loose-fitting, loosely woven, light-colored clothing (preferably fabrics like cotton that "breathe," not nylon or acrylic), and in the sun cover your head with a wide-brimmed hat.

Mountain Sickness: Hazards of High Altitudes

In recent years mountain climbing and high-altitude vacations have enjoyed an explosive popularity, with millions trekking, flying, or driving to towering peaks throughout the world.

Soaring along with this quest for peak experiences is the incidence of illness that results from the body's reaction to the reduced oxygen pressure at high altitudes. Although the serious, potentially life-threatening effects of high-altitude sickness are largely preventable, many climbers fail to take the proper precautions and don't recognize or heed the early warning signs. Too often, when trouble is obvious, the wrong treatment is applied, endangering the victim's health and life.

Example: In the mid-1970's on Alaska's Mount McKinley, which stands 20,320 feet above sea level, nearly two dozen climbers became severely — some fatally — ill in the rarefied atmosphere on North America's highest mountain.

Example: Every winter in the Colorado Rockies, many skiers who ordinarily dwell at or near sea level become headachy, nauseated, lightheaded, or weak, and some develop pneumonialike symptoms while working the slopes at an altitude of about 9,500 feet.

Example: Climbers ascending to the snowcapped peaks of Kilimanjaro, 19,340 feet above sea level, commonly get irritable and sometimes downright hostile, with their mood reverting to normal as they descend Africa's highest mountain.

Half or more of those who go above 10,000 feet suffer symptoms of mountain sickness. For some, symptoms appear at altitudes as low as 7,000 feet, and deaths have occurred in previously healthy persons at 10,000 feet.

Symptoms of Mountain Sickness

The more common mild symptoms of acute mountain sickness include headache, irritability, forgetfulness, mental sluggishness, insomnia, weakness, light-headedness, loss of appetite, nausea and vomiting, intestinal gas, passing pains in the chest or back, palpitations, and rapid, difficult, or irregular breathing. Small hemorrhages under the surface of the eyeball may also occur; they usually cause no permanent damage and clear up without treatment.

The more severe symptoms include shortness of breath, cough, gurgling breathing sounds, blue skin color, frothy or bloody sputum, hallucinations, unsteadiness, inability to coordinate movements, paralysis, seizures, and loss of consciousness. These result from excessive accumulations of water in the lungs and brain (pulmonary and cerebral edema) which occur when the body tries to adapt rapidly to a reduced oxygen supply. Other symptoms include blood clots, pulmonary embolism, blurring of vision, double vision, and hemorrhages in the retina.

A victim of mountain sickness may get any combination of the above symptoms. They commonly appear twelve to twenty-four hours after a rapid ascent. Don't let a brief, uneventful visit to a mountaintop lead you to believe you are invulnerable to high altitude problems. Most who visit Pikes Peak, for example, drive up, take a look around, snap a few pictures, and then leave, with few staying long enough to begin to feel sick.

High altitude alone can induce the symptoms of mountain sickness, but strenuous exercise — climbing, skiing, and the like — can speed up the appearance and enhance the severity of symptoms by increasing the body's need for oxygen (that is why there were objections to holding the 1968 Olympics in Mexico City, about 7,800 feet above sea level).

In response to reduced oxygen at high altitudes, breathing and heart rates increase to get more oxygen from the air into the lungs and in turn into the blood. The physiological adjustments found in persons who live permanently at high altitudes do not occur fast enough to help newcomers.

There is no sure way to predict who will and who will not get mountain sickness. It is not related to prior physical training or fitness. For unknown reasons, persons under twenty are more susceptible than those between twenty and forty-five.

How to Avoid Altitude Problems

These problems need not discourage those who yearn to scale majestic peaks. Rather, they should encourage a healthy respect for the hazards of high altitudes and adoption of an intelligent, health-saving plan to reach them. The vast majority of climbers who get into trouble do so because they have gone too high too fast, subverting the body's ability to adapt to the stresses of high altitude. Mountain sickness is in a sense a disease of modern technology and high-speed life-styles.

Dr. Charles S. Houston, a University of Vermont researcher into the effects of high altitude, has observed, "The modern climber is usually in a hurry, flying from home to mountain base and thence rapidly by small plane to a landing above 10,000 feet. In the next few days he climbs — usually with a heavy pack — faster than adaptation can keep up, and trouble begins."

Dr. Houston, who at age sixty-five was still doing studies at 18,000 feet on Mount Logan in the Yukon Territory, says the primary precaution is a leisurely ascent. He wrote in the *New England Journal of Medicine*, "The climber who wishes to fly to 10,000 feet is well advised to rest there for a day or two admiring his surroundings, and to budget one day for each thousand feet climbed to 14,000 feet and two days per thousand feet thereafter." In an interview from his mountain camp Dr. Houston said that it would be best for climbers to go no higher than 8,000 feet from sea level in one day. Even then, he said, some develop symptoms.

People with serious heart or lung diseases face an additional hazard because they are already short of oxygen at sea level. Dr. Houston recommended that anyone with symptoms at sea level (such as shortness of breath or angina) should stay below 5,000 feet. Most of those who are well at sea level can ascend safely to 8,000 feet, the doctor said.

A drug called acetazolamide (Diamox), taken starting two days before the climb, can help prevent mountain sickness by enabling the body to move more air in and out of the lungs without disrupting the blood's acid-base balance. Consuming a lot of liquid, but avoiding excessive salt intake, is also helpful, Dr. Houston said.

What to Do When Symptoms Occur

If mild symptoms appear en route to a high altitude, the doctor said, the climber should stop his ascent and rest, but not take to his bed (except to sleep for brief periods) because lying down may worsen the situation. If alarming symptoms develop, the climber should descend to a lower altitude immediately; that usually leads to a rapid recovery.

Another physician-climber, Dr. Peter H. Hackett, has pointed out that "acute mountain sickness is generally a harmless, transient and self-limiting syndrome, cured immediately by descent. Sixty-three percent of our own cases were able to continue their ascent, dosing themselves with mild analgesics and sleeping pills for headache and insomnia. The remaining 37 percent, however, had to stop where they were for two to three days before proceeding or, more often, they descended, occasionally to reascend later."

Climbing companions should not go for help leaving behind a very ill or semiconscious victim of mountain sickness since death can occur in minutes. Nor should they attempt to bring the victim to a nearby but higher base camp. Getting the victim down fast and, if possible, giving oxygen en route are the most crucial steps to saving the person's life and preventing permanent brain damage.

Once you've had acute mountain sickness, it's important to treat altitude with more respect, the doctors advised. But you need not be banished forever from mountaintops. A one-time victim will not necessarily get it again — especially if a sensible climbing schedule is followed.

Keeping Warm:
How to Fight Winter's Cold

Human beings evolved as semitropical animals: We are comfortable unclothed in calm, dry air at a temperature of 85 degrees Fahrenheit. Our bodies are better equipped to cope with hot weather than with cold. Therefore, in winter in northern climes we must take extra precautions to prevent excessive exposure to cold and extra steps to help our bodies conserve their own heat.

Some people think — incorrectly — that they can check the thermometer or step outside briefly and determine how to dress. Temperature is by no means the only important factor, and when you first go from a heated house into the cold outdoors, it's likely to feel colder than it really is.

The following tips should help you to be comfortably and healthfully warm in winter weather.

What to Wear

Those who complain, "It's not the cold, it's the wind," are right. Wind removes the layer of air your body has heated around you to keep itself warm. A mere five-mile-an-hour wind can carry away eight times more body heat than still air. The so-called wind-chill factor measures the increase in cooling power of moving air, whether it's wind that is blowing or you who are moving rapidly and in effect creating a wind against you. At 20 degrees in a twenty-mile-an-hour wind, the cooling effect is equivalent to calm air at minus 10 degrees. [See diagram, opposite.] The amount of clothing you'd need to keep you warm when you're sitting still at 70 degrees would be enough at 40 degrees if you were walking briskly or at minus 5 degrees if you were running.

For anyone out in the cold, it's far better to wear layers of relatively light, loose clothing than one thick, heavy item. Between each layer there's a film of trapped air which, when heated by your body, acts as an excellent insulator. Avoid tight clothing (and tight shoes and boots) since they leave no room for trapped air. Layered clothing is especially important if you're going out to exercise or do heavy work. A doctor-jogger who suffered penile frostbite urges extra protection for the groin when running.

Wetness increases the loss of body heat. Air is a very poor conductor of heat, but water is an excellent one. If your skin or clothing gets wet, your body will lose heat much more rapidly. Even at 50 degrees you can suffer ill effects of cold if you are wet. To reduce wetness from perspiration, avoid overdressing. In wet weather wear water-repellent (not waterproof) outer garments that will keep you dry on the outside and still "breathe" enough so that moisture from your body can escape.

Body heat is most likely to be lost from parts that have a lot of surface area compared to total mass — namely, the hands and feet. Keep them warm and dry. For the hands, mittens are better than gloves. Better yet, wear thin gloves under mittens so that if you need finger dexterity, you can take the mittens off briefly and not totally expose your hands. On your feet, it's best to wear looser-fitting shoes and two pairs of socks

— either both wool or a cotton pair underneath and a wool one on top. Also helpful are boots that are lined or bought a half size larger and worn with a pair of socks underneath. Remember, if your feet get wet, they will lose heat rapidly, so waterproof your shoes and boots.

If all the rest of your body is covered, as much as 90 percent of the heat you lose can come from your head, so be sure to wear a hat, and on very cold or windy days wear a scarf or ski mask on your face. Vaseline on your nose and lips will help reduce heat loss and prevent drying. Don't be fooled by pink cheeks: In the cold, they don't mean your skin is hot. Rather, they result from a slowdown of metabolism in skin cells in response to cold. The skin looks pink because very little oxygen is being removed from the blood and red, oxygenated blood is moving through your surface veins.

Babies and small children have a lot of surface area compared to mass and therefore lose heat more rapidly than adults. A baby sitting in a stroller needs to be bundled up and perhaps even wrapped in a blanket in cold weather. But parents commonly overdress small children who are out running and playing hard. They get overheated and perspire, and

WIND CHILL FACTOR CHART

Estimated wind speed (in mph)	Actual thermometer reading (in degrees Fahrenheit)							
	50°F	40°F	30°F	20°F	10°F	0°F	−10°F	−20°F
	EQUIVALENT TEMPERATURE							
Calm	50	40	30	20	10	0	−10	−20
5	48	37	27	16	6	−5	−15	−26
10	40	28	16	4	−9	−24	−33	−46
15	36	22	9	−5	−18	−32	−45	−58
20	32	18	4	−10	−25	−39	−53	−67
25	30	16	0	−15	−29	−44	−59	−74
30	28	13	−2	−18	−33	−48	−63	−79
35	27	11	−4	−20	−35	−51	−67	−82
40	26	10	−6	−21	−37	−53	−69	−85

(Wind speeds greater than 40 mph have little additional effect.)

LITTLE DANGER (for properly clothed person). Maximum danger of false sense of security.

INCREASING DANGER
Danger from freezing of exposed flesh.

GREAT DANGER

NOTE: Hypothermia, trenchfoot, and immersion foot may occur at any point on this chart.
SOURCE: Patient Care.

when they stop to rest, they get chilled and shivery. The mother of such a child who comes home with his teeth chattering may say to herself, "I guess I didn't dress Johnny warmly enough," when in fact she overdressed him. Better to send children out to active play in layers of light clothing (but with hands and feet well protected) so that they can shed a layer or two while exercising and put them back on when they stop.

As for fabric, wool is superior to cotton because it can trap a lot of air and it readily regains its thickness after being compressed by body movements. Goose or duck down, the natural insulator of these water birds, is an excellent fill that provides warmth with little weight. Synthetic fabrics that spring back into shape after compression are good, too. When damp or wet, polyester fiber fill is a better insulator than goose or duck down. However, after being wetted repeatedly, polyester loses some of its airiness and therefore some of its insulating properties.

Fur is nature's insulator for mammals (the goose bumps you get when you're cold represent the evolutionary vestiges of an attempt to fluff out the fur for extra warmth), and wearing fur is the next best thing to having some. A lot of dead air is trapped between the hairs, forming a warm blanket around you. But before you invest in expensive fur or down, be sure you are not allergic to it.

What to Do — and Not to Do

Don't drink alcoholic beverages before going out or while you are out in the cold. The initial sensation of warmth you get from alcohol is deceptive. It results from an expansion of the surface blood vessels; this counters the body's natural heat conservation mechanism of constricting surface vessels (which diverts heat to the body's vital internal organs). Thus, alcohol increases the loss of body heat. It's also wise to avoid smoking cigarettes since nicotine decreases the blood supply to the far reaches of the body and interferes with warming of the arms, legs, hands, and feet.

Avoid staying in one position for too long when it's cold. Exercise generates body heat by contracting the muscles. Shivering represents an involuntary effort — albeit a meager one — to generate heat by rapid muscle contraction when voluntary efforts have failed to keep the body sufficiently warm. If you start to shiver, that's the signal to get in out of the cold as quickly as possible. If you have to stand around in the cold, flail your arms, stamp your feet, jog in place, clap your hands — do anything reasonable to get your muscles working.

In extreme cold, inhale through your nose and exhale through your mouth. Inhaled air is warmed in the nasal passages before reaching the lungs. A scarf or face mask over the nose and mouth will help to warm the air you breathe in. People with respiratory diseases should avoid going out in very cold weather because the cold air may trigger bronchial spasms and cause breathlessness. Even healthy people might be wise to avoid very strenuous exercise that results in panting in the cold since this may allow inadequately warmed air to reach the lungs and cause internal chilling and respiratory spasms.

Warm-up exercises are especially important before you exercise in the cold. Cold air causes the arteries around your heart to constrict, and this reduces the supply of oxygen-containing blood to your heart. Do at least five minutes of warm-ups indoors to get the blood flowing to your muscles and to dilate the arteries around your heart. A scarf worn across the chest will help to prevent arterial constriction caused by cold air and winds. Avoid sudden exertion, like lifting a heavy shovelful of snow. Pick up only small amounts of snow, and better yet, push small amounts without lifting at all, and take frequent rests. Don't overdo.

When you sleep, be sure to use adequate covers, even if you think you won't need them. Internal heat production falls off during sleep, and you may wake up cold and shivering.

Avoid overheating your house. It's much healthier to have indoor temperatures in the 60's than the 70's. The less extreme the differences are between inside and outside temperatures, the better. Also, overheated houses get very dry, and your respiratory passages become parched, destroying their first line of defense against invading microorganisms such as cold viruses. (Cold weather, incidentally, doesn't cause colds. Rather, when it's cold, you're more likely to be indoors and exposed to someone else's viruses. Even the stress of becoming chilled doesn't seem to enhance the likelihood of catching a cold, according to one study in which volunteers were placed in chilled rooms and cold baths.)

If the humidity in your house drops below, say, 20 percent in winter, you may want to use a humidifier. Adding moisture to the air is especially important for persons with respiratory conditions. However, humidifiers can be a source of allergy-provoking microorganisms (bacteria, fungi, and protozoa) and may cause more problems than they solve. Cool-mist vaporizers are less likely to be a problem than those that heat the water. Steam vaporizers are not a problem because the microorganisms cannot grow in boiling water. But any humidifier should be regularly and thoroughly cleaned with a detergent (once a week for the console models) to remove all mineral deposits and microorganisms. However, adding bleach, Lysol, copper sulfate, or other disinfectants to the water in the humidifier has no effect on the hazardous microorganisms. [See chapter on humidifiers, page 372.]

Hypothermia and Frostbite: Preventing Cold Injury

With growing millions of Americans participating in outdoor winter activities and with household temperatures being lowered to conserve costly fuel, injuries and deaths caused by cold are becoming increasingly common. Yet, experts say, by understanding the causes of cold injury, knowing the early signs and appropriate first-aid measures, and adopting some simple preventives, serious and deadly consequences can usually be avoided.

Example: Five-year-old Jimmy was having so much fun making snow statues with his friends in Minnesota that he never noticed the painful tingling in his fingers under his soaked-through mittens. By the time he got home his fingers were numb — frostbitten. Although no surgery was needed, the fingers remained stunted like a small child's while Jimmy grew to be a strapping six-footer.

Example: A seventy-six-year-old widow who lived alone in a drafty New York apartment lay down for a nap late one bitter cold January afternoon and never got up. By the next evening, when someone thought to check up on her, she was dead. The cause, accidental hypothermia, a precipitous drop in body temperature.

Each year tens of thousands of elderly Americans, along with hunters, hikers, and motorists stranded in storms, succumb to overexposure to the cold. Surprisingly many of these deaths occur when the outside temperature is between 30 and 50 degrees Fahrenheit. Cold injury at relatively warm winter temperatures is particularly likely to occur during wet weather since wet clothing conducts heat away from the body.

When Body Temperature Drops

The New York widow was clearly a likely candidate for developing hypothermia. She was old, she had thyroid problems that interfered with her body's ability to regulate its temperature, and she hadn't been eating well. Other circumstances that set the stage for accidental hypothermia include the use of alcohol and drugs, such as barbiturates and certain tranquilizers (chlorpromazine and other phenothiazine derivatives), inadequate clothing, inactivity, insufficient sleep, little body fat, and various endocrine, heart, and blood vessel diseases.

Although your hands and feet may be able to withstand a drop of 30 to 40 degrees below normal body temperature, when your internal, or core, temperature drops just 10 to 20 degrees, the result may be death. The body tries to preserve internal heat by constricting surface blood vessels (alcohol expands these vessels and contributes to heat loss) and by burning more body fuel to increase heat production.

Warning signs. Shivering, an involuntary contraction of the muscles to generate heat, is usually the first sign that the core temperature has begun to drop, and it should be a signal to do something right away. If you are outdoors, get to a nearby shelter quickly. Wet clothes should be removed. Warm liquids and a quick-energy food like chocolate or raisins can be given to the conscious victim of hypothermia. To hasten warming, the victim and one or two companions should be wrapped together unclothed in blankets or a sleeping bag. In mild cases, when the victim is fully conscious, a warm — but not hot — bath may be used, but a bath could be dangerous in more advanced cases, which require hospital treatment.

The warning signals of hypothermia in the elderly are less apparent. Older victims usually do not shiver and may not even say that they feel cold. But their speech and movements may become sluggish, and they may feel drowsy and get dizzy when changing position. If you suspect hypothermia in an older person (on the basis of symptoms or if a fever thermometer fails to rise above 94 degrees), call the doctor immediately. Don't try to warm the limbs because this may further reduce core temperature. Blankets and warm drinks (but not alcohol) are the best first-aid remedies.

Prevention. To prevent hypothermia among the elderly, experts recommend that indoor temperatures be kept at 65 degrees or above at all times for people aged sixty-five to seventy-five, and at 70 degrees for people over seventy-five. People who work or play outdoors in winter should be certain to dress adequately — in several layers, with hands, head, and ears well covered and feet protected by two pairs of socks and waterproof shoes or boots. In wet weather, wear water-repellent outer garments. Blue jeans are about the worst garments for keeping you warm and dry. [See chapter on keeping warm in winter, page 347.]

Avoid getting overheated since the moisture of perspiration carries away body heat. Don't overdo strenuous exercise on very cold days because the cold air inhaled into your lungs may eventually overwhelm your body's ability to warm itself. Get plenty of rest, eat a diet high in fats and carbohydrates (which provide ready fuel for the body), don't smoke or drink alcohol and don't wear yourself out with activity. If you get chilled, stay indoors for several hours to rewarm and rest before going out again.

Preventing Frost Injury

Similar preventive measures can help ward off frostbite. In addition to covering their bodies well, skiers and snowmobilers should remember to protect their faces from the freezing winds. Those pink cheeks (ears, fingers, and toes as well) are not a sign of robust health but, rather, indicate that cells near the body surface are not working and therefore don't remove oxygen from the blood.

Touching bare hands to cold metal, or to gasoline or other volative products stored outside when it is very cold, can cause immediate severe frostbite.

In frostbite, fluid between the cells freezes and the cells themselves become dehydrated. The resulting cell damage may cause death of the tissue. Sometimes the damage is so severe that a digit must be amputated.

The warning signs of frostbite are a feeling of extreme cold and pain in the affected part — usually the fingers, toes, ears, or nose — followed by a burning sensation. The part then becomes hard and numb, and the skin takes on a white, yellow-white, or mottled blue-white color.

Treatment. For a century and a half the first-aid treatment of frostbite followed the methods devised by Napoleon's officers during their icy retreat from Moscow. This suggested rubbing the frozen part with snow or ice. Now doctors know better. *Frozen tissue must be rewarmed rapidly, preferably by being placed in warm water (no hotter than 108 degrees) or, if warm water is unavailable, by being tucked into a warm area of the body, such as the armpit or between the thighs.* But don't rub it: that can cause severe tissue damage and increase the chances of infection. On the contrary, the part should be handled very gingerly. Don't put the frozen part near a fire or hot stove or under hot water. The high temperature can cause severe burns.

If normal color and sensation don't return to the frozen part within twenty minutes of first-aid treatment, a doctor should be seen. If there is any danger of refreezing, do not rewarm the part yourself. It is far better to leave the tissue frozen and get the victim to medical care, keeping the frostbitten part protected en route by padding it with a soft thick cloth.

Rewarming a frostbitten part can be very painful, and a painkiller or sedative may be needed. Following treatment, dark blisters may form, and the skin may becomed blackened and eventually slough off. This is part of the healing process. Surgery is usually not necessary, at least not at first, and amputation can usually be avoided. Some of the most grotesque-looking frostbite injuries eventually heal with minimal permanent effects. But once frostbitten, the tissue may remain permanently supersensitive to cold.

Getting Painless Pleasure from the Sun

Until about half a century ago a lily-white or peaches-and-cream complexion was revered among women of means, who wore wide-brimmed hats and carried parasols to protect themselves from the sun. Only farmers and laborers who could not avoid being out in the sun sported suntans and eventually developed the leathery, prematurely wrinkled skin and weather-beaten look associated with chronic exposure to the sun's ultraviolet rays.

In recent decades sun worshiping has become a national cult. A richly tanned skin is popularly regarded as a sign of beauty and robust health. Some even go so far as to "paint" on a tan if they can't get one naturally. While millions bask in the summer sun and follow the sun south in winter, tanning booths, which use artificially produced tanning rays, have made year-round suntans possible even for stay-at-homes.

For some the sun is indeed health-giving. Aside from its psychological benefits, it can help relieve such conditions as psoriasis, acne, asthma, and aching joints. The sun is also a major source of vitamin D, which is made on our skin under ultraviolet light.

The Sun's Health Risks

Unfortunately for most people the sun is also an insidious troublemaker. We have already begun to pay the price of our sun worship with increasing rates of skin cancer, more rapidly aging skin, and a wide range of bizarre reactions to sun exposure.

A healthy appreciation of the sun's potential for harm as well as good is long overdue. While few dermatologists expect Americans to abandon their sun god overnight, most hope that a better understanding of the sun's effects on human skin and some tips for self-protection will inspire a safer form of worship.

Sensitive skin types. Not everyone is equally susceptible to sun damage. A lot has to do with how readily you tan since tanning is nature's way of trying to protect the skin from ultraviolet light. In *Between You and Me* (Boston: Little, Brown, 1978), Drs. John A. Parrish, Barbara A. Gilchrist, and Thomas B. Fitzpatrick point out that those who are fair-skinned and never tan tend to get sunburned in just ten or fifteen minutes. Such people, with Skin Type I, are also at greatest risk of eventually developing cancerous lesions, freckles, and pigmented, loose, dry, wrinkled skin. This cumulative, irreversible damage, which may not show up for decades, begins at birth and cannot be forestalled by any kind of cosmetic ablution.

Those with Skin Type II, who usually burn but may sometimes acquire a faint tan, are also highly susceptible to sun damage. Type III skin, which usually tans but sometimes burns, and Type IV skin, which almost never burns and always tans well, are much less at risk of developing chronic sun damage. But no one, not even the darkest black, is immune to sunburn, skin cancer, or premature aging of the skin from the sun.

The burning rays. Two types of ultraviolet ray are important to the sun's effects. The shorter rays (UVB) are the main cause of sunburn. They are most intense in the middle of the day — between 10:00 A.M. and 2:00 P.M. (11 to 3, daylight savings time). The longer UVA rays, which predominate in the morning and late afternoon hours, are considerably less potent in terms of sunburn, but they are the primary cause of photosensitivity reactions, and recent evidence indicates that UVB and UVA can activate each other's harmful effects. Those who get a moderate burn at noon and go out again in the late afternoon can become badly burned because their skin has been sensitized to ultraviolet light.

You don't need a hot, sunny summer's day to get a good dose of ultraviolet light. Up to 80 percent of ultraviolet rays can penetrate haze, light clouds, or fog. A big hat or beach umbrella is not surefire protection since ultraviolet rays can be reflected upward from the ground, sand, and water. Snow is one of the best reflectors, sending more than 85 percent of the rays back up. You can even get sunburned while sitting in the shade because some rays are reflected sideways.

A sizable percentage of ultraviolet rays may penetrate lightweight summer clothing. They can also hit you while you're swimming underwater, and they readily pass through a wet T-shirt. Don't be fooled by a cool breeze or low air temperature. You can get just as burned on a sunny June day whether the temperature is 50 degrees or 90 degrees. In fact, because you miss the warning of feeling too hot, you're more likely to get broiled on a cooler day.

Suntan and sunburn. People with Skin Types I and II (about one-third of the population) should not try to get tan. For those with darker complexions, the best way to acquire a pleasing tan is slowly, during the UVA part of the day and only for fifteen minutes a day at first. Gradually build up exposure to forty-five minutes a day, but always try to avoid the middle of the day.

Don't judge how much sun you have gotten by how burned or tan you look while you're out. It takes four or more hours after exposure for the full sunburn to show.

If you should suffer a sunburn, the best immediate first aid is cold compresses and aspirin (for adults, three to start, then two every five hours thereafter) to relieve pain and reduce swelling. Calamine lotion may also relieve the agony of sunburn, but avoid Caladryl, which contains an antihistamine that could cause an allergic reaction. Severe sunburn requires a doctor's attention and prescription medication. Don't try to treat raw, blistering skin yourself.

Sunburned skin loses its ability to sweat normally for two weeks after healing. So if you suffer an extensive burn, avoid getting overheated for a few weeks.

Sun damage. In addition to the acute effects of sunburn, exposure to the sun's ultraviolet rays can cause chronic damage, permanently destroying the elastic fibers that keep the skin tight and young-looking. After years of sun exposure, the elastic fibers begin to snap, and the skin becomes loose, wrinkled, and old-looking. The layers of skin cells also thicken in response to repeated sun exposure, causing a hard, leathery texture. If you want to know what the skin on your face would look like today if it had only rarely been in the sun, take a look at your buttocks.

Ultraviolet radiation also damages the DNA, or genetic material, in skin cells. Eventually, accumulated DNA damage can result in the formation of cancerous cells. Sun exposure is the primary cause of superficial types of skin cancer, which are highly curable. It is also a cause of the usually fatal skin cancer called melanoma, which is becoming increasingly common on sun-exposed parts of the body.

Sunlight is responsible for a number of photosensitivity reactions, which result from an inherent susceptibility or an underlying disease or from the use of a particular drug or cosmetic. Sun reactions commonly are triggered by the use of deodorant soaps; perfumes; antibiotics like tetracycline, sulfonamides, and griseofulvin; thiazide diuretics; tranquilizers; and oral contraceptives.

A confusing array of products — lotions, creams, oils, gels, sprays — making an even more confusing series of claims, confront the unsuspecting consumer. The types of sun products include the following:

● **Sun-blocking agents,** which are opaque and deflect the ultraviolet rays. These may contain zinc oxide, titanium dioxide, or talc. While cosmetically not pleasing, they are useful for areas that burn very easily, such as the lips, earlobes, and nose.

● **Sunscreens,** which selectively absorb UVB or varying proportions of UVB and UVA. According to *The Medical Letter*, a drug advisory for doctors, there are now available for over-the-counter sale a wide range of sunscreen products that are rated according to the degree of pro-

A GUIDE TO SUNSCREENS

Skin Type	SPF Range	Products	Absorbs
I Very fair. Always burns, never tans.	10-15	Super Shade 15	UVB, UVA
		Piz Buin Exclusiv Extrem Creme	UVB, UVA
		Total Eclipse	UVB, UVA
II Fair. Usually burns, sometimes tans faintly.	6-12	Eclipse	UVB
		Pabanol	UVB
		Piz Buin 6	UVB, UVA
		PreSun	UVB
III Sometimes burns, usually tans.	4-6	A-Fil	UVB, UVA
		Maxafil	UVB, UVA
		Pabafilm	UVB
		Pabagel	UVB
		Partial Eclipse	UVB
		Piz Buin 4	UVB
		Pro Tan	UVB
		RV Paque	UVB, UVA
		Sea & Ski 6	UVB
		Solbar	UVB, UVA
		Sundown	UVB, UVA
		Sungard	UVB, UVA
		UVAL	UVB, UVA
IV Almost never burns, always tans.	2-4	Coppertone 2	UVB
		Piz Buin 2	UVB
		RVP	UVB, UVA
		Sundare	UVB

UVB: Stronger, midday rays that are the main cause of sunburn.
UVA: Less potent in terms of sunburn.
Credit: Adapted from *The Medical Letter*, June 1, 1979.

tection they can give against ultraviolet radiation (see table, page 357). The most effective sunscreens contain the chemical PABA or benzophenone or both. Ultimate effectiveness depends on which formulation is used, the base in which the chemicals are mixed, and their concentration.

Contrary to popular belief, sunscreens do not prevent tanning or burning; they merely slow the process. Most block out the burning UVB rays but let some or all of the tanning UVA through. The higher the Sun Protection Factor rating, the more ultraviolet light (particularly UVB) the product keeps out. If, for example, a product has a Sun Protection Factor rating of 4, it means that it should quadruple the amount of time you can stay in the sun without burning. It does not guarantee that you won't burn. If you stay out long enough, the effect will be the same as if you had used no protection at all.

To be effective, sunscreens should be applied twenty to forty-five minutes before you go out in the sun and reapplied every two hours and after washing, swimming, or heavy sweating. They should be used by everyone who goes out in the sun, regardless of skin type. Very light-skinned and sun-sensitive persons are advised to use a sunscreen with a Sun Protection Factor of 10 to 15 daily as a matter of routine to build up a protective layer in the skin. There are now products with an SPF of 20 available.

358

Sunscreen chemicals themselves can sometimes cause bad reactions, including allergies and dermatitis. It's a good idea to test a small area of skin before you apply a new product widely.

● **Suntan lotions,** which offer little or no protection against ultraviolet light and sunburn. Nor do they "promote tanning," as some claim. What they contain are oils that change the optic properties of the skin and speed up the sun's effect. Some lotions contain a chemical that reacts with the skin to produce a fake tan. This coloring can last for days or weeks but offers little protection against sunburn.

[For information on protecting your eyes in the sun, see the chapter on eye injuries, page 406.]

Lightning: Be Prepared for the Not-So-Improbable

"May lightning strike me dead" is a popular way of conveying the extreme improbability of an event. Yet lightning strikes are not as unlikely as this expression suggests. According to the National Oceanic and Atmospheric Administration, lightning strikes the earth 100 times each second. While the vast majority of these strikes do nothing more than create spectacular light displays, at least 125 Americans are killed by lightning each year, two to three times that number are seriously injured, and many more narrowly escape death or serious harm.

For example, in the spring of 1979 a fourteen-year-old New Jersey boy died when he and a companion were struck by lightning during soccer practice. A week before, two Texas cowboys and their horses died of a lightning strike while herding cattle during a storm. A month before that, lightning struck an oil tanker docked in Texas, killing one man and injuring thirty-three.

Most deaths and injuries from lightning are preventable if you know what to do when a thunderstorm is approaching. Unfortunately many people do just the wrong thing — such as run for cover under the nearest tall tree — and ignore the safest measures immediately at hand. In a recent analysis, 11 percent of lightning deaths involved people who were taking shelter under trees, 8 percent were on open water, 7 percent were riding tractors, and 4 percent were playing golf.

What Lightning Is and What It Does

To appreciate the importance of recommended safety measures, it helps to understand some things about the nature of lightning and the objects it strikes.

A bolt of lightning is a gigantic spark with an electrical potential of up to 100 million volts (for comparison, ordinary household current, which can deliver quite a shock, carries 120 volts). The spark occurs when a negatively charged thunderstorm cloud induces a positive charge on the ground below for several miles around. The difference between the positive and negative charges gradually builds until enough of an electrical potential exists to overcome the insulation provided by the miles of intervening air, which is a poor conductor of electricity.

The usual lightning strike is a flow of electrical current from the cloud to the ground. Thunder, incidentally, is the noise caused by the explosive expansion of air as it is heated by the intense current passing through. The lightning is seen first because it travels at the speed of light, whereas the thunder approaches at the much slower speed of sound.

Lightning can strike in a wide area around a thunderstorm, so measures to protect yourself and your family should begin as soon as thunderclouds are seen or heard nearby. *Do not wait until it starts to rain.* In fact, a bolt of lightning can come "out of the blue." It can jump out of the side of a thunderstorm and strike the ground miles away. Just such an event resulted in injuries to five boys in Ames, Iowa, when they resumed their Little League game after a storm had moved north.

Lightning always follows the path of least resistance. It tends to choose the closest — usually the tallest — object when it strikes: an isolated tree, a person in an open field, a house on a hilltop, a telephone pole or wire, an antenna, a fishing pole. In general, you are safer from lightning injuries in the city than in rural or suburban areas because tall buildings attract the lightning charge and carry it safely into the ground. Lightning also chooses the most conductive pathway — for example, metal or water rather than air. This is why you should get out of or off the water and put down your fishing rod and golf clubs at the first sign of an impending thunderstorm.

Lightning does not have to strike directly at you or the object you are in, on, or holding to cause injury and death. Although direct strikes are the most dangerous, the most frequent injuries result from the spreading of the electrical current after it has struck. That's why it is so dangerous to stand under a tall tree. If the tree is struck, fingers of electric current spread along the ground. The same thing can happen if you're in the water when lightning strikes nearby.

How to Protect Yourself

The following lightning safety rules were developed by the National Weather Service. They should be applied as soon as a storm approaches.

● Get inside — a house, large building, or all-metal vehicle (not a convertible with a nonmetallic top) with the windows and doors completely closed. Your car is one of the safest places to be because the metal box gives the lightning a preferred pathway to the ground. Do not lean against the doors or hold onto metal parts or use your CB radio (except in an emergency) until the storm ends. If you are in a house, it is safe to watch the storm from a closed window. If windows or doors are open, the lightning can come in and strike whatever might be in its path.

● If you are inside, avoid using the telephone (again, except in emergencies), especially in rural and suburban areas where telephone poles are frequently struck by lightning. The current can travel through the telephone wire and burn your face and damage your hearing. However, it is usually not necessary to discontinue use of electrical appliances unless you are living in a house that is isolated (for example on a hilltop) or lightning has come in through your electrical outlets in the past. Otherwise, the risk of lightning's coming into the house through the electrical system is extremely small.

If you are outside and unable to get to safety in an automobile or building, observe these precautions:

● Do not stand beneath a natural lightning rod such as a tall, isolated tree. You are safer if there are a whole lot of trees, but it is best to take shelter under a thick clump of small ones. If you are camping in a tent inside a forest, you are relatively safe when you are not near a tall, isolated tree or in an open area. If possible, it's best to wait out the storm in your car.

● Do not make yourself into a natural lightning rod by projecting yourself above the surrounding landscape. If you are in an open field or on a beach, get down on your knees, put your hands on your knees, and tuck your head down. This diminishes your vertical height and minimizes your contact with the ground, reducing the chance that you will be hit by current spreading through the ground as well as by a direct bolt. In a boat, get as low as you can (below deck if there is one), and stay away from the mast of a sailboat.

• Get out of and away from water.

• Get away from anything that's metal, including golf clubs, motorcycles, tennis rackets, bicycles, fishing rods, aluminum baseball bats, metal clotheslines or fences, farm equipment, and metal sheds. Do not try to get the clothes off the line at the last minute.

• If you feel an electric charge that causes your hair to stand on end or your skin to tingle, lightning may be about to strike you. Immediately drop to the ground on your knees as described above.

If all else fails and someone is struck seemingly dead by lightning, a bystander should immediately begin mouth-to-mouth resuscitation (if breathing has stopped but the heart is still beating) or cardiopulmonary resuscitation (CPR) if both breathing and the heart have stopped. These first-aid techniques are taught by the American Red Cross and many other groups around the country. [See chapter on CPR, page 426.] The electric jolt can disrupt the rhythm of the heart, which runs on electricity, but this does not mean the person is beyond saving. Immediate resuscitation can make the difference between life and death. You cannot get electrocuted by handling someone who's been struck by lightning; the body does not retain the electrical charge.

Passive Smoking:
A Danger to All

A Los Angeles businessman asked the airline agent to give him a seat "as far as possible from the smoking sections because smoke makes me cough." A woman asked the headwaiter at an elegant New York restaurant to "please tell the gentlemen at the next table to put out their cigarettes or move to a different table."

Throughout the country "passive smokers" are speaking out. Growing numbers of nonsmokers are trying to rid their environment of a pervasive pollutant that is a general nuisance to most and a genuine health hazard to some. In dozens of communities their individual efforts are now supported by legislation that restricts smoking in public places either by banning it entirely or by segregating smokers the way airlines and railroads have done for years.

Although inhaling the smoke from other people's cigarettes has not yet been proved to cause heart disease, there is some evidence that it can cause lung cancer, and many other actual and potential hazards of passive smoking have been delineated by researchers here and abroad. Passive smoking can injure the health and threaten the lives of nonsmoking wives, children, infants, and unborn babies as well as people with chronic heart and lung diseases and allergies to tobacco smoke.

Some studies have been criticized because they involved artificial settings in which the smoke levels exceeded usual normal situations, but certain facts about passive smoking are undisputed.

The American Lung Association points out, for example, that two-thirds of the smoke from a burning cigarette enters not the smoker's lungs, but the general environment. A smoker inhales for an average of twenty-four seconds per cigarette, but a cigarette burns for about twelve minutes.

In many respects the sidestream smoke, which escapes into the air between puffs, is worse than the mainstream smoke that the smoker inhales directly. Although it is diluted by air, sidestream smoke starts out with more cadmium, twice the amount of tar and nicotine, three times more of the cancer-causing agent 3,4-benzopyrene, five times more carbon monoxide, and fifty times more ammonia than mainstream smoke. Sidestream smoke also contains such noxious substances as cancer-causing nitrosamines, nitrogen dioxide (an irritating gas that can damage the lungs), formaldehyde, hydrogen cyanide, arsenic, and hydrogen sulfide (the chemical that smells like rotten eggs). In addition to sidestream smoke, the nonsmoker gets the residual mainstream smoke that the smoker exhales.

The air is likely to be heavily polluted in any enclosed space where smoking is permitted. At a typical campus party, for example, the level of particulates in the air from cigarette smoke is forty times above the United States air quality standard. After spending thirty minutes in a smoky room, nonsmokers have higher than usual heart rates and blood pressure and high levels of carbon monoxide in their blood, high enough to impair their ability to judge time intervals or distinguish relative brightness, such as from oncoming cars. Studies suggest, in fact, that nonsmokers in a very smoky room could inhale enough nicotine and carbon monoxide in an hour to equal the effects of their having each smoked a cigarette. Most urban nonsmokers have measurable amounts of nicotine in their body fluids, and the only way it gets there is through passive smoking.

Animal studies suggest that exposure to "secondhand" smoke can cause illness. Dogs developed lung tissue breakdown after breathing air laden with cigarette smoke ten times a week for a year. Rabbits exposed to the sidestream smoke from twenty cigarettes a day for two to five years developed emphysema. And rats exposed to tobacco smoke for forty-five minutes a day for two to six months developed twice the number of lung tumors as nonexposed rats.

For obvious ethical reasons, similar studies cannot be done with people, but the normal practice of the smoking habit has provided some natural experiments.

The most dramatic of the natural experiments involves unborn babies, who are the passive recipients of what their smoking mothers inhale. Among pregnant women who smoke, there is an increased risk of suffering a miscarriage or having a stillborn baby. In addition, babies of smoking mothers are twice as likely to be smaller than normal at birth, and they face a third higher risk of dying soon after birth.

The prenatal effects of smoking probably result from the fact that the amount of oxygen reaching the fetal organs is reduced because nicotine is a powerful constrictor of blood vessels and because in both the mother's and the baby's blood carbon monoxide from the cigarette smoke replaces some of the oxygen needed for normal growth and development. Even if just the father smokes, a German study of 14,774 pregnancies showed, the baby is more likely to be born dead or afflicted with a birth defect, perhaps because nicotine damages sperm.

According to a British study involving 13,000 children, the effects of passive smoking during fetal life, and probably during childhood as well, are apparent at age eleven, when the average reading score is three months behind and the children are on the average three-fourths of an inch shorter than if their mothers had not smoked.

Studies in Britain and Israel showed that the infants of smoking parents have nearly twice the risk of being hospitalized with pneumonia or bronchitis. And a study in Detroit among hundreds of families that have been followed for years showed that schoolchildren exposed to tobacco smoke at home have twice the expected number of respiratory infections. Tobacco smoke can also trigger asthma attacks.

The health effects of passive smoking apparently continue throughout life, although they are somewhat harder to measure in adults. A study in San Diego of nonsmoking workers who each workday inhaled the sidestream smoke of their colleagues showed a significant impairment in the nonsmokers' lung function.

A study in Erie County, Pennsylvania, revealed that the nonsmoking wives of men who smoke die on the average four years younger than women whose husbands are also nonsmokers. A large Japanese study indicated that the nonsmoking wives of smoking men faced a fourfold increase in their own risk of developing lung cancer, and a Greek study also showed a significantly increased lung cancer risk among nonsmoking wives.

If a person's circulatory or respiratory system is already crippled by disease, tobacco smoke can seriously aggravate the condition. The American Medical Association estimates that at least 35 million Americans have respiratory ailments that are made worse by tobacco smoke. People with angina pectoris (chest pains that result from an insufficient supply of oxygen to the heart muscle) are likely to become incapacitated by their pain at lower levels of exercise if they are first exposed to cigarette smoke. A study by Dr. Wilbert S. Aronow of the Long Beach, California, Veterans Administration Hospital showed that in patients with heart disease the amount of exercise they could do before angina symptoms developed was decreased by 22 percent after passively smoking fifteen cigarettes in two hours' time in a well-ventilated room and by 38 percent in a room that was not ventilated. In addition, the patients' resting heart rates and blood pressures increased, and they were more likely to develop abnormal heartbeats that sometimes presage a heart attack.

Dr. Aronow's study suggests that people who have suffered heart attacks might be wise to avoid places that are heavily polluted with tobacco smoke.

What to Do About Passive Smoking

Short of locking yourself up in an airtight room, there are a number of steps you can take to reduce or avoid exposure to someone else's tobacco smoke.

● Let the people you associate with know that you are bothered by cigarette smoke. Politely tell people, strangers included, that their smoking is bothering you. If necessary, put no-smoking stickers in your office, car, and home, or wear a button thanking people for not smoking.

● Check on your local laws on where smoking is prohibited, such as in elevators, stores, and theaters, and be firm with people who violate the law.

● Patronize restaurants that segregate smokers, and encourage your favorite restaurants to do the same.

● Check on the smoking rules in movie theaters before you buy your ticket; most forbid smoking in all or part of the theater. Tell the usher if someone violates the rules.

● Always sit in nonsmoking sections on planes, trains, and buses. If you have a confirmed reservation and arrive at the proper check-in time, an airline must provide a no-smoking seat for you if you want it or risk a fine of up to $1,000.

● If you belong to organizations or attend meetings or conferences, you might propose that smoking be prohibited in the meeting room or, if the room is large enough and well ventilated, that smokers be segregated in back of the room.

Noise:
A Ubiquitous Health Risk

You are awakened at 3:00 A.M. by a fire siren. No sooner do you doze off again than the rattle and roar of garbage collection disturb your sleep once more. At 7 the alarm puts an end to your fitful night, and although you feel irritable and tired, you get up to start your day — only to confront the electric razor, the hair dryer, the morning news, the electric blender, the whistling tea kettle, a crying child.

You leave the house to hear jackhammers, a motorcycle, an ambulance, rush-hour traffic, the subway. At work the clamorous machines vie with hammering workmen and banging in the air-conditioning ducts. Back home again to raucous youngsters, the garbage disposal and dishwasher, a blaring television, and an even louder stereo. You try escaping outdoors only to encounter a portable radio at full volume.

Noise. It's everywhere, disturbing your peace, jarring your nerves, damaging your hearing, and — a growing body of evidence indicates — contributing to a wide array of serious ailments and perhaps shortening your life. Despite increasing attention to this insidious and pervasive pollutant, it is generally agreed that the environment of most people — both in and out of their homes — is noisier today than ever.

Although all the health effects of noise have not yet been clearly defined, there is no question that noise can cause physical and psychological injury. While much environmental noise is beyond an individual's control, there are things you can do to reduce the noisiness of your surroundings and to protect yourself and your family from the damaging effects of noise.

The Harmful Effects

Damage to hearing. More than 16 million Americans have already suffered noise-caused hearing loss, and another 40 million, not counting workmen, are currently exposed to hazardous noise levels. Noise injuries eventually destroy the delicate hair cells in the inner ear which detect the different frequencies of sound and transmit them to the brain's auditory center. The louder the noise, the less exposure it takes to cause permanent hearing loss, which begins with the upper frequencies. The damaging effects of noise start at 75 decibels, about the level of traffic noise at a major intersection. Chronic exposure to 75 decibels for about forty years causes hearing loss.

The current standard for work environments is an eight-hour average exposure to 90 decibels, which is two and a half times louder than 75. At 90 decibels you have to shout to be heard a few feet away. It results in hearing loss in a significant proportion of workers in just a few years. Attempts to lower this standard to 85 decibels, which would halve the number of workers injured, have been contested as too costly.

For the sake of comparison, other common sources of noise are a jet plane at 500 feet, 110 to 120 decibels; a rock band or discotheque, 115; a motorcycle revving up, 110; a subway train and an electric blender, 90 to 100; a power lawn mower, 96; an electric shaver, 90; a vacuum cleaner, 85, and ordinary conversation, 60.

Youngsters who ride minibikes or who listen to a lot of loud rock music have been shown to suffer permanent hearing loss in the upper frequencies. A study in a New York City public school, one side of which abuts an elevated subway, showed that children in the noisy classrooms had a harder time learning verbal skills than comparable children in quieter classrooms.

The warning signs of impending noise injury are a prolonged inability to hear well after the noise has stopped, discomfort in the ears or actual pain if the noise is very loud, and ringing in the ears. Early signs of damage include difficulty in hearing high-frequency sounds like ticking clocks, telephone bells, and chirping birds; difficulty distinguishing the speech sounds *s, sh, ch, p, m, t, f,* and *th*; and difficulty hearing normal speech clearly. [See the chapter on hearing loss, page 309.]

Sleep disturbances. No one needs to be told that it is distressing to be awakened in the middle of the night by noise, but you may not realize that even if the noise is not loud enough to waken you, it can still be disturbing. Studies have shown that noise causes a disruption in normal sleep and dream patterns even if the person remains asleep. Brain waves show that noise disruption results in a more wakeful stage of sleep. These disturbances may cause a person to feel tired, tense, and forgetful the next day.

Psychological damage. Noise makes people tired, nervous, and irritable, says Dr. Jack C. Westman, a psychiatrist at the University of Wisconsin. Excessive noise, his studies have shown, aggravates family tensions and is a common factor in family arguments. This is particularly a problem for people who spend the workday in a noisy environment and come home looking for peace and quiet, only to find chaotic noise.

Physiological damage. A fear of loud noises is one of the two instinctive fears people are born with. It triggers a fight-or-flight reaction, causing the heart to beat faster, the blood pressure to rise, and the blood to flow preferentially to the brain and muscles.

According to Dr. Westman, the sound levels produced by common kitchen appliances can cause dilation of the pupils, drying of the mouth, loss of skin color, muscular contraction, a reduction in the flow of gastric juices, and diminished motility of the digestive tract. There is also evidence that noise can increase cholesterol levels in the blood and interfere with sugar metabolism.

The sum of such effects may be an increased risk of developing heart disease, high blood pressure, peptic ulcers, and perhaps diabetes. While a person may learn to "tune out" chronic noise psychologically, he can never completely adapt to the physical effects of noise.

Noise damage may actually begin in the womb. Unborn babies respond to even moderate noises by moving about and increasing their heart rates. Two studies of babies born to mothers living in high-noise areas near airports showed an increased rate of birth defects among them.

Are You Protected Against Noise?

A number of cities and states have some antinoise ordinances, but outside the occupational area there is no overall national noise control law. The Environmental Protection Agency is authorized to regulate environmental noise and to label consumer products as to their noise level. National noise regulations are in effect for motorcycles, medium and heavy trucks, garbage trucks, and interstate railroads, and the agency has proposed regulations for buses and earth-moving equipment. Consumer products like vacuum cleaners and air conditioners do not yet have noise ratings, but noise control items like hearing protectors (earmuffs and ear plugs) are now rated for effectiveness.

Noise experts say that consumers should complain (loudly) about products that are too noisy and, better yet, refuse to buy them. They point with dismay to an effort some years ago of a manufacturer that produced a quiet vacuum cleaner. Housekeepers didn't like it because they equated its noiselessness with lack of power.

Workers who are exposed to damaging noise levels should be certain to protect their ears as well as to demand improved noise controls from their employers. Professional earmuffs and plugs are available, but putting a piece of cotton in your ears does little good.

SOURCES OF NOISE POLLUTION

Here are some examples of the noise levels, in decibels, of common sources of noise pollution. Decibels are measured on a logarithmic curve, so that the higher on the scale you go, the greater the difference between one number and the next. Thus, although the noise of a Concorde (120 decibels) is only 5 decibels greater than that of a conventional jet (115 decibels), it is more than twice as loud. The smallest change of sound intensity that the human ear can detect is approximately 1 decibel, no matter what the original intensity.

Pain level

Close-in jet plane takeoff, 150 decibels (brief period of exposure can permanently damage ears); large pneumatic riveter at four feet, between 120 and 130.

Discomfort level

Thunderclap, 120; four-engine jet aircraft at 500 feet, between 110 and 120; rock-and-roll band, 100 or more, depending on distance.

Annoyance level

Inside subway train, between 90 and 100; occasional volume of buses, 95; jackhammer, 94; electric blender, 93; a shout, a truck, a sports car, heavy traffic, occasional peak kitchen noise, 90; noise that interferes with telephone conversation, 80; automobile, 70; automatic dishwasher at close range, between 60 and 70.

By comparison, conversation at three feet generates about 60 decibels, a "quiet" room about 40, and a whisper about 20.

Dr. Westman suggests a number of ways to reduce noise in the home. Improved insulation and the use of air conditioners can help to block out street noise. The kitchen, which is the noisiest room in a typical home (in addition to its noisy appliances, it contains smooth hard surfaces that sounds bounce off), can be designed with washable carpet on the floor, acoustical tiles on the ceiling, baffles around appliances, and even fabric on the walls. All these absorb, rather than reflect, sound.

In addition, Dr. Westman suggests, some sensible controls can be applied to reduce people noise. Since young children are noisy by definition, they should be given a place to play that is remote from the rest of the family, where they can make all the noise they want without disturbing adults. Instead of yelling at a child to quiet down, get up and do something about it, quietly. Also, there should be well-enforced ground rules about when and how loud the television and stereo can be played.

If you want to preserve your hearing, limit your stay at discos, bowling alleys, and other such noisy environments to two hours at a time. Wear hearing protectors when you use power tools, lawn mowers, or other noisy machines, and cover your ears when you deplane in an open area.

Indoor Pollution: Is It Safe to Breathe?

The air you breathe in your home or office may be more harmful to your health than the outdoor air in the most polluted of cities. Many people don't realize that their "perpetual cold" or other nagging symptoms may be caused by the air in their own homes, at school, or on the job. Some have been plagued for years and have visited doctor after doctor in a vain attempt to uncover the cause of their problem. Once the real culprit is suspected or identified, many sources of indoor pollution can be greatly reduced and perhaps prevented entirely.

Indoor air pollution has been linked to a wide variety of adverse health effects, including headaches, respiratory problems, frequent colds and sore throats, chronic cough, skin rashes, eye irritation, lethargy, dizziness, and memory lapses. Long-term effects may include an increased risk of cancer. Though children, the elderly, and people with chronic ailments like asthma, allergies, heart and lung diseases seem especially vulnerable, symptoms may also occur in otherwise normal, healthy individuals.

Virtually every household and office building is a potential source of excessive amounts of one or another toxic pollutant — nitrogen dioxide, carbon monoxide, hydrocarbons, formaldehyde, radon (a radioactive product of radium), sulfur dioxide, asbestos, not to mention the chemicals in hair sprays, deodorants, oven cleaners, paints, pesticides, laundry aids, floor and furniture polishes, glue, and, ironically, air fresheners. Your kitchen range, fireplace, heater, rugs, walls, furniture, clothing, even the sheets you sleep on can be significant sources of indoor air pollutants.

The levels of potentially hazardous substances in indoor air often exceed those allowed outside and are sometimes as great as or greater than permissible industrial exposures. Yet, a study by the Environmental Protection Agency showed, the average person spends about 90 percent of his or her time indoors, and most of that time is spent at home. The average industrial exposure is only forty hours a week, but an infant is exposed to home pollutants for nearly twenty-four hours a day.

The Value of Ventilation

The pollution problem is most serious in homes tightly sealed to keep out the winter cold. In a typical "leaky" house, all the air is exchanged with fresh outdoor air about once an hour, but a well-sealed house may take four to ten times longer to replace the indoor air completely. This allows an enormous buildup of potentially harmful substances in the air.

Therefore, better ventilation — not sealing up the house too tightly and proper use of venting systems — is the main key to solving problems with indoor pollution. A side benefit of a not so tight house may be a reduction in indoor humidity, which means less growth of mold spores, a common cause of allergic reactions.

Though not perfect, heat exchangers — duct systems in which the incoming outdoor air picks up most of the heat in the stale indoor air as it is vented outside — can greatly improve the air exchange in a tightly sealed home without much increase in energy cost. Electrostatic air cleaners can filter out many air pollutants in the home, but they also create ozone, itself a respiratory irritant. The effectiveness of ion exchangers as air cleaners is controversial.

The Major Indoor Pollutants

Following is a description of the major indoor pollutants identified so far, their sources, their effects, and what you can do to protect yourself and your family from exposure to them.

Formaldehyde. This ubiquitous chemical is by far the most worrisome indoor pollutant. It seeps out of urea formaldehyde foam insulation (not polyurethane foam); particle board used in walls, partitions, and virtually all the cupboards and furniture made in recent years; rugs and carpets made from synthetic fibers; drapes; permanent press clothing and linens; and many drugs and cosmetics.

A study by Seattle researchers of the occupants of more than 400 mobile homes (which use particle board and are made tight) and 200 regular homes with formaldehyde insulation revealed a high concentration of formaldehyde in the air and complaints from a large proportion of occupants of eye irritation, frequent upper respiratory infections, chronic headaches, periodic memory lapses or drowsiness, and, in the elderly, chest pains and heart problems. A study in laboratory rats showed a high rate of nasal cancers developed in those animals that chronically breathed formaldehyde at levels often found in mobile homes; on the basis of this and other findings, the Consumer Product Safety Commission banned urea formaldehyde foam insulation (the ban covers insulation installed after August 1982).

Studies have shown that a sensitivity to formaldehyde can develop through repeated exposure. To protect yourself against this chemical, wash new permanent press items several times before using them; avoid products made from particle board (or coat them with a sealant); check the ingredients list on cosmetics before you buy them; and don't use formaldehyde foam to insulate your house. If you are considering buying a new house in the summer, when it's harder to detect the smell of formaldehyde, ask for a warranty against formaldehyde fumes in the purchase agreement.

Nitrogen dioxide. As a major by-product of combustion, this irritating air pollutant is commonly found in homes with gas (both natural and liquid propane) cook stoves and heaters at levels far higher than outdoors. A Harvard study showed that children living in homes with gas stoves had a significant reduction in lung function. A British study revealed an increase in colds and bronchitis among children whose homes had gas ovens. Nitrogen dioxide has been implicated in long-term respiratory problems and possibly heart disease and cancer.

A gas range should be fitted with a hood that is vented to the outside, and the vent should be turned on whenever a burner is lit or the oven is used.

Carbon monoxide and hydrocarbons. These chemicals are also released into the air when substances burn. Carbon monoxide is an insidious pollutant that can cause drowsiness, headache, impaired heart function, and even death in high concentrations. The hydrocarbons, such as benzopyrene, cause cancer in laboratory animals and can damage the liver, respiratory system, and nerve tissue. Indoors the main sources of these pollutants are tobacco smoke, wood- and coal-burning stoves, fireplaces, gas ranges, self-cleaning electric ovens, pesticides, and automobiles in garages attached to or beneath the house.

Studies have shown that the children of smoking parents have more respiratory infections and asthmatic symptoms than other children. People who work next to smokers are more likely to have impaired lung function. The nonsmoking wives of men who smoke die on the average four years sooner, and according to a controversial Japanese study, such women may face a significantly greater risk of developing lung cancer than they would if their husbands did not smoke. [See chapter on passive smoking, page 361.]

To reduce the hazards of passive smoking, restrict smoking in your home, and agitate at work for a smoking ban (or at least for placing all smokers together in a well-ventilated area). If a family member smokes, ask that all smoking be done as far from others as possible, preferably near an open window, in the basement, or, even better, out of doors.

Self-installation of wood- or coal-burning stoves invites disaster. Experts should be consulted on proper ventilation. Follow the manufacturer's operating guidelines, and make sure the draft is set properly before the stove is lit. The safest stoves are those that are airtight. Fireplace flues should be cleaned periodically, and the damper always opened before the fire is lit. When operating the self-cleaning device on an oven, open the kitchen window, leave the room, and close the door.

Radon. This radioactive gaseous element comes from radium in the soil, rocks, bricks, concrete, and water (primarily well water) in and around many homes throughout the country. Levels in homes often exceed those outdoors and may reach the amount in a uranium mine. Although as yet it has not been directly linked to specific health risks, radiation experts estimate that thousands of lung cancer cases result each year from exposure to household radon.

Proper radon measurements are not readily available to the public. They require a monthlong measurement on a film that registers radioactivity. A home found to be heavily contaminated can be protected by applying epoxy or other sealant to the basement floor and walls and sealing all cracks between the basement and first floor and around utility intakes.

Household chemicals. The toxic effects of substances in household products are many and varied. Few are fully labeled as to their potentially hazardous contents. But all tell the consumer how to use the product safely. Be sure to follow instructions, using adequate ventilation and perhaps a face mask when working with products like oven cleaners, paints and paint removers, floor and furniture waxes, and pesticides. Fewer irritating fumes result from oven cleaners that do not require heating the oven to do the job. If you are unwilling to open a window wide in the winter, it may be safest not to use these volatile products until warmer weather arrives.

Humidifiers: More Risk than Benefit?

When cold weather descends and the humidity drops indoors and out — sometimes to the level of the Sahara — skin gets dry and itchy, lips chap, and mouths and throats become parched. Many people blame their propensity for wintertime colds and coughs on the discomforting dryness of winter air. In the wake of the energy crunch, humidifying indoor air has been promoted as a means of increasing comfort at lower room temperatures. Consequently many American homes now have humidifiers.

In the old days people placed pans of water on radiators and stoves to counter indoor dryness, which also desiccates furniture and increases static electricity. In recent years more efficient and expensive humidifiers have been installed in millions of homes and offices. The units may be centrally attached to the furnace in buildings heated by forced air. Or separate consoles may be used to moisten the air in individual rooms. During bouts of respiratory illness, vaporizers spewing forth cool mist or hot steam have long been used.

Do Humidifiers Benefit Health?

Several studies have suggested that breathing humidified air in winter decreases the likelihood of upper respiratory infections, especially in people with nasal allergies. A study of Canadian schoolchildren showed a 20 percent reduction in absenteeism when the humidity in the school was increased from 22 to 35 percent. A United States Army study showed fewer upper respiratory infections among soldiers when humidification was added to the heating system in the barracks.

However, other studies have indicated otherwise. Humidified air may enhance perceptions of comfort, but, these studies show, for ordinary healthy people it appears to make little or no difference to health. Sometimes, in fact, humidifiers themselves have been the cause of distressing and confusing respiratory symptoms that, in rare cases, can lead to irreversible and potentially fatal lung damage, according to studies by Dr. Jordan N. Fink of the Medical College of Wisconsin and numerous other researchers in the United States and Britain.

Other experts in allergic and respiratory diseases say that evidence for the health benefits of increasing indoor humidity is meager. Dr. Donald Proctor of Johns Hopkins Medical Center, who has studied the effects of various indoor environments on the nose, says that dry air has no harmful effect on the nasal passages of healthy people. "Raising the humidity does nothing to enhance the health of the normal nose, and it's an open question as to whether it's of benefit to sick people," he reports.

Although it is commonly asserted among pulmonary physicians that a generous level of humidity is desirable for persons with respiratory illnesses, there's no strong evidence to support this belief, reports Dr. William R. Solomon, allergist at the University of Michigan. In fact, patients with obstructive lung diseases often feel worse when it's humid, according to Dr. Anne Davis, thoracic specialist at New York University and Bellevue Hospital.

Dr. Proctor has found that the nose is a highly efficient air-conditioning system that warms incoming air to body temperature and saturates it with water vapor before it reaches the bronchial passages. Even when the air is very dry, the nose is an effective humidifier, he and his fellow researchers in Denmark have found. "For persons who are mouth breathers, the mouth is also a fairly good humidifier," Dr. Proctor says. "Besides, almost no one is an exclusive mouth breather — some air passes through the nose as well."

Studies of people who work in buildings that are artificially humidified have shown them to be no healthier than those who work in drier air, Dr. Proctor says. As for the supposed increase in feelings of warmth when cool air is humidified, Dr. Proctor's studies in a controlled environmental chamber have shown little effect. "Cold air feels colder only if it's extremely dry, much drier than you would get inside a home," he reports. His studies suggest that reports of upper respiratory irritation that are commonly attributed to dryness are more likely due to the high levels of pollutants that can build up in indoor air when windows are kept shut and homes are tightly sealed to keep down heat loss. [See chapter on indoor pollutants, page 368.]

The main benefit of increasing humidity, according to Dr. Steven Horvath, physiologist at the University of California at Santa Barbara, is psychological. "When people breathe dry air, they think they're less comfortable than when they're breathing moist air. But from a physiological standpoint, it really makes no difference. Humidity is important physiologically only when it's hot because high humidity reduces evaporation and interferes with the body's ability to cool itself."

The Association of Home Appliance Manufacturers makes no medical claims for humidifiers because, an association spokesman said, "we do not have evidence of medical benefit." However, the association said, manufacturers do maintain that humidifiers help plants and furniture.

The Risks: Humidifier Fever

Without a clear-cut demonstration of benefit to health, some specialists question whether humidifiers, especially those centrally installed, are worth the potential risks. Numerous cases of allergic lung disease, called hypersensitivity pneumonitis, have been linked to organisms that thrive in humidifiers, particularly the centralized units through which warm air passes. Outbreaks of humidifier fever, as the syndrome is called, have occurred among groups of workers in a centrally humidified office. Distress is usually at its worst on Mondays after a weekend away from the contaminated humidifier, abating somewhat as the week progresses and possibly disappearing over the weekend.

Symptoms of humidifier fever may include shortness of breath, cough, fever, and malaise. If the disease is not detected early in its course, permanent damage may occur as lung tissue is gradually and irreversibly destroyed. Yet the symptoms are easily confused with those of other disorders and may continue for years before they are linked to the heat-loving bacteria and fungi that can thrive in humidifiers. British researchers have found that certain protozoa that grow in humidifiers can also cause humidifier fever.

Dr. Harriet Burge of the University of Michigan, who has made a systematic study of microorganisms that grow in home humidifiers, suggests that central units be kept free of scale (mineral deposits from water) on which the organisms grow. In hard-water areas this may require cleaning the unit as often as every week. The drain-through type of centralized humidifier, which has no stagnant water, is less likely than the reservoir type to be a problem; it also requires far less frequent cleaning to keep the unit free of microorganisms.

Console humidifiers should be thoroughly cleansed with detergent at least weekly, Dr. Burge recommends. Empty and wash cool-mist vaporizers daily, rather than merely replace the water that's sprayed out. Adding bleach, Lysol, copper sulfate, or other disinfectants to humidifiers has no effect on hazardous organisms, she found, although such substances may reduce odor problems.

Steam vaporizers are not associated with humidifier fever because microorganisms don't grow in boiling water. However, they can be a shock and burn hazard. They should not be used around small children and should always be kept clear of the household traffic pattern.

How to Combat Dry Skin

Dry skin is caused by a lack of moisture, not of oil. To prevent peeling and cracking of skin during the low-humidity winter months, Dr. Hillard H. Pearlstein, a dermatologist associated with the Mount Sinai School of Medicine in New York City, recommends daily use of a body oil, an emollient, or a water-based moisturizer to help keep the skin hydrated.

Oil reduces evaporation of moisture from the skin and is best applied immediately after a bath or shower has saturated your skin with moisture. Ordinary baby oil is inexpensive and as effective as fancier and costlier products. If you wish to use a bath oil, first soak in the tub for ten or fifteen minutes, then add the oil. If the oil is put in first, it will coat your body and prevent full hydration of your skin, Dr. Pearlstein says.

Ordinary soap is very drying because it removes both oil and water from the skin. For dry skin problems, a superfatted soap (available in pharmacies) should help. Excessive bathing also dries the skin by removing oil. Don't overdo bathing in winter — no more often than once a day, Dr. Pearlstein says, followed by application of an oil or moisturizer.

IX.
Safety

You undoubtedly have insurance that provides monetary compensation in case of fire, theft, accidental injury, or death. But are you willing to take out what is clearly the most desirable and rewarding kind of insurance — adoption of the safety measures that prevent most disasters from occurring in the first place? Many people who think of themselves as stable and sensible in fact live very dangerously.

More often than not the stimulus to safer living is an accident that results in injury or worse: the child who swallows poison, the drowning death of a friend, the fatal injuries of an unbelted driver. Many of us are also unwilling to anticipate accidents by learning the first-aid measures that can often make the difference between minor and serious injury, even between life and death. The odds against your ever needing them may be long, but if and when something happens to you, a one-in-a-million chance occurrence becomes one-in-one.

Anticipating emergencies does not mean you are a morbid soul who expects the worst, and safe living is not dull, expensive, or particularly time-consuming. Rather, it's smart to be, as the Boy Scouts say, prepared, if you value life and health — your own and those of the people you love.

Basic First Aid: Techniques You Should Know

Accidents and emergencies are by definition unexpected events. But a little planning for the fact that such things happen to everyone sooner or later can do a lot to minimize their adverse effects, to make life more pleasant for the victim, and perhaps even to save a life.

Most of the commonly needed first-aid techniques are easy to learn and easy to remember. Here are recommendations from the American Red Cross and other safety experts for handling common emergencies.

What to Have on Hand

Your medicine chest. [See also the chapter on medicine cabinet, page 467.] A home cabinet stocked for safety should contain the following items:

● For ingested poisons — activated charcoal to absorb the poison; syrup of ipecac to induce vomiting (but used only on the advice of a physician or poison control center); and Epsom salts to speed the excretion of the poison.

● Band-Aids of various sizes; a roll of adhesive tape; sterile dressings (preferably 4-inch-by-4-inch gauze pads); a roll of 4-inch gauze to hold the dressings; and a pair of blunt-end scissors.

● Sodium bicarbonate — mix a pinch with a quarter teaspoon of salt in a quart of water, and drink for heat exhaustion.

● Aspirin for pain relief.

● Antibacterial swabs or an antiseptic first-aid spray (but no peroxide, iodine, Mercurochrome, or alcohol).

● Calamine lotion to relieve itching.

● A quick-reference first-aid guide (free guides are available from Metropolitan Life's Health and Welfare Department, 360 Park Avenue South, New York, New York 10010).

Your car. The glove compartment of your car should contain the same items, but in smaller quantities. You can buy a commercial auto first aid kit or, for much less money, make up your own. Your car should also have flares, a reflective sign saying *Disabled*, a flashlight with extra batteries, extra fuses for the car's electrical system, and a couple of dimes for phone calls.

On an outdoors trip, you should add a snakebite kit (if you will be more than half a day from a hospital), Swiss army knife, portable radio with extra batteries to keep abreast of the weather, insect repellent, suntan lotion, and an adequate supply of any medication you must take regularly.

What to Do in Case of . . .

Drowning. If you are not trained as a lifesaver, stay out of the water. Instead, extend a stick or towel, throw out a flotation device, or row to reach the victim. Once you have the victim onshore or in a boat, if he or she is unconscious, tilt his or her head back, and check to see if the person is breathing. Watch for the rise and fall of the chest, listen for breathing noises, and feel for breath with your cheek. If the victim is not breathing, begin **mouth-to-mouth breathing:** Pinch his or her nose, seal your lips around his or her mouth, and keeping his or her head tilted back, give four quick breaths.

Check again to see if the victim has started breathing, and if not, resume mouth-to-mouth breathing — giving one breath every five seconds for an adult and one puff of air every three seconds for a child. [See also chapter on water safety, page 402.]

Choking. If the victim cannot breathe or talk, get behind him or her and wrap your arms around him or her above the waist. Make a fist with one hand, place it just beneath the upside-down V of the rib cage, grasp the fist with the other hand, and give four hard upward thrusts. [See also chapter on choking, page 422.]

Bad cuts. Raise the cut above the heart, and using gauze pads, an article of clothing, or your bare hand, apply pressure directly on the cut. If this doesn't control the bleeding, press on the appropriate pressure point: For a leg wound, press the heel of your hand against the femoral artery on the front center of the thigh just at the crease of the groin; for

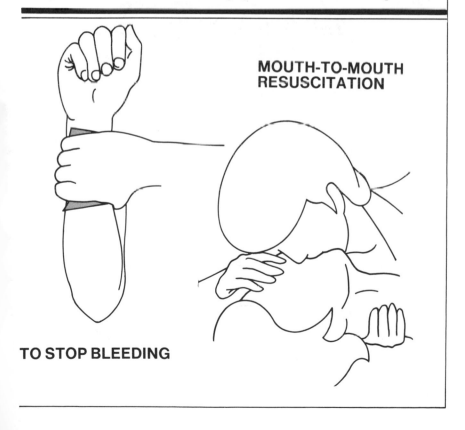

MOUTH-TO-MOUTH
RESUSCITATION

TO STOP BLEEDING

an arm wound, use the flat surface of your fingers, and press against the artery on the inside of the upper arm about midway between the armpit and the elbow (in the groove between the large muscles). Do not use the pressure point technique any longer than necessary to stop the bleeding. *Do not use a tourniquet unless there is no other way to control severe bleeding and the victim's life is threatened.* Once applied, a tourniquet must be left tight and removed only by a physician.

Puncture wounds. If the wound is more than one-eighth of an inch deep, dress it and see a doctor. Do not try to make it bleed. If the victim is impaled on an object, such as a picket fence, do not try to remove the victim from the object. Instead, cut the object (if necessary, call the fire department), and get the victim with the object in him or her to the hospital.

Eye injury. For chemical burns, turn the victim's head and bend it over so that the injured eye is facing down; then flush the eye with water for at least five minutes. To remove a cinder, use a clean handkerchief or piece of gauze.

WASHING THE EYE

Fracture or sprain. Immobilize the injured limb, and take the victim to the hospital, or if the neck or spine may be injured, call an ambulance.

Burns. First-degree (redness) and second-degree (redness and blistering) burns should be immersed in cold water for about twenty minutes. For sunburn, take a cold bath. Do not use grease on burns. [See also chapter on burns, page 398.]

Fishhooks. If the hook is stuck in past the barb, push it through in the direction it entered the skin until the barb end comes out the other side; then clip off either end with a wire cutter, and pull out the remaining piece.

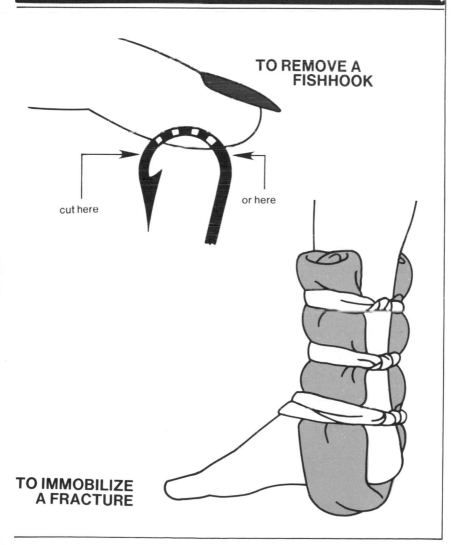

TO REMOVE A FISHHOOK

cut here

or here

TO IMMOBILIZE A FRACTURE

Insect bites and stings. If stung by a bee, remove the stinger by scraping without squeezing the venom sac. For stings by wasps, bees, hornets, or ants, cleanse with soap and water, and apply ammonia to reduce swelling. Or apply a paste of meat tenderizer. If the victim develops symptoms of an allergic reaction, get him or her to a doctor or hospital fast. Treat tick bites by covering the insect with a heavy oil; half an hour later carefully remove the tick with a tweezers; then scrub the area with soap and water. For itchy bites, apply calamine lotion. [See also chapter on insect stings, page 412.]

Poison plants. Wash with brown soap or ammonia, apply calamine lotion to relieve itching, and bandage any open wounds. [See also chapter on poison plants, page 409.]

Snakebites. A nonpoisonous snake leaves a set of teeth marks, but no fang marks. Have a doctor look at it and get a tetanus shot. A poisonous snake leaves one or two fang marks with or without teeth marks. Most of the first-aid remedies you may have learned in the past — tying off the bitten part, applying ice, and sucking out the venom — can actually do more harm than good. The best first aid is to do nothing (do not give the victim anything to eat or drink) and get the victim to a hospital as quickly as possible. Only if you are more than twelve hours from a hospital should the wound be suctioned, using the suction cup from a snakebite kit.

Summoning Emergency Aid

Emergency numbers. Know the phone numbers for the poison control center, police and fire departments, and ambulance in the area in which you live or where you are staying on vacation. At home these numbers should be posted on or near every phone.

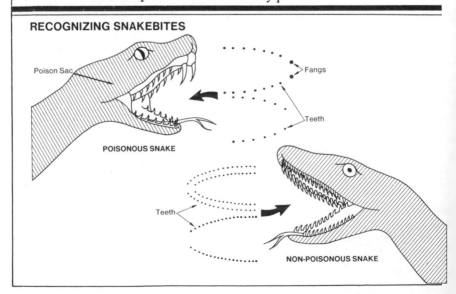

RECOGNIZING SNAKEBITES

Poison Sac

Fangs

Teeth

POISONOUS SNAKE

Teeth

NON-POISONOUS SNAKE

Calling an ambulance. Give the specific location — intersection, street address, and apartment number — and have someone wait for the ambulance at the location you gave. Give your name and the phone number you're calling from. Tell specifically what is wrong — for example, chest pain, not breathing, abdominal pain, bleeding (from where and how badly) — since the victim's symptoms may determine how sophisticated a rescue vehicle you will get.

While waiting for the ambulance, gather the patient's medications and, if possible, prepare a medical history, including doctor's name, known allergies, and past hospitalizations. Pay attention to the patient's symptoms so you can accurately describe them to the ambulance attendant. Have the patient's clothing ready to go to the hospital with him or her, but don't try to dress the patient.

For Further Reading and Information

If you are interested in taking a basic or advanced first-aid course, contact your local chapter of the American Red Cross. Useful manuals include:

American Medical Association. *Handbook of First Aid and Emergency Care.* New York: Random House, 1980.

American National Red Cross. *Standard First Aid & Personal Safety,* 2nd ed. New York: Doubleday, 1979.

Arnold, Peter, with Edward L. Pendagast, M.D. *Emergency Handbook.* New York: Doubleday, 1980.

Hartley, Joel, M.D. *First Aid Without Panic.* New York: Hart, 1975.

Smith, Bradley, and Gus Stevens. *The Emergency Book: You Can Save a Life!* New York: Fireside/Simon & Schuster, 1978.

Weiss, Jeffrey, ed. *The People's Emergency Guide.* New York: St. Martin's Press, 1980.

381

How to Make Your Home Safe to Live In

Many people breathe a deep sigh of relief upon returning home "safe and sound" from a trip. But few realize that the chance of accidental injury or death in the "safety" of their own homes may be as great as, or greater than, in a plane or on the road.

Home accidents receive little public attention because they are less dramatic than a plane or auto crash and, except for fires, rarely attract outside interest. But their toll in dollars and health is very high. From bedroom to backyard, you and those you live with may risk injury from falls, fires, poisons, electrical shock, suffocation, drowning, flying missiles, or cuts.

Each year more than 4 million Americans are disabled by home accidents, and 27,000 die of their injuries. Although the highway toll is higher, unlike most away-from-home mishaps, the overwhelming majority of home accidents are preventable. They are neither acts of God nor the fault of a stranger, but rather careless mistakes on the part of some family member.

It may be impossible to achieve a 100 percent guarantee of home safety, but the following area guide should help to raise your accident consciousness and "hazard-proof" your house or apartment. Remember, when it comes to home accidents, in all likelihood the life or limb you save will be your own or that of someone you love.

In the Kitchen

In addition to the everyday hazards associated with stoves and knives, many kitchens today are equipped with high-speed electrical gadgets, such as blenders and food processors, capable of inflicting injuries as serious as those caused by an industrial wood-planing machine. Yet, unlike factory workers, few cooks are well-schooled in the safe handling of their instruments. Be sure to read the manufacturers' operating instructions carefully, and don't take shortcuts.

Do not wash an electrical gadget while it is still plugged in, and unplug all such gadgets between uses. A utensil (wood or metal) in the jar of a blender that is turned on can create high-speed missiles of wood, glass, or plastic. To avoid burns, do not poke a utensil into a toaster before you unplug it.

Keep your knives well sharpened (you're more likely to cut yourself trying to use a dull knife), and cut away from you against a firm surface. Hold foods you are cutting with a curled hand, rather than with extended fingers.

At the stove be sure all pot handles are turned inward (but not extending over a hot burner), and always use a potholder. Do not wear blousy clothing (especially loose sleeves) or highly flammable fabrics like nylon while cooking. To avoid steam burns, lift lids like a shield, tilting them so that the steam escapes away from you. Never use water on a grease fire. Rather, use salt or baking soda or a small chemical fire extinguisher, which you should keep in the kitchen, readily accessible but not near the stove, and know how to operate. Be extremely careful taking hot food out of wall ovens, the shelves of which should not be above the user's chest.

To prevent falls, climb only on step stools, not on chairs or counters, and wipe up all spills immediately. Avoid highly polished floors (use a nonskid wax), and if you have an area rug or mat, be sure it has a nonslip backing and lies flat on the floor.

Keep all cupboard doors and drawers closed. If you have small children, keep knives and other sharp utensils out of sight in closed drawers, and store all cleaning compounds (especially dishwasher soap and oven cleaner) and poisons in a cupboard secured with a childproof lock. Do not leave plastic food bags lying about; small children can suffocate by putting such bags over their heads. And do not store cookies or

382

other childhood delights in cupboards above the stove.

In the Bathroom

Here, like the kitchen, the hazards center on burns, shocks, and falls. Keep your water heater set no higher than 120 degrees, and always test the water temperature before entering a shower or tub. The tub floor should have a nonslip mat (with suction cups that are kept firmly fixed to the tub) or, better yet, nonskid strips or patches that are permanently attached. Next to the tub, use a nonskid mat, or cover the entire floor with a washable carpet (but discard it when the nonskid backing wears out). Grab rails next to the tub and toilet can help avoid falls, especially among the elderly and infirm. Never leave a young child alone in the bathtub, even for a moment; children can drown in just a few inches of water.

It's best not to use electrical appliances like razors, hair dryers, and radios in the bathroom; if you do, be sure to plug them into individual insulated sockets, not multiple plugs, and stay away from water while you're using them. If you use a space heater, it should be one of an approved design that prevents contact with the heating element and preferably is mounted on the wall.

All medicines should be well labeled and, if there are young children at home, stored in a locked cabinet. Never tell a child that medicine is or tastes like candy or syrup. If small children spend any time in your home, keep all medicines — prescription and over the counter — in vials with child-resistant caps. Discard all leftover medication prescribed for temporary conditions. Drugs used for chronic or recurring health problems should be labeled with an expiration date and discarded when they reach it. Never take medicine — not even aspirin — in the dark, and always read the label to determine the right dosage. [See chapter on the medicine cabinet, page 467.]

383

In the Bedroom and Living Room

Do not run electrical cords under rugs or furniture where they could become worn or frayed and where you may not notice the wear. Avoid overloading outlets and trailing wires where they may be tripped over. Electric irons should be unplugged after each use.

Keep a lamp (and your glasses) on a table right next to your bed, or leave a small night light on. Do not wear loose-fitting, smooth-soled slippers, lest they function as befits their name. Rubber or plastic soles are preferable to leather in the house.

If you have small children, cut the loops of shade cords to prevent the possibility of strangulation. Windows accessible to children should have metal guards, or else they should be fitted with locks that keep them from being opened more than a few inches. Window screens are not adequate protection.

Always use a fire screen with a fine mesh in front of the fireplace. Be sure to have chimneys and flues cleaned and inspected annually. Keep matches out of the reach of children and provide guests with stable ashtrays. Never, never smoke in bed or while resting in your favorite easy chair or on the sofa.

Keep a smoke detector, with an active battery, in the bedroom or hallway (use two detectors in a two-story home). Make sure everyone in the family knows various escape routes in case of fire. A fireladder in an upstairs bedroom is a good insurance policy.

In Stairways and Entrances

All stairways, indoors and out, should be well lit, in good repair, and equipped with sturdy handrails, preferably on both sides. The steps should have nonskid strips or well-fitted carpeting. Never leave anything on the steps; you may save a trip up or down the stairs and end up with one to the hospital instead.

Don't carry loads that are too awkward or heavy or that block your vision. Keep gates with childproof latches at the top and bottom of all stairways if you live with a mobile infant or toddler.

House and room entrances should have light switches that you can operate before you enter the room. Switches should never be partially blocked with furniture.

In the Garage and Basement

Do not store old newspapers, oil-soaked rags, or other flammable materials. Keep all chemicals out of the reach of children in their original containers and clearly labeled. Hazardous tools should be unplugged after use and put away.

If you have a basement workshop, be sure it is well lit and well ventilated. All electrical workshop appliances and extension cords used with them should have heavy utility cords and grounding plugs. Carefully read instructions for safe use. Wear safety goggles when sawing, sanding, chipping paint, or spraying paint or chemicals. Don't let children stand nearby while you're working.

Block the wheels front and back when servicing your car. Never run the motor if the garage door and window are closed. Store flammable liquids (gasoline, fire starter, etc.) in safety cans, and store gasoline outside, never in the garage or basement, where the slightest spark could ignite escaped vapors.

In the Garden

Before mowing the lawn with a power mower, clear away all rocks, sticks, toys, etc. that could become lethal missiles. Keep small children indoors, and never allow a child to operate a power mower. Read operating instructions carefully. Electric lawn mowers should never be used on wet grass or in the rain. Push — never pull — a power mower, wear shoes with good traction, and mow across — not up and down — slopes. Never refuel a hot power mower, and always turn off the motor to clear the grass chute.

Never leave garden tools and hoses lying about to be tripped over; hang them up on a secure rack or hook. Keep the cord of electric hedge clippers over your shoulder while working. Follow instructions on the use and disposal of pesticides; always spray downwind, and avoid spraying altogether on blustery days. Store all pesticides in their original containers in locked cabinets.

Pools and ponds should be fenced and well latched, with children allowed near them only when accompanied by a responsible adult. Poles, ropes, buoys, and life belts should be kept nearby. Wells, cisterns, septic tanks, and cesspools must be kept properly covered at all times.

Don't barbecue on windy days or while wearing loose clothing. Keep proper tools and mitts nearby, as well as a container of water or sand to throw on the fire should it blaze up.

Never squirt lighter fluid, kerosene, or any other flammable liquid onto a lit fire, even one that is just smoldering; the flame can shoot up the liquid to the can and cause an explosion. Better to use an electric starter, but not in the rain or while standing on wet ground; be sure to unplug it immediately after use. Or use paper or solid fire starter to kindle charcoal. When using paper, crumple it, pile the briquets on top, and then light the paper. Never burn charcoal indoors; the coals release hazardous amounts of carbon monoxide.

For Further Reading

Lee, Richard V., M.D., and Tony Smith, M.D. *Accident Action.* New York: Viking, 1979.
Weiss, Jeffrey, ed. *The People's Emergency Guide.* New York: St. Martin's Press, 1980.

Seat Belts:
They Do Save Lives

"Buckle up and live." — You've undoubtedly heard this or a similar slogan a dozen times. Yet only one in ten Americans heeds its advice. If anything, use of seat belts is declining (one in eight automobile occupants used them as recently as 1978) at a time when the motor vehicle injury and fatality rate is rising.

Automobile accidents are a leading cause of death among Americans under sixty-five. In children aged one to fourteen, accidents of all types cause half the deaths, and motor vehicle accidents lead the list, claiming some 2,000 young lives each year in this country. In a recent study of children killed in crashes, Baltimore researchers found that infants under six months of age had the highest death rate among vehicle occupants. Although infants accounted for only 2 percent of the children involved in crashes, they represented 15 percent of the child fatalities.

Many such deaths — and many serious nonfatal injuries — could be prevented if both adults and children were properly secured in safety seats or seat belts while riding in cars. One estimate holds that 91 percent of deaths and 78 percent of injuries suffered by children under five in car accidents could be prevented by the use of existing safety devices. In adults the fatality rate among auto passengers could be cut in half by the consistent use of lap-and-shoulder seat belts.

Protecting the Young Passenger

Children loose in a car are more likely than adults to become flying missiles during a crash. An infant weighing 15 pounds would be flung with a force of 300 pounds in a crash at twenty miles per hour. Children unharnessed in the far rear of a station wagon or the back of a truck are not safe. If seated in the lap of an adult, the child is likely to be crushed during a crash by the force of motion of the adult's body even if the adult is wearing a seat belt. More often than not, when parents hold children on their laps, the youngsters become cushions that protect the parents from colliding with the dashboard or windshield. Instead, the children receive the brunt of the crash, often suffering severe head injuries as a result.

Studies by the Insurance Institute for Highway Safety show that children are least likely to be injured in a crash if they are restrained in the back seat (preferably in the middle of the seat), and are most likely to be injured if unrestrained in the front seat. In the rear of the car the child is less likely to strike hard interior surfaces.

Although it is best to begin using car restraints right after a child is born, it's never too late to start protecting your children. Tell them the car seat is a special present to keep them alive and healthy, and suggest

386

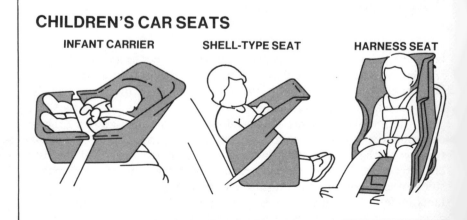

CHILDREN'S CAR SEATS

INFANT CARRIER   **SHELL-TYPE SEAT**   **HARNESS SEAT**

they pretend to be astronauts. Show them that adults also protect themselves with seat belts, and buckle up yourself every single time you get in the car.

Infants. Before a child can sit up securely when unsupported, he or she should ride in an infant car seat in a semireclining position facing the rear of the car. The device should have energy-absorbing padding and its own harness system, with the entire setup held in place by the car seat belt. Car beds and ordinary infant seats that are not designed for crash safety give no protection in a car and should not be used.

Children under four. After early infancy and until the age of about four (or when the child weighs forty pounds and stands forty inches tall), he or she should ride in a safety-tested child car seat. The best kind is made of hard molded plastic with a shield in front, energy-absorbing padding, and harness straps for the shoulders, lap, and crotch. Like the infant seat, it is held in place by the car seat belt.

Most car seats also have a tether strap at the top to prevent the child's head from flying forward in a crash. Unless the tether is used (attached to the metal frame of the car or to the rear seat belt if the car seat is in the front), the device offers inadequate protection. Some child seats are designed to prevent forward motion without the use of a tether, but if the device comes with a tether, it must be used to be fully effective.

Improved testing standards for car seats are now in effect on items manufactured after January 1, 1981. For seats made before that date, choose one that has been tested in simulated crashes using child-sized dummies. These are called dynamic or impact sled tests. The cheapest available devices are those least likely to pass such tests, although they often met the old standards of the U.S. Department of Transportation. Contact the company or the Public Affairs Office of the U.S. Department of Transportation (Washington, D.C. 20590, 202-426-9550) before you buy if you are uncertain about the kind of testing done.

If on some occasion (such as a rented car out of town) you have no choice but to use a standard car seat belt to restrain a very young child, use only the lap belt, and place it across the child's thighs rather than abdomen.

Children over four. After the car seat has been outgrown, the child can use a standard lap seat belt. But the shoulder harness should not be used until the child is more than fifty-five inches tall. Before that, the shoulder belt would run across the child's neck. Two children or a child and an adult should not be strapped in with one seat belt.

Protecting Adults

While far from perfect and somewhat lacking in comfort and ease of use, the shoulder-and-lap belts now found in American and most foreign cars offer much more protection than many people realize. Belted accident victims are half as likely to die from injuries as those who are not buckled in. In a study of 1,126 accidents in which one or more victims were hospitalized, those wearing seat belts had 86 percent fewer life-threatening injuries. Only 28 percent of unbelted occupants escaped injury, compared with 42 percent of those wearing seat belts. Nearly a quarter of those thrown from the vehicle were killed (they accounted for half the deaths in the study), and severe injuries to the head and spine were twice as common among those not wearing belts.

Unbelted vehicle occupants not only endanger themselves, but also can injure other passengers. A Michigan study of more than 4,000 accidents showed that occupant-to-occupant collisions caused or aggravated injuries in 22 percent of the crashes. Thirteen percent of the human collisions contributed to severe or fatal injuries.

Studies have shown that the people who most need seat belts (as judged by their accident rates) are least likely to use them, namely, drivers who take risks. In a study by Johns Hopkins University, drivers who ran red lights were less likely to buckle up. Another study conducted by General Motors showed that drivers who tailgate other cars on freeways are less likely to wear seat belts.

Unjustified fears. People who try to justify their unwillingness to use seat belts often express fear of being trapped in a car that bursts into flame or sinks in water. In fact, these are rare occurrences that are far outweighed by the protection afforded by seat belts in more frequent kinds of accidents. Others cite cases in which the occupant would have been killed had he or she *not* been thrown from the car. Again, the far more frequent event is a fatality or crippling brain or spinal injury when the force of a crash ejects the occupants or throws them against the windshield.

Still others cite injuries caused by the seat belts themselves. These include damage to abdominal organs, broken ribs, and injury to the spinal column and pelvis. In a study of 3,325 car occupants wearing belts

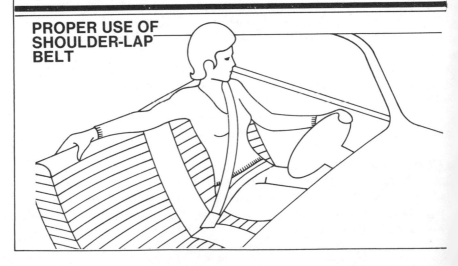

PROPER USE OF SHOULDER-LAP BELT

at the time of an accident, 30 percent sustained some injury, but in fewer than 1 percent were the injuries severe. In many of the cases the seat belt victims would have been severely injured or killed in the accident had they not been wearing belts. Although seat belt injuries have occurred to the fetus when pregnant women were involved in accidents, a study by the University of Oklahoma Medical School showed that fetal and maternal death were far more likely to occur if pregnant women did *not* use seat belts.

Proper use. Many seat belt injuries are caused by improper use. The lap belt should be worn like a bikini — at or below the protrusion of the hipbone. The belt should be comfortably tight and not twisted or snagged on the seat. The diagonal shoulder belt should never be worn without the lap belt.

Accidental Poisonings: How to Prevent and Treat Them

When our children were born, my husband and I systematically poison-proofed our home. Cupboards were arranged with poisons in the back of shelves, out of ready reach of a quick-moving toddler when the doors were opened. On the door of every cupboard that enclosed a potentially lethal substance — the pantry (with its soy sauce, salt, cooking sherry, and what-have-you) and liquor cabinet, medicine chest, housecleaning bin, gardening shed, and laundry room — we installed a childproof lock that no preschooler in my experience has yet been able to open.

But as careful as we were, our two-year-old was among the more than 500,000 children accidentally poisoned each year. He drank medicine that had just been purchased and was still in its bag among the groceries, instead of safely locked in the medicine chest. Fortunately he decided it was "yukky" before he did real damage. But other children have been less fortunate.

Susie, aged three, had to be rushed to the hospital after she fed herself and her doll party "soda" from a pop bottle she found under the sink, not knowing that the original contents of the bottle had been replaced by turpentine. A one-year-old girl spent nine days in the hospital after swallowing charcoal lighter that her family had left in the yard.

Peter, also aged one, grabbed a fingerful of detergent from the dishwasher, severely burned his mouth, and nearly died when the resulting swelling cut off his air passages. An eighteen-month-old boy did die after drinking floor cleaner containing a petroleum distillate, and another succumbed after being given a spoonful of "mineral oil" from a bottle that had been refilled with carbon tetrachloride.

There is no better time than the present to review how well you and your children are protected from being injured by the quarter of a million potentially poisonous household items on the market: Drugs, vitamins, cleaning agents, pesticides, petroleum products, polishes, paints, and even perfumes are on the long, lethal list.

How to Prevent Accidental Poisonings

To protect your family against poisoning, you need to know where potential hazards lurk and how to treat these substances with the care they require. You must arrange the household, where three-fourths of poisonings occur, in such a way as to minimize the risk of accidental poisoning by young and old, and you must know what to do if, despite your efforts, a poisoning accident should occur.

If small children live in your house or visit you, these precautions are essential:

● Store all household cleaning materials, from bleach to bowl cleaner, out of reach of small children (definitely not under the sink) in a locked closet. Do the same for toxic substances kept in the garage and basement.

● When using substances that can produce hazardous fumes, such as oven or drain cleaner, cleaning fluid, paint, or paint remover, be sure that no children are around and that one or more windows or doors are opened wide. Always read instructions and warnings on the label before using such products.

● Keep all drugs, vitamins, birth control pills, cosmetics, and hair preparations in a high, locked cabinet. Never refer to medicine as "candy" or as being "delicious." Don't take drugs in front of small children; they are great imitators, especially of their parents. Remember, small children will eat anything, even if it doesn't taste good.

● Be sure all drugs and hazardous household products are packaged in child-resistant containers. For the aged and handicapped, one size of such products can be sold legally in ordinary containers, but they must be labeled "Not recommended for use in households with young children." Child-resistant, incidentally, does not mean childproof, so don't leave such containers around to tempt a youngster. He or she just may figure out how to open them. Be certain to keep the products in their child-resistant containers, and close them properly after each use, securing the safety feature.

● Take care in discarding poisons. Flush leftover drugs down the toilet, rinse the containers, and then discard them. If you throw out the remains of hazardous household products, be sure children have no access to the garbage.

● Never transfer a hazardous substance out of its original container, and don't put such a substance in a bottle or jar that once held food, drinks, or medicine. Be sure warning labels stay on the container until the product is used up or discarded.

• Never leave small children unattended around hazardous substances, even for just a minute to answer the door or phone. If you are interrupted while using a hazardous substance, take it with you. Be especially alert during the peak poisoning time — the so-called arsenic hour — between 4:00 and 6:00 P.M., when children get hungry and cranky and parents are preoccupied preparing supper. When traveling, check out unfamiliar surroundings where a child may have access to hazardous substances he or she is protected from at home.

• Don't use mothballs in your closets. Small children love to ferret around in dark places and pop round, hard things in their mouths.

Even if children never cross the portals of your home, most of the above precautions can help protect your family and friends from accidental poisoning. In addition, never store poisons in the same cabinet with food items, always follow directions on the label, use only recommended amounts of drugs and cleaning agents, check the label in bright light before taking any medicine, and don't take medicines prescribed for

WHAT TO DO IN POISONING CASES

If exposed to:	Immediate action	Secondary action
Poisonous gas	Protect yourself from being overcome. Get victim into fresh air. If breathing stopped, give mouth-to-mouth resuscitation.	Identify cause. Call poison control center, hospital emergency room, or physician.
Substance in eye	Flush thoroughly with gentle stream of lukewarm water for fifteen minutes, holding eyelids apart.	Identify cause. Call poison control center, hospital, or physician for further treatment.
Ingested poison	If victim is conscious and not convulsing, give one glass of water to drink. Identify cause, and call poison control center, hospital, or physician, if possible giving details on substance, amount ingested, and victim's size, age, and symptoms.	If induction of vomiting is recommended, give victim one or two glasses of water, then syrup of Ipecac; or make victim gag, and collect vomitus. If hospital treatment is recommended, take whole container of suspected poison and vomitus with you.

Warning:
It is always best to get medical advice before you institute first aid for an ingested poison. However, if you cannot obtain such advice quickly, and if the victim is conscious and not convulsing, give him or her water to drink. Then induce vomiting unless a strong acid or alkali has been swallowed.

Source: Based on information from the National Poison Center Network, Pittsburgh, Pennsylvania.

someone else or for a previous illness without consulting a physician first.

What to Do If Poisoning Occurs

Know the signs that someone has been poisoned: an open drug or chemical container, stains on clothing, odor on breath, abnormal behavior, nausea, excessive stimulation or drowsiness, shallow or difficult breathing, loss of consciousness, convulsions, dizziness, and burns on the mouth or hands.

Keep the phone numbers of the local poison control center, the nearest hospital emergency room, your family physician, and your pediatrician next to your telephone. Eighty-five percent of poisoning accidents can be treated at home, so don't make a frantic trip to the emergency room before calling your physician. In all cases of ingested poisons, obtain medical advice, if possible, before treating the victim with anything but a glass of water.

Have on hand a one-ounce bottle of syrup of ipecac (about $1 at most pharmacies); this is a safe and effective way to induce vomiting, but it should be used only after medical advice. Do not use salt water to induce vomiting; use a blunt instrument, like the back of a spoon or your finger — also only after medical advice — to make the victim gag if no ipecac is available.

Do not induce vomiting if a corrosive substance — a strong acid or alkali like bowl and drain cleaners, ammonia, bleach, and strong detergents — has been swallowed or if the victim is unconscious or having convulsions. Corrosive material can do further damage when it is regurgitated, and an unconscious or convulsing victim could inhale vomitus. Be sure to hold the victim's head down when he or she vomits, catch the vomitus in a basin, and keep the contents for the doctor.

Purchase a bottle of activated charcoal, to be used to prevent absorption of some poisons. But don't use burned toast for this purpose. Neither ipecac nor charcoal should be used without the advice of a poison control center, hospital, or doctor.

There are no pat rules for treating poisoning cases. Exactly what first aid is desirable will depend on the type of poison, how much was ingested, the victim's age, size, health status, and your capabilities and knowledge. First-aid recommendations are continually being revised on the basis of new findings. You cannot always depend on the advice given on product labels since it may be outdated.

For Assistance and Further Information

There are approximately 580 poison control centers around the country, with varying degrees of competence and service. About 90 million Americans are served by the National Poison Center Network, with regional and satellite centers staffed twenty-four hours a day and meeting specified standards.

The network uses the bilious green symbol of Mr. Yuk as an educational tool. To obtain Mr. Yuk stickers (which include the phone number of a network poison control center if there is one in your area) for labeling household poisons, send a stamped, self-addressed envelope stating your hometown to National Poison Center, Children's Hospital of Pittsburgh, 125 DeSoto Street, Pittsburgh, Pennsylvania 15213.

The network has also prepared a home advice table on poisoning and its treatment called "Danger Lurks," available by sending 25 cents to Order Department, OP-304, American Medical Association, 535 North Dearborn Street, Chicago, Illinois 60610.

Food Poisoning: It Can Happen to Anyone Who Eats

Although food poisoning is not as common as it was when every picnic was packed in a wicker basket, there's still many an outing that brings along an unwelcome guest invited by poor choice and improper handling of picnic foods. Food poisoning can also occur at home, the result of improper handling and cooking of foods (especially turkey and pork) and the use of incorrect home canning techniques.

The symptoms of food poisoning usually last at most a few days and need only ordinary home remedies: a bland diet and lots of fluids and perhaps an antidiarrheal drug. But some forms can be fatal. If symptoms are severe or if the victim is very young, very old, or sick to begin with, prompt medical attention is advisable.

If you suspect food poisoning, report it to the health department, and warn others who may have eaten the same food. If possible, save the suspect food in the refrigerator for a health department inspector, and make sure no one else eats it. Remember, tainted foods don't always look, taste, or smell bad.

The Common Culprits

The most common food poisoning culprits are three bacteria that like the very same foods picnickers and holiday celebrants do — potato salad, ham, fried chicken, egg salad, stuffed turkey, meats of all sorts. They are:

Salmonella. Salmonellosis, affecting an estimated 2 million people each year, is considered one of the nation's most important communicable diseases. At least 150 different species of *Salmonella* are known to attack the human digestive tract. It is a common contaminant of foods from domestic animals, especially eggs, poultry, meats, and dairy products, as well as fish and shellfish.

Salmonella bacteria are destroyed by the heat of normal cooking — temperatures of at least 140 degrees for ten minutes or more, depending on the nature of the food, or higher temperatures for shorter times. But they can multiply rapidly if the food is held at between 44 and 115 degrees for any length of time. In a few hours at such temperatures, millions of salmonella bacteria may contaminate an ordinary portion. Yet ingestion of a mere half million organisms can make an otherwise healthy adult sick.

Eight people who went to a family birthday party landed in the hospital with salmonella poisoning from eating chicken that was thawed unrefrigerated, fried too quickly to destroy all the bacteria, and then held on the stove until dinner several hours later.

Symptoms of salmonella poisoning include severe headache, vomiting, diarrhea, abdominal cramps, and fever. They usually appear within six to forty-eight hours after the contaminated food has been consumed, and last two to seven days.

Staphylococcus aureus. This organism commonly gets to food from the nose, throat, or pimples of those who handle or prepare food. The symptoms — vomiting, diarrhea, prostration, and abdominal cramps — are caused by ingestion of toxin produced by the bacteria. The illness may start thirty minutes to eight hours (usually two to four hours) after tainted food has been eaten; it lasts for one to two days.

Although staph bacteria are destroyed by normal cooking, the toxin is not. Therefore, it is crucial to prevent growth of the organism to begin with. Cured meats, sandwich spreads, salads, milk, and cream-filled cakes are excellent breeding grounds and can become laced with toxin if contaminated food is left unrefrigerated for a few hours.

In one episode of staph poisoning, the sneeze of the hostess contaminated the knife used to slice a ham, which then sat on a table for several hours and resulted in the entire party's getting sick.

Clostridium. *Clostridium perfringens* also produces a toxin that can cause illness, usually diarrhea but not vomiting or fever, which starts nine to fifteen hours after the tainted food has been eaten and lasts about a day. *C. perfringens* forms spores that may survive ordinary cooking; the spores can germinate and produce toxin if the food is left standing at temperatures of between 45 and 120 degrees.

A relative of this organism, *Clostridium botulinum*, produces a deadly nerve toxin, causing nausea and vomiting, blurred vision, difficulty in swallowing, weakness, paralysis, and possibly death. The symptoms appear two hours to as many as eight days afterward. The difficult-to-kill botulinum spores germinate in the absence of oxygen when little acid is present and the temperature is above normal refrigeration temperatures.

The usual source of botulinum toxin is improperly prepared home-canned foods, especially low-acid vegetables, meats, poultry, and fish. To avoid this problem, these foods must be canned in a pressure cooker according to established times and procedures. All low-acid home-canned foods should be boiled for ten minutes before they are tasted or eaten. [See methods, page 395.]

Trichinella spiralis. This parasite causes trichinosis, a more common form of serious food poisoning than botulism. The tiny trichinella worms come from eating infected, undercooked meat, usually pork but sometimes beef. The worms invade via the intestinal tract, moving first into the blood and then the muscles. They cause fever, swelling (especially around the eyes), muscle pains, and diarrhea three to thirty days after infected food has been eaten.

How to Prevent Food Poisoning

• Keep cold foods cold and hot foods hot. On picnics, use a portable icebox, thermos bottles, or dry ice to keep foods cold. All milk, meat, poultry, fish, fruit juices, and foods containing uncooked or quick-cooked eggs should be kept cold. At home in summer, it is best to refrigerate all cheeses, eggs, and root vegetables.

• Don't take picnic foods made with eggs or milk products or home-made mayonnaise unless they can be refrigerated until served. (Studies have shown that commercial mayonnaise is too acid to permit the growth of food poisoning organisms.) Leave home the custards, cream-filled or meringue pies, the potato salad, and the chicken, ham, tuna, and egg salad sandwiches. The safest picnic foods are simply prepared, cooked at the time of eating, dry or acid — bread, cookies, crackers, raw fruits and vegetables, fruit juices, cooked vegetables and stewed fruits, dry cereal, hard cheese, peanut butter, canned fish, canned baked beans, hard-boiled eggs in their shells, jellies.

• Handle picnic food as little as possible until it is served. Make sandwiches at the picnic site unless they can be refrigerated. Don't take fancy foods that require a lot of handling to prepare.

• Don't overstock your refrigerator or cooler. The food reaches a lower temperature if air can circulate around it. When packing the cooler, start with refrigerated food. An hour or so later you can test the temperature by placing a food thermometer on or in the food that is farthest from the ice.

• Be sure to cook thoroughly barbecued foods like chicken and pork. Bacon should be grilled at least five minutes, a one-inch-thick pork chop twenty minutes per side, a pork roast twenty to thirty minutes per pound, until there is no sign of pink.

• Don't leave food standing on the table while eating your picnic. Keep hot foods hot and put cold foods back in the cooler immediately after serving them. The same goes for foods prepared at home; don't leave foods that should be refrigerated standing on the counter or table for longer than you're working with them.

• Thaw all meats and poultry in the refrigerator. For faster thawing, put the food in a plastic bag and hold under cold running water, or if you must, place it in a double paper bag without water. The idea is to have the temperature high enough to thaw but low enough to prevent bacterial growth on the food surface.

• After cutting up raw meats or poultry, be sure to wash the cutting surface and knife thoroughly before using them to make sandwiches or other prepared food. Don't place cooked food on an unwashed platter that had raw meat on it.

• Always wash hands carefully before handling food, and avoid preparing food if you have an infected cut or sore.

• After cooking, don't cool foods on the stove or counter. Put them into the refrigerator immediately, or cool them quickly by immersing them in an ice bath, and then refrigerate them.

How to Can Safely

Many people who have been "putting up" foods for years, following canning methods handed down from previous generations, may not be using safe methods. Many persons new to canning fail to realize that there is a right way and a wrong way to do it. Some recently published "back to nature" books give incorrect canning instructions.

The basic idea in canning is to destroy or prevent the growth of all microorganisms — yeasts, molds, and bacteria — that could cause food spoilage, while you preserve as best as possible the taste and texture of good-quality foods. Under no circumstances can you afford to sacrifice safety for the sake of appearance, but proper canning techniques will allow you both in most cases.

The organisms that can spoil food can be destroyed by boiling (212 degrees Fahrenheit at sea level) for a sufficient length of time. However, although most organisms are killed in a reasonable length of time, ordinary cooking (specifically less than six hours) does not destroy the spores of *Clostridium botulinum.*

Since *C. botulinum* will not grow in high-acid foods (below a pH of 4.6 — tomatoes, for example, have a pH of about 4.2), it is not necessary to destroy botulinum spores in foods that are high in acid. These can be safely canned in boiling water at 212 degrees. But low-acid foods must be processed at higher temperatures, achieved only by the use of a pressure cooker, to kill the spores. The foods most commonly involved in botulism outbreaks are beans, corn, spinach, peppers, and asparagus.

The particular method of canning to use depends on the nature of the food you are preserving. Here are three accepted safe methods of canning:

Open-kettle canning. The food is cooked and then packed hot into hot sterilized jars and sealed (with paraffin) with no further cooking done. This method is safe only for jellies (not jams or preserves) made with sugar. If mold grows under the wax during storage, discard the entire jar.

Water-bath processing. Jars filled with raw or partially cooked food are capped, covered with water, and boiled in a large kettle for a specified period of time. This method is safe only for high-acid fruits and vegetables, such as tomatoes, cherries, strawberries, and dill pickles, and for jams and preserves made with sugar. It should never be used for meats, for low-acid vegetables like corn, green beans, or peppers, or for low-acid fruits like pumpkin or figs. So-called low-acid tomatoes are safe to can this way. Only four tomato varieties — Garden State, Ace, 55VF, and Cal Ace — need to be pressure-canned.

Pressure canning. Jars filled with raw or partially cooked food are covered and cooked under pressure for a specified period of time. In this way a temperature of 240 degrees, which is necessary to destroy the botulinum spores, can be reached. All low-acid fruits and vegetables and all fish and meats must be canned under pressure to be safe. All combinations of foods that contain one or more low-acid items must also be canned this way. At high altitudes, water boils at lower temperatures, and the recommended pressure for canning must be adjusted accordingly — add one pound of pressure for every 2,000 feet above sea level.

It is not safe to can in an oven, dishwasher, microwave oven, or slow cooker because proper canning temperatures cannot be reached.

Some Safe Canning Tips

When canning, be sure to follow the instructions in an up-to-date authoritative canning guide, such as the Ball "Blue Book," available for $2.50 from the Ball Corporation, 1509 South Macedonia Street, Muncie, Indiana 47302. In addition, the United States Department of Agriculture sells reliable food preservation guides (see box below). The following precautions should help to assure you of safe home-canned foods:

• Don't cheat on the recommended processing time. The time depends on the nature of the food, the size and shape of the jar, the size of the pieces of food, and the ratio of solids to liquid.

• Be sure to leave the specified amount of headspace (half an inch for most fruits and vegetables, one inch for very starchy foods); overpacking the jars can lead to underprocessing.

WHERE TO GET CANNING BOOKLETS

The following Department of Agriculture booklets on food preservation can be obtained from the Superintendent of Documents, U.S. Government Printing Office, Washington, D.C. 20402:

Order Name and Number	Price
Home Canning of Fruits and Vegetables G-8	45 cents
Home Freezing of Fruits and Vegetables G-10	75 cents
Freezing Combination Main Dishes G-40	40 cents
How to Make Jellies, Jams and Preserves at Home G-56	55 cents
Making Pickles and Relishes at Home G-92	45 cents
Freezing Meat and Fish in the Home G-93	55 cents

• Use only jars, cans, and lids made specifically for home canning (not mayonnaise or coffee jars). Do not reuse sealing lids (but the canning rings used to secure the lids can be recycled), and do not use jars that are cracked, chipped, or nicked.

• Do not use overripe fruits (especially tomatoes) since they lose acidity, and don't process fruits or vegetables with bruises or soft spots.

• Avoid canning combinations of foods, such as meat with vegetables. It is better to can each item separately and combine them before serving. If you do can a combination, be sure to process the jars according to the ingredient that requires the highest temperature and longest time.

• Adjust processing time and temperature for altitude.

• After the jars have cooled, test the seal according to the instructions on the box of lids. Store jars in a cool, dry place.

• Do not use or taste any canned foods that show signs of spoilage, such as bulging lids, leaks, off odors, or mold. Because mold can cause a loss of acidity and allow botulinum to grow and produce toxin, it is not safe to scrape off mold and eat the remaining food. Destroy all suspicious canned foods out of the reach of children and pets. Canned foods that float in the jar do not indicate spoilage.

• Canned foods are best consumed within a year or two of processing. However, they will still be safe after longer storage if they have been properly prepared and stored and the jar has not been damaged.

• To be on the safe side, boil all canned low-acid foods and all vegetables — acid or not — for ten minutes before serving them. This will destroy any botulinum toxin that may be present.

Burns:
How to Prevent and Treat Them

A toddler yanks on the tablecloth and dumps his mother's hot cup of coffee over his head, causing severe facial burns. An elderly woman slips in the shower and, trying to right herself, accidentally turns off the cold water and scalds herself on tap water that exceeds 150 degrees. A space heater left on all night starts a house fire that claims the lives of two children and causes disfiguring burns of their parents, who tried in vain to rescue the youngsters.

Each year an estimated 2 million Americans suffer serious burns. More than 100,000 burn victims must be hospitalized for treatment, and 12,000 die (a third of them are children under fifteen) from their injuries or ensuing complications.

Treatment of burn victims has improved greatly in recent years with the establishment of specialized burn centers and the development of lifesaving techniques, such as temporary skin grafts. But it is far better to prevent them since treatment and rehabilitation may take years and the victim may still be left with life-limiting deformities.

Most burns are the result of "accidents just waiting to happen" — situations that would not occur if you or someone else had thought ahead and observed reasonable precautions. In addition, the severe consequences of some burns can be avoided by following proper first-aid procedures (see box, page 401).

Contrary to popular belief, applying butter or greasy ointments or sprays is not the first thing you should do for a burn. Rather, no matter how serious the burn, flushing with or immersing the burned part in cold water or, in some cases, applying a cold compress (but not ice) is the proper first step. The cold water, which should be applied as soon as possible for up to thirty minutes, diminishes swelling and fluid loss, limits the extent of the damage, and helps to counter infection and pain. The folk remedy aloe (sometimes called the burn plant) was shown in experiments in the 1930's to promote healing of some burns, but further testing is needed to determine its current usefulness.

Types of Burns

A burn can result from heat, chemicals, electricity, or radiation. According to the American Red Cross, the most common causes of burns are carelessness with matches and lighted cigarettes (especially smoking in bed); scalds from hot liquids; defective heating, cooking, and electrical equipment; the use of open fires (especially when one wears flammable clothing); improper use of flammable household liquids; immersion in overheated bathtubs; and accidents with chemicals like lye, strong acids, and strong detergents.

The severity of a burn is determined by its depth (how many layers of tissue are injured) and its extent (how big an area of the body is involved). A relatively minor burn involving a large part of the body surface can be more serious than a deep burn of only a small area.

In general, a minor burn involves the outermost layers of skin and less than 10 percent of the body and causes reddening and pain, but not blistering or swelling. The injured cells will peel off, and the skin heals without scarring usually in a week or two. In more severe burns injury to deeper layers prolongs healing time, but the skin can still regenerate if proper medical care is obtained. In the most severe burns all the skin layers are destroyed and the wound cannot heal without skin grafts.

Any burn of the face, eyes, hands, feet, and genitals is considered serious and in need of prompt medical attention. Hospital care is needed for all burns involving more than 20 percent of an adult's body surface or 10 percent of a child's body.

There is much more to a burn than destruction of skin tissue. The skin is the body's barrier against loss of vital fluids and its protection against infection. Burn victims can suffer extreme fluid loss, resulting in shock. Infection is a common and often devastating complication, and proper antibiotic therapy can be lifesaving. For seriously burned people, temporary skin grafts, often involving pig skin or skin donated by close relatives, may offer lifesaving protection against fluid loss and infection until it is possible to graft the patient's own skin permanently.

Burns greatly increase the victim's metabolic rate, and malnutrition can result if enough calories and nutrients are not given. Feeding through a stomach tube or into a major vein can greatly improve chances for survival and speed recovery. Every major organ system can be damaged by the effects of a serious burn. If a fire was involved, smoke inhalation may cause lung injury.

In addition to physical pain, a burn victim can suffer extreme emotional agony. The fear of disfigurement, the social isolation, the sense of loss, the guilt if personal negligence caused the accident, and the struggles against the physical complications can cause severe emotional shock.

How to Prevent Burns

The best way to deal with burns is to prevent them. The following measures are among those recommended by the Red Cross and public health officials:

● Never smoke in bed or when you are feeling sleepy.

● Make sure heating equipment and chimneys are cleaned annually, and don't store oily rags or papers in confined areas or near the furnace.

● Don't leave space heaters on all night, and don't use one in the bedroom of a small child who could walk into it or knock it over.

● Keep pot handles turned inward and clean grease from cooking surfaces promptly. Never cook while wearing blousy or loose clothing, and make sure curtains cannot blow across cooking surfaces.

● Don't keep cookies and other childhood temptations in cupboards near or above the stove.

● Use heat-resistant potholders (not dish towels or bare hands) when handling hot pots, even if the pot has a heatproof handle. When opening the cover, raise the edge that is farthest from your body to prevent a steam burn.

● Make sure your house is properly wired to handle the numerous high-powered electrical appliances now common in American homes. Don't overload electrical circuits. When a manufacturer recommends that an appliance be grounded (usually by a three-pronged plug with a grounding wire in a three-hole outlet), follow the advice.

● Unless your television set is designed to be installed in an enclosed space, make sure it has adequate ventilation.

● If you have toddlers at home, don't leave cups of hot liquid on accessible surfaces or tubs of hot water into which a child could fall.

FIRST AID FOR BURNS

The proper emergency treatment for a burn depends on its cause and severity. Conflicting advice is given in the many first-aid books currently available. The following recommendations are derived from one of the newest guides, *The American Medical Association's Handbook of First Aid and Emergency Care* (New York: Random House, 1980). For any and all burns, this book cautions against applying grease, butter, sprays, ointments, or home remedies.

Minor burns. These involve redness and pain and sometimes mild swelling, but no blistering. They are commonly caused by sun, brief contact with hot objects, hot water, or steam.

1. Place burned area immediately under cold running water, or apply a cold-water compress using a clean cloth, until pain subsides.

2. Cover with sterile or clean bandage.

Serious burns. In addition to redness, swelling, and pain, these usually involve blisters and/or a moist, oozy appearance to the skin. They commonly result from deep sunburn, hot liquids, and flash burns from gasoline or other flammable substances.

1. Put burned area in cold (not ice) water, or apply clean cold-water compresses.

2. Pat dry and cover with sterile or clean bandage.

3. Raise burned arms or legs above the level of the heart.

4. Get medical attention.

5. *Do not* try to break blisters.

Severe burns. The skin appears white or charred. Little or no pain may be felt because nerve endings are destroyed. Fire, prolonged contact with hot substances, or electrical burns are common causes.

1. Make sure victim is breathing.

2. Place cold cloth or cool water (ice water can intensify shock reaction) on burns of the face, hands, or feet.

3. Cover burned area with a thick sterile dressing, such as clean linens or a disposable diaper.

4. Call for an ambulance immediately. Even with a small severe burn, medical care is necessary.

5. Elevate burned hands, legs, or feet, higher than the heart if possible. A person with burns of the head or neck should be propped up with pillows and checked often for breathing difficulties.

6. Treat for shock: Keep victim lying down unless head or neck is burned. Raise feet eight to twelve inches unless victim is unconscious or has severe facial injuries. Such victims should be placed on their sides, with the head and shoulders slightly raised if they have difficulty breathing. Keep victim warm with a blanket or coat. If medical help is more than two hours away and victim is conscious, give a solution of one teaspoon salt and one-half teaspoon baking soda mixed into one quart of water: four ounces every fifteen minutes for an adult; two ounces for a child aged one to twelve; one ounce for an infant. Clear juices may also be given.

7. *Do not* try to remove clothing that is stuck to the burn or put ice or ice water on burn. Don't give the victim alcohol, and don't give any fluids to an unconscious victim.

Chemical burns.

1. Immediately put burned area under cold running water for at least five minutes. At the same time remove clothing from burned area.

2. Then follow instructions on container of the responsible chemical, if available.

3. Cover with clean bandage (use a cool, wet dressing for pain), and seek medical attention.

4. In case of a chemical burn of the eye, immediately flush eye under running water for about ten minutes. Place face under faucet with injured eye nearest sink basin to prevent chemical from washing into the other eye. Be sure to hold eyelids open, lifting them to get water to all parts of the eye. Alternatively, place affected half of face in basin of water, and move eyelids up and down. *Do not* rub eye. Cover with clean bandage with lids closed and seek immediate medical attention, preferably from an ophthalmologist.

Never leave a small child unattended in a tub or near an open fire.

• Make sure the tap water in your house or apartment building is no higher than 120 degrees. At this temperature it would take ten minutes of exposure to adult skin to cause a severe burn. For every degree above 104, the time it takes to get a scalding burn diminishes rapidly. At 140 to 150 degrees, the temperatures preset at the factory on most water heaters, in two to five seconds of exposure an adult's entire skin layer may be destroyed by severe burns.

• Use nonflammable cleaning fluids and read the labels, heed the warnings, and follow the instructions for proper use of all chemical sprays (including hair sprays and deodorants), detergents, pesticides, and other household and garden products. Store such products in cool, well-ventilated areas.

• Install a smoke detector or two in your home, and make sure it always contains live batteries. Keep small fire extinguishers near the furnace and in the kitchen, and make sure everyone knows where they are and how to use them. Keep near the sink a piece of hose that could be attached quickly to the faucet.

• Establish and practice an in-case-of-fire escape plan that includes two ways to get outdoors from every room in your home. You may want to install a folding fire ladder in an upper-story window of a private house that has no fire escape.

• If fire breaks out, first get everyone out of the house; then call the fire department. In escaping from a burning building, stay close to the floor, and using your palm, touch each door before opening it. If it feels hot, use another escape route, or wait by a slightly opened window, hanging out an article of clothing or sheet to signal rescuers. If someone's clothing catches fire, smother it with a coat or blanket or by rolling the victim on the floor or ground.

Water Safety:
How to Prevent Drowning

Although he had lived in Minnesota, the Land of 10,000 Lakes, for all his forty-six years, Don P. never learned to swim. Nonetheless, one hot summer day he decided to join his family on an inner-tube trip down a Wisconsin river. Suddenly a woman near him fell off her tube and began floundering in the churning water. Don leaped to her rescue and quickly lost his footing on the slippery rocks. He was in water only chest-high, but he could not right himself. If not for an alert bystander who dived in to help, both Don and the woman probably would have drowned.

Each year in the United States 6,000 to 8,000 people die from drowning, and more than 1 million have close calls like Don's. Small children wander off and fall into unattended pools and ponds. Boats overturn; fishermen lose their footing; swimmers panic when struck by a cramp or caught in a current; young and old alike swim out farther than they should.

The majority of these drownings and near-drownings are avoidable. If people understood the risks of water sports, followed some basic rules of safety, and learned how to save themselves when in trouble, the joys of a refreshing swim or a relaxing boat ride need not be marred by tragedy. Here are some tips on making a splash safely.

When Swimming . . .

● If you can't swim or are a weak swimmer, don't go into calm water deeper than shoulder height. The rougher the water or stronger the current, the more cautious you should be. Children who do not swim well should never be allowed to float out over their heads on a raft or in a tube. The device might deflate, or the child slip off. Children who cannot swim should wear life jackets whenever near water. Many drown after falling off docks.

● Never swim alone. Even a strong swimmer should have a companion along when swimming in deep water. If you are in the water alone, stay near the shore, and be sure that someone onshore who is a good swimmer is watching. At beaches and public pools swim only when and where there is a lifeguard on duty, and even then small children should be supervised by a responsible adult.

● Don't swim right after eating a meal. An hour's wait is a good general rule. After eating, your blood tends to pool in your gastrointestinal area, causing a relative shortage of blood in the muscles of the limbs. This increases the likelihood that cramps will develop in your arms or legs. Abdominal cramps may also result from too vigorous exercise soon after eating.

● Don't plunge directly into very cold water. This causes the blood vessels in your arms and legs to constrict and may cause cramping. Instead, slowly acclimate your body to the cold water by vigorously rubbing your extremities with the water and jiggling your arms in the water up to your elbows. No matter what the water temperature, leave the water when you begin to feel cold or tired; children with chattering teeth should come out of the water.

● Horseplay, shouting, or phony cries for help should never be allowed in the water. One ten-year-old boy drowned when his swimming companions thought his call for help was a fake since he'd teased them with it so often before.

● Don't do deep-breathing exercises before taking a swim underwater. While such exercises can increase the time you can swim without seeming to require a breath, they can also fool your body into thinking your brain has enough oxygen when it doesn't. As a result, you may black out suddenly, without warning, and drown.

• Don't dive into water of unknown depth or bottom. Many an unwary diver has been permanently crippled by striking his head on a submerged boulder or tree trunk. Aboveground pools are too shallow for safe diving. Dive only into water that is six or more feet deep.

• All pools should be protected by a high fence or gate (preferably six feet high and a type that can't be scaled by a child) that can be locked when not in use. If you plan to be away for an extended period, the pool should be emptied or covered securely.

• Your pool should be clearly marked with depths at various points, and a buoyed rope placed across the middle. If a diving board is in use, swimmers should stay clear of the diving area.

• Stay out of the water in a thunder storm. [See the chapter on lightning, page 358.] Also, keep portable electrical equipment away from poolside.

• Don't attempt water sports like skiing or scuba diving without lessons from a qualified instructor.

404

• At the beginning of the swimming season children should not assume they can swim as well or as far as they did at the end of the previous season. At any time every swimmer should know the limits of his ability and endurance and not try to exceed them.

• Children should be taught to swim early, preferably before they enter school, but swimming programs for children under three years old are not advised. According to the American Academy of Pediatrics, infants may be able to learn to swim and to keep their heads above water, but they cannot be taught water safety and proper reactions to an emergency. Very young children rarely can swim far because they don't learn how to breathe properly. Swimming instruction for older children and adults is available at Ys, Red Cross chapters, many public pools, camps, and schools.

• At any pool or swimming area keep some sort of rescue equipment handy, such as a long pole or shepherd's crook and a life ring on a rope. You can make an excellent rescue device by attaching a gallon plastic jug to about forty feet of rope and filling the jug with an inch or so of water for ballast.

Ideally as many people in the family as possible should learn basic first aid and lifesaving. Such courses are taught through Red Cross chapters, at Ys, and at schools throughout the country. At the least, everyone over the age of twelve should know how to do mouth-to-mouth resuscitation. In one study, 75 percent of the drownings were witnessed by someone who was old enough to have saved the victim, but who unfortunately did not know what to do.

When Boating . . .

- Never overload a boat. If there is no stated loading capacity, a good rule is one person to a seat. In calm water, in a small craft there should be at least six inches of freeboard above the water. In rough water or waves, a larger freeboard allowance is necessary to prevent swamping. The boat should be balanced from side to side and from fore to aft.

- A boat should be operated only by someone totally familiar with how it works and how to handle it under a variety of conditions. The boat should be in top working order, but small motorboats should always be equipped with oars, just in case.

- There should be a life preserver or safety cushion on board for each occupant, and anyone who is not a good swimmer should wear a Coast Guard-approved life jacket at all times. Life belts or jackets should always be worn by water skiers.

- Be aware of and guided by weather conditions before going out in a boat. If a storm approaches, get back to shore immediately. If necessary, wait out a storm before attempting to return home.

- Know boating rules of the road to avoid collisions.

- If your boat should swamp or capsize, stay with it unless it is heading toward danger (such as a dam), the water is very cold, or safety is near enough to swim to. Know how to swim to shore in or on a capsized or swamped boat.

405

How to Keep from Drowning . . .

The most common cause of drowning is panic. A swimmer struck

DROWNPROOFING

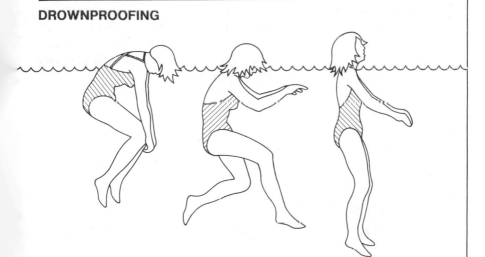

Take a deep breath and hold it. (1) Place face in water with arms and legs dangling. When ready to breathe: (2) Raise arms and spread legs. (3) Lower arms, bring legs quickly together, exhale, raise head just enough to clear surface, and inhale. Repeat as needed.

by a cramp, tumbled by a wave, caught in a current, or too exhausted to continue will stop thinking and perform motions that accomplish little and waste remaining energy. The panicked swimmer swallows and inhales water and drowns.

• To relieve a cramp, float on your back (your body's natural buoyancy will keep you up), relax, and try to massage the cramped area. Avoid stretching a cramped limb until the pain eases.

• If you are tumbled by a wave, don't fight it. You'll soon resurface right where you started from since the water in a wave does not move in and out but rather up, down, and around in a circle.

• Don't try to fight a current. If an ocean current is carrying you out, swim parallel to the beach until you escape its pull. Or let the current carry you out some distance until it dissipates. In a river always swim diagonally across the current in the direction of its flow, and walk back along the shore to reach your destination.

• A person rescued from a near-drowning must be brought to a hospital for observation for at least twenty-four hours. Many "saved" people die from delayed effects of near-drowning, which can be detected and treated effectively only in a hospital.

• Learn and use a technique called drownproofing. It allows you to stay afloat for very long periods with minimum expenditure of energy. It is much easier than treading water or even floating horizontally. It is a skill that every swimmer should learn and practice. Here's how it's done:

Floating upright (vertically) with your arms dangling at your sides, take a deep breath, hold it, and hang there with your face underwater. When you need a breath, exhale slowly through your nose, raise your arms, and cross them in front of your face. Then move your arms apart, and when they are fully extended, push downward with your palms, tilt your head back, and when your mouth comes out of the water, take a breath. Then lower your head and arms again and bob until you need another breath. When you feel able, you can move into a horizontal position and start kicking toward shore, repeating the drownproofing technique whenever needed.

For Further Reading

American Red Cross. *Lifesaving Rescue and Water Safety.* Washington, D.C.: 1974.

Eye Injuries: Protecting Your Most Precious Sense

A young squash player from Massachusetts had her eye cut open when her opponent's racket struck and smashed her glasses. A New York tennis player was struck in the eye by a ball smashed across the net, causing near-blinding tears of the retina, bleeding, and scarring. Two young women using a sun lamp suffered extremely painful burns of the cornea.

Every year millions of Americans participate in activities that endanger the most valued of their five senses, sight, and thousands suffer eye injuries that can impair vision. Though prompt and proper treatment often saves sight, hospitalization and multiple operations may be needed. And for many, even the best therapy cannot preserve useful vision.

Eye specialists have noted an alarming increase in eye injuries in recent years, especially during the summer months. The causes range from sports like tennis, baseball, hockey, cycling, basketball, and swimming to such activities as gardening, do-it-yourself projects, sunbathing, and setting off fireworks. Sports and recreational activities alone account for more than 35,000 eye injuries a year that require emergency hospital treatment.

Yet, according to the National Society to Prevent Blindness, 90 percent of all eye injuries can be prevented with proper precautions, which usually involve nothing more elaborate than observing a few simple rules of safety and wearing appropriate protective glasses or eyeguards. A number of inexpensive products that can help to save your sight are available.

Preventing Sun Damage

The most common summer eye problem, says Dr. Robert J. Crossen of the American Association of Ophthalmology, is sunburn of the sensitive areas around the eye. Burns of the eye itself, in which ultraviolet rays of the sun or a sun lamp damage the cornea, are less common but more serious. They often do not show up for twelve to twenty-four hours, and the victim may awake in the middle of the night with searing pain and a feeling of sand grains in the eyes.

Immediate treatment by an eye doctor (an ophthalmologist, not an optometrist) can usually prevent permanent damage, but sometimes the cornea remains scarred, impairing vision. Prolonged exposure to sunlight can also cause a temporary diminution in night vision that may interfere with the ability to drive home safely after a day outdoors. Over the years repeated, extended exposure to ultraviolet light may increase the risk of developing cataracts. [See chapter on cataracts, page 328.]

To prevent sun damage to the eyes, be sure to wear sunglasses during prolonged or intense exposure to the sun. If you wear prescription glasses, get your prescription ground into sunglasses; clip-ons, though cheaper, are less effective.

Choose your sunglasses with practical considerations, not fashion, uppermost in mind. Examine the light transmission factor on the label. The glasses should transmit no more than 30 percent of the light; select those that transmit only 10 to 15 percent for use on the beach, water, or snow. Sunglasses should be dark enough so that you cannot see your eyes through them when you look in a mirror.

Some, called gradient density lenses, are made darker on top of the lens and may be useful for driving or just walking around on a bright day. For driving or boating, polarizing lenses can help to reduce glare. For intense glare, mirrored lenses are best. Phototropic lenses that adjust to the light intensity cost more but may serve well under a wider variety of light conditions. Choose those that are still quite dark even when in their faded state.

Gray or smoke-colored lenses are least likely to distort color. Green and brown lenses are also good. But stay away from high-fashion colors like pink, orange, yellow, and blue; they distort color perception and usually let through too much light.

Never wear sunglasses indoors or after dark; this habit can lead to permanent impairment of night vision. Sunglasses are not adequate protection in a tanning hut or under a sun lamp, where you must wear sun goggles. Only a few minutes under the intense light of a sun lamp can burn your eyes, even with sunglasses on.

Impact Injuries

Even though all eyeglass lenses must now be made from impact-resistant glass or plastic, regular glasses or sunglasses are usually not strong enough to withstand the force of a stone thrown by a lawn mower or a smashed tennis ball or a swung racket. Contact lenses offer no protection at all. To protect your eyes adequately, these and related activities demand the use of special eye guards — sports eye protectors or industrial safety lenses. Mandatory use of face protectors for hockey players, it was found, reduced eye and face injuries to 1 percent of the number of injuries suffered by unprotected players.

Performance standards for sports safety eyewear are now being developed. In the meantime, the National Society to Prevent Blindness recommends:

● Industrial-quality safety glasses, which can be obtained either with noncorrective lenses or with lenses ground to your prescription. These glasses should have plastic lenses and bear the insignia Z87.1, 1979, indicating that they meet the current requirements of the American National Standard Practice for Occupational and Educational Eye and Face Protection. These can be obtained through opticians, eye doctors, or suppliers of safety equipment. Without prescription lenses, they usually cost between $10 and $15.

● Sports eye protectors, which are a goggle type of molded eyeguards, with or without lenses. These can also be made with prescription lenses, but they cost more than industrial safety glasses. For activities like badminton, cycling, yard work, and do-it-yourself ventures, a full lens is recommended. They can be purchased from opticians, eye doctors, sporting goods stores, and racket clubs.

According to Dr. Paul F. Vinger, a Lexington, Massachusetts, ophthalmologist who has studied sports injuries to the eyes, the best protection is given by optical-quality polycarbonate lenses, which can withstand very high-intensity blows. One such product, Action Eyes by Bausch & Lomb, sells for about $25. Another, Pro-tek Gargoyles, retails for about $40. They are injection-molded (one-piece), wraparound, lightweight, shatterproof eye protectors with clear or sunglass tint, useful for skiing and cycling as well as for racket sports.

Dr. Vinger also urges better court manners to prevent injuries. Shots should never be fired in anger or frustration, nor should more than one ball be in play at one time.

Safety goggles should also be worn when you trim shrubs, use a power mower or workshop tools, or spray pesticides or paint. Goggles can protect your eyes from the irritating smoke of a barbecue as well. As for fireworks, the best defense is not to fool with them or stay around anyone who is. Each year, Dr. Vinger says, more than 1,000 Americans suffer eye injuries from fireworks.

Water Hazards

Heavily chlorinated pools can cause a mild chemical burn of the cornea, resulting in a scratchy feeling in the eyes. The condition usually clears up in a few days without treatment. Cold packs may help reduce the irritation, and sometimes treatment with a topical antibiotic is used. Some people are extremely sensitive to chlorine's effects and suffer eye irritation even from lightly chlorinated water. When you swim in ponds, especially at camps and resorts, eye infections like conjunctivitis, or pinkeye, are common hazards that require treatment with antibiotic ointments.

The best way to protect your eyes from water damage is to wear watertight swim goggles (they cost $3 to $5 and are available at most sporting goods stores) and to refrain from sharing towels, to prevent the spread of infection.

Poisonous Plants: "Leaves of Three," Etc.

Peter was fishing from a riverbank. Georgina was picking wild strawberries. John and his father were cutting dead trees for firewood. Grace was collecting rocks for her garden. Along with what they went for, all came away with an unexpected "gift" from a native American — poison ivy.

Sensitivity to poison ivy — along with its less common relatives poison oak and poison sumac — is really an allergy. Four out of five Americans eventually become sensitized to the lacquerlike chemical urushiol, which is present in all parts of these plants: leaves, stem, berries, bark, and roots. Most people seem to need more than one exposure before a noticeable reaction occurs, but it appears that if exposed often or heavily enough, even the most resistant person will get it.

Anyone who, boasting resistance, blithely traipses through patches of the poison plants is simply inviting disaster — if not that time, then the next or the time after that. Therefore, it is wise for everyone who ventures outdoors where wild things grow (including your own backyard) to learn to recognize — and avoid — poison ivy, oak, and sumac in their various guises.

Recognizing the Troublemakers

"Leaves of three, let them be . . ." The familiar warning refers to the one fixed characteristic of poison ivy and poison oak, the fact that each leaf always consists of three leaflets. Other than that, poison ivy or oak leaves may vary in length from one to five inches, be hairy or hairless, elliptical or egg-shaped, with margins that may be saw-toothed, deeply cut, gently or deeply lobed, or entirely smooth. The leaves are usually glossy green in spring and summer, but in fall they turn an inviting pink, yellow, or scarlet that may seduce gatherers of fall foliage. Many of the plants bear clusters of small whitish green flowers in spring that mature into white berries in August.

The plants themselves may grow as short ground cover, bushy shrubs, sturdy vines, or even, according to one report, trees. Poison ivy plants grow well in moist woodlands and along the tree-shaded edges of lawns, but they can also survive in dry, rocky areas and are found throughout the United States except in the California area, where poison oak reigns.

Poison sumac forms a tall shrub or small tree. Rather than three leaflets, each sumac leaf consists of seven to eleven leaflets — one at the tip and the others arranged in pairs along a red axis. The leaflets are bright green and come to a point, but unlike their nonpoisonous relatives, they have smooth rather than sharply pointed edges. Poison sumac is a less common cause of plant allergy because it grows in wet areas — swamps, bogs, and such — where fewer people tread.

Preventing Exposure

If you cannot avoid walking in or near areas where these plants grow, be sure to wear long pants and sleeves, shoes and socks, and even gloves. Afterward, wash the clothing thoroughly in detergent. You can get these plant allergies not just from direct contact with the plants but also from touching clothing, tools, pets, golf clubs, doorknobs, and whatever might have been contaminated with the plant resin.

Urushiol, the oily allergen (allergy-provoking substance) in these plants, is so potent that as little as one-thousandth of a milligram can produce the typical rash. It is also highly resistant to destruction. Contact with a tool or an article of clothing that was contaminated by urushiol years before can cause an allergic attack, unless the object was thoroughly cleansed with strong soap or detergent and water.

If poison ivy or one of its relatives grows on your property, the best thing to do is kill it. It cannot be destroyed by being pulled up or dug into the soil. Only herbicides that kill the roots will keep the plants from coming back.

The Brooklyn (New York) Botanic Garden recommends the following herbicides — 2,4-D, silvex, amitrol, or ammonium sulfamate — one or more of which should be available at most garden centers. The spray can formulation is said to be most effective. If there are other patches of poison plants in the vicinity, birds may resow them on your property, so the treatment should be repeated if you see the plants come up again.

After the plant has died, urushiol will remain potent for a time. If you leave the dead plants where they are, avoid the area for several weeks. If you gather them up, don't touch them with bare hands, and dispose of them in sealed plastic bags. You may also bury the dead plants in the soil. Be sure to wash all tools and clothing thoroughly when you're done. But whatever you do, don't burn the plants. The urushiol will become airborne on particles of soot and can cause a severe allergic reaction in your eyes, nose, and mouth as well as all over your body.

411

POISONOUS PLANTS

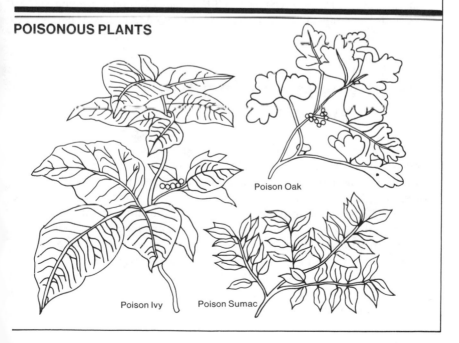

Poison Oak

Poison Ivy   Poison Sumac

How to Treat Exposure

If you are exposed or think you were exposed to a urushiol-containing plant, remove contaminated clothing and wash your skin thoroughly and immediately (preferably within five, and at most ten, minutes) with a strong laundry (alkali) soap and water. This does not guarantee no reaction, but if done soon enough, it will reduce the severity of the reaction and also prevent you from spreading urushiol to other parts of your body.

The symptoms of these plant allergies generally appear within a few hours of exposure, but they may show up as long as two days later. Symptoms include headache, a rash characterized by redness, blisters, swelling, burning and itching, and in some cases a very high fever.

To relieve discomfort in milder cases, apply calamine or some other soothing lotion, or a poultice of baking soda or Epsom salts, or an over-the-counter hydrocortisone cream, lotion, or ointment. Two folk remedies — rubbing with the crushed leaves of the common plantain or jewelweed, a native wild flower related to the garden impatiens — are also said to bring relief. More severe cases may need prescription cortisone ointments and a doctor's attention. Scratching should be avoided in all cases because it encourages infection, but it cannot spread the attack unless you still have urushiol on your skin.

There is no effective way to desensitize a person who is allergic to urushiol (as most of us are) except by avoiding all contact with it. Currently available desensitization treatments can produce unpleasant and sometimes dangerous reactions. A recommendation a few years ago by the late natural foods advocate Euell Gibbons to desensitize yourself by eating the leaves is not only ineffective but also dangerous. It can lead to a severe irritation of the digestive tract and possibly death.

Insect Pests: Avoiding Bites, Stings, and Allergic Reactions

Among the arthropods are the human species' oldest, most prolific, and persistent enemies. They bite, sting, suck, swarm, buzz, crawl, and sap the pleasure from picnics, camping trips, fishing expeditions, summertime hikes, and strolls in the setting sun. Just when you think you've found the perfect site to pitch a tent or build the summer cottage of your dreams, along come the blackflies to drink your blood, or the wood ticks to bury their heads in your flesh, or the chiggers to dissolve your skin — not to mention the ubiquitous hordes of hungry mosquitoes.

While we have never succeeded in completely controlling the multitudes of six- and eight-legged creatures that plague us, many ways have been found to discourage these pests from feeding on our flesh and blood. Understanding the habits of people-loving insects, mites, and spiders can help you to outwit them. Or if that fails, it helps to know how to relieve the misery they inflict.

Chemical Protection

First, a general word about repellents and insecticides. The most effective repellent yet developed is a substance called deet, or diethyl-meta-toluamide. Deet is present in various concentrations in several leading repellents, including Cutter, 6-12, and Off! Other effective chemicals are dimethyl carbamate, dimethyl phthalate, ethylhexanediol, and butopyronoxyl.

One application of repellent generally lasts several hours. It should be reapplied after swimming, after heavy sweating, or where the skin is rubbed. Don't spray repellent directly on your face; spray it on your hand, and then apply it to your face, being careful to keep it out of your eyes. If repellent gets in your eyes, flush them immediately and thoroughly with plain water.

Outdoor aerosol sprays are of limited value unless used in an enclosed area. The safest ones contain pyrethrin as the active ingredient. An hour before an outdoor party you might try spraying with a pyrethrin fogger, but don't expect freedom from buzzing and biting friends to last the entire evening.

The Common Culprits

Mosquitoes. Mosquitoes are opportunists. Ninety-five percent of the biting mosquitoes in the United States breed in temporary pools of water. Following a rain, eggs are laid in puddles, or previously laid eggs hatch into larvae and mature into adults. The adult males are vegetarians, but the females use animal blood to produce the next batch of eggs.

Therefore, the first line of defense against mosquitoes is to eliminate places around your home where rain pools may form. Fill in ditches and low spots; clean gutters; empty plant saucers; keep fish (which eat mosquito larvae) in ponds and decorative pools. Keep windows and door screens in good repair. When camping, avoid sites near stagnant water.

Make yourself unattractive to mosquitoes, which are drawn to body warmth and moisture and dark colors. Keep cool; bathe often; wear light, dull colors and don long sleeves and pants in the evening and early morning, when females feed; and use a repellent on exposed parts of the body. If you stay near someone the mosquitoes like better than you, you will be relatively shunned. Mosquitoes generally find men more attractive than women, and adults more attractive than children.

Mosquito bites swell and itch because the insect injects an enzyme to keep her blood meal from coagulating. For relief, try a cold compress or ice cube, an anesthetic first-aid or sunburn spray, calamine lotion, or, for more severe reactions, an over-the-counter hydrocortisone cream.

Chiggers. These are not insects but rather red mites about one-two-hundredth of an inch long that crawl in moist soil and up grasses and shrubs and onto hapless humans. The larva stops to feed on a person when it finds a soft spot or an impediment, such as a belt or sock top. When it pierces the skin, it releases a digestive enzyme that liquefies the skin cells, and then it consumes the liquid. It goes deeper and deeper, eating for a week to ten days, and then falls off, leaving behind a welt that can itch intensely.

From New England to Minnesota to the Gulf of Mexico, you can expect to find chiggers in fallow fields and cutover lands, where tall weeds and small animals are abundant. For protection (for example, when you go berry picking), use a chigger repellent on your clothing as well as on exposed skin, and tie your pants at the cuffs and your shirt at the wrists. Don't sit directly on the ground.

Following exposure to chiggers, take a long bath with sulfur soap, preferably scrubbing with a brush. Try coating bites with clear nail polish. Ice cubes bring relief; scratching invites infection.

Ticks. A cousin to the chigger, the tick also inhabits damp, weedy areas. Sometimes the tick carries a paralyzing toxin that could be fatal if the tick is not removed very carefully. In some parts of the country, including parts of the East Coast, ticks carry Rocky Mountain spotted fever. Small, oval, and crablike in appearance, the tick surreptitiously attaches itself to its host with its teeth, swelling larger and larger as it feeds on blood.

Don't try to remove a tick forcibly. Instead, coat it with petroleum jelly, heavy oil, grease, turpentine, or gasoline; wait half an hour; and then try to lift it gently with tweezers, taking care not to squeeze it. If the tick is still in tight, place a heated needle or lighted match or cigarette close to the tick to force it to release its grip. After removal, wash the area for about five minutes with soap.

If you live in or visit tick territory, check your body for ticks daily (especially the scalp, behind the ears, and places where clothing is tight, such as under bra and underwear bands), and check children twice a day. Use of repellents and wearing clothing that is tightly tied at the ankles and wrists help.

Biting flies. Unlike the common housefly, the stable fly, horsefly, deerfly, blackfly, sand fly, and biting midge are bloodsuckers. Each stabs its victims with a bayonetlike proboscis and injects substances to break down tissue. They range in size from the large horsefly (up to an inch long and often called a greenhead for its huge, brightly colored eyes) and the deerfly (spotty-eyed with banded wings and bodies) to the tiny sand fly and midge, only a few millimeters long and capable of penetrating screens and mosquito nets (the infamous "no-see-ums").

Blackflies, with black bodies and iridescent wings and an extremely painful bite, are active during the day, usually in isolated woody areas near water. Sand flies feed only at night, and midges at sunset. Horseflies and deerflies love warmth and sunlight and rarely bite on cool or cloudy days. Flies are generally attracted to dark clothing, like blue jeans. Wash fly bites thoroughly to prevent infection.

Stinging hymenoptera — bees, wasps, hornets, ants. The sting of these insects is dangerous to the 1 to 2 million Americans who are allergic to the injected venom. If extreme local swelling or any generalized reaction — such as hives, wheezing, tightness in the throat, cramps, nausea or diarrhea, painfully swollen joints — occurs, get to a doctor or hospital immediately. A person who is highly allergic may go into shock and die within minutes of being stung.

People with known allergy to insect stings should at all times carry with them a sting kit containing a preloaded syringe of adrenaline, an inhaler of adrenaline, liquid antihistamine, and a tourniquet. Such a kit, which costs a few dollars, can be purchased at a pharmacy with a prescription from a physician, who should provide instructions for its proper use. Recent studies have shown that desensitization treatments using pure venom from the responsible insect can protect against life-threatening allergic reactions. Such treatments should be started about three months before the insect season. Treatments with whole-body extracts of the offending insect are far less effective, if they work at all.

Because hymenoptera are attracted to bright colors, flowery prints, perfumes, sugary syrups, and meat, to avoid being stung, stick to light-colored clothing; don't use hair spray, setting or shaving lotion, perfume, or heavily scented deodorant; and don't wear flowers in your hair. Even some suntan lotions are troublesome. Keep picnic foods covered except for what you are eating and dispose of refuse immediately. Don't walk barefoot outdoors.

Don't flail wildly at hovering hymenoptera. Stay still, or move away slowly. Don't chase those that land; either leave them alone or kill them with one swift blow. Carry an aerosol can of insecticide in the car; pull over, stop the car, and spray at a trapped insect rather than swat at it. And don't touch a freshly killed wasp or hornet because it may still be able to sting.

If stung, apply an ice cube to reduce swelling and a dilute solution of household ammonia or sodium bicarbonate (baking soda) paste to the bite to relieve the pain. Or you might apply a paste of meat tenderizer, which contains an enzyme that destroys the protein in the venom.

Spiders. Few American spiders are harmful, but the bite of the black widow or the brown recluse can be fatal. The black widow, about fifteen millimeters long with a shiny black body and red hourglass marking on the underside, produces a dull, numbing pain that can progress to severe abdominal pain and pains in all the skeletal muscles, spasm of the diaphragm, nausea, and fever. The effects of a spider's venom are instantaneous and usually self-limiting. There is little point in applying a tourniquet or trying to suck out the venom. Ice packs will help to relieve the pain and slow the absorption of venom. Keep the victim still, and call a doctor or get to a hospital.

The brown recluse is violin-shaped, comes in all shades from tan to dark brown, and commonly inhabits outbuildings and storage closets in the southern and western parts of the country. A bite produces pain hours later, and a blistering wound that takes about three weeks to heal develops. Children may suffer severe reactions. Immediate medical attention is advised.

Nonpoisonous spider bites should be washed thoroughly with soap and water, treated with an antiseptic, and bandaged. To prevent spider bites, be careful when handling woodpiles or objects that haven't been moved in a long time. Shake out all stored clothing thoroughly before wearing it. When camping, brush out your sleeping bag before you get in it, and shake out your shoes and socks before putting them on.

Dog Bites and Other Pet-Caused Ailments: Minimizing the Risks

Pets are an important part of American life. More than half of American households own one or more dog or cat. The Humane Society of the United States estimates that there are at least 100 million owned, free-roaming (once owned but now wild), and feral dogs and cats in the country.

Pets — which include birds, hamsters, gerbils, rabbits, fish, snakes, mice, rabbits, frogs, monkeys, and other animals — fill important needs for millions of people. They are a source of pleasure and amusement; provide companionship and friendship for the lonely, isolated, and bereaved; act as substitutes for children, spouses, parents, or friends; help teach children responsibility; and help prepare adults for parenthood.

But when improperly chosen or cared for, pets can also be a source of serious bites and sometimes baffling and debilitating illnesses. At least forty different diseases can be transmitted from pets to people. They may be acquired from direct contact with an infected animal or from the animal's excrement. Sometimes just breathing the air in the vicinity of an infected pet can cause illness. Pet-transmitted diseases are more often a problem in urban areas, where pets are permitted to wander about and defecate and urinate in areas where children play.

An Epidemic of Dog Bites

Seven-year-old Michael was playing Frisbee on the sidewalk in front of his house when a neighbor approached with his Great Dane on a leash. Michael ran to make a catch just as the dog passed by. Suddenly, for no apparent reason, the huge animal lunged at Michael and tore an inch-long hole in his cheek.

Michael was lucky. Stitches closed the wound, and the scar is small and neat. Other children have lost eyes, noses, chins — sometimes half their faces — as a result of dog bites. Some have died. Yet simple precautions on the part of dog owners and potential victims could prevent most of these attacks.

As more and more urban and suburban residents around the country purchase large dogs, the problem of dog bites is reaching frightening proportions. Some experts call it an unrecognized epidemic — a far more serious threat to health and life than the unsightly and unscently problem of dog feces and urine, which has prompted loud outcries from concerned citizens in many communities.

Public health officials estimate that nationwide more than 1 million people (and probably as many as 2 to 3 million) are bitten by dogs each year, resulting in about a dozen deaths. More than half the victims are children. The cost of medical care for dog bites exceeds $100 million a year.

As pet dogs get larger and more aggressive, the bites get more serious, and an increasing proportion of them occur on the faces of young children, many of whom stand head to head to a large dog like a German shepherd or Great Dane. Although shepherds represent about 10 percent of all dogs, they are responsible for about 40 percent of all bites.

Three out of four dog bites are unprovoked. Like Michael, the victim does nothing untoward to anger or annoy the dog. Rather, the dog is "nervous" or seems to interpret some ordinary human activity as a threatening or inciting gesture. In nearly 80 percent of cases the bite is inflicted not by a stray, but by a dog whose owner is known — usually a neighbor or friend or the victim's own family.

Most dog bites occur between 3:00 P.M. and 7:00 P.M., when children and dogs are outside in the greatest numbers. After being cooped up in a house or apartment all day, many large dogs are irritable and snappish and more likely to take out their frustrations on a small moving object like a child.

How to Prevent Dog Bites

Doctors and veterinarians who have studied the dog bite problem recommend the following preventive measures:

● People living in cities and suburbs should think twice before buying a large dog for a pet. Guard dogs trained to attack are absolutely unsuitable as pets. Large dogs need a lot of room and exercise and are inappropriate for areas where many children play. If you live in a congested area with a large dog, make sure it gets plenty of exercise each day (but without endangering strollers, bikers, and joggers).

• Always keep your dog on a leash outside the house, and walk the dog at hours and in places that are relatively free of children. If you see children playing on the sidewalk, take the dog into the street. Dogs allowed to roam free near their homes often establish "territories" and may bite strangers who invade their turf.

• Keep high-strung dogs away from children entirely, and destroy any dog that has bitten a person without provocation. In many cities a dog is allowed three reported bites before the animal must be destroyed. If you are bitten, be sure the incident is reported to the local health department and the owner informed. If the attack was vicious and unprovoked (even if it was the dog's first), you should press a complaint to have the animal destroyed.

• Teach children — and adults for that matter — to be cautious around dogs. Children should not be allowed to pet strange dogs. When entering a house where there is a dog, ask the owner to tie it up or hold it before you go in until the dog has gotten used to you. Especially avoid watchdogs and guard dogs. In New York City guard dogs must wear yellow tags indicating they are a "biohazard."

• If you are being pursued by a dog, stop. Stop running, or riding, or jogging. Hold your ground, point at the dog, and say in an authoritative voice, "Go home." If you are with a child, do not pick the child up. Instead, push the child behind you and order the dog home.

How to Treat a Dog Bite

If you are bitten, Dr. William P. Graham and his colleagues at the Milton S. Hershey Medical Center in Hershey, Pennsylvania, emphasize the importance of prompt and proper treatment to prevent infections and unsightly scars. If the injury is a scratch, Dr. Graham recommends that you thoroughly cleanse the wound with soap and water and rinse it well a couple of times a day.

A puncture wound or a bite that tears open tissues should be washed with soap and water as soon as possible and kept under running water for at least five minutes to wash out the animal's saliva. Cover the wound with sterile gauze, and go immediately to a physician or hospital emergency room. Antibiotics are usually prescribed for five or more days (penicillin, or erythromycin for those with penicillin allergy). If stitches are needed to close the wound or to produce a neat scar on an exposed part of the body, they are best done by a surgeon, who is trained to minimize scarring.

If the victim has had a tetanus shot within the last year, another shot is not necessary unless the injury is severe, Dr. Graham maintains. As for rabies, the need for immunization if you are bitten by an unknown dog that cannot be found depends on the incidence of rabies among the dogs and nearby wild animals in your area.

In New York City, for example, there has been no case of rabies in a dog since 1954, and rabies immunization for the victim of a dog bite is considered unnecessary unless the dog may have come from another area. In the United States as a whole, the last confirmed case of rabies from a dog bite occurred in 1963. But this may be partly because more than 35,000 victims of dog bites undergo the series of painful injections each year. A new rabies vaccine that is less hazardous and involves fewer injections is now available.

Protect Your Pet Against Rabies

Because so few cases of human rabies from domestic dogs and cats now occur, many people have become overly complacent about this disease, which is nearly universally fatal. Only about 40 percent of the approximately 40 million dogs that live in the United States are properly immunized against rabies, and a far smaller proportion of domestic cats are protected.

Reported cases of rabies among wild animals have increased dramatically in recent years. These animals could easily infect pet dogs and cats that live in rural and suburban areas, not to mention people who wander into fields and woods for recreation. If you own a dog or cat, make sure that the animal is immunized against rabies and that the immunization is kept up-to-date. The first shot should be given to a puppy or kitten at three months of age and again at one year. Depending on the vaccine used, dogs should get booster shots every year or every three years; in cats, boosters are given annually.

If you are bitten by a stray dog or cat, it should be killed immediately and its brain examined for rabies. If the animal is a pet dog or cat that appears to be healthy, it should be confined (securely in a kennel, since a rabid animal may try to run away), observed for ten days, and examined by a veterinarian before it is released from confinement. If any sign of illness develops during confinement, the animal should be killed and its brain examined for rabies.

Rabies immunization of the bite victim should be started immediately if the animal is found to be infected or if the animal appears sick at the time the bite occurred. A ten-day wait before the shots are started is considered safe if the animal appears healthy at the time of the bite. If the animal cannot be found, a physician — perhaps after consulting public health experts — should decide if immunization is wise.

Other Pet-Caused Diseases

Roundworm. Most puppies are infected with roundworms, the eggs of which are excreted soon after birth. These eggs can be carried to the animals' coats when their mother licks them. About 20 percent of adult dogs are also infected with roundworms. Cats can also transmit roundworms.

The usual human victims are young children, who may swallow the eggs after contact with infected animals or while playing in dirt contaminated with their excrement. After ingestion the eggs hatch, and the larvae can travel to many organs, including the lungs, liver, heart, and eyes. The infection, called visceral larva migrans or toxocariasis, produces a flulike illness with recurrent fever, cough, loss of appetite, weakness, night sweats, and lung congestion. A mild infection will cure itself, but severe cases are treated with worm-killing drugs.

To prevent roundworm infections, all puppies and any infected adult animals should be dewormed.

Heartworm. Although once confined to the eastern seaboard, this dog parasite has spread in recent years through the Mississippi Valley and Great Lakes region. It is transmitted from dog to dog to people by the bites of mosquitoes. Human infections produce no symptoms. But the worms, which cannot survive in a human host, migrate to the lungs and die, forming a lesion that looks like cancer on an X ray. Thus, victims must undergo a surgical biopsy to permit a proper diagnosis.

Heartworm in dogs can be prevented by daily doses of a drug called Hetrazan before, during, and for two months after the mosquito season.

Toxoplasmosis. This parasitic disease can be transmitted to people by ingestion following contact with the feces of infected cats. In most people it causes mild symptoms that are usually passed off as flu. But in pregnant women the infection can have devastating effects on their unborn children, resulting in blindness, mental retardation, and other birth defects.

To protect the fetus, a pregnant woman should always wash her hands after handling a cat. The litter box should be emptied daily, but by someone else, and the feces flushed down the toilet. Also, a pregnant woman should be wary when working in a garden that cats may have used as a toilet, and all vegetables harvested from such a garden should be thoroughly washed.

Psittacosis and other bird infections. Psittacosis, a lung infection that causes headache, chills, loss of appetite, fever, and a hacking cough, is spread by parakeets, parrots, canaries, pigeons, and other psittacine birds. The usual route of human infection is through inhalation, for example, of the cage dust. Following diagnosis via a blood test, the infection is usually treated with tetracycline.

An infected bird appears droopy, eats poorly, and has ruffled feathers. Such birds should be taken to a veterinarian for treatment or destroyed.

Other diseases transmitted by birds include cryptococcosis, a fungus that most commonly causes meningitis; histoplasmosis, a fungus often confused with tuberculosis; and an allergic disorder called hypersensitivity pneumonitis (or pigeon breeder's disease).

Salmonellosis. Particularly common around Easter time, this bacterial infection, which produces symptoms of food poisoning, is commonly contracted from the feces of pet chicks. For this and other reasons (the chicks nearly always die soon after Easter), chicks should not be given as pets.

Salmonella contamination was so prevalent among pet turtles that in 1975 the Food and Drug Administration banned their sale. Frogs and aquarium snails may also carry the bacteria, which cause vomiting and diarrhea. The illness is best prevented through careful hygiene: Always wash after handling aquarium pets or water, and don't keep pet birds in rooms where food is prepared or eaten since the organisms readily multiply in foods kept at room temperature.

Cat-scratch fever. Most often contracted following the scratch or bite of a young cat, this disease is caused by a virus for which there is as yet no specific treatment. The symptoms — swollen lymph nodes, high fever, loss of appetite, and weakness — may appear weeks after the scratch and eventually will subside on their own.

The disease is uncommon among cats confined to the house but can be picked up easily by cats that spend part of the time outdoors. However, as a precaution, immediately after all cat scratches, the wound should be washed with an antiseptic cleansing agent like alcohol. Infected cats appear healthy.

Pasteurella. Cat and dog scratches and bites may also transmit a potentially dangerous infection with *Pasteurella multocida*, a bacterium that lives in the mouths of up to 50 percent of healthy cats and dogs. The infection can cause local tissue destruction and, in more severe cases, bone infection and blood poisoning. Antibiotics, usually penicillin, are used to treat it and are recommended as a preventive after a deep scratch or bite.

Fleas, ticks, and mites. Although people are hardly their preferred hosts, bloodsucking parasites that live on pets can sometimes be transmitted to their owners. Often the fleas invade humans after their animal hosts have died or run away.

Cat and dog fleas can cause far more itchy, painful distress to people than to their rightful hosts. Sometimes fleas carry serious diseases, like tularemia, tapeworms, and, very occasionally, bubonic plague.

Infested pets and the areas where the pets commonly reside should be treated with appropriate insecticides. Be sure to apply the treatment to nooks and crannies, around baseboards, under rug edges, and in other dark, protected places where flea larvae may thrive.

Dog ticks can be vectors of Rocky Mountain spotted fever, a usually mild but sometimes serious infection that is now prevalent throughout the country, particularly in suburban and rural areas. Ticks should be removed promptly but never touched with bare hands. Use tweezers at the tick's head, and avoid squeezing the body. Then burn up the tick, and discard it. Antibiotics, usually tetracycline, should be given to any-

421

one who develops the characteristic rash of Rocky Mountain spotted fever.

People are often afflicted with human scabies (mites), but sometimes the dog mite (a cause of mange) also seeks a human host, burrowing into the skin and producing such symptoms as rash, hair loss, and intense itching. The likely infested areas are forearms, chest, belt line, and thighs, where contact with an infested dog is most likely. Mites are treated with the same insecticides used against lice. They usually disappear from humans after they have been eradicated from the infested dog.

Protect Yourself from Pet Diseases

A number of precautions can help protect you and your family from pet-borne diseases.

- Acquire pets only from a reliable dealer who practices good sanitation. Do not attempt to take wild or sick animals or monkeys as pets.
- Have a new pet checked over by a veterinarian, who can also provide needed immunizations (rabies, distemper, hepatitis, and leptospirosis for dogs; rabies and respiratory virus for cats).
- Keep your pet clean and properly housed. Litter boxes should be emptied daily.
- Practice good hygiene. Always wash your hands after handling a pet, don't let it lick your face, keep the pet's eating utensils separate from those of the family, and keep pets out of people's beds.
- Keep your tetanus shots up to date, and see a doctor if any animal bite breaks the skin.

422

Choking:
You Can Easily Prevent Death

Each year 2,500 to 3,900 Americans choke to death. Choking is the sixth leading cause of accidental fatalities in this country, more common than deaths in air crashes and by firearms. In children under the age of six, choking is the leading cause of accidental death in the home. Adult diners-out are frequent victims.

Example: A woman was having lunch with a friend in a San Francisco restaurant when she suddenly got up from the table and, without a word, tottered to the ladies' room, where she slumped to the floor and died. The autopsy revealed that a large piece of hamburger had blocked her bronchial tubes, asphyxiating her.

Example: A thirty-three-year-old man had had several drinks prior to his steak dinner in a Florida restaurant. He collapsed at the table; the rescue squad and the physician in the emergency room where he was taken assumed that he had suffered a heart attack. In fact, this victim of a "café coronary" had choked to death; a large piece of meat had wedged itself against the opening to his windpipe, preventing him from breathing.

A person who cannot breathe has only about four or five minutes before death or irreversible brain damage occurs. There is no time to summon a physician or ambulance. On-the-spot rescue is essential.

Through the years a number of first-aid remedies have been suggested for victims of choking, ranging from sharp raps on the back to plastic tweezers to cutting a hole into the trachea. In most cases these approaches were unsuccessful. Some could be downright dangerous.

The Heimlich Maneuver

Then, in 1974, a controversial surgeon from Cincinnati proposed, on the basis of studies of dogs, an entirely new approach, one that could easily be taught to the general public. The method, known as the Heimlich maneuver after its inventor, Dr. Henry J. Heimlich (now at Xavier University in Cincinnati), has since been learned by millions of American children and adults.

Four years later Dr. Heimlich reported that at least 2,500 lives were saved by his technique, and most of the rescuers were lay persons. Since that time countless more individuals have owed their lives to the Heimlich maneuver and its prompt and proper use by a bystander.

While it cannot be said with certainty that every one of these cases involved persons whose airways had been completely blocked and who would have died without the Heimlich maneuver, it's clear that it has saved many lives. Among them:

• A six-year-old child who choked on a piece of wax candy. The child's mother was driving when she heard screams from the back seat, where her two children were sitting. She turned to see the six-year-old choking and turning blue. As she pulled to the curb, her eight-year-old applied the Heimlich maneuver, which he had learned in school, and the candy flew out of the younger child's mouth.

• A woman who had served on the staff of former Governor Nelson A. Rockefeller of New York and who choked on a piece of chewing gum while dancing. She was given the Heimlich maneuver by a fellow dancer who saw that she could neither speak nor breathe. The gum popped out of her mouth.

• A nine-month-old infant who choked on a piece of foam rubber that he had gouged out of a mattress cover. His mother performed the maneuver, and the wad came out of the child's throat.

• A New York editor at an afternoon tea who choked on a chunk of cucumber. Another woman who had seen the Heimlich maneuver demonstrated on television rescued her.

How To Do It

The technique is easy to learn (according to one report, a four-year-old used it to rescue his two-year-old sibling, who had choked on a piece of chicken skin), and analyses of many hundreds of cases have shown that it can be properly and safely applied by lay rescuers of all ages. The method can even be used by the victim and to save people whose lungs have filled with water as they have begun to drown. The technique is basically this:

The rescuer places his or her fist with the thumb against the victim's abdomen, slightly above the navel, but below the rib cage. The rescuer then grasps the fist with the other hand and presses into the abdomen with a quick, upward thrust.

The thrust pushes up the diaphragm and forces a large volume of air up from the lungs to the site of the obstruction. The resulting pressure and flow of air expel the obstructing object.

The maneuver can be repeated several times if it doesn't work at first. If the victim is standing, the rescuer stands behind him or her to apply the maneuver. If the victim is seated, the rescuer kneels or squats behind the chair.

If the victim has collapsed on the floor, a different hand position should be used: Place the heel of one hand on the abdomen just below the rib cage, and cover it with the other hand. Then sit astride the victim at the thighs, and with the victim's face turned upward, apply the technique.

If the rescuer is too small or too weak to reach around the victim from behind, or if the victim is obese, the maneuver can be performed effectively only if the victim is lying on his or her back.

When rescuing an infant, instead of a fist, use the forefinger and middle finger of one hand to apply the abdominal thrust.

To rescue yourself, place your fist in the correct position, grasp it with the other hand, and do the upward thrust.

To prevent breaking ribs and injuring internal organs, it is extremely important that the rescuer not squeeze or hug the victim. *The chest should not be compressed.* Also, if the victim is lying down, the rescuer must straddle the person, not kneel alongside.

Recognizing a Choking Victim

It is important not to panic and to take a few seconds to assess the situation before attempting a rescue. If a person's airway is completely blocked, he or she will not be able to speak, breathe, or cough normally. A choking person may motion frantically and have a terrified look on his or her face.

In a few minutes the victim may turn blue and lose consciousness, but don't wait for the victim to collapse to attempt a rescue. A person who is suffering a heart attack will, unlike a victim of choking, be able to talk and breathe at first.

The circumstances are also a clue. Most choking deaths occur while the victims are eating or are in or near a dining area. In one study of deaths in Florida restaurants, fifty-five of fifty-six persons who died suddenly had choked on food. Only one "café coronary" was actually a heart attack.

In the typical case the choking victim was talking or laughing while eating and had consumed a fair amount of alcohol. To help identify a choking victim further, Dr. Heimlich suggests the use of a universal sign — the victim grasps his or her throat with a hand if he or she is choking and cannot talk or breathe.

However, if the victim is coughing, the windpipe is only partly obstructed, and the person can get in enough air to prevent death. In this situation, wait a minute. If it becomes obvious that the victim is weakening and cannot clear the obstruction alone, apply the Heimlich maneuver.

Dr. Heimlich is convinced that whether the obstruction is partial or complete, the victim should not be slapped on the back. However, the choking rescue taught by the American Red Cross and endorsed by a National Academy of Sciences committee on emergency procedures includes four back slaps (between the shoulder blades, using the fleshy part of the hand) before the Heimlich maneuver is applied four times.

HOW TO DO THE HEIMLICH MANUEVER

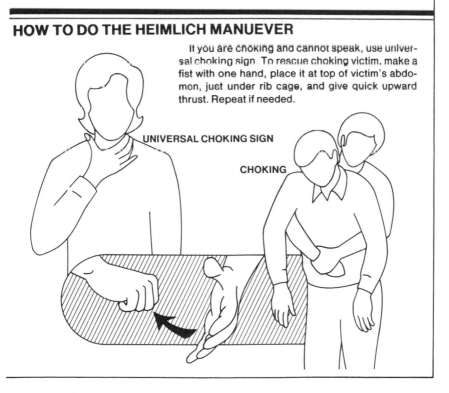

If you are choking and cannot speak, use universal choking sign. To rescue choking victim, make a fist with one hand, place it at top of victim's abdomen, just under rib cage, and give quick upward thrust. Repeat if needed.

UNIVERSAL CHOKING SIGN

CHOKING

The academy committee cited one study indicating that the back slaps produce a sharp spike of pressure in the windpipe that dislodges the obstructing object, which can then be expelled by the abdominal thrust.

How to Keep from Choking
- Don't talk or laugh with food in your mouth.
- When eating solid food, take small bites, and chew each one well before attempting to swallow. Eat slowly. People who wear dentures should be certain to chew their food thoroughly.
- Don't drink excessively before eating.
- Don't perform vigorous activities when you have food, gum, or candy in your mouth.
- Keep a baby's playing and sleeping areas clear of small objects that can be put in the mouth.
- Don't give peanuts or hard candy or foods with small bones or seeds in them to very small children.
- Check your baby's toys and your own clothes for small loose parts — buttons, pins, jewelry, doll eyes, etc. — that can be pulled off and put in the mouth.

CPR: Saving Hearts
Too Good to Die

In 1976 Federal District Judge John J. Sirica suffered a massive heart attack while delivering a speech. Although the former Watergate judge had no heartbeat and was "legally dead" for four minutes, a deputy federal marshal saved his life and his brain by immediately doing mouth-to-mouth breathing and chest compression until hospital rescuers arrived.

Six months before, a thirteen-year-old New Jersey girl — who had just learned the technique, called cardiopulmonary resuscitation, or CPR, in her eighth-grade class — saved her father's life. The fifty-year-old man had collapsed with his second heart attack. His breathing and his heart had stopped, and while his daughter performed CPR, his wife summoned an ambulance.

The federal marshal and the New Jersey eighth-grader are among more than 1 million medical and lay people in the United States who have been trained to perform this lifesaving technique. The goal is to train everyone, from teenagers up, who is willing and able. The reason is that heart attacks are the most common life-threatening medical emergency in this country.

Each year some 1.5 million Americans suffer heart attacks, and 700,000 die as a result — half before the victims ever reach a hospital and

100,000 within the first five minutes of their attack. Rarely is the victim lucky enough to collapse moments away from competent medical assistance. Yet 3 out of 4 sudden deaths are witnessed by bystanders, few of whom know what to do to help save the victim's life. Experts estimate that more than 100,000 lives could be saved by CPR each year if enough people mastered the technique.

What CPR Does

To be performed effectively, CPR must be learned from a qualified instructor and practiced on a mannequin that has been wired to record how well the "rescuer" is doing. While not as simple as learning the ABCs, ABC is, in fact, the clue to effective CPR technique: A for opening the victim's *airway* (breathing passage), B for restoring *breathing* with mouth-to-mouth resuscitation, and C for *cardiac compression,* a rhythmic pressure applied to the chest wall to squeeze blood out of the heart and into the general circulation.

CPR is a holding action, an artificial way to get oxygen-containing blood flowing to the brain and other body tissues when the heart has stopped beating. If the brain's sensitive tissues are deprived of oxygen for more than five minutes, brain death or permanent damage usually occurs. CPR must be started immediately if a victim is unconscious, is not

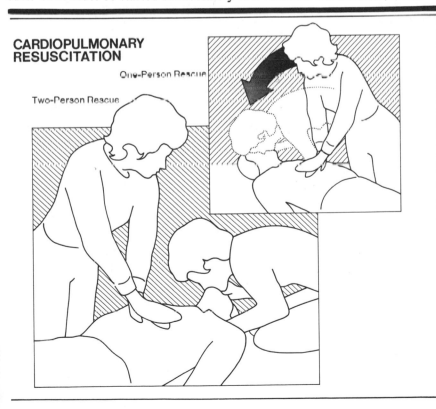

CARDIOPULMONARY RESUSCITATION

One-Person Rescue

Two-Person Rescue

breathing, and has no pulse. It must be continued without halt until the arrival of more sophisticated life support equipment that can restart the heart or maintain it mechanically.

Many victims of sudden death have what cardiologists call "hearts too good to die" — undamaged hearts that could have gone on beating for years if the victims' circulation had been maintained until medical techniques could restore their hearts' normal pumping action.

A study in Birmingham of nineteen consecutive patients taken to a hospital after suffering cardiopulmonary collapse shows the potential of CPR. Eleven of twelve patients for whom CPR was *not* begun within five minutes of their collapse arrived at the hospital in a coma; six died, and five of the six survivors suffered brain damage. By contrast, only two of seven patients for whom CPR was begun within five minutes arrived in a coma; only one died, and only one of the six survivors had brain damage. The five others resumed normal lives, and one took CPR training himself and became a CPR instructor.

In addition to heart attack victims, CPR can rescue victims of drownings, electric shocks (including lightning strikes), drug overdoses, and suffocation.

CPR cannot save all people whose lungs and heart stop functioning. In some, so much heart muscle is damaged by the attack that the heart can no longer be an effective pump. Or the attack may irreversibly damage the heart's electrical conduction system. Sometimes the victim dies despite effective CPR because vomit is inhaled, and other times it is difficult or impossible to transport the CPR-maintained patient to a place where advanced medical care is available.

Since CPR is considered an emergency medical procedure covered by Good Samaritan laws throughout the country, lay rescuers face no liability for damage incurred, unless their intent was clearly malevolent.

CPR was actually proved effective more than twenty years ago, but not until the early 1970's did medical groups like the American Red Cross and the American Heart Association decide to encourage lay people to learn the technique. Now it is recognized that the only way CPR can save a significant number of lives is if millions of ordinary citizens know how to do it.

Some people hesitate to take CPR because they are repulsed by the idea of putting their mouths on a stranger's mouth, but those who have done CPR rescues say that this revulsion disappears instantly when you are faced with a real life or death emergency. Others may think they are not big or strong enough to do CPR, but in fact, anyone who weighs 90 pounds or more can become an effective rescuer.

What and Where to Learn

Even before you have learned CPR, there is one step in the rescue technique that can be learned simply by reading about it, and that may sometimes be all that is needed to restore breathing. This is called the head tilt: With the victim on his or her back, you place one hand under the victim's neck and the other on the forehead, and tilt the jaw up and head back. This keeps the tongue from blocking off the airway and should be the first thing you do when you come upon an unconscious person, unless there is a possibility that the victim's neck is broken.

CPR courses ranging from about six to twelve hours in length are being taught throughout the country. The best way to find out about such courses is to contact your local hospital, Red Cross chapter, or local division of the American Heart Association. It is especially important for those who live with a heart patient to learn the technique.

X.
Medical
Care

The medical care system is admittedly an awesome and intimidating enterprise. It is also often mystifying, especially to lay people who understand neither the language nor the methods used by physicians and other medical care personnel and institutions.

Out of ignorance and reluctance to question those to whom you trust your health care, you may jeopardize the very health and life you are anxious to preserve. You should know that often the best treatment is *no* treatment, just reassurance that nothing serious is wrong and that time will heal you. The doctor who buys time and provides reassurance instead of a prescription may be doing you a real favor.

Although the axiom of Western medicine is "First, do no harm," harm does indeed result from many medical ministrations and inappropriate choices. Doctors, after all, are human, and the institutions and techniques they must rely on are necessarily imperfect.

Learning how to confront the system, select appropriate care, and ask the right questions can go a long way toward improving your chances for a long and healthy life. Further progress toward better health demands that you become an active participant in your own care.

How to
Choose a Doctor

One of the most important health decisions you'll ever make is the choice of a man or woman to oversee your medical care. Most Americans devote more time and thought to buying a new car than to selecting the physician they will depend on to keep them alive and well. Even those who do some searching around before they decide on a doctor often use the wrong criteria, and as a result, some end up with a "lemon."

Several of the traditional guidelines to finding a good physician — such as asking friends, checking credentials, and calling the local medical society — are no guarantee of quality medical care, and some may be next to useless. You may find a superbly trained doctor to whom you could never relate, or you may find one who is highly personable but medically incompetent. What you should get is a doctor who combines the virtues of both — a sensitive, empathetic human being with good training who practices scientific medicine.

To compile a list of possibilities, call the nearest hospital that is affiliated with a medical school or that has a residency training program, and ask the department of internal medicine or family practice for names of doctors on the staff who have private practices in your area. In many areas the county medical society can also provide a list of names. Ask the local pharmacist, as well as colleagues, friends, or neighbors whose opinions you trust, for the names of their personal physicians.

Factors to Consider

Select a doctor while you're healthy. Few people think about doctors when they feel perfectly healthy. Actually this is just when you should select a physician who can help preserve your health as well as oversee any future medical needs. When you're sick and anxious, you have little time or physical and emotional energy to devote to the steps outlined below. Chances are, you'll go to the first doctor you find who will see you immediately, or you'll be forced to use a hospital emergency room.

Choose a primary care physician. Too many people fragment their medical care by seeing only specialists — a dermatologist for a skin rash, an allergist for a perpetual runny nose, a urologist for a urinary tract infection, an orthopedist for a sprained ankle, etc. Many women improperly use their gynecologist as a general practitioner since he or she is often the only doctor a woman sees on a regular basis.

While there is clearly a need for medical specialists under certain circumstances, there is a far greater need for someone who sees you as a total person, not as an organ housed in a body. Your regular physician should be either a family practitioner or an internist (both undergo years of specialty training to become "generalists") who keeps track of all aspects of your health care and determines when another specialist's care may be needed.

Ideally the same doctor should look after you and your spouse and, in the case of a family practitioner, perhaps your children as well. This gives the doctor a better idea of family influences on the health of individual members and often helps in diagnosing an ailment that may afflict more than one family member. For example, for years doctors had been telling my husband that the itchy, painful rash he had on his hands was eczema, but not until a doctor saw both him and our son at the same time was it apparent that both have psoriasis.

Consider the doctor's age and sex. Generally speaking, look for a doctor who is neither very young nor very old. Dr. George D. LeMaitre, author of *How to Choose a Good Doctor* (see reading list below), suggests that you select someone who is under sixty years of age and not likely to retire or die before you are ready to move on. A younger doctor also is more likely to know the latest medical developments, although an older doctor has more clinical experience.

If you are a man, would you feel comfortable with a woman doctor? If you're a woman, would you prefer a female physician?

Check on training, credentials, and hospital affiliation. Choose a doctor who has obtained certification in an American specialty board — either internal medicine or family practice — or who is board-qualified (completed specialty training but not yet passed the examination). You can obtain this information from the doctor's office or the local medical society or at a large public library from the *Directory of Medical Specialists* or the *American Medical Directory*.

The doctor should have admitting privileges at a good nearby hospital (one fully accredited by the Joint Commission on the Accreditation of Hospitals), preferably a hospital affiliated with a medical school or with a specialty training program. Such physicians are likely to know the latest techniques and have access to highly qualified specialists if needed.

Consider such practical matters as accessibility and fees. A doctor who is hard to get to (for example, for reasons of distance, traffic, or parking), who is available only during hours when you could not conveniently get there, who keeps you waiting too long, or who charges more than you can comfortably pay is not a doctor you're likely to get much use of. If you are housebound, look for a doctor who makes house calls. Ask who covers for the doctor when he or she is out of town. Is the doctor's answering service efficient and reliable?

Evaluate the doctor's attitude and manner. As important as a doctor's knowledge is the way in which he or she relates to patients. Medicine is as much an art as a science. Are you seen as a person with a life outside the doctor's office and a human being beyond the ailment in question? Do you feel comfortable trusting this person with your life (it may someday come to that)? Does the doctor treat you warmly and un-hurriedly? Do you feel comfortable about asking questions and relating intimate matters? [See chapter on how to talk to your doctor, page 435.]

Spurn doctors who practice assembly-line medicine, flitting from patient to patient in a series of examining rooms, or continually inter-rupting your visit to take phone calls that aren't urgent. Good medicine takes time, concentration, and hard work.

The attitude of office personnel is often a good clue to the doctor's manner. When you call, are you treated courteously, and are your ques-tions fully answered?

Does the doctor "play God" rather than willingly admit to uncer-tainty? Are you made a party to decisions about your care? Does the doc-tor readily seek or welcome a second doctor's opinion when in doubt or confronted with a difficult medical decision?

Look for an emphasis on preventive medicine. "The most up-to-date, highly trained doctor can be useless to his patient if he doesn't cover the big picture by teaching his patients about good health and how to maintain it," Dr. LeMaitre says. Your doctor should inquire about your diet, exercise habits, smoking and drinking habits, occupational risks, and hobbies and should make appropriate health-promoting recommendations. Preventing illness is the most important aspect of medical care, especially since most serious ailments are not curable.

Avoid red herrings. Doctors who have a long list of famous patients or who must schedule appointments weeks or months in advance are not necessarily the best doctors and may actually have little time for "ordi-nary" patients.

Beware of doctors who routinely make telephone diagnoses, who immediately order batteries of expensive (and possibly hazardous) tests, or who are too quick to prescribe antibiotics, tranquilizers, or other po-tent drugs before exhausting simpler remedies. Most routine ailments brought to a doctor's attention are viral in origin and not amenable to antibiotic therapy. Except in highly select circumstances, tranquilizers are inappropriate solutions for someone having difficulty coping with the normal stresses of life.

For Further Reading

Belsky, Marvin S., M.D., and Leonard Gross. *How to Choose & Use Your Doctor.* New York: Arbor House, 1975.

LeMaitre, George D., M.D. *How to Choose a Good Doctor.* Andover, Mass: Andover Publishing Co., 1979.

Levin, Arthur, M.D. *Talk Back to Your Doctor.* New York: Doubleday, 1975.

Talking to Your Doctor: Key to Good Care

Most of us at one time or another have suffered from the same disease: inability to talk to our doctors. We have been told things by doctors that we didn't understand, and not wanting to appear stupid or to question the doctor's judgment or to take up too much of his or her valuable time, we went home worried or confused.

Among the many common fears:

● If you ask your doctor what he means by hypertension, fibroid, edema, or any other medical terms he may use, he will think you're stupid.

● If you ask the doctor how she arrived at her diagnosis, she will think you're challenging her judgment.

● If you tell him it hurts when he examines you, he will think you're a complainer.

● If you call to tell her about side effects of the medication she prescribed, she'll think you're never satisfied.

● If you tell the doctor about your drinking problem, he'll think you're no good and won't want to treat you.

All the above statements are false — or at least they should be. If not, there's something wrong with the doctor — and possibly with the patient as well.

It's very easy to be intimidated by doctors. Clearly they know a lot more than we do. Time is short, and there's a waiting room full of people with problems perhaps worse than ours. And since most of our interactions with doctors occur when we are sick and frightened and highly vulnerable, we often welcome the opportunity to regard the doctor as an omniscient healer who will take over and make us well.

The time has come, though, for doctors to stop playing God and for patients to stop worshiping their physicians. While it is important for patients to have confidence in the men and women to whom they entrust their medical care, the doctor-knows-best, let-the-doctor-do-all-the-talking-and-make-all-the-decisions attitude can be counterproductive to good medical practice and may even endanger the patient's life.

Dr. Marvin S. Belsky, a New York internist, tells of one uncritical patient who was lulled into inaction by her well-known doctor's mistaken assurances. She repeatedly visited the doctor to have a lump on her breast examined, and each time he reassured her that it was nothing. Nine months later, when the lump was finally biopsied, it was found to be cancer.

You can help to shatter the medical mystique by learning what to say to your doctor and when and how to say it. You can learn when to speak up, to be assertive without being offensively aggressive, to participate in decisions about your care without telling the doctor his or her business, to assess your interaction with the doctor and to evaluate critically the care he or she gives you without becoming a doctor-hopper.

Improving Patient-Doctor Communication

The following guidelines can help you get the most out of your communication with doctors and improve the efficiency and quality of the medical care you receive.

● Always check your understanding of what the doctor has told you about your condition and its treatment. Repeat to the doctor in your own words the nature of the problem and what you're supposed to do about it. Even better, write it down right there in the doctor's office. Some doctors deliberately use medical jargon to impress their patients. Most use it inadvertently, forgetting that not everyone understands that, for example, hypertension means "high blood pressure" and not "high-strung" or "under stress." Ask doctors to define any word or phrase they use that you're not certain you understand.

● Tell your doctor *all* details about your health, including your personal and your family's medical history ("crazy" relatives and all), stressful factors in your life, illnesses that you may regard as shameful, drugs you may use or abuse (including alcohol). It's not your job to decide what is and what is not relevant to your condition. Tell your doctors everything and let them decide.

● It is no virtue when consulting with a doctor to deny the facts of your illness. When a neighbor on the street asks, "Hi, how are you?" you may reply, "Fine," even if you're really falling apart. But when your doctor asks that question, it's your duty to tell him or her that you've been having trouble sleeping, or your back hurts, or your marriage is on the rocks, or whatever ails you mentally or physically. Half or more of the physical problems brought to doctors turn out to have an emotional basis, so if your doctor is going to be able to arrive at a proper diagnosis and treatment, he or she needs to know what is going on in your head as well as your body.

● Prepare for your visits to the doctor by carefully observing your condition and by making a list of what you want to tell or ask him or her. Be concise, but give detailed information — not "I get stomachaches," but "I get a sharp pain on the right side of my abdomen an hour or two after eating a big meal." You might even rehearse beforehand how you will discuss a particularly delicate matter such as an embarrassing problem or your desire to see a consulting physician.

● Be sure your doctor explains the benefits and risks of and alternatives to the treatment recommended. If he or she suggests surgery, for example, ask what other treatments might be tried first or what would happen if you decided not to have an operation at this time. [See chapter on surgery, page 451.]

• If a drug is prescribed, what are the side effects you might experience and how should you cope with them? Too many patients fill the prescription, take a few pills, decide the cure is worse than the disease, and, without telling the doctor, stop taking the medicine or change the dosage. Side effects (known or suspected) that disturb you should be reported immediately to your doctor, who may modify how you take the drug or prescribe another less troublesome medication. [See chapter on drugs, page 457.]

• You should request a consultation with another physician under the following circumstances: If your doctor is unable to make a definite diagnosis within a reasonable length of time, say, two or three visits; if the doctor says you have a serious chronic or potentially fatal illness, such as diabetes or cancer; if the doctor diagnoses a very rare illness; if the doctor says your illness has an emotional basis; or if surgery is recommended as the treatment or to aid in diagnosis.

• Tell the doctor if you are unhappy about the way you are being treated by office assistants, the answering service, or the doctor himself or herself. Say so if you feel rushed, brushed aside, talked down to, if you think the doctor isn't hearing what you're saying or has given you a treatment regimen that you know will disrupt your life in a way that will greatly reduce your chances of following it.

Your doctor doesn't have to be as sympathetic as your best friend, and you don't have to "love" him or her. But your doctor should be someone you feel listens to you — to both your verbal and your nonverbal messages — and in whom you can confide about matters that may affect your health. If you have no rapport with your doctor or he or she fails to take the time to "see" you as a whole person as well as a collection of organs, you might want to consider finding another physician.

Before You Call the Doctor . . .

In their book, *How to Talk to Doctors* (see "For Further Reading," page 438), Dr. John Verby of the University of Minnesota Medical School and Jane Verby recommend the following steps before you call your doctor about an illness:
1. Take your temperature, and record it.
2. Jot down the things that bother you, such as headache, dizziness when standing, sore throat, aching ear.
3. Recall when your condition began and if other symptoms may have preceded your present ones.
4. List the order in which your symptoms appeared.
5. Know what medications you are now taking, how much and how often.
6. Decide what you want from the doctor — an appointment to discuss your condition and decide on a treatment; a complete physical

examination; advice over the phone; a decision on how to proceed from here.

7. Consider how urgent your need is to see the doctor and what days and hours are best for you to make an appointment. Be sure to call if you find you cannot get to the doctor at the appointed time.

For Further Reading

Belsky, Marvin S., M.D., and Leonard Gross. *How to Choose and Use Your Doctor.* New York: Arbor House, 1975.

Levin, Arthur, M.D. *Talk Back to Your Doctor.* New York: Doubleday, 1975.

Preston, Thomas, M.D. *The Clay Pedestal: A Reexamination of the Doctor-Patient Relationship.* Seattle: Madrona, 1981.

Verby, John, M.D., and Jane Verby. *How to Talk to Doctors.* New York: Arco, 1977.

Routine Medical Checkups: What and How Often?

Perhaps nothing is more of an institution in American medicine than the annual checkup. Millions of Americans have them, and millions more suffer twinges of guilt because they think they *should* have them but don't. However, growing numbers of physicians are questioning the advisability, need, health benefits, and cost effectiveness of this medical ritual. Several specialists say routine checkups should be abandoned altogether because, they maintain, the examinations rarely reveal presymptomatic illness where the start of early treatment actually makes a difference in the outcome. Others urge a significant variation on the annual theme, with the frequency of examination geared to the individual's age and likely health problems.

Still others defend the annual routine checkup as the best value for your health dollar, able to detect unsuspected conditions such as high blood pressure, diabetes, and curable cancers of the cervix and colon before symptoms arise and complications develop. The periodic checkup has been shown to reduce deaths and disability from a number of "postponable" diseases, including the effects of high blood pressure and certain cancers. Proponents of the annual checkup also say it is the best way to establish a friendly and informed relationship with the "quartermaster" of your body, the doctor whom you may need to call on during the rest of the year for telephone consultation, emergency treatment, prescription refills, or medical advice.

The questions of whether, where, and how often to have a checkup, as well as what kind of checkup to have, who should do it, and how much it should cost, are becoming increasingly pertinent as hundreds of automated health testing centers and prepaid health maintenance organizations spring up around the country and as medical insurance companies restructure their coverage with a greater emphasis on preventive care.

What's in a Checkup?

A checkup can range from a half hour $30 computer analysis of blood, urine, and other test results to a three-day $500 executive-style examination at a major medical clinic. However, most examinations today take about forty-five minutes to an hour, cost $50 to $150 and are done by private physicians — internists, family practitioners, and pediatricians — or specially trained nurse practitioners who are supervised by physicians.

Some doctors recommend annual checkups for all adults; others recommend a checkup every five years in early adulthood, gradually increasing in frequency until the examination finally becomes yearly after, say, the age of sixty or later. Most doctors recommend, at the least, a complete baseline examination early in adult life, say, by age 30.

According to Dr. Arthur Levin, author of *Talk Back to Your Doctor* (see "For Further Reading," page 442), the baseline examination should include a thorough history (fifteen to thirty minutes), in which the doctor asks about your social, occupational, and medical history, your family's medical history, and the functioning of all your body parts and organ systems (eyes, heart, bowels, skin, emotions, and so forth); a physical examination (ten to fifteen minutes) in which the doctor examines your entire body by observing, feeling, thumping, or listening through instruments to appropriate parts; and laboratory tests, including complete blood count, urinalysis, TB skin test, Pap smear (for women) and stool test for hidden blood. Other tests may be done on the basis of your physical examination, symptoms, or personal or family history.

439

A chest X ray is not a necessary part of the examination unless you have respiratory symptoms or are exposed to substances, such as cigarette smoke or asbestos, that can cause lung disease. Most cardiologists believe that an electrocardiogram is of limited value unless it is done as a stress test while the patient is exercising on a treadmill or stationary bicycle. [See chapter on exercise stress testing, page 95.]

The ostensible purpose of a periodic checkup is to maintain health. While most doctors do examinations and tests — such as taking blood pressure, checking for sugar in the urine, or examining the cells of the cervix (Pap smear) — that can reveal early signs of curable or controllable illness, many neglect factors such as personal habits, nutrition, safety precautions, and emotional stresses that can be reshaped to help you prevent illness.

Dr. Lester Breslow, dean of the School of Public Health at the University of California, Los Angeles, and Ann R. Somers, community medicine specialist at Rutgers Medical School in New Jersey, have outlined a "lifetime health-monitoring program" that is widely regarded as a reasonable and practical way to do periodic checkups to maintain good health. Their recommendations for adults are described in the chart on page 441. If your doctor neglects the counseling and educational component of your periodic checkup, you are not getting your money's worth.

What to Consider

Here are other factors you should take into account when submitting to a checkup, whether once a year, once every five years, or once in a lifetime:

Time and timing. Dr. Isadore Rosenfeld, a New York cardiologist who wrote *The Complete Medical Exam* (see "For Further Reading," page 442), says that a half-hour exam is not enough. He warns against going to a doctor who has a very busy practice treating sick people because such a doctor is unlikely to give the checkup the time and undivided attention it should have. Dr. Rosenfeld also suggests avoiding late-afternoon and early Monday morning appointments, when the doctor may be distracted or tired.

The examiner. If possible, Dr. Rosenfeld says, avoid relying on a superspecialist — one who is devoted to the care and healing of a particular organ system — who may give relatively short shrift to the rest of your body. You might also think twice before going to a distant clinic or an automated health testing center because these will not provide you with the one unquestioned benefit of a routine checkup: the establishment of a continuing relationship with a physician. However, a completely adequate examination can be done by a nurse practitioner who works for your doctor.

The cost. Ask first what the examination is likely to cost, and check your insurance policy to see what it covers. Most policies do not reimburse for routine examinations of healthy people. If any abnormality is found in the course of your examination, make sure your doctor records it on your insurance claim form. That way you may get something back.

Preparation. Do not try to "whip yourself into shape" in the days or weeks before your examination, Dr. Rosenfeld warns. A crash diet can throw off the lab tests, and a sudden spurt of exercise can precipitate serious, even fatal illness. When you make the appointment, ask whether you should follow any special diet or clean out your bowel before arriving at the doctor's office.

The history. Your medical and family history, which preferably should take about half an hour the first time the doctor takes it, is the most important part of a checkup. More than 50 percent of internal illnesses can be picked up on the basis of the history alone (20 percent by the physical examination and another 20 percent by lab tests). The doctor should quiz you about your habits, occupation, leisure activities, family and job stresses, and family medical history as well as your present symptoms and past medical history. Tell him or her all pertinent facts about your health, including emotional, marital, or sexual problems. You may be asked to complete a lengthy questionnaire, which the doctor should review with you before doing the physical exam.

Disrobing. For the physical examination, you should undress completely and be given a sterile gown or sheet to cover you between parts of

HEALTH-MONITORING PROGRAM FOR ADULTS

Age	Frequency of Exams*	Services to Be Provided
18 to 24	Once	Complete physical, medical and behavorial history. Tetanus booster. Tests for syphillis, gonorrhea, malnutrition, cholesterol and blood pressure. Health education in nutrition, exercise, study, career, job, occupational hazards, sex, contraception, marriage and family relations, alcohol, drugs, smoking, and driving.
25 to 39	Twice at about 30 and 35	Complete physical. Tests for blood pressure, anemia, cholesterol, cervical and breast cancer. Instruction in self-examination of breasts, skin, testes, neck, and mouth. Counseling in nutrition, exercise, smoking, alcohol, marital, parental, and other aspects of behavior and life style related to health.
40 to 59	Four times, once every five years	Complete physical and medical history. Tests for chronic conditions (high blood pressure, heart disease, diabetes, cancer, vision, and hearing impairment). Immunizations, as needed. Counseling in changing nutritional needs, physical activities, occupation, sex, adjustment to menopause, marital and parental problems, use of cigarettes, alcohol, and drugs. For those over 50, annual tests for blood pressure, obesity, and certain cancers.
60 to 74	Every two years	Complete physical. Tests for chronic conditions (see above). Counseling regarding changing life style related to retirement, nutritional requirements, absence of children, possible loss of spouse and probable reduction in income and physical resources. Annual flu shot. Periodic podiatry treatments, if needed.
75 and over	At least once a year	Complete physical, medical, and behavorial history. Counseling regarding changing nutritional requirements, living arrangements, limitation on activity and mobility. Annual flu shot.

*For healthy persons.

Note: Most services listed above can be effectively rendered by specially trained nurse practitioners or other paramedical personnel under a physician's supervision.

Source: Based on "Lifetime Health-Monitoring Program" by Dr. Lester Breslow and Anne R. Somers, *New England Journal of Medicine,* March 17, 1977.

441

Aftermath. To get the most for your money, prepare yourself mentally to act on some or all of the doctor's recommendations to maintain your health, whether it means losing weight, reducing the salt and fat in your diet, cutting back on alcohol or addicting drugs, quitting smoking, exercising, or using seat belts. Ask the doctor to explain the potential health value of his or her recommendations (you may also request some pertinent literature) and to outline a sensible approach to making the necessary changes in your life.

As Dr. Richard C. Bates, a Lansing, Michigan, internist, wrote in the magazine *Medical Economics*: "I regard the [routine] exam as an exercise not to find disease but to prevent it. Heart attacks, accidents, emphysema, cirrhosis, and lung cancer are very rare diseases among my clientele because I care about the way they care about themselves."

For Further Reading

Levin, Arthur, M.D. *Talk Back to Your Doctor.* New York: Doubleday, 1975.
Rosenfeld, Isadore, M.D. *The Complete Medical Exam.* New York: Simon & Schuster, 1978.

Laboratory Tests: What They Are and What They Mean

A forty-five-year-old friend proudly announced that he had just had a complete checkup and had been told that his cholesterol level and blood pressure were "normal." When I asked what the readings were, he responded, "Well, I don't know. The doctor didn't tell me, and anyway, they wouldn't mean anything to me."

Few people understand the significance of laboratory and other health tests, and even fewer can interpret their results. Yet knowing how you fared on various tests and what the results mean can make you a more effective partner in your health care.

The results of laboratory tests are not diagnoses, but clues to possible abnormalities. In most cases an abnormal finding can reflect any number of possible disorders involving various organs or body functions.

All tests require interpretation by a physician, and Dr. Mike Oppenheim, a Los Angeles general practitioner writing in *Woman's Day*, cautions against having a battery of tests (such as in a multiphasic health screening program) without first consulting a physician. Too often — Dr. Oppenheim estimates 5 percent of cases — the test battery turns up one or more falsely abnormal results that set in motion a chain of further tests, needlessly alarm the patient, and add to the cost of medical care.

Whenever a test result falls out of the normal range, the test should be repeated before any assumptions are made about its health significance. Even the best of medical laboratories sometimes make mistakes, or an error may be made in collecting the specimen, or some other unusual circumstance may have skewed the result.

If you are tested, the doctor should explain to your satisfaction what the results may mean. Too often, though, people are content to accept their doctors' verdict without question and fail to realize that for some test results, such as cholesterol and blood pressure, what is "normal" from an American perspective may be abnormal if you take a more global view.

Test results can be distorted by diet (that is why some are done only after an eight-hour fast), vigorous exercise, over-the-counter and prescription drugs (including aspirin, vitamins, and birth control pills), alcohol, lack of sleep, stress, fear, or anxiety. Be sure to tell the doctor about the drugs you are taking and anything unusual about your current life.

Always record the results of important tests like cholesterol and blood pressure, and keep them, properly dated, as part of your personal health record.

In their booklet "A Self-Health Guide to Medical Laboratory Tests" (see "For Further Reading," page 445), Dr. Gary R. McIlroy and Marlene Travis point out that medical tests can alert the doctor to a hidden disease, assist in diagnosing a suspected problem, or warn of a potential risk. But, they add, it's also important to realize that no series of laboratory tests can certify you as healthy.

The Common Tests

Here is what you should know about common medical tests:

Cholesterol. Cholesterol, a waxy alcohol found in the blood, can become part of the deposits that clog the arteries. [See chapter on fats and cholesterol, page 14.] The usual serum cholesterol measurement reflects the total amount found in 100 milliliters of blood serum and is represented as so many milligrams percent or as ml per dl (for deciliter). High levels of serum cholesterol have been linked to an increased risk of heart disease.

However, more important than total cholesterol are the relative contributions of the different types — HDL, or high-density lipoprotein, cholesterol, which helps to *protect* against heart disease; and LDL, or low-density lipoprotein, and VLDL, or very-low-density lipoprotein cholesterol, both of which contribute to cardiac risk. You should have at least one measurement made of your cholesterol fractions, and if you are found to have high total cholesterol and low HDL levels, follow your doctor's advice about eating less fat and cholesterol, increasing the amount you exercise, and losing weight.

Do not be content with a doctor's statement that your cholesterol level is "normal." Most doctors regard a reading of up to 260 milligrams percent as "within the normal range" and some go as high as 300 milligrams in defining "normal." Yet such levels are associated with a relatively high risk of developing heart disease. In countries where heart attacks are rare, the average (that is, "normal") cholesterol level is well below 200.

Blood pressure. Your blood pressure reading is represented by two numbers: The higher one, systolic pressure, represents the force generated when your heart pumps; the lower number, or diastolic pressure, is that between beats. Since many factors, including anxiety and fear, can distort your true blood pressure, at least three measurements, preferably on different days and at different times of day, should be made before the existence of an abnormally high pressure is assumed. (Low blood pressure is not a hazard, unless you get dizzy when you stand up.)

A reading of 120/80 (the numbers refer to millimeters of mercury) or lower is considered normal. For adults, 140/90 is considered the border line between normal and high. However, even a lower reading in youngsters and young adults may be cause for concern because it signals a potential future problem. Your blood pressure should be taken at every medical visit.

Treatment of even mild high blood pressure can be lifesaving. Treatment measures include achieving normal weight, maintaining a diet low in salt and other sources of sodium, and, possibly, the use of diuretic or other drugs. [See chapter on high blood pressure, page 631.]

Glucose. Too much sugar in the blood or urine can be a clue to existing or impending diabetes as well as to other health problems. Tests for excess sugar are best done following a fast since food significantly alters the results. A reading of 60 to 115 milligrams per 100 milliliters of blood is considered normal. [See chapter on diabetes, page 660.]

Many people have been incorrectly diagnosed as suffering from low blood sugar, or hypoglycemia, on the basis of a glucose tolerance test. A proper diagnosis of hypoglycemia must be based on a dramatic fall in blood sugar that is *simultaneously* accompanied by such symptoms of low blood sugar as weakness, headache, and nausea. [See chapter on low blood sugar, page 509.]

Urinalysis. Normally urine is sterile and contains few, if any, cells or nutrients. A single urine sample can be used to check for many factors — including sugar, protein (albumin), blood, crystals of chemicals, bilirubin (resulting from an excessive breakdown of red blood cells), bacteria, and pus — that could signal kidney or other diseases or infection. Urine is also checked for its color (very dark urine may indicate dehydration or illness), odor, clarity, and acidity.

Blood tests. A complete blood cell count can be done on a few drops of blood from a single pinprick. The test examines the volume of red blood cells, which carry oxygen to body tissues. A deficiency may indicate anemia, possibly the result of hidden blood loss or excessive menstrual bleeding. An excess may also indicate illness.

An excess of white blood cells occurs as a result of infection, leukemia, or allergy; other conditions, such as exposure to radiation or toxic chemicals, can cause deficiencies. A precise diagnosis is based in part on which of the five types of white blood cells is present in abnormal amounts.

The most common indicators of anemia are the amount of hemoglobin (the oxygen-carrying pigment in red blood cells) in the blood or, even better, the hematocrit — the percentage of the total blood volume that is composed of blood cells (mostly red blood cells). A normal hematocrit is 40 to 55 percent (slightly lower in women).

The blood can also be analyzed for chemical substances in addition to glucose: enzymes (SGOT and SGPT from the liver and muscles, LDH from muscles and red blood cells, and alkaline phosphatase from liver or bone); blood urea nitrogen (BUN), a measure of kidney function; thyroxine (measured as T4), the thyroid hormone; creatinine, a measure of muscle and kidney function; uric acid, a possible indicator of gout; and sodium, potassium, and chloride, the electrolytes that are essential to normal cell function. The blood sedimentation rate measures how red blood cells settle in a test tube, a possible indicator of infection.

For Further Information

For detailed information about the hundreds of medical tests, their possible significance and factors that can distort the results, you may want to consult *The Encyclopedia of Medical Tests* by Cathey Pinckney and Edward R. Pinckney, (New York: Wallaby Pocket Books, 1978). Try your library, or contact Facts on File, 460 Park Avenue South, New York, New York 10016.

The booklet ''A Self-Health Guide to Medical Laboratory Tests'' by Dr. Gary R. McIlroy and Marlene Travis can be purchased from Healthstyles Publications, 4005 West Sixty-fifth Street, Minneapolis, Minnesota 55435.

X Rays:
Reducing the Risks of Radiation

Inhabitants of the modern world are surrounding themselves with an ever-increasing number of sources of radiation — from such consumer items as CB radios, microwave ovens, smoke detectors, and sun lamps to environmental sources like communication towers, high-tension electrical lines, and nuclear power plants.

In recent years public concern has mounted about the hazards of being exposed to these and other sources of radiation over a period of many years, particularly since they are added to the unavoidable background, or natural, radiation from sky and earth.

At the same time, however, lay people have paid relatively little attention to the most common nonnatural source of potentially harmful radiation in today's world — medical and dental X rays. Together these account for more than 90 percent of the public's exposure to man-made sources of radiation.

In a year, two-thirds of the population undergoes one or more X ray examinations or treatments, with the typical examination involving five separate X ray films. The number of X ray examinations received by the average American is now growing by what some experts consider an alarming rate.

While in most cases the benefits of these X rays clearly outweigh the hypothetical risks, studies have shown that many health-related X ray exposures are inappropriate or frankly unnecessary. Of those X rays that are needed, some expose the individual to far more radiation than they should. By being alert to the possibility of abuse and by asking a few pointed questions, you can do much to protect yourself from avoidable radiation risks.

There are two kinds of radiation: ionizing (X rays, cosmic rays, radiation from radioactive materials, and shortwave ultraviolet radiation from sunlight and sun lamps) and nonionizing (radiowaves, microwaves, infrared and longer-wave ultraviolet radiation). Ionizing radiation is the more damaging of the two, capable of disrupting atoms by knocking off electrons and causing injury to the cells or genetic material of living tissues.

Nonionizing radiation is relatively low in energy, and instead of damaging the atoms in living tissue, it changes their energy level and generates heat. This is the mechanism by which microwave ovens operate. The potential hazards of prolonged exposure to low levels of nonionizing radiation are as yet unknown.

The risks of ionizing radiation, on the other hand, have been well studied. It can produce mutations, or inheritable changes, in the genetic material and thus can cause birth defects and cancer. Its effects are cumulative; repeated exposure to low doses can add up to the damage wrought by a single large dose.

Large doses of X rays (such as might be used in therapy) to the reproductive organs can cause sterility or, in less extreme cases, may damage sperm or eggs and result in the birth of malformed children. X ray exposure during pregnancy may increase the risk that leukemia and other cancers will develop in the offspring. Certain tissues — for example, the thyroid gland and the breasts — are more sensitive to radiation effects than others, and cancers have developed in these tissues many years after radiation treatments to nearby organs.

The much lower radiation doses involved in diagnostic X rays have not yet been directly linked to an increased cancer risk except if exposure occurred prenatally. Nonetheless, there is no such thing as a "safe" dose of ionizing radiation. Thus, whether you are pregnant or not, it is clearly in your best interest to be sure that your exposure to X rays is kept to an essential minimum and that in each case the expected benefits of the examination justify the possible risks.

How to Reduce Your Radiation Exposure

A consideration of the following questions should help you achieve this goal.

Is this X ray necessary? Ask the physician or dentist what the X ray can be expected to show and how this may help in your care. Make sure you understand the explanation well enough to know that the X ray is not being taken just to protect the doctor. Ask whether other less hazardous tests would yield similar information or whether X rays taken at a previous time can be used.

Often when people change physicians or dentists or see a specialist as a consultant, they fail to mention that they have already had X rays taken. In many cases, the old set is adequate or needs only supplementation, rather than a repeat of the whole series.

Routine chest X rays are no longer considered appropriate or necessary. They, like other X rays, should be done only when medically justifiable. A chest X ray is not an essential part of a routine medical exam unless, for example, you are a cigarette smoker or have worrisome respiratory symptoms. Neither are routine dental X rays recommended at every visit or even every year. They should be done only when there is a clear-cut need and no other way to obtain the information.

Do you keep an X ray record? Just as you should keep a record of immunizations, you would also do well to record all X rays: the date, type, and name of the doctor who would have the films. This will help you keep track of your total X ray exposure as well as avoid repeating X rays already taken. You may also request copies of your X rays (for a small additional fee) that you can keep. Free X ray record cards can be obtained by writing to X rays, Food and Drug Administration, Rockville, Maryland 20857. Take your record with you when seeing a physician or dentist for the first time, and ask that the information about your previous X rays be included on your chart.

Are you pregnant or think you could be? Doctors and X ray technicians often fail to ask this crucial question before exposing a woman of childbearing age to X rays that could reach the abdomen. If the X ray is medically necessary, it should be done if the woman is pregnant or not, and a protective lead shield should be used over the abdominal area if this does not interfere with the needed picture. Another alternative may be an ultrasound examination instead of an X ray.

Many X ray examinations, such as preemployment back X rays or dental X rays, are elective and could easily be postponed until after childbirth. Or if you are planning a pregnancy, it might be wise to obtain all needed X rays (such as dental X rays) at least two months before you try to conceive. To avoid inadvertent radiation exposure of a pregnant

447

woman, many physicians and dentists abide by the "ten-day rule" when X-raying a woman of childbearing age. According to this rule, all non-emergency X rays are done within ten days of the start of the menstrual cycle, when pregnancy is highly unlikely.

Are you protected against X ray scatter? Since the reproductive organs are highly vulnerable to radiation damage, the genital area of men and boys and the lower abdomen of girls and women of childbearing age should always be protected by a lead shield or apron during an X ray examination, even of the mouth. For men, a gonad shield gives adequate protection.

Is the X ray dose as low as possible? You are most likely to keep your radiation dose to a minimum if a medical X ray examination is done in the office of a full-time radiologist or in a hospital X ray department, rather than in the office of an ordinary physician. One of the major causes of excess radiation exposure is error on the part of the technician, necessitating a repeat of the film.

All dentists and dental hygienists are trained in proper X ray techniques. But make sure your dentist's machine is fitted with a long, cylindrical X ray cone; the old short, pointed cones deliver far more scattered radiation.

Also check on when the X ray equipment was last inspected. The date should be posted on or near the machine. If inspection was more than two years earlier, you may want to have the X ray taken elsewhere. The older the equipment, the higher the dose it is likely to deliver. The newest mammography (breast X ray) machines, for example, use far less radiation than was the case in the past.

Immunizations: Shots for Good Health

Iron lungs may be long forgotten, but polio and other serious childhood diseases remain a threat to millions of young children who are not adequately immunized against them. All fifty states now require certain immunizations before a child can start school, and schools in many states have begun enforcing tougher laws about proof of immunization for all school-age children, regardless of grade level.

Keep a Record

Many parents are unable to produce concrete evidence that their children are fully immunized against the seven common highly contagious diseases for which effective vaccines are available: diphtheria, pertussis (whooping cough), tetanus, polio, measles, mumps, and rubella. (Experimental vaccines against chickenpox, the remaining plague of childhood, are being tested.) Although most parents probably start off with good intentions and conscientious record keeping, few are able to produce complete and up-to-date immunization records after the first few years of a child's life.

At the same time many parents are confused about how long the vaccines work, how many doses are required for full protection, and the need in some cases (but not others) for periodic booster shots to maintain immunity.

The best way to keep track of your own and your child's immunizations is to obtain an official state immunization record form from your city or county health department and take it with you at every medical checkup so that the doctor can record each vaccine dose as it is given, along with the correct date.

Risks of Complacency

Ironically, successful use of the various vaccines has created the current complacency about immunizations. These days parents just don't think much about measles, for example, when no child they know is af-

---

Recommended Immunization Schedule for Children

The following schedule is advised by the Immunization Division of the Center for Disease Control in Atlanta, a part of the United States Public Health Service.

At this age:	Your child should receive:
2 months	diphtheria, tetanus, pertussis (DTP, first dose) oral polio (first dose)
4 months	DTP (second dose) oral polio (second dose)
6 months	DTP (third dose)
15 months	measles* mumps* rubella*
18 months	DTP (fourth dose) oral polio (third dose)
4 to 6 years (at school entry)	DTP (fifth dose) oral polio (fourth dose)
14 to 16 years and every 10 years thereafter	tetanus-diphtheria booster

*These three may be given combined in a single injection.

flicted with the disease. Others improperly conclude that it is dangerous to have their children immunized because they hear rumors or reports that the risks associated with some vaccines may be greater than the chances of getting the diseases naturally.

In fact, the infrequency of natural infections has bolstered — not diminished — the need for artificial protection through immunization. No longer do millions acquire immunity to these diseases by developing a very mild or an inapparent case through exposure to others who are ill. As long as even a few cases of a disease occur in the population, children who are not immunized are likely to catch it.

Smallpox vaccination is no longer required because the disease has been eliminated in this country and, more recently, in the world, public health officials have concluded. The current goal is to wipe out measles from American soil. Until that is accomplished, every child must be immunized against measles.

Side effects of vaccinations are common, but nearly always mild: a sore arm, slight fever, or mild rash are the usual ones. Only rarely do severe reactions occur, and even less often does an immunized person acquire the disease from the vaccine (for example, 1 in 4 million people who receive oral polio vaccine get polio as a result). The principle of immunization is to trigger the person's immune system, causing, in effect, very mild disease that stimulates the immune system to produce defensive antibodies, just as it would do naturally if the individual had gotten the full-blown disease.

While cases of the preventable diseases are at an all-time low, thousands of youngsters are still threatened each year with one of these infections. In fact, cases of paralytic polio still occur among American children.

Getting the Proper Doses

The following tips for safe and effective immunizations come from the nation's official Advisory Committee of Immunization Practices:

● Most of the commonly administered vaccines can be given simultaneously without compromising their effectiveness or increasing the seriousness of side effects. Thus, an infant may safely receive vaccines for diphtheria, tetanus, and pertussis, (collectively known as DTP) along with oral polio vaccine.

● For full protection, some vaccines, such as those for diphtheria, pertussis, tetanus, and polio, require several doses that are best given a certain number of months apart (see table with recommended schedule). However, if the schedule of doses is interrupted, it is not necessary to start the series again from the beginning or to give extra doses of the vaccine.

● Persons suffering from diseases (such as leukemia) or receiving treatments (such as radiation therapy or corticosteroids) that impair their immunological responses should not be given vaccines made from live, modified viruses because they may develop the full-blown disease. Oral polio vaccine should not be given to household contacts of such individuals because vaccine recipients may transmit the virus.

● Generally, to avoid possible harm to an unborn child, live-virus vaccines — especially rubella, measles, and mumps — should not be given to pregnant women or to women likely to become pregnant within three months. However, there is no known harm from vaccines made from killed viruses (such as the Salk polio injections), bacteria, or toxoids (modified bacterial toxins, such as are used in diphtheria and tetanus vaccines).

● Only one shot is needed to provide complete (and probably life-long) protection against measles, mumps, and rubella, and these three can be given in one combination vaccine. Four doses of oral polio vaccine and five doses of DTP are recommended for full protection. In addition, tetanus and diphtheria boosters should be given every ten years (or, in the case of tetanus, ten years after a dose has been given following a wound that might be contaminated with tetanus bacteria). More frequent tetanus boosters may increase the severity of side effects.

● Now that millions of Americans have taken up outdoor activities or become do-it-yourselfers, it is especially important that everyone maintain full tetanus immunity since the responsible bacteria are ubiquitous in soil and dust. Although the disease, which is fatal in more than 60 percent of cases, is most commonly associated with deep puncture wounds, it has also occurred following the prick of a rose thorn and garden-variety scrapes and scratches. Yet experts estimate that more than three-fourths of adults are not adequately protected against tetanus.

Surgery:
What to Know About Operations

The examination of Eli's coronary arteries indicated that he was a prime candidate for a heart attack. At age fifty-two, with one child entering college and another starting high school, Eli was hardly ready to consider his life over. So, when his internist recommended an operation to bypass the partly obstructed arteries feeding the right side of his heart, Eli was ready to go ahead with it.

The procedure was described to him, and he was shown a movie on what the surgery would be like. But not until he was hospitalized the day before surgery did anyone tell Eli what he really wanted to know: Would it improve his chances of averting a heart attack and premature death?

The surgeon told him that for people with his particular problem the statistics thus far showed no increase in life expectancy or diminished chance of heart attack. Eli canceled the operation, checked out of the hospital, and went home to think about it some more.

Each year some 20 million Americans undergo surgery. Only about 20 percent of these operations are emergencies in which neither patient nor doctor has a real choice about whether or when to operate. Emergency surgery is performed, for example, to control severe bleeding, for suspected appendicitis, to relieve severe pressure on the brain, or to deliver a baby that cannot be delivered safely the usual way. The remaining 80 percent of operations are elective cases, in which the patient, basing a decision on a doctor's advice, chooses to have surgery.

Sometimes the choice involves a life and death matter, as in surgery to remove a cancer, but it is not a medical emergency; there is time to consider alternative therapy and to decide how, when, where, and by whom the operation should be done.

In the vast majority of operations the decision does not involve a life-threatening situation but, rather, a condition that affects the patient's quality of life. Will you stick to a rigid diet and put up with occasional discomforting attacks, or should you have your gallbladder removed? Should you undergo a hysterectomy for those bothersome fibroids? Back surgery to remove a sometimes painful disk? A tonsillectomy for recurrent sore throats? A face-lift to get rid of telltale wrinkles?

Americans are the most operated-on people in the world. We have the highest ratio of surgeons to population, and most of us have insurance that pays most or all of the direct costs of surgery. Surgery is so commonplace that many people fail to realize that all operations are serious and potentially life-threatening and should not be undertaken lightly. They forget that sometimes people die or suffer permanent disability as a result of a so-called routine or minor operation.

Consider Safety and Necessity

Here are some guidelines to help you determine the necessity and desirability of any operation you may be considering and to help assure that any surgery you undergo is performed by a well-qualified physician under circumstances that would favor a healthful outcome.

● Avoid using a surgeon as your regular physician or as the first doctor you see about a problem. A surgeon is someone to consult if an internist, a family practitioner, or some other physician thinks surgery may be warranted. A surgeon is less likely than an internist to give equal consideration to nonsurgical approaches to treatment.

● You should know what is supposedly wrong with you and how

the doctor arrived at the diagnosis. If the explanation is unclear, ask questions until you understand.

• Discuss the alternatives to surgery. You may want to give one of them a try before deciding to go ahead with an operation.

• Choose a surgeon who has been certified by the appropriate American specialty board — for example, obstetrics and gynecology, general surgery, otolaryngology, etc. Just as you wouldn't select a banker to install plumbing, you wouldn't want an orthopedic surgeon to remove your uterus or a general practitioner to operate on your back. About 55 percent of doctors who perform surgery are board-certified surgeons. While that is no guarantee of excellence, it means the doctor has had at least two years of special training and has passed a rigorous examination.

• The surgeon should operate in a hospital accredited by the Joint Commission on Accreditation of Hospitals. If the surgery is complicated or the patient's condition makes an otherwise straightforward operation particularly dangerous or difficult, it may be best to have the operation at a teaching hospital (one affiliated with a medical school). In other cases a good community hospital can provide excellent care. Either way, ask who will actually do the surgery: the doctor you hire or someone else.

• The surgeon should also explain, to your satisfaction, just what benefits you're likely to gain from surgery and what risks you will face. Ask specifically about complications and death rates.

• Ask the surgeon about his or her personal experience with the operation. How many has the surgeon done? What percent succeeded? What are the complications, major and minor, and what percentage of patients developed them?

• Choose a surgeon who is skilled at the operation you will undergo, someone who operates frequently — say, several times a week — but not one who does assembly-line surgery all day long. The busiest and richest surgeons are not necessarily the best.

• Whenever considering surgery, get a second opinion from another qualified surgeon. This is particularly important for operations that are commonly done unnecessarily. These include hysterectomies, gallbladder surgery, tonsillectomies, disk surgery, hemorrhoidectomies, removal of varicose veins, and hernia repairs. [See chapters on hysterectomy, page 232, gallbladder disease, page 595, tonsillectomy, page 306, backaches, page 524, hemorrhoids, page 530, varicose veins, page 561, and hernia, page 619.] If you tell the consultant you already have a surgeon, any financial considerations that might influence the consultant's judgment would be removed. Many insurance plans now cover the cost of a second surgical opinion.

The consultant should review tests already done, repeat those that are in doubt, and perhaps order others that were overlooked. The consultant should examine you and take a complete history of your condition. If the original surgeon and the consultant disagree on the advisability of an operation, you may want a third opinion. Most policies that cover consultations also cover a third opinion in the case of a disagreement.

• Find out what the surgery will entail, how you can expect to feel afterward, how long you are likely to be hospitalized, what kind of assistance you may need when you get home, and when you can expect to be able to resume normal activities. The more such facts you have beforehand, the fewer the surprises and the less psychological and physical discomfort you're likely to feel afterward.

• Ask the surgeon about the fee *before* the operation. Also, check on the hospital's rates and the anesthesiologist's fee. Find out what part of the costs your insurance will cover.

• Ask who will administer the anesthesia. For most elective operations, the anesthesia presents the greatest risk, yet less than half the anesthetics are administered by a physician who has received special training in the field. Often the "anesthetist" is not even a specially trained nurse. While local anesthesia is usually less hazardous than general anesthesia, it can also present serious risks and should be administered only by a well-trained professional, such as a nurse-anesthetist.

• Don't insist on an operation if your doctor advises against it. Some people actually prescribe their own unnecessary surgery. If one doctor doesn't want to operate, they shop around until they find someone who will.

Like Eli, many people fail to ask the questions that will help them to decide whether they really want to undergo a particular operation — if to them, the potential benefits would outweigh the possible risks. Sometimes risks, including the risk of death, are not even considered in the decision to undergo surgery. Many people accept without question a doctor's recommendation for surgery. However, one doctor may be able to treat a condition surgically while another physician may be able to cure that condition with drugs, diet, rest, exercise, or simply time. By checking into alternatives, you can sometimes avoid an unnecessary operation.

For Further Reading

Crile, George, Jr., M.D. *Surgery: Your Choices, Your Alternatives.* New York: Delacorte, 1978.

Denney, Myron K., M.D. Second Opinion. New York: Grosset & Dunlap, 1979.

Isenberg, Seymour, M.D., and L. M. Elting, M.D. *The Consumer's Guide to Successful Surgery.* New York: St. Martin's Press, 1976.

Kra, Siegfried J., M.D., and Robert S. Boltax, M.D. *Is Surgery Necessary?* New York: Macmillan, 1981.

454

Ambulatory Surgery: Cheaper and Safer

Joann, thirty-five-year-old mother of two, was scheduled to undergo a sterilization operation. She arrived at the hospital at 8:00 A.M., was through with surgery by 10, and was home in time to lunch with her sons. She recalls, "It made all the difference not having to spend the night in the hospital. I wasn't sick, and I'm sure I recovered a lot faster at home than I would have in a sterile hospital room."

Ambulatory — or outpatient — surgery is a fast-growing phenomenon in the United States. When appropriate, one-day surgery in a hospital outpatient facility, freestanding surgical clinic, or doctor's office can save time and money, prevent family disruptions, and greatly reduce the psychological and physical trauma of having an operation.

Years ago minor surgery was often done in doctors' offices. Then, as the surgical profession assumed responsibility for most operations, more and more surgery was moved into heavily equipped and well-staffed hospital operating rooms. Regardless of how healthy they may have been to start with, postoperative patients often spent a week or more "resting" in a hospital bed and frequently left the hospital quite debilitated, invalided more by "hospitalitis" than by the actual effects of surgery.

The Benefits

Surgeons now realize that patients recover faster if they get out of bed and out of the hospital as soon as possible. The less time spent in the hospital, the less likely the patient is to acquire a hospital-based infection and the mental attitude of a sick person. Furthermore, the cost saving, if not directly to the patient, then to the patient's insurance company (and ultimately the patient's insurance costs), ranges from 50 to 75 percent. Ambulatory surgery reduces delays in waiting for a hospital bed and lessens the chances of getting bumped from scheduled surgery when emergencies take priority.

Some 700 different operations — a third of all surgery — can now be done in an outpatient setting. In addition to sterilization operations (both male and female) and some hernia repairs, commonly done one-day procedures include breast biopsy, tonsillectomy, cataract removal, eye muscle surgery, removal of cysts and other growths, D and C (dilatation and curettage), oral surgery, and various forms of plastic and orthopedic surgery.

What to Expect

If you are scheduled for an outpatient operation, the preoperative work-up — including a complete physical, blood and urine tests, and a chest X ray — will most likely be done a day or more in advance at the doctor's office, surgical center, or outpatient clinic. You will be told not to eat or drink anything after midnight before your surgery (violation of this prohibition could result in a life-threatening reaction to anesthesia).

At the time of surgery you will be given a light, quick-acting anesthetic (general, regional, or local, depending upon the nature of the operation) and/or a strong pain-killer. After surgery, when you have become fully alert and are recovering normally, you can be discharged with a responsible adult to care for you and a set of written instructions about what to do to enhance your recovery, when and whom to call if problems develop, and when to return to have stitches removed.

How Safe?

Studies of many thousands of outpatient operations have proved their safety as long as the patients treated on an ambulatory basis are properly selected. In general, patients are required to be in good health (though some centers will accept patients with serious underlying diseases like a previous heart attack, diabetes, or high blood pressure), below the age of sixty or so, and with relatives or friends who can care for them postoperatively.

Information gathered from forty-nine freestanding surgical clinics in 1978 indicated that only 7 in 10,000 patients required hospitalization because of emergency or life-threatening complications. A study published in 1980 of 13,433 patients operated on at Northwest Surgicare Ltd., a freestanding clinic in Arlington, Illinois, revealed that only 106 patients suffered serious postoperative complications and that only 16 required transfer to a hospital for further care.

The most frequent problems involved hemorrhage (74 cases) and infection (10 cases). The authors noted that this was a "remarkably low incidence of infection" as operations go and that overall "there is no evidence that the complication rate is related to the choice of surgical setting, i.e., outpatient vs. inpatient." Of 403 patients with serious underlying diseases, only 3 suffered serious complications — a rate no higher than that for healthier persons.

Before deciding on outpatient surgery, check your medical insurance policy to be certain the procedure is covered if no overnight hospitalization is involved. Although in recent years major insurance companies (Blue Cross-Blue Shield and private insurers) have pressed for more ambulatory procedures, not all procedures and facilities are covered. Medicare generally restricts payment to hospital-based clinics.

Take care, too, in selecting the facility. There are now about 100 freestanding surgical centers, and a recent survey of hospitals in metropolitan areas revealed that 70 percent now have ambulatory surgical facilities. If you are considering surgery in an office-based facility or freestanding clinic, ask what arrangements it has for transferring patients to a hospital in case of an emergency. Many patients prefer the more hotel-like atmosphere and camaraderie of a freestanding clinic. Others like the security of a hospital-based facility since the full range of services are available should they be needed.

For Further Information

Ambulatory facilities that have been in operation for longer than a year are eligible for accreditation by the Accreditation Association for Ambulatory Health Care, Inc., 4849 Golf Road, Skokie, Illinois 60077. You can write to the association for a list of approved centers. Or contact your state's department of health services or local Health Systems Agency for the names of licensed facilities.

Drugs:
What to Know About Those You Take

Americans swallow nearly 40 billion doses of tablets, capsules, elixirs, and other medicinal potions each year. Seven prescriptions a year are filled for every man, woman, and child. On top of that, Americans dose themselves with various combinations of the half million over-the-counter remedies. We take medicines for headaches, birth control, upset stomachs, anxiety, colds, allergies, sleeplessness, and somnolence, often washing them all down with another popular drug, alcohol.

While many extol the relief and healing that drugs can bring, few realize the extent of their potential dangers. In some cases the cure can be far worse than the disease.

Every drug — even aspirin or an antacid — can sometimes cause unwanted side effects. Drugs can also interact with one another or with certain foods or drinks to cause serious reactions. Each year some 300,000 Americans suffer such severe adverse drug reactions that they have to be hospitalized, and 18,000 patients who are given drugs while in the hospital die from the side effects of their medication.

In addition, many patients fail to get the full, if any, benefit from the drugs they take because no drug was needed to begin with, or because the wrong drug was prescribed, or because the drug was taken improperly. Thus, they face the risk of an adverse reaction without any compensating benefit. For example, an estimated 10,000 Americans annually suffer life-threatening reactions from antibiotics that were needlessly prescribed.

Guide to Safe and Effective Use

You can help to protect yourself and your family from such risks by gaining a healthy respect for the potential hazards as well as the benefits of drugs and by learning what to tell your doctor about you and what questions to ask about the drugs precribed. The following guidelines have been suggested by various physicians and pharmacists, medical organizations, and consumer groups:

● Ask your doctor the purpose of the prescription. The doctor should tell you the diagnosis of your condition, how it was arrived at, and how the prescription might be expected to help you. For example, if you have a sore throat, the doctor should take a throat culture to determine the cause before prescribing an antibiotic since antibiotics are useless against virus infections, the most common cause of sore throats.

● No matter how sick you may feel, don't pressure the doctor into giving you a prescription if he or she thinks none is needed. Sometimes the best medicine is none at all, but you have a right to ask the doctor the reason for this decision.

● Ask if the drug might be prescribed in generic form instead of as a more costly brand name. Generics can often save half the cost of medication with no loss in effectiveness. In some cases, though, your doctor may have a good reason for preferring a particular brand.

● Ask the name of the drug and what side effects it might have, and which of them, if they should happen to you, should be reported to your doctor immediately. While the doctor can't be expected to tell you every last adverse reaction that has been reported, you can and should be told the more common side effects patients experience, including effects on your sexual performance and possible alarming effects — such as the fact that a drug may turn your urine blue — that may or may not cause physical discomfort.

The doctor should ask you in advance of writing the prescription whether you have had any bad reactions to similar drugs in the past. If you have unpleasant effects from one drug, the doctor can often substitute another equally effective drug that causes you little or no difficulty.

● Find out precisely how the drug should be taken and what, if any, precautions you should follow in taking it. Too often the doctor rattles off instructions which the patient only half hears or completely misunderstands. Then the doctor writes some hieroglyphic on a prescription blank, and the patient leaves the office confused. Ask the pharmacist to write both the name of the drug and directions for taking it on the label. "Take as directed" is hardly helpful if you never knew or have forgotten the directions.

The activity of some drugs is reduced by the presence of food in the stomach or too much water or juice, so it is important to know when in relation to meals the drug should be taken. Also, some drugs interact with certain foods, alcohol, and other drugs, producing a toxic reaction or canceling out the drug's effect. For example, milk reduces the effectiveness of the antibiotic tetracycline. Antidepressants called MAO inhibitors react with a substance in cheese, wine, and other foods to cause a potentially life-threatening reaction. Anticoagulants can interact with a variety of drugs, including some antibiotics and aspirin, to produce an enhanced blood-thinning effect that could result in hemorrhage.

• The doctor should tell you when to expect results from the medication and how soon to call if no improvement occurs. The doctor may want to substitute a more effective drug or reconsider the diagnosis. Ask whether you will need another appointment to find out if your ailment has cleared up or improved.

• Be sure to take the medication your doctor prescribes according to the schedule, amount, and time designated. As many as half of patients fail to take prescriptions at all, and another large proportion take them sporadically or stop too soon. A drug may do little good unless a certain amount is present in your blood and tissues at all times. In the case of a bacterial infection you may feel well after a few days on an antibiotic, but to destroy the organisms completely and prevent a recurrence, you may have to take the drug for days or weeks longer.

• Don't take drugs that were left over from a previous illness or that were prescribed for someone else unless the doctor tells you to. Many drugs lose effectiveness during storage, the dosage may be inappropriate, or the drug may be hazardous for you, even though it was safe for the person it was prescribed for (or for you at the time it was originally prescribed).

• Even if the doctor doesn't ask, give all the facts he or she needs to write a rational prescription. Are you pregnant? (Many drugs can damage the unborn child.) What other drugs — including over-the-counter preparations and vitamin or mineral megadoses — do you take? Have you had a bad drug reaction in the past? Do you have any chronic illnesses, such as heart or kidney disease, or have you had past illnesses, such as hepatitis, that could be complicated by a drug? Do you drink alcoholic beverages?

• If you use the same pharmacist to purchase all your medications, both prescription and over the counter, and the pharmacist keeps records of customer prescriptions, he or she may be able to alert you to a possible hazard associated with the drug you are about to buy.

• Take care in storing your drugs. Although most people have their medicine chest in the bathroom, this is actually the worst possible room in which to keep drugs. [See chapter on the medicine cabinet, page 467.] The heat and humidity can cause rapid deterioration of many drugs. Choose a cool, dry place out of direct light or sun. Remove the cotton from a new bottle and discard it. Many drugs have expiration dates, so be sure to ask the pharmacist how long a drug may be kept. If you have young children in the house, be sure that all medications are in childproof containers and that you replace the tops properly each time. [See chapter on poisons and poisoning, page 389.]

• Take advantage of the various aids that can inform you about the drugs you may take. A number of books and guides that explain in layman's terms the essential facts about widely used drugs have been published recently (see "For Further Reading" below).

The federal Food and Drug Administration has mandated patient package inserts on the effects, precautions, and side effects of some prescription drugs. These inserts are now distributed along with prescriptions for oral contraceptives, hearing aids, all estrogen and progestin drugs, and for IUDs. Ask your pharmacist about them.

For Further Reading

About Your Medicines. Prepared and distributed by the United States Pharmacopeial Convention, Inc., 12601 Twinbrook Parkway, Rockville, Md. 20852. The USPC also publishes bimonthly the *About Your Medicines* newsletter, available on subscription.

Benowicz, Robert J. *Non-Prescription Drugs and Their Side Effects.* New York: Today Press/Grosset & Dunlap, 1977.

Bressler, Rubin, et. al. *The Physicians' Drug Manual: Prescription and Nonprescription Drugs.* New York: Doubleday, 1981.

Graedon, Joe. *The People's Pharmacy.* New York: Avon, 1980.

Long, James W., M.D. *The Essential Guide to Prescription Drugs,* rev. ed. New York: Harper & Row, 1980.

Silverman, Harold, and Gilbert I. Simon. *The Pill Book.* New York: Bantam, 1979.

Strauss, Steven. *Your Prescription and You.* Available from Medical Business Services, Butler and Maple Avenues, Ambler, Pa. 19002.

Wolfe, Sidney M., M.D.; Christopher M. Coley; and the Health Research Group. *Pills That Don't Work.* New York: Farrar, Straus & Giroux, 1981.

Drugs and the Elderly: Special Considerations

Accidental drug abuse and misuse by elderly men and women are far more common than even most professionals realize. They always compromise medical care, often cause confounding illness, and sometimes threaten life.

Example: An elderly Minnesota man was taking five different drugs, although the only one he could identify was a sleeping medication. After suffering a heart attack, he was sent home with two new prescriptions, which he began alternating with the old drugs so that none would be "wasted." Fortunately his bizarre drug combination was discovered in time because it could have been fatal.

Example: An anticonvulsant was prescribed for an elderly woman who suffered from dizziness and hand tremors. One side effect of the drug is depression, so the woman was also taking antidepressant medication, which numbered among *its* side effects unsteadiness and tremors.

Dorothy Lundin, a retired nursing professor from the University of Minnesota, uncovered many such cases among elderly men and women whose drug-taking habits and knowledge she studied. Though all lived independently and were responsible for their own health care, fewer than 5 percent of those taking prescription drugs knew enough about the medications to ensure their safe use. Confusion about the purpose and proper dose and schedule for each drug was commonplace. Sometimes patients deliberately reduced the dose to make the drug last longer and save money.

There is much that individual elderly patients and their families can do to maximize the benefits and minimize the risks from needed drugs and to avoid unnecessary and potentially hazardous medication. Being well informed about the purpose and proper use of drugs can help to ward off medical crises and reduce the costs of medical care. Yet the Minnesota study showed that elderly people were generally reluctant to ask their doctors about drug use because they thought the doctor was too busy or not interested.

Hazards Change with Age

People over sixty-five take three times more drugs than younger people primarily because the elderly have more chronic illnesses. Often elderly patients will have two or more doctors treating them for different conditions. It's not unusual for an older person to be taking several different potent prescription drugs on a regular basis, plus one or more over-the-counter preparations — for example, a diuretic to lower blood pressure, an antidiabetes drug, a heart-rhythm regulator, aspirin to counter arthritic pain, and a laxative to treat constipation.

Such multiple drug use harbors the potential of producing severe and sometimes life-threatening reactions, especially if a single physician is not overseeing the use of all the drugs. One study showed that patients between the ages of seventy and eighty experienced twice as many adverse drug reactions as patients aged forty to fifty. Ironically, the side effects of drugs are sometimes mistaken for symptoms of a new disorder, prompting the doctor to write yet another prescription. In some cases, drug-induced effects mimic symptoms of mental deterioration, which are incorrectly assumed to be signs of senility about which nothing can be done.

Changes in the body with age make the elderly more susceptible to complications caused by individual drugs and their interactions. A drug dose that is safe and effective in a younger person may cause severe toxic reactions in an eighty-year-old. For example, Tim R. Covington, professor of pharmacy at the West Virginia University Medical Center, notes that the aged "are hypersensitive to morphine and other opiate derivatives such as codeine. From these drugs the aged can expect more than the normal amount of sedation, mental confusion and lack of coordination." Sensitivity to tranquilizers like Valium and Librium also increases in old age.

On the other hand, sometimes the normal adult dose of a drug is inadequate to treat an older person. In some cases elderly people react to a particular medication in a fashion diametrically opposite to that of a young person.

As you age, the proportion of your body that is water and lean muscle tissue decreases and the percentage that is fat increases. This means a drug that is soluble in water will reach a higher concentration in an older person unless the dose is adjusted accordingly. By the same token, a fat-soluble drug can accumulate to higher levels in the body of an elderly person and thus have more prolonged effects.

The liver, which is responsible for metabolizing (breaking down) most drugs, and the kidneys, which excrete the metabolites (breakdown products), function less efficiently in older people. Their decreased efficiency slows the rate at which drugs leave the body. A person with impaired kidney function may run into trouble with potassium supplements, digoxin, penicillin, tetracycline, and some medications for high blood pressure, among other drugs, Dr. Covington says.

Preventing Drug Mishaps

The following steps can help prevent drug-related mishaps at any age, but especially for the elderly:

● Tell the doctor about all other medications, both prescription and over the counter (including vitamins, laxatives, and home remedies), that you are currently taking. If you don't know their names, take the vials with you to the doctor's office, or call your pharmacy for the information. Tell the doctor about any reactions you've had in the past to particular drugs.

● Bring a pad and pen to the doctor's office, and write down the name of each drug, its purpose, and when, how, and for how long it is to be taken. If you cannot write it, ask the doctor or nurse to do so — legibly. The Minnesota study and others like it showed that very few older people remember verbal instructions about drugs.

● If the doctor doesn't tell you, ask whether the drug should be taken with food or on an empty stomach, whether certain foods or drinks (like alcohol) should not be consumed while you are on the drug, and whether certain activities (like driving) should be avoided.

● Ask about common side effects and interactions with other drugs you may be taking and which reactions should be reported promptly to the doctor. Very often a change in the dose or the way a drug is taken can minimize reactions without loss of benefit. In some cases a different prescription is needed. But don't stop taking a drug because you don't like its effects without first consulting the doctor.

● If you have a complicated medication schedule to follow or your memory is poor, devise a drug diary or calendar to help you remember what to take when. Check off each dose as you take it; even young people often can't recall when or whether they've taken the last dose. Some people are helped by setting out the day's individual drug doses each morning in paper cups or an egg carton labeled with the time and method of administration. But mixing the entire day's drugs in a pillbox is an invitation to error and may cause some drugs to lose potency.

• Ask the pharmacist to write the name of each drug and the treatment schedule and instructions on the vial. If your vision is poor, you may have to make your own labels. Keep all drugs in their original containers since this reduces the chances of taking the wrong medication or dose. If you have difficulty opening childproof containers, ask the pharmacist to use regular vials, but be sure to keep them out of the reach of children (including occasional visitors).

• Try to use the same pharmacy to fill all your prescriptions and to supply your over-the-counter medications as well. That way the pharmacist will be more likely to spot potentially dangerous combinations.

• Don't keep old medications around, and don't take drugs prescribed for someone else unless the doctor tells you to. Ask the pharmacist how best to store your prescriptions; the bathroom medicine chest is often the worst place because the warmth and dampness speed deterioration of many drugs. [See chapter on the medicine cabinet, page 467.]

• Take all medications according to the schedule prescribed (every six hours four times a day may mean getting up during the night to take a dose) for the entire time recommended. If you stop too soon, you may suffer a relapse.

• You may be able to reduce your reliance on some drugs, and hence your chances of adverse reactions, by making changes in your eating and exercise habits. For example, a walk after supper, a glass of warm milk before bed, or relaxation exercises may substitute for sleep-inducing medications. A low-sodium diet, weight loss, and a daily exercise program may help lower blood pressure to normal without drugs. Ask your doctor about life-style therapies in lieu of drugs for chronic ailments.

For Further Reading

A useful booklet, "Using Your Medicines Wisely: A Guide for the Elderly," has been prepared by the National Institute on Drug Abuse. Free single copies can be obtained by writing to Elder-Ed, P.O. Box 416, Kensington, Maryland 20795.

Aspirin, etc.:
Is the Competition Really Better?

Bufferin, the ads claim, acts "twice as fast as aspirin" without upsetting your stomach. Anacin is said to have "more of the pain reliever doctors recommend most." Alka-Seltzer is supposed to help you overcome both the stomach upset and headache precipitated by stress, fatigue, or overindulgence. We've been told that only Excedrin, the "extra-strength pain reliever," can conquer an "Excedrin headache," whatever that may be. Another ad maintains that "doctors recommend Tylenol more than all leading aspirin brands combined" and insists that Tylenol is "safer than aspirin."

Beset by such conflicting and confusing claims, the consumer is hard put to know what to take for the fevers, aches, stresses, and strains of life. Should you pay more for a famous brand name that claims superiority over its competitors, or will plain old generic aspirin at one-sixth the price do the job just as well? Is aspirin as dangerous as some competitors suggest? Is anything really safer?

The facts are these: Most over-the-counter pain relievers are really dressed-up aspirin, and most claims for superiority over regular aspirin are based on poor or incomplete data. There is little justification for the combinations of ingredients in some products. In carefully controlled studies aspirin has outranked both over-the-counter and leading prescription drugs as a pain reliever. No drug, not aspirin or any of its look-alikes, is completely safe. And aspirin's main comptitor, acetaminophen (Tylenol, etc.), is not the drug most doctors recommend.

The Various Products

Yet the consumer's head has clearly been turned by paid publicity. In 1972 *Consumer Reports* noted that four-fifths of every dollar spent on over-the-counter pain remedies went for aspirin's more costly competitors. Here's what the buyer got:

Buffered aspirin (aspirin plus very small amounts of antacid). A National Academy of Sciences drug panel found little evidence to support the claim that this amount of buffering reduces the frequency of stomach irritation that sometimes results from aspirin. At least two studies showed no decrease in stomach irritation as a result of substituting a buffered product for plain aspirin. Although the buffered product is absorbed somewhat faster, the panel said no evidence showed that this results in quicker pain relief, and the Federal Trade Commission ordered the maker of Bufferin to run a disclaimer to that effect in future ads.

You can counter some of plain aspirin's irritating effects on your stomach by taking it with a full glass of water or milk, perhaps with a pinch of baking soda added to the water. Or crush the aspirin and mix it in a glass of warm water. Also, avoid taking aspirin on an empty stomach. Another alternative is to buy enteric-coated aspirin, which doesn't dissolve until it gets to the small intestine and thus doesn't irritate the stomach. To counter the extra cost, ask the pharmacist for generic coated aspirin.

Brand-name aspirins (plain aspirin with a company trademark). The consumer pays handsomely for the cost of advertising a product that may be no different from the unadvertised cheap store brands. However, sometimes cheap aspirin is poorly manufactured, leaving an acid residue, or it may be allowed to deteriorate on the shelf. Open the bottle, look, and smell. If the product appears yellow or smells like vinegar or contains a number of broken tablets, don't buy it.

Aspirin combinations (aspirin mixed with other pain relievers and/ or caffeine.) Anacin, for example, contains 20 percent more aspirin than a regular 5-grain (325-milligram) aspirin tablet, plus the amount of caffeine in half a cup of coffee, which has no proven pain-relieving value except perhaps for persons suffering from a caffeine-withdrawal headache. You can get the extra potency in an Anacin tablet much less expensively by taking one and a quarter tablets of plain aspirin in place of each Anacin tablet.

Excedrin contains aspirin, acetaminophen (another pain reliever as effective as aspirin), salicylamide (a pain reliever vastly inferior to aspirin), and caffeine. Its total analgesic value is estimated to be no greater than plain aspirin. Here, too, the Federal Trade Commission called for corrective advertising to disabuse the public of the unproven notion that Excedrin is a better pain reliever than aspirin.

Alka-Seltzer is aspirin (five grains per tablet) plus a strong antacid. Its value as an antacid is sorely compromised by the inclusion of aspirin, a known stomach irritant. As a pain reliever it is absorbed faster because it enters the stomach already dissolved, and it may be useful for those whose stomachs get very upset by aspirin. For everyone else, Alka Seltzer is a very expensive way to take aspirin.

Cope (aspirin, caffeine, and two buffers) and Vanquish (aspirin, acetaminophen, caffeine, and two buffers) have 28 percent more aspirin or aspirin equivalent than plain aspirin. You can get the same pain-relieving value by taking one and a quarter plain aspirin tablets. The same is true for Empirin, which has three and a half grains of aspirin, two and a half grains of phenacetin, and caffeine. Phenacetin is comparable to aspirin as a pain reliever, but it has been associated with serious kidney damage and is no longer used by most manufacturers.

In general, combination drugs — aside from having no proven value over plain aspirin — increase the chances of side effects and interactions that could result in their doing more harm than good.

Acetaminophen (a pain-reliever comparable in potency to aspirin but lacking aspirin's anti-inflammatory properties). The lack of anti-inflammatory action can be important because pain is frequently the result of inflammation. But to its advantage, acetaminophen also lacks some of aspirin's more serious side effects — namely, stomach irritation, gastrointestinal bleeding, and reduced ability of the blood to clot. Thus, it is a useful pain reliever for people with ulcers or bleeding disorders and those taking anticoagulants. A further advantage of acetaminophen is its stability in liquid form, making it easier to administer to small children. Many pediatricians prefer it to aspirin to reduce fever in children. However, acetaminophen is not totally free of hazard. Overdoses can cause serious and sometimes fatal liver damage.

Acetaminophen is sold as Tylenol, Datril, Anacin-3 ("100 percent aspirin-free"), Bayer acetaminophen, and a variety of cheaper unadvertised store brands. Anacin-3, extra-strength Tylenol, and extra-strength Datril have the strength of one and a half aspirin tablets; the other products have the same potency as aspirin.

The Placebo Effect

Why, then, you ask, does one product seem to work better than another? If none is superior to plain old aspirin, why don't you get the same relief from the cheapest and plainest form of this ancient drug? The answer lies not in the ingredients found in the other products, but in a time-honored remedy: the placebo effect. If you are led to believe that one treatment is better, faster, or more potent than another, the power of suggestion can add to its true power. If plain, undisguised aspirin got the same Madison Avenue hype as its more expensive competitors, it would undoubtedly work as well.

The Mayo Clinic put aspirin and several of its over-the-counter and prescription competitors to a properly controlled test against moderate cancer pain. When all the drugs were cloaked in the same blue capsules, aspirin outperformed even the prescription drugs codeine, Darvon, Ponstel, and Talwin as well as over-the-counter acetaminophen and phenacetin preparations. Included in the test was plain sugar, not known to have any specific pain-relieving effect. Yet 22 percent of patients were significantly helped by it. This is a measure of the power of the placebo effect. It's what you pay for when you choose the high-priced tablets instead of aspirin.

Aspirin: Some Important Don'ts

Aspirin, although far and away the nation's leading drug and one of the most useful medications known, is not for everyone. Because of its various side effects, for some people or under some circumstances, it should not be taken or should be used only with caution under a doctor's guidance. In most of the following circumstances, acetaminophen can be used in place of aspirin for the relief of pain and fever.

● Aspirin should not be used by anyone with stomach ulcers, or a past history of ulcers, gout, or bleeding disorders. If you find that taking aspirin increases menstrual bleeding, acetaminophen or some other drug made for menstrual pain can be used instead.

● Don't use aspirin in feverish children who have been dehydrated by vomiting or diarrhea or by the failure to drink enough liquids, unless it is recommended by a doctor who knows the circumstances.

● Don't mix aspirin with alcohol (this rules out taking Alka-Seltzer to relieve the agonies of overindulgence). Alcohol irritates the stomach lining and increases the amount of internal bleeding that aspirin can cause.

● Don't take aspirin if you are also taking any of the following medications: anticoagulants, strong prescription drugs for arthritis, oral diabetes drugs, or antigout drugs (except Zyloprim), unless told to by a doctor who knows what else you're taking. Aspirin can interact with all these and possibly cause serious reactions. Aspirin also interacts with vitamin C; the vitamin slows the excretion of aspirin, possibly causing a toxic buildup of the drug if you take several doses.

● Unless advised by your physician, don't take aspirin during the last three months of pregnancy or within a week of a scheduled operation. Aspirin can prolong or delay labor and, if taken too close to delivery, can cause bleeding problems in the mother and infant. It can also increase blood loss during surgery.

● Don't take aspirin if you are among the approximately 2 in 1,000 people with an allergic reaction to it. The allergy can sometimes be life-threatening. People with asthma are more likely than others to develop hypersensitivity reactions to aspirin and therefore should not take the drug without a doctor's advice.

Your Medicine Cabinet: Hindrance or Help?

When did you last look — I mean, *really* look — in your medicine cabinet? You'd probably be amazed at what you find: leftover antibiotics from that strep throat you had five years ago, an assortment of outdated tablets and capsules, miscellaneous vitamins, a mostly evaporated vial of merthiolate, the remains of various painkillers, decongestants, antacids, cough syrups, ointments, and salves, the purposes of which you've long since forgotten.

Chances are, too, that your cabinet is poorly equipped and even more poorly arranged to help much when you need it most. Doubtless on more than one occasion you've searched frantically for that thermometer, eye cup, or burn ointment, but they were hard to spot among the shampoos, cotton balls, curlers, shaving creams, and sprays. And why didn't you have syrup of ipecac on hand when little Johnny decided to eat a fistful of sugar-coated tablets that you'd failed to put in a childproof container?

"Your family medicine cabinet is something like fire, an excellent servant but a horrible master," notes Byron G. Wels in his book *The Medicine Cabinet* (see "For Further Reading," page 470). "It can be a panacea when an emergency arises, provided that you have it properly prepared and equipped to handle such emergencies. At the same time, if it or the items inside it are misused, it can be deadly dangerous."

Mr. Wels, whose book was written in consultation with William M. Weinstein, professor of pharmacy at the Rutgers College of Pharmacy, points out that "too many people wait until a crisis develops before they equip their medicine cabinets to meet that unexpected emergency." And, he adds, the usual "hit-or-miss method of buying medications offers no assurance that sufficient medication of the type you may need will be there when you need it." Here's how to make your medicine cabinet serve you well.

How to Arrange It

Take an inventory. Unless you're starting fresh with an empty new medicine cabinet, the best approach to setting up a truly useful one is to take a complete inventory of what you have and prepare yourself to discard most of it. Set out the entire contents on a clear tabletop. All prescriptions left over from an illness long past should be emptied down the toilet. Keep only those prescribed for a chronic or recurring ailment, such as high blood pressure or hay fever. Also discard over-the-counter drugs that have passed their expiration date (check the label or vial for a date) or have been in your cabinet for more than a year.

Most drugs deteriorate or change with time and exposure to air, moisture, or light. After a while they lose potency, and some may decompose to produce toxic ingredients. Instead of alleviating pain or illness, they may actually make matters worse.

Of course, any item that has lost its label or purpose should be thrown out regardless of age. You should also discard old tubes of ointments and creams that have hardened or separated; liquids that have become cloudy, discolored, or formed gunk at the bottom of the containers; tablets that are crumbly, capsules that have broken or melted, and tinctures from which much of the alcohol has evaporated.

Mark what you keep. Place the date of inventory on all drugs that you're keeping. From here on, label all new drug acquisitions with the date of purchase. Make sure the pharmacist writes the name of the drug on the label (you might add your own label stating its purpose), and secure all labels with a good-quality transparent tape.

To help prevent accidental overdoses, Mr. Wels suggests fixing a strip of adhesive, sticky side out, or sandpaper around the vials of drugs that can be abused, such as narcotic pain-killers, sleeping pills, and tranquilizers.

Establish a system. It's best to reserve your bathroom cabinet to store the items you most frequently use in the bathroom: cosmetics, soaps and shampoos, razors, lotions, syrups, tissues, enema and douche bags, hot-water bottle, first-aid remedies, etc.

Drugs really don't belong in the bathroom since heat and dampness hasten their decay. They are best kept in a separate small cabinet or closet (one you can lock if you have small children in the house) outside the bathroom. A few should be stored in the refrigerator; they would say so on the label.

The shelves of both the bathroom and the drug cabinets should be clearly marked for category of item — "First Aid," "Hair Items," "Skin Items," etc. — to help you find what you need fast and to help keep order. Both cabinets should be well lighted to reduce the possibility of error. Inside the door of the bathroom cabinet, you might post a card of emergency information, including what to do in case of poisoning, and phone numbers of your local emergency medical service or ambulance squad, poison control center, hospital, pharmacy, and physician. A similar list of numbers should be posted near each telephone in the house.

What to Keep

The items you keep in your medicine cabinet will in part depend on the size and ages of your family members and their particular health problems. But pharmacists and emergency medical personnel recommend certain standard items. Often, if you are well equipped at home, you can avoid a stressful and costly trip to a hospital emergency room or physician's office. Here's what you would find in a well-stocked medicine cabinet.

First-Aid Essentials:

• For cuts and scrapes: plain soap and water, the best antiseptic for superficial wounds (antiseptic and antibiotic sprays, alcohol and hydrogen peroxide are not needed in such cases, and more extensive wounds should be seen by a physician); adhesive bandages (Band-aid type) of various sizes.

• For eye injuries: a prepared eyewash and eyecup. Don't use dry cotton, tissue, or cloth to remove something from the eye.

• For burns: a burn ointment or spray, to be applied after first-aid treatment with cold water. Never use butter, and don't put a burn ointment on a large or deep burn that requires medical attention. [See chapter on burns, page 398.]

• For skin problems: a hydrocortisone cream (now sold over the counter) to be used externally or calamine lotion to relieve minor itches and rashes, such as reactions to insect bites and poison ivy; petroleum jelly; antifungal powder or spray for athlete's foot; a sunscreen to prevent sunburn and a sunburn spray for relief; insect repellent. Antibacterial swabs or antiseptic first-aid spray are optional; their effectiveness in countering infection is questionable.

• For swallowed poisons: syrup of ipecac to induce vomiting after swallowed poisons (except when the poison is a strong acid or alkali — call the poison control center first if you're not sure); activated charcoal to adsorb poisons that should not be regurgitated; and Epsom salts to speed the elimination of poisons. [See chapter on poisons and poisoning, page 389.]

• Miscellaneous: surgical tweezers, perhaps with a built-in magni-

469

fier, for removing splinters; sterile cotton balls and gauze pads; blunt-end scissors for cutting tape and gauze; an elastic bandage for sprains; ice bag to reduce swellings; hot-water bottle and heating pad for various aches and pains; aspirin and acetaminophen (an analgesic for those who cannot take aspirin) for pain relief and fever reduction; sodium bicarbonate for heat exhaustion and bee, ant, and wasp stings; and a thermometer, oral and/or rectal (for young children).

Useful "patent" medicines:

Many over-the-counter drugs, as those sold without a prescription are now called, are of questionable usefulness. This is probably the case for most such drugs found in the average American medicine chest. Yet, if you select the right ones, they often can spare you considerable discomfort and possibly a doctor's bill. Your selection should reflect the kinds of problems you and your family are likely to encounter.

• For occasional gastrointestinal problems: a simple antacid, such as Maalox or Amphojel or generic or store brand combinations of aluminum hydroxide and magnesium hydroxide; simethicone or activated charcoal for excessive flatulence (charcoal should not be used regularly since it can interfere with absorption of essential mineral nutrients); and perhaps a bulk-forming laxative (such as psyllium or dietary bran) or a stool softener for constipation (eating a bran cereal would also do the trick). Antinausea drugs are of questionable usefulness, except for those taken in advance to prevent motion sickness. Antidiarrheal medications are also questionable; simple diarrhea is best treated by dietary restriction, and severe or persistant diarrhea should be evaluated by a physician.

• For respiratory symptoms: a nasal decongestant spray, to be used no more often than the label recommends, or an oral decongestant to relieve nasal and sinus congestion. Cough medications are of questionable effectiveness; if you insist on using one, stick to those that are not suppressive. [See chapter on coughs, page 503.] Antihistamines can relieve allergic reactions and runny noses, although their usefulness for most symptoms of a cold is questionable.

For Further Reading

Wels, Byron G., with William M. Weinstein. *The Medicine Cabinet.* Maplewood, N.J.: Hammond, 1978.

Informed Consent:
Let the Buyer Beware

When you call a repairman to fix a costly machine, such as a dishwasher or television set, you're likely to ask for a "diagnosis" of the trouble, what would be required to fix it, how long it will take, and how much it will cost. But when your body breaks down and requires "fixing" by a physician, chances are you're not nearly as inquisitive as you might be about a broken TV, even though your life may be at stake.

While it is certainly important for you to trust the physician who cares for you, trust should be based on something more than blind faith. You have a right — in fact, some say an obligation — as a patient to know what is wrong, how it might be corrected, and what the chances for success are. In many medical malpractice suits today patients claim that they were "never told" beforehand about possible complications or the likelihood that the treatment would fail.

Studies have shown that being well informed is clearly to your benefit. Patients who know what to expect usually do better. They tend to cooperate more in their own care, recover more rapidly, suffer less emotional anguish, and require less pain-relieving medication.

Each year tens of millions of Americans undergo surgery or complex diagnostic tests, receive hazardous treatments, or participate in research studies for which they are asked to give their "informed consent." They acknowledge, usually on a form they sign (which is kept by the hospital or clinic), that they understand the nature of their illness; the proposed operation, treatment, or test; its risks and benefits; and its possible alternatives.

The Purpose and Pitfalls of Consent

Consent procedures are intended to protect people from serving as unwitting subjects in intentional or unintentional medical experiments. They provide patients with an opportunity to know more about what they're buying in the way of medical care. They help to clarify the trade-offs involved and prevent unrealistic expectations. And they give patients the right to refuse the care in question.

However, numerous studies have shown that for most patients, their understanding of what is about to happen and why is usually inadequate and sometimes completely wrong. For example, in a recent study in Pennsylvania, 200 cancer patients were asked on the very day they signed treatment consent forms if they knew what their treatment would involve. Only 60 percent did; only 59 percent knew why it was being done; only 55 percent knew at least one possible complication, and only 27 percent could name any treatment alternative. Yet all had just given their "informed consent" to the potentially hazardous therapy by signing forms that outlined all the above factors.

In fact, Dr. Barrie R. Cassileth and colleagues at the University of Pennsylvania Cancer Center reported, 80 percent of these patients misunderstood the purpose of the consent forms, thinking they were "legal documents to protect the physician's rights." Fewer than half thought they had something to do with the patient's rights or served to explain the nature of the treatment. And 28 percent thought incorrectly that they had no choice but to sign a consent form.

Actually the way most consent forms are written, they really *are* more for the doctor's and hospital's benefit than the patient's. Most forms are prepared by doctors and lawyers who are accustomed to technical language. The forms usually contain many multisyllabic words, long and complex sentences, and concepts unfamiliar to the average lay person.

A Better Approach

Even under the best of circumstances, a patient's ability to understand and remember information during the stress of illness or hospitalization is likely to be diminished, notes Dr. Gary R. Morrow, a psychologist at the University of Rochester Medical Center who analyzed sixty consent forms from five national cancer centers where experimental treatments are used. He found that patients who take the completed consent forms home before signing possess more information about the proposed procedure than patients who simply read and immediately sign the forms in the clinic.

No form — or any audiovisual technique — is an adequate substitute for a conversation between the physician and the patient in which the patient can ask questions and acknowledge his or her understanding or lack of it. To obtain truly informed consent, the conversation should take at least twenty minutes, says Dr. George Robinson, cardiovascular surgeon at the Montefiore Hospital in the Bronx, New York. It should cover the following points:

- The diagnosis and nature of the illness
- The proposed operation, treatment, or test
- The risks of the procedure
- The potential complications
- The benefits of the proposed procedure
- Possible alternative methods of managing the problem

In addition to making certain that the patient knows what is about to happen and why, this personal approach to obtaining consent fosters rapport between the doctor and patient and increases the probability that medical care will be a cooperative, rather than an adversary, proceeding. Informed consent is as much the patient's obligation as the physician's. It is up to the patient to ask questions and be sure they are answered in an understandable fashion before agreeing to the procedure in question.

Medical Insurance: How Well Are You Covered?

There's probably nothing that more people have, yet know less about, than their medical insurance. Too often people learn what is — and, more important, what is *not* — covered by their policies the hard way: when faced with a staggering bill for medical services they thought were covered.

In other cases people miss out on services and/or reimbursement because they don't realize what is due them or how to file and follow through on a claim. For example, a national survey by the Rand Corporation published in 1981 revealed that when the policy had a deductible (in which the insurance company starts paying after, say, the first $100 of expenses in a year), only about half the families knew they were entitled to reimbursement for outpatient physician services and prescription drugs, perhaps because in most years medical expenses did not exceed the deductible.

Still others who think they are adequately covered could face financial ruin because their policies have failed to keep pace with soaring increases in medical care costs. Those policies that reimburse patients a specified amount for each hospital day may no longer be adequate now that the average hospital charges well over $100 a day for a semiprivate room.

Even those covered by Medicare, the federally financed insurance program for people over sixty-five, can incur staggering bills that are not reimbursed, and supplemental policies purchased to fill in Medicare gaps are often not what they are thought to be.

All told, even though more than 60 percent of the population has at least $250,000 in benefits for "catastrophic" medical expenses, only 30 percent is protected from potential financial insolvency by a policy that puts a ceiling on out-of-pocket medical expenditures. At this point you would become eligible for Medicaid, a state and federal assistance (not insurance) program for the medically indigent.

To be sure, medical insurance policies, like income tax forms, are often unintelligible to the average person. Also, few people like to delve into matters like insurance that they hope they'll never have to use. For fire and theft insurance, this may be true. But medical care at some point in life is as inevitable as death and taxes, so it pays to understand what you have and what else may be available and desirable. If you are covered under a group policy through your job or association, check with your personnel adviser to see if any gaps exist that warrant coverage through the purchase of a low-cost personal supplemental policy.

For those in the market for a new policy, it's important to appreciate the different choices available so that you can select what will be best for you and your family.

The type of coverage chosen not only affects your pocketbook but can also influence the kind and quality of medical care services you receive, particularly how much attention is paid to keeping you healthy and not in need of costly medical "repairs."

Be wary of bargains. While a costly policy does not guarantee good coverage, a cheap one almost certainly assures against it. Group health insurance, such as through your job, your union, or some other organization you belong to, is cheaper than an individual policy offering the same benefits. If it is possible to continue a group policy after you retire, it's to your advantage to do so. If you're shopping for a new policy, look for a guarantee that only you, not the company, can cancel it.

The processing of medical claims can be a hassle for patients, who may feel they have no recourse but to accept the companies' reimbursement decision. Just as accountants are often needed to help people file income tax returns, there are now companies that help you process medical insurance claims, a testimony to a system desperately in need of simplification and reform.

Basic Types of Coverage

Basic hospitalization. More than 90 percent of the population has this kind of insurance, which covers such hospital charges as room (semiprivate), food, X rays, lab tests, drugs, operating room fees, etc. Usually, as in the case of Blue Cross, you are fully covered for a specified number of days — such as 120 — in the hospital, with the time available renewed after a certain number of months have elapsed. The longer the coverage, the more expensive the policy. Other policies have a system of indemnity benefits in which a specified amount per day is paid toward hospital room and board, perhaps leaving you with a large bill to pay on your own.

For all elective procedures, be sure to check your policy first to see whether they are covered. Cosmetic surgery, for example, usually is not, unless it is needed following an accidental injury or to repair a birth defect. However, certain outpatient procedures, such as kidney dialysis, emergency room care, and radiation therapy, may be fully covered.

Basic medical/surgical. This (like Blue Shield) covers doctor bills incurred as a result of surgery or hospitalization and sometimes also doctor's services at a private office or in your home. The reimbursement allowance may fall short of the doctor's actual fees, requiring you to pay the difference. Some policies say they pay "up to" a certain amount for a particular procedure; this does not mean you will get the maximum allowed in your case. A medical/surgical policy is often offered in combination with basic hospitalization; both are considered highly desirable.

Major medical. These policies are in effect "catastrophic" health insurance that pick up where basic hospitalization/medical/surgical policies leave off. They are almost a necessity these days if a major illness should strike. However, policies vary widely in what they cover and what they cost. The typical policy covers hospitalization; surgery; diagnostic techniques; doctors' fees; private-duty nursing; home medical care; prescribed drugs, therapies, and medical devices; and rehabilitation services.

However, few policies cover routine checkups for ostensibly healthy people. You can often get around this limitation if your doctor investigates a particular health complaint you may have at the time of your visit.

There may be a waiting period before a policy takes effect. Some policies exclude coverage (for a prescribed time, at least) for preexisting medical conditions. Some pay the first dollar of expenses, but most have a deductible (usually $100 to $1,000) that the patient must first satisfy before insurance steps in. The larger the deductible, the lower the cost of the insurance, so if you are buying an individual policy, it may pay to take the largest deductible you can afford. Though the deductible covers expenses incurred during a calendar year, you may be allowed to apply bills from the last three months of the previous year to satisfy your deductible.

Beyond the deductible, the insurance usually reimburses you for 75 or 80 percent of your costs. You pay the rest. As care gets more expensive, your share of the costs does, too.

Look for a stop-loss limit in the policy which specifies a maximum amount you would have to pay per year for an individual or for the family. Beyond that amount the insurance would pay all costs up to the total maximum amount for which you are insured. Most experts suggest a lifetime maximum of $250,000, but as medical costs continue to rise, this, too, should rise. Many people now have a $1 million maximum, and some have no limit to their protection. In some cases the maximum applies to each separate illness, a further advantage.

Neither major medical nor other medical insurance policies cover income lost because of a disability. For this, you would need a separate disability insurance policy. Here again, the benefits vary greatly; look for noncancelable, long-term (until age sixty-five) coverage for disability caused by both accidents and illness.

But experts caution against insurance for specific diseases, such as cancer; your policy should cover you no matter what costly illness might strike.

The health maintenance organization, or HMO. This is really not insurance as such but rather a prepaid group practice in which the individual or family pays so much a month to receive all or nearly all needed medical services free (some groups charge a minimal fee per visit). Since the group's only income is usually the "premiums" paid by members, it is in the doctors' interests to hold down costs by keeping members healthy. Thus, more attention may be paid to preventive health practices and periodic examinations, which are rarely covered by conventional insurance.

Other advantages of an HMO include "one-stop shopping" since most specialists and special tests are available in the same building or complex; greater predictability of annual medical care costs; twenty-four-hour, seven-day-a-week availability of medical care from a doctor who has ready access to your records; greater continuity of care; and possibly less reluctance to seek medical help when you are uncertain of the need.

Disadvantages include having to use only those doctors who are members of the group, though allowances may be made if you need treatment far from home. HMO membership may cost more than other kinds of insurance, and if your policy is through your employer, you may have to pay extra. HMO benefits may vary widely from group to group, so check carefully before you join.

Medicare. While clearly better than nothing, Medicare is far from a guarantee that elderly Americans will not be devastated by the costs of medical care. In fact, today the average senior citizen pays more out of pocket for medical care than he or she did before Congress authorized Medicare.

Medicare covers all people over sixty-five who are eligible for Social Security or Railroad Retirement Benefits as well as younger people who are disabled or who have chronic kidney disease. Others over sixty-five can purchase Medicare insurance.

Medicare comes in two parts, and all who are eligible should have both. Part A, which is free, is hospital insurance that helps to pay for the costs of a hospital stay and after-hospital care in a skilled nursing home or through a home health agency. It does not cover doctor bills or custodial nursing home care. Part B, which costs participants a small monthly fee, helps to pay doctor bills, outpatient hospital services, and the costs of various medical services and supplies. It does not cover such typical needs of the elderly as eyeglasses and hearing aids and the examinations for their prescription, flu shots, drugs, dentures and dental care, private nursing, routine foot care, custodial nursing home care, or treatment in a foreign country. Also not covered are acupuncture, cosmetic surgery, most chiropractic services, and routine physicals.

Medicare A and B both have deductibles, which can go up every year. In 1982 the hospital deductible was raised to $260; beyond sixty days in the hospital the patient must contribute to the cost ($65 a day through the ninetieth day). Part B pays for 80 percent of "reasonable" medical costs, which may be considerably less than what your doctor charges. Therefore, it pays to find a doctor who will accept Medicare's payment schedule, charging you no more than the remaining 20 percent.

You might also investigate purchasing a private supplemental policy to fill in at least some of Medicare's gaps and take over where it leaves off. But note that most such policies still follow Medicare's fee schedule and pick up the remaining 20 percent of "reasonable" costs, leaving you to foot the rest of the doctor's bill.

When Medicare awards you much less than your doctor charges, you might consider appealing the decision, which is often in error. A call to your local congressman may be a shortcut to quick action.

For Further Reading

Those who wish to make more sense out of Medicare coverage might consult *How to Recover Your Medical Expenses,* by Kal Waller. New York: Collier Books, 1981.

Home Care: Alternative to Hospital and Nursing Home

One winter, after seventy-five years of independent living, Norma, a widow, fell on an icy road and and broke her hip. She was depressed by the prospect of spending months as an invalid in a nursing home while her hip mended. She brightened when she learned that with the help of a local home care program, she could return to her own home to recover.

At home Norma surprised the doctor with how quickly she mended and was up and around again. Thanks to visiting nurses, a special van that took her to the hospital for periodic checkups, and wonderful meals prepared by friends, relatives, and a part-time homemaking assistant, Norma maintained her independence and her usual good spirits. By June she was even able to tend the vegetable garden her grandsons planted for her.

Home care, as an alternative to costly and prolonged hospitalization or residence in a nursing home, is a growing phenomenon in medicine today. It is being used for patients with illnesses like heart attack that involve a lengthy recovery period; for patients who are chronically ill, for example, disabled by a stroke; for patients who are terminally ill; for children for whom a long hospital stay can be extraordinarily stressful; and for the elderly who are too ill or disabled to function entirely on their own.

The American Public Health Association has estimated that at least 10 to 25 percent of people in institutions could live at home if adequate services were available. Former Secretary of Health, Education and Welfare Joseph Califano has estimated that one in seven patients now cared for in hospitals could be treated as well or better at home. Ironically, the home care movement is a return to traditional medical practices; until relatively recently, sick and dying people were cared for primarily at home. Prolonged hospitalization was the exception rather than the rule.

The Advantages

Although prompted more by economics than humanitarian considerations, home care is proving to be emotionally and medically advantageous to patients and their families. Among the benefits that have been noted:

- Wounds heal faster at home since the patient's state of mind, an important factor in recovery, is likely to be much more positive at home.
- Patients feel better and eat better when they are surrounded by familiar people and objects and given food prepared to their liking.
- Patients take more responsibility for their own care when removed from the dependency fostered by institutional care.
- Fewer sleeping pills are needed when sleep is not disturbed by unfamiliarity and the noises of hospital personnel and other patients.
- The family is less disrupted by the need to make frequent trips to the hospital.
- Home care costs less.

The kinds of services available at home are expanding rapidly and the number of home care providers, both nonprofit and private, is growing as well. According to "Home Health Care" (see "For Further Reading," page 480), a Public Affairs Pamphlet by Theodore Irwin, in many communities throughout the country you can participate in home care programs that provide nursing care; transportation to the hospital or physician for periodic treatments or follow-up examinations; rehabilitative therapies such as occupational, physical, respiratory, speech, and nutritional therapy; counseling by a social worker; medical equipment; various tests and treatments, such as blood tests, intravenous drug therapy, and kidney dialysis; and homemaking services like shopping, cooking, and light housework.

Programs vary widely in the quality and extent of services provided and in how much of their cost is covered by medical insurance. Twenty-five states now regulate home health care agencies, and in seven states insurers are required to make home care benefits available to their clients.

Before Opting for Home Care . . .

- Check first to be sure your insurance or Medicare or Medicaid will cover your home care expenses. Although your policy may reimburse home care costs at a lower rate than hospital costs, it still could cost you less than being in the hospital. But often it personally costs you more to be treated at home, even if total overall costs are much less.
- Is your home situation suitable for such care, in terms of both physical layout and ability and willingness of other family members to provide what help is needed?
- Is the patient's condition of a type that would respond to home care, or would the security of round-the-clock institutional care be more appropriate?
- What about the patient's personality? A patient who is extremely

nervous, demanding, or crotchety could make matters worse for the family at home.

• Are the kinds of care needed available in the community?

For Further Information and Services

To determine what services can be obtained at home, check with one or more of the following: the physician in charge, the hospital's social services department, the local Visiting Nurses Association, or the Yellow Pages listing under home health agencies. Other sources of information include: the National Council for Homemaker-Home Health Aide Services, 67 Irving Place, New York, New York 10003, which maintains a nationwide listing of home care services; the National League for Nursing, 10 Columbus Circle, New York, New York 10019; and the Home Health Services and Staffing Association, Suite 205, 1101 Fifteenth Street NW, Washington, D.C. 20005, which maintains a listing of proprietary home care services.

For Further Reading

Baulch, Evelyn M. *Home Care.* Millbrae, Calif.: Celestial Arts, 1980.
Irwin, Theodore. "Home Health Care: When a Patient Leaves the Hospital." Public Affairs Pamphlet No. 560, 1978. Available for 50 cents from Public Affairs Pamphlets, 381 Park Avenue South, New York, N.Y. 10016.

Nursing Homes: How to Get Good Care

Nursing homes have been the subject of considerable public scandal and private agonizing in recent years. The number of these facilities mushroomed in response to Medicare and Medicaid reimbursement, which made nursing home care a possibility for growing numbers of aged, ailing Americans who can no longer care for themselves or be cared for at home. Today well over 1 million Americans, 90 percent of them over age sixty-five, are residents of nursing homes.

Clearly there have been abuses — often at the patient's expense — as a relatively unmonitored industry emerged. In contrast with hospitals, 80 percent of which are nonprofit institutions, more than three-fourths of nursing homes are privately owned and in business to make money.

While profit and good care are not necessarily incompatible, tales are legion of nursing home patients who are overly sedated, poorly fed and cared for, and left to languish in bed or in front of a TV set. Furthermore, according to various estimates, between 10 and 50 percent of nursing home residents really don't belong in such an institution but are there simply because they have no place else to go.

Thus, it is hardly surprising that the decision to send a relative — in most cases, a parent — to a nursing home commonly stirs up strong feelings of guilt and fear. These feelings are often compounded by grief over the realization that the move may be the "beginning of the end" for a loved one. As the Senate Special Committee on Aging put it, "To the average older American, nursing homes have become almost synonymous with death and prolonged suffering before death."

The Benefits of a Nursing Home

Yet the nursing home can be — and often is — the best solution for all concerned, especially the patient. It can alleviate loneliness, provide essential physical and medical care, fulfill basic daily needs, and offer security and protection, particularly for confused or self-destructive patients. The nursing home experience does not have to be disastrous if a home that can best meet the patient's needs is selected.

Some basic facts may help put the matter of nursing homes into a better light. Only one in twenty persons over sixty-five is in a nursing home, and, on the basis of current statistics, 80 percent of us who reach that age will not spend any time in such a facility. Nor is the nursing home necessarily a dead end. Through coordinated rehabilitative efforts, more than half the residents of a skilled nursing home can be discharged to live independently once again.

As noted by Irving R. Dickman in the Public Affairs Pamphlet "Nursing Homes: Strategy for Reform" (see "For Further Reading," page 484), most nursing home residents have not been abandoned by their families. In fact, only one in five is placed in a home by a family member or enters on his or her own. More than two-thirds are sent by a hospital or welfare agency. In most cases nursing home patients lack any close relatives to help care for them. Their average age at entrance is eighty-four, with nine in ten patients over age sixty-five, and four in ten over eighty-five. Eighty percent are poor. The average length of stay is eighteen months.

Types of Homes

The type of home selected should match the patient's need for nursing and other services. These should be determined by a physician who performs a complete physical examination to evaluate the patient's medical requirements and rehabilitative potential. Types of facilities include:

Residential. This is a group living situation that provides overall supervision and a protective environment, including room and board and planned activities. It is ideal for people who need help in dressing, cooking, shopping, eating, bathing, or other daily activities, but not special medical or nursing services. Such homes are not covered by Medicare or Medicaid.

Intermediate care. Here a minimum of medical service, primarily in the form of nursing care, is provided for patients who may need help with medical treatments ordered by a physician. Although twenty-four-hour nursing care is supposed to be available, often these facilities, which may receive Medicaid reimbursement, provide little more than custodial care. They represent the bulk of nursing homes.

SELECTING A NURSING HOME

If possible, the patient should participate in the choice of a home. Location is important if there are family or friends in the area who might want to visit.

Several resources can help you compile a list of appropriate facilities in the chosen area: the patient's physician, the local medical society, social services department, community welfare or aging council, Social Security office, and the state chapters of the American Health Care Association (for proprietary homes) and the American Association of Homes for the Aging (for nonprofit homes). Ask for the names of licensed facilities that are eligible for the type of reimbursement you expect to rely on.

The next step is to visit the homes, both on an official tour and, if possible, as an ordinary visitor of a patient. The following checklist will help you evaluate what you find. Take it with you, and don't hesitate to ask questions about anything that is not immediately apparent.

Institutional factors

- Is the home licensed by the state or local agency? Ask to see the certificate. Is it accredited by the Joint Commission on Accreditation of Hospitals?
- Is a medical examination required before or immediately after admission? This is *de rigueur* in good nursing homes.
- Is there an arrangement with a nearby hospital for transfer and care of any patient who needs hospitalization?
- Is the facility clean and relatively free of bad odors?
- What are the visiting hours, and who can come?
- Does each bedroom have a window and open onto a corridor?
- Is there room to maneuver a wheelchair?
- How many beds to a room? Four should be the maximum.

Costs

- Is the home eligible for Medicare and/or Medicaid reimbursement?
- What is covered under the basic rate? What is extra? To guard against surprise charges, get a signed statement about coverage from the home you choose. Remember, however, that while the better homes tend to charge more, higher costs do not guarantee better care.
- Are there refunds on advanced payments should the patient leave the home?
- Does the patient's insurance policy cover any or all charges?

Safety

- Is the building fireproof or fire-resistant, and are there a sprinkler system and clearly posted emergency exit routes?
- Are there ramps for wheelchairs, and are the halls wide enough to permit two chairs to pass?
- Are the floor coverings nonskid and the hallways well lit?
- Are there grab bars in the halls, bathrooms, and elevators and call bells at bedside and in the bathrooms? Do they work?

Staff

- Is there a doctor and a registered nurse on call twenty-four hours a day?
- Is there provision made for regular dental care? What about an ophthalmologist,

podiatrist, or any other specialist the patient may need? How often are they available?
● Is the nursing staff trained in basic rehabilitation techniques? Is there a full-time physical therapy program directed by a qualified physical or occupational therapist?
● Is there a social worker available to handle family and patient concerns and negotiations with other community resources?
● Is the staff friendly and efficient in responding to patient calls? If possible, talk to a few current residents.
● Does the staff encourage patients to be independent?
● Are patients overtranquilized or restrained to minimize staff harassment? Often the patients who are the best candidates for rehabilitation are the most heavily sedated since they are more active and demanding than others.

Food
● Are the meals varied, well balanced, well cooked, and appetizingly served? Are special likes and dislikes taken into account?
● Is there a dietician who prepares meals for patients on special diets?
● Are the menus prepared a week or more in advance, and does the food served match what's on the menu?
● Are patients encouraged to eat in a group, or do they dine alone in their rooms?
● Do those who need help in feeding get it, and get it promptly, before the food gets cold?
● Is the dining room attractive and accessible to patients in wheelchairs?

Activities
● Is there a recreation program?
● Are there rooms for socializing, physical therapy, and occupational therapy?
● Are the grounds well kept, and are patients who are able to go outside encouraged to do so daily?
● Do volunteers from the community work with and visit patients regularly?
● Are patients kept busy and occupied? Are there activities like card games, knitting and sewing, conversation?
● Are outings scheduled?

Personal factors
● Are patients treated with dignity and respect, or are they talked down to as if they were small children?
● Do patients have privacy — for dressing and undressing, phone calls, visits?
● Are any personal possessions, such as a favorite rocking chair, allowed, and is there room for keeping personal belongings?
● Are there arrangements for religious observances?
● Are a barber and a beautician available?
● Are patients allowed to wear their own clothing? Are they kept clean and well groomed?
● Can patients leave for special outings or home visits?

You may find after you've selected a home that there is a long waiting list, especially for patients who do not pay full fees. Sometimes a "philanthropic" contribution (some call it a bribe) to the home helps to short-circuit the wait. In any case put the patient's name on the list and explore temporary alternatives, such as various home care services. [See chapter on home care, page 478.]

Skilled nursing. Round-the-clock nursing services are available, and preventive, rehabilitative, social, spiritual, and emotional care are provided as needed on a regular basis. These facilities are recognized for coverage by Medicare and Medicaid and are eligible for accreditation by the Joint Commission on Accreditation of Hospitals.

Extended care. Round-the-clock nursing care and medical supervision are supposed to be available in these facilities, which provide an extension of hospital care on a long-term but not necessarily permanent basis. Medicare and sometimes private health insurance covers such care (but benefits may have a time limit), and the facilities are eligible for accreditation.

How to Complain

If, after the patient has been placed in a nursing home, you are unhappy with the treatment, Mr. Dickman advises that you speak first to the administrator and, if you get no satisfaction, then to the local senior citizens group or any local pressure group interested in nursing homes. All complaints should also be brought to the local Social Security office and to the state's nursing home ombudsman, who can direct your complaint to the right state agency. You may also want to contact the American Health Care Association, 1200 Fifteenth Street NW, Washington, D.C. 20005 (for proprietary homes), or the American Association of Homes for the Aging, 1050 Seventeenth Street NW, Suite 770, Washington, D.C. 20036 (for nonprofit homes).

483

For Further Reading

Dickman, Irving R. "Nursing Homes: Strategy for Reform." Public Affairs Pamphlet No. 666. Available for 50 cents from Public Affairs Pamphlets, 381 Park Avenue South, New York, N.Y. 10016.

XI.
Symptoms

When you're ill and someone asks how you are feeling, you are likely to answer in a way that really isn't an answer: "I have a cough (fever, sore throat, pain in my shoulder)." For while these conditions certainly have significance to you, the sufferer, they are merely *symptoms* — clues to any of a very wide variety of underlying ailments. And unless their cause is uncovered and properly treated, you may gain only temporary relief from self- and physician-prescribed ministrations.

Though they usually represent short-lived, minor ailments, occasionally a symptom like a cough, a sore throat, a pain, and even an itch can be a sign of a life-threatening illness. In other cases, like low blood sugar, the symptoms may be a lot of "sound and fury, signifying nothing."

It is important to know when to take your symptoms seriously and seek professional assistance rather than rely on your own devices, over-the-counter remedies, or Father Time. It is also important to be able to assess the quality of a doctor's evaluation when you bring a symptom to his or her attention.

Pain:
Almost No One Escapes It

"Americans are probably the most pain-conscious people on the face of the earth. For years we have had it drummed into us — in print, on radio, over television, in everyday conversation — that any hint of pain is to be banished as though it were the ultimate evil. As a result, we are becoming a nation of pill-grabbers and hypochondriacs, escalating the slightest ache into a searing ordeal."— Norman Cousins, in *Anatomy of an Illness.*

In the course of a year more than 45 percent of Americans seek medical treatment for pain. Most are at least temporarily frightened by their discomfort. For some 10 million Americans, pain is a day-in and day-out affair that cripples their lives. Only a relative handful of people — about 100 in all, according to medical records — have been born without the ability to feel physical pain.

Pain is a wholly personal experience. No one can feel another's pain, and probably no two people experience pain in precisely the same way. Nor can any instrument or test measure the dimensions of a person's pain, the way a thermometer measures fever or a blood test reveals cell numbers.

Pain is thus completely subjective. When dealing with a patient in pain, a doctor must rely totally on the person's description of the discomfort. Pain can be sharp, throbbing, or dull; mild or severe; transient or prolonged; continuous or intermittent. Sometimes a pain is referred — that is, felt in an area of the body different from where it originates.

Despite its universality, misunderstandings about pain — among both lay people and physicians — abound. Few doctors are taught anything about pain beyond the descriptions of pains that are symptoms of specific diseases. When doctors cannot find an organic cause for pain, they tend to dismiss the symptom as irrelevant and regard its victim as a malingerer. Many nonmedical persons share these misconceptions. When told by a doctor that there is no apparent physical explanation for a pain, they conclude that the discomfort must be imagined.

In fact, *all pain is real,* whether caused by a tumor pressing on a nerve or by tension that tightens muscles or by fear that constricts arteries. Gastrointestinal cramps triggered by anxiety can be just as painful — and are just as real — as those due to amebic dysentery or colitis. The only "fake" pain isn't pain at all — it's a deliberate lie told by a malingerer.

What Is Pain?

In simplest terms, pain is a sensation that begins when certain nerves are stimulated, probably by chemical pain substances (bradykinin is one) released when cells are injured. The nerves transmit the pain message through the spinal cord to the brain, which processes the information and tells you that you hurt somewhere.

Most of the time pain is a protective signal. It may call attention to some underlying organic disorder, for example, painful urination that results from a bladder infection or angina pains from diseased coronary arteries. Or it may result from an injury, like a cut or a broken bone, protecting the person from further damage by making it too painful to use the injured part. Pain can act as a warning to avoid future injuries; a child who touches a hot stove quickly learns to keep hands off hot things.

Physical pain can also warn of disorders that originate in the mind or emotions. A nagging headache or chronic low back pain may result from tension, anxiety, stress, or fear that needs to be recognized and dissipated in a less damaging way. Such pains are called functional or psychogenic — originating in the psyche — but that doesn't make them any less real or life-disrupting than pains that are organic in origin, the result of a physical disorder.

People with psychogenic pain fully deserve medical attention, and should not feel guilty about their misery or about "imposing" on a doctor's time. The main problem is that few doctors are equipped to recognize and treat the causes of psychogenic pain, and tend, instead, to prescribe pain-killers that may mask the pain temporarily but don't cure the underlying cause.

Many pains have both a physical and an emotional component. The pain of a disease or injury may trigger fear, tension, or anxiety that makes the pain worse. This fact accounts for the pain relief many people get when they are told by a doctor that the cause of their discomfort is "nothing serious." Or conversely, an emotionally induced pain can result in damage to a tissue that produces even more pain.

Types of Pain

There are two basic kinds of pain: *acute* and *chronic*. Acute pain tends to start suddenly, is often sharp, and is short-lived. Acute pain is usually the result of an injury, surgery, infection, or internal disease that heals within days, weeks, or a few months at most. Usually treatment is directed at the underlying cause, perhaps with a mild pain-killing drug to ease the way.

Chronic pain, on the other hand, is persistent, lasting many months or years. It has outlived its usefulness as a warning (or never had any in the first place) and instead become an all-consuming, life-disrupting phenomenon that fogs the mind, interferes with the ability to perform everyday functions, and causes psychic misery.

Chronic pain may start with an acute ailment that then takes on an emotional component, causing the pain to linger for many months or years after the initial ailment has been resolved. Sometimes the origin of chronic pain is totally emotional. Or it may result from an incurable disease, such as advanced cancer, arthritis, or nerve disease. Whatever the origin, the longer the pain lasts, the more important psychological factors become. The patient's entire outlook, personality, and conduct of life may be changed by persistent pain. Unemployment, divorce, and suicide are common among victims of chronic pain.

Many experts say chronic pain is a disease in itself that should be treated by a team of pain specialists, such as are found in pain clinics at medical centers throughout the country. Certainly it is a widespread and costly problem, afflicting an estimated 10 million Americans and costing some $60 billion a year in medical care costs and lost productivity. According to specialists at pain clinics, many victims hop from doctor to doctor, who may prescribe dozens of potent drugs and perform needless operations, all of which can jeopardize the patient's health without providing lasting relief of the pain.

Perceptions of Pain

Many factors influence whether you notice a pain at all and, if you do, how much it hurts. Since the pain message is received and interpreted by the brain, competing messages may block it, or other factors may enhance the intensity of a painful sensation.

The pain threshold — the point at which a person reports feeling pain — can be raised as much as 45 percent by a loud noise, hypnosis, or other distractions. Fully one-third of all pains can be relieved by a placebo, or sugar pill, if the patient thinks it is an active pain-killing drug. Recent studies suggest that placebos work by triggering the release of the body's own morphine, endorphins. The fact that a pain can be dissipated by a placebo does not mean it was a fake or emotional in origin.

Excitement or preoccupation with an activity may block perception of pain. The stories of athletes who don't realize they've broken a bone until the end of exciting competition are legion. The mother who distracts a hurt, crying child with another activity is accomplishing the same thing. On the other hand, anxiety, depression, fatigue, fear, or stresses totally unrelated to the condition at hand may greatly magnify pain.

Studies have shown that pain is lessened if patients are told in advance what to expect. Telling children who are about to undergo a painful procedure that "it won't hurt a bit" may actually make the experience more, not less, painful. On the other hand, anxious anticipation of pain to come can make it worse.

Cultural factors have a major influence on pain sensitivity. Studies have shown that the Irish tend to deny pain, and "Yankees" take a matter-of-fact attitude toward it. Italians tend to be vociferous about their discomfort and want it relieved immediately. Jewish patients are also vocal about their pains but worry more about the significance of the pain than its alleviation.

Parents, by adopting an overzealous or casual attitude toward pain, can greatly influence how their children react to it. So can religious attitudes. Those who accept pain as "just punishment" for sins or view it as an opportunity to share Christ's suffering may hurt less than persons who regard pain as undeserved. Age and sex also affect pain perception. As you get older, your sensitivity to pain is likely to decline. Women tend to have lower pain thresholds than men.

Pain Relievers

Throughout history, incantations, prayers, exorcisms, tattoos, talismans, and charms have been used to rid the human body of life-disrupting pain. Many of the pain remedies used by ancient peoples are still with us today: herbal brews, opium, heat, cold, massage, surgery, and even electrical shock (using a torpedo fish). As far back as 3000 B.C., in fact, acupuncture was used in China to relieve pain.

Modern pain relief borrows from all these techniques, refining and extending them to apply to specific pain situations. Though all problems of severe, chronic, or recurrent pain are hardly solved, patients in pain today have a far better chance of getting substantial or complete relief than they did as little as fifteen years ago.

Pain relievers work in one of two ways: locally, at the site of origin, by reducing or totally blocking the transmission of a pain signal, or centrally, in the brain, by blocking the reception or perception of the pain signal.

After years of regarding pain relief as a treatment the physician administers to the patient, pain specialists today realize that much help can come from within the person in pain. This is especially true for persons with chronic pain that no longer has an organic cause, such as many chronic back ailments.

At pain clinics throughout the country, where as many as seventeen different medical specialists — including an orthopedist, a neurologist, a psychologist or a psychiatrist, and a physical therapist — may be involved in diagnosing and treating a patient in pain, such techniques as self-hypnosis and behavior modification have brought dramatic relief to many long-suffering patients.

The major methods of pain relief in use today include the following:

Anesthesia. General anesthesia, administered by inhalation or injection, deadens the brain, including those portions that support vital functions. Thus, it is used only for a limited time, as during surgery. Local anesthesia, like Novocain or spinal block, deadens the nerves in the region of the pain. Since it numbs all sensation, it, too, is used only in limited circumstances, such as during surgery or childbirth.

Sometimes, in the treatment of chronic localized pain, such as that resulting from cancer, neuralgia, or chronic pancreatitis, a local anesthetic will be injected into a particular nerve. This therapy, called nerve block, has proved especially helpful for treating the pain of shingles. In fact, nerve block treatment of the initial attack often results in rapid healing of this viral nerve infection and prevents the long-lasting pain that sometimes follows it.

Analgesics and other drugs. There are two basic types of analgesic drug: narcotics, which work on the central nervous system, and nonnarcotics, which work locally. Narcotics — morphine, codeine, methadone, and meperidine (Demerol), among them — do not block out pain but rather make it less distressing to the victim. Because they are addicting and patients develop a tolerance that leads to ever-increasing doses to achieve the same relief, narcotics should be used for only a limited time, such as after surgery or a severe injury. In addition, morphine may be given for an indefinite period to patients with intractable pain caused by terminal cancer. However, narcotics are often misused in patients with other kinds of chronic pain, resulting in addiction and the need for drug withdrawal treatment.

Nonnarcotic analgesics include such over-the-counter remedies as aspirin and acetaminophen and several prescription drugs (like Darvon). In cases where anxiety or depression is causing or exacerbating pain and in cases of nerve pain (such as tic douloureux), tranquilizers, antidepressants, or other psychoactive drugs may provide pain relief. A third or more of pain patients benefit from a placebo, which works on the patient's own psychological resources and triggers the release of endorphins, natural substances many times more powerful than morphine.

Nerve surgery. This is a drastic approach, to be used only when other methods of pain relief fail. It involves severing the nerve pathways that transmit pain sensations. It is used primarily for cancer patients and persons with tic douloureux who cannot otherwise be helped. In the latter case, a preferred approach is destruction of the responsible facial nerve by the use of radio waves. Nerve surgery for back pain rarely provides lasting relief and may complicate the patient's problem.

Transcutaneous nerve stimulation (TNS). A portable instrument the size of a cigarette pack can generate electricity that stimulates nerves which block out pain. Electrodes are placed on the skin at "trigger" points, and the instrument is turned on by the patient when needed. Hours of relief may follow as little as five to thirty minutes of use. TNS is often used to treat neck and low back pain, phantom limb pain, and pain following nerve injury or infection.

Acupuncture. This ancient pain remedy apparently works similarly to TNS, by stimulating nerves that suppress pain perception, and also by triggering the release of endorphins. Needles the size of fine hair are inserted through the skin into predetermined points (often the same as those used in TNS) near to or distant from the painful area. The needles are either twirled manually or stimulated by an electric current. A single treatment lasts twenty to thirty minutes, and several treatment sessions may be needed for maximum benefit. Acupuncture has proved especially helpful in treating chronic low back pain, but its usefulness in areas other than pain relief remains highly questionable.

Hypnosis. Contrary to what many people think, hypnosis works best at aborting pain caused by organic illness. It is rarely helpful — and may even be harmful — to those with emotionally induced pain. It works at least in part by focusing the person's attention on something other than the pain, thereby blocking out perception of pain. Patients can be taught self-hypnosis to use whenever needed. It is especially useful for persons with migraine headaches, burns, cancer pain, and the pain of labor and childbirth.

Biofeedback. People can learn to control ordinarily automatic body functions, such as involuntary muscle contractions or blood vessel constriction, by being given a visual or sound signal about them. Through a series of training sessions over a period of weeks or months, a victim of tension headaches can learn to relax the muscles that cause pain. Or patients with migraine headaches can learn to warm their hands (through dilation of blood vessels), which somehow constricts the blood vessels in the head that cause migraine pain. The technique is often practiced at home, with the patient using a portable biofeedback device. Eventually the patient can exercise control on his or her own, without the aid of a device, although an occasional refresher treatment session may be needed. Relaxation exercises (yoga, meditation, and others) may produce benefits similar to biofeedback but without use of a machine.

491

Behavior modification. This technique can be highly effective in treating chronic pain that has a strong emotional component. Often pain persists long after the cause is gone because the patient is somehow "rewarded" for his discomfort, perhaps by being relieved from chores, receiving special attention and sympathy, and being discouraged from doing anything that might "worsen" the pain.

Both patient and family must cooperate in efforts to change a patient's pain-enhancing behavior. To get the treatment started, the patient may have to be hospitalized for a week or more, especially if withdrawal from narcotics is also needed.

In behavioral treatment the patient's pain complaints and other pain-related behaviors are ignored or discouraged, and statements and activities that reflect a healthy existence are rewarded. In some cases a local anesthetic is used temporarily to enable the patient to undergo physical therapy and do exercises to build up long-underused muscles. Behavior modification has been especially helpful to people with chronic back pain.

When and Where to Get Pain Treatment

It's wise to seek medical attention if you experience a sudden severe pain or a recurring pain or if you develop a pain you haven't had before. An internist or a family practitioner is generally the best kind of specialist to consult initially. The doctor's task will be to determine the likely cause of the pain and, if possible, treat it directly or refer you to another specialist for treatment.

Patients with long-standing, or chronic, pain may benefit from a visit to a reputable pain clinic, where specialists from many different disciplines participate in the diagnosis and treatment. The clinic approach is far better than hopping from doctor to doctor, trying one thing after another, and perhaps becoming hooked on drugs or maimed by surgery along the way.

Dr. Richard A. Sternbach, director of the Pain Treatment Center at the Scripps Clinic and Research Foundation in La Jolla, California, warns against what he calls the "Ma-and-Pa Pain Centers" that have sprung up around the country, offering "cures" through one or another technique but rarely paying attention to the whole person and the emotional factors surrounding the pain.

Most reputable clinics are affiliated with a major hospital or medical center. They usually take patients who are referred by other physicians (although self-referral is possible in some cases). They are staffed by specialists from several different disciplines, have a team of consulting specialists, and offer comprehensive diagnosis and treatment, using a wide variety of techniques.

Treatment at a pain clinic can cost anywhere from $1,000 to $3,000 as an outpatient, and much more if hospitalization is required. Costs vary widely, as does insurance coverage, which may depend on the nature of the clinic, the diagnosis, the need for hospitalization, and the type of treatment ultimately used. It's wise to check on costs and coverage before you commit yourself to clinic care.

Dozens of good clinics now exist. Your doctor or a nearby medical school may know of one in your area. If not, your doctor can contact the American Society of Anesthesiologists' Committee on Pain Therapy, which annually produces a detailed descriptive directory of pain clinics.

For Further Reading

Bogin, Meg. *The Path to Pain Control.* Boston: Houghton Mifflin, 1981.
Bresler, David E., M.D. *Free Yourself from Pain.* New York: Wallaby/Simon & Schuster, 1979.
Mines, Samuel. *The Conquest of Pain.* New York: Grosset & Dunlap, 1974.
Whitbread, Jane. *Stop Hurting! Start Living!* New York: Delacorte, 1981.

Fatigue: The Cause
Is Usually Emotional

Fatigue is one of the most common complaints brought to doctors, friends, and relatives. You'd think in this era of labor-saving devices and convenient transportation that few people would have reason to be so tired. But probably more people complain of fatigue today than in the days when hay was baled by hand and laundry scrubbed on a washboard. Witness these typical complaints:

"It doesn't seem to matter how long I sleep — I'm more tired when I wake up than when I went to bed."

"Some of my friends come home from work and jog for several miles or swim laps. I don't know how they do it. I'm completely exhausted at the end of a day at the office."

"I thought I was weary because of the holidays, but now that they're over, I'm even worse. I can barely get through the week, and on the weekend I don't even have the strength to get dressed. I wonder if I'm anemic or something."

"I don't know what's wrong with me lately, but I've been so collapsed that I haven't made a proper meal for the family in weeks. We've been living on TV dinners and packaged mixes. I was finally forced to do a laundry because the kids ran out of underwear."

493

The causes of modern-day fatigue are diverse and only rarely related to excessive physical exertion. The relatively few people who do heavy labor all day long almost never complain about being tired, perhaps because they expect to be. Today, physicians report, tiredness is more likely a consequence of underexertion than of wearing yourself down with overactivity. In fact, increased physical activity is often prescribed as a *cure* for sagging energy.

Kinds of Fatigue

There are three main categories of fatigue:

Physical. This is the well-known result of overworking your muscles to the point where metabolic waste products — carbon dioxide and lactic acid — accumulate in your blood and sap your strength. Your muscles can't continue to work efficiently in a bath of these chemicals. Physical fatigue is usually a pleasant tiredness, such as that which you might experience after playing a hard set of tennis, chopping wood, or climbing a mountain. The cure is simple and fast: You rest, giving your body a chance to get rid of accumulated wastes and restore muscle fuel.

Pathological. Here fatigue is a warning sign or consequence of some underlying physical disorder, perhaps the common cold or flu or something more serious like diabetes or cancer. Usually other symptoms besides fatigue are present that suggest the true cause.

Even after an illness has passed, you're likely to feel dragged out for a week or more. Take your fatigue as a signal to go slow while your body has a chance to recover fully even if all you had was a cold. Pushing yourself to resume full activity too soon could precipitate a relapse and almost certainly will prolong your period of fatigue.

Even though illness is not a frequent cause of prolonged fatigue, it's very important that it not be overlooked. Therefore, anyone who feels drained of energy for weeks on end should have a thorough physical checkup. But even if nothing shows up as a result of the various medical tests, that doesn't mean there's nothing wrong with you.

Unfortunately too often a medical work-up ends with a battery of negative test results, the patient is dismissed, and the true cause of serious fatigue goes undetected. As Dr. John Bulette, a psychiatrist at the Medical College of Pennsylvania Hospital in Philadelphia, tells it, this is what happened to a Pennsylvania woman who had lost nearly fifty pounds and was "almost dead — so tired she could hardly lift her head up." The doctors who first examined the woman were sure she had cancer. But no matter how hard they looked, they could find no sign of malignancy or of any other disease that could account for her wasting away. Finally, she was brought to the college hospital, where doctors noted that she was severely depressed.

They questioned her about her life and discovered that her troubles had begun two years earlier, after her husband died. Once treated for depression, the woman quickly perked up, gained ten pounds in just a few weeks, then returned home to continue her recovery with the aid of psychotherapy.

Psychological. Emotional problems and conflicts, especially depression and anxiety, are by far the most common causes of prolonged fatigue. Fatigue may represent a defense mechanism that prevents you from having to face the true cause of your depression, such as the fact that you hate your job. It is also your body's safety valve for expressing repressed emotional conflicts, such as feeling trapped in an ungratifying role or an unhappy marriage. When such feelings are not expressed openly, they often come out as physical symptoms, with fatigue as one of the most common manifestations. "Many people who are extremely fatigued don't even know they're depressed," Dr. Bulette says. "They're so busy distracting themselves or just worrying about being tired that they don't recognize their depression."

One of these situations is so common it's been given a name — tired housewife syndrome. The victims are commonly young mothers who day in and day out face the predictable tedium of caring for a home and small children, fixing meals, dealing with repairmen, and generally having no one interesting to talk to and nothing enjoyable to look forward to at the end of their boring and unrewarding day. The tired housewife may be inwardly resentful, envious of her husband's job, and guilty about her feelings. But rather than face them head-on, she becomes extremely fatigued.

Today, with nearly half the mothers of young children working outside the home, the tired housewife syndrome has taken on a new twist: that of conflicting roles and responsibilities and guilt over leaving the children, often with an overlay of genuine physical exhaustion from trying to be all things to all people.

Emotionally induced fatigue may be compounded by sleep disturbance that results from the underlying psychological conflict. A person may develop insomnia or may sleep the requisite number of hours but fitfully, tossing and turning all night, having disturbing dreams, and awakening, as one woman put it, feeling as if she "had been run over by a truck."

Understanding the underlying emotional problem is the crucial first step toward curing psychological fatigue and by itself often results in considerable lessening of the tiredness. Professional psychological help or career or marriage counseling may be needed.

What You Can Do About It

There is a great deal you can do on your own to deal with both severe prolonged fatigue and those periodic washed-out feelings. Vitamins and tranquilizers are almost never the right answer, sleeping pills and alcohol are counterproductive, and caffeine is at best a temporary solution that can backfire with abuse and cause life-disrupting symptoms of anxiety. Instead, you might try:

Diet. If you eat a skimpy breakfast or none at all, you're likely to experience midmorning fatigue, the result of a drop in blood sugar, which your body and brain depend on for energy. For peak energy in the morning, be sure to eat a proper breakfast, low in sugar and fairly high in protein, which will provide a steady supply of blood sugar throughout the morning. Coffee and a doughnut are almost worse than nothing, providing a brief boost and then letting you down with a thud. [See chapter on breakfast, page 72.]

The same goes for the rest of the day: Frequent snacking on sweets is a false pick-me-up that soon leaves you lower than you were to begin with. Stick to regular, satisfying, well-balanced meals that help you maintain a trim figure. Extra weight is tiring both physically and psychologically. Getting your weight down to normal can go a long way toward revitalizing you. [See chapter on permanent weight control, page 72.]

Exercise. Contrary to what you may think, exercise enhances, rather than saps, energy. Regular conditioning exercises, such as jogging, cycling, or swimming, help you to resist fatigue by increasing your body's ability to handle more of a work load. You get tired less quickly because your capability is greater.

Exercise also has a well-recognized tranquilizing effect, which helps you work in a more relaxed fashion and be less dragged down by the tensions of your day. At the end of a day exercise can relieve accumulated tensions, give you more energy in the evening, and help you sleep more restfully. [See chapter on the benefits of exercise, page 86.]

Sleep. If you know you're tired because you haven't been getting enough sleep, the solution is simple: Get to bed earlier. There's no right amount of sleep for everyone, and generally sleep requirements decline with age. Find the amount that suits you best, and aim for it. Insomnia and other sleep disorders should not be treated with sleeping pills, alcohol, or tranquilizers, which can actually make the problem worse. [See chapter on insomnia, page 557.]

Know yourself. Try to schedule your most taxing jobs for the time of day when you're at your peak. Some are "morning people" who tire by midafternoon; others do their best work in the evening. Don't overextend yourself, trying to climb the ladder of success at a record pace or to meet everyone's demands or expectations. Decide what you want to do and what you can handle comfortably, and learn to say no to additional requests. Recognize your energy cycles and plan accordingly. Many women have a low point premenstrually, during which time extra sleep may be needed and demanding activities are particularly exhausting.

Take breaks. No matter how interesting or demanding your work, you'll be able to do it with more vigor if now and again you stop, stretch, and change the scenery. Instead of coffee and a sweet roll on your break, try meditation, yoga, calisthenics, or a brisk walk. Even running up and down the staircase can provide refreshment from a sedentary job. If your job is physically demanding, relax in a quiet place for a while. The do-something-different rule also applies to vacations; "getting away from it all" for a week or two or longer can be highly revitalizing, helping you to put things in perspective and enabling you to take your job more in stride upon your return.

Fever:
An Important Clue

One of the special characteristics of mammals is their ability to maintain a stable body temperature despite a wide range in environmental temperatures. This is what it means to be warm-blooded. A tiny section of the brain called the hypothalamus houses the body's thermostat, which in people is normally set at about 98.6 degrees Fahrenheit, give or take a degree or two.

When it's cold outside relative to our internal temperature, our surface blood vessels contract to reduce heat loss and our muscles quiver (shiver) to produce more heat. When it's hot, our surface blood vessels dilate and we lose body heat through the evaporation of sweat. We can assist the workings of our natural heat control system by putting on or taking off clothes or heating or cooling the surrounding air.

Sometimes, however, the internal controls seem to go awry, resulting in a rise in body temperature — or what is commonly called fever. Fever is a symptom that can have a number of causes, some more serious than others.

Fever may result from a resetting of the body's central thermostat triggered by an infectious organism or toxic chemical, including certain drugs. It can follow an inability of the body's cooling mechanisms to keep up with internally generated or externally imposed heat, such as from exercising vigorously in hot, humid weather, overdressing, or staying too long in a sauna. Or it can result from a defect in the body's heat loss mechanisms, such as that caused by a bad sunburn and certain antidepressant drugs. In heat stroke the uncontrolled rise of body temperature can be fatal if it is not reduced promptly. [See chapter on heat disorders, page 342.]

The most common cause of fever is an infection by some noxious microorganism. Recent evidence indicates that in cases of infection, fever may play an important role in helping to defend the body against disease. Fever-inducing microorganisms cause the white blood cells to release a protein called endogenous pyrogen. Pyrogen travels to the brain, where it stimulates the resetting of the body's thermostat at a higher level. For unknown reasons an infection-caused fever almost never rises higher than 106 degrees, and techniques used to reduce a high fever do not lower it below "normal" body temperature.

Fever has a number of unpleasant effects. It dehydrates and enervates. It may cause headache, loss of appetite, nausea, and vomiting. It often causes chills; you shiver because your thermostat is now set higher than usual relative to the surrounding air and your body must generate more heat to maintain that higher temperature.

Fevers above 103 degrees in an adult may upset mental processes temporarily, causing a lack of judgment, confusion, or even delirium.

HOW TO READ A THERMOMETER

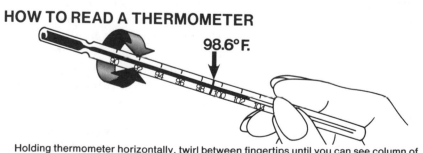

Holding thermometer horizontally, twirl between fingertips until you can see column of mercury clearly. Long vertical lines represent whole degrees; short lines represent 0.2 degree. Temperature shown is 98.6.

Young children can suffer convulsions from a very rapid rise in body temperature, but once a high fever develops, convulsion is unlikely. According to the best available evidence, these febrile convulsions, though frightening, are not dangerous and do not cause brain damage.

The higher your fever, the worse you're likely to feel. But it doesn't necessarily follow that you're more seriously ill when your fever is high than when it's only a degree or two above normal. Babies and young children have incompletely developed heat-regulating systems, so they tend to run high temperatures even from minor infections.

A child with a strep throat that requires medical treatment may have a temperature of only 100, whereas a flulike illness that needs only symptomatic care may send the temperature soaring to 104. Premature infants and elderly people, on the other hand, rarely run high fevers. In fact, they can have serious infections and no fever at all.

When to Take a Fever Seriously

Many parents overreact to low-grade fevers in their children. A temperature is not considered "high" until it reaches 105, and harm from fever does not begin until the temperature is 106 or 107. The child's other symptoms are more important than the fact that temperature is 100 or 103. In children, any of the following circumstances should prompt a call to the doctor:

• If a temperature above 101 orally or 102 rectally persists for more than a day.

• If a fever of 104 or higher lasts for four hours and doesn't go down in response to fever-reducing drugs.

• If any fever, even a low one, persists for four or more days.

• If the child is less than four months old.

• If there are other worrisome symptoms, such as rash, sore throat, earache, bad cough, breathing difficulties, extreme lethargy, vomiting, diarrhea, or stiff neck.

An adult should also check out a persistent temperature or one associated with possibly serious symptoms such as the above.

In reporting a fever to the doctor, note the time of day, how the temperature was measured, and any trends. Body temperature normally fluctuates during the day — usually lowest first thing in the morning, highest in the late afternoon or evening. A child sent to school with a normal temperature in the morning may come home feverish at 3 P.M. If a child has been sick with a fever, it's usually wise to keep him or her home for one extra day after the temperature returns to normal.

Should Fever Be Treated?

Recently specialists have begun to question the wisdom of treating most fevers (as opposed to treating their underlying causes). Some doctors suggest that the side effects of the medications used may actually increase a feverish patient's discomfort. If fever is caused by an infection, drugs like aspirin which have anti-inflammatory properties may delay healing and increase contagiousness. When pain relief is needed, other drugs that lack aspirin's anti-inflammatory properties (including acetaminophen and various prescription drugs) might be used. [See chapter on aspirin, page 463.]

Furthermore, fever may aid recovery since an increased body temperature inhibits the growth and reproduction of many disease-producing organisms. In some cases, such as when the doctor wants to see if an antibiotic is working, it may be preferable to let a fever run its course. Artificially lowering the body temperature may also make it difficult to know when an illness is really over.

A person racked with fever-induced chills is likely to curl up under a pile of covers. According to Dr. J. Franklin Donaldson, a fever expert affiliated with the Tufts University School of Medicine, keeping the patient comfortable with the use of warm clothing, blankets, warmed room air, and warm liquids is advisable when a fever is developing. However, if sweating occurs, the patient has become overheated, and some sources of warmth should be removed.

It is also important to give plenty of fluids — preferably clear liquids — to a person with fever, to replace the water lost from the body through evaporation and to facilitate sweating. A feverish body burns

499

HOW TO MEASURE BODY TEMPERATURE

Feeling the forehead with your lips or hand does not give an accurate reading, or even a good guess, of body temperature. You must use a fever thermometer — oral or rectal — and shake it down to at least 96 degrees before you use it.

Rectal temperatures are most accurate. Oral temperature readings, usually a degree lower than the rectal temperature, can be thrown off by mouth breathing, recent consumption of hot or cold foods, or smoking. It's difficult to obtain an accurate reading orally from a young child, and an oral thermometer has too fragile a bulb to be used rectally.

Don't worry if a thermometer breaks in the mouth and the mercury is swallowed. Thermometers contain only a tiny amount of metallic mercury, which is much less hazardous than mercury salts.

If you cannot measure it by other methods, body temperature can also be measured in the armpit, using any type of fever thermometer.

If you're taking the temperature of a very young or uncooperative child, it's a good idea to use a thermometer that registers within a degree of the actual temperature in less than a minute. Otherwise, you should leave the thermometer in for three minutes rectally or five minutes orally. In taking a rectal temperature, lubricate the bulb first with petroleum jelly or cold cream.

To read the thermometer, hold the glass end, and slowly twirl it until you can see the silvery column of mercury. Each small line on the scale represents two-tenths of a degree. Thus, if the column of mercury ends at the third line after the 100 mark, the temperature is 100.6. After reading the temperature, shake the thermometer down, wash it with cool water and soap, and store it in its container in a safe place.

extra calories, but the adage about starving a fever may still be wise since sick patients are likely to have difficulty digesting or retaining solid food. If fever is prolonged, however, a vitamin supplement may be helpful.

Given the new understanding of the role of fever, many doctors now give fever-reducing drug treatment only when a child's temperature rises above 102 degrees (some say over 104) or the child is very uncomfortable. The most effective treatment for reducing fever caused by illness is aspirin or acetaminophen, both of which lower the set point of the body's thermostat. Without such "centralized" lowering, other measures to bring down fever, such as tepid sponge baths, increased fluids, and light covers, are futile in the long run since the temperature is likely to rise again quickly. However, such measures can greatly enhance comfort.

The drug treatment should be repeated every three or four hours, as directed, to keep the thermostat at its new lower setting. If vomiting prevents treatment by mouth, rectal aspirin suppositories are available at pharmacies. Acetaminophen, which can be obtained in liquid form, may be easier to administer to a very young child; it is also less likely than aspirin to upset the stomach.

In addition to blocking the action of pyrogens on the body thermostat, fever-reducing drugs stimulate sweating and dilation of surface blood vessels, which help to cool you down. This is the familiar sensation of the fever's "breaking"; it commonly occurs during the night, and you may wake up soaked with sweat but feeling a lot better than when you went to sleep.

Caffeine raises body temperature and can block the effects of fever-reducing drugs, so it may be wise to avoid drinking coffee, tea, and cola and taking caffeine-containing drugs (for example, Anacin and Excedrin) when you are trying to reduce a fever.

If lowering a seriously elevated body temperature is the goal, it is better to wear only light clothing, use a sheet or thin blanket as a cover, and keep the room temperature low (70 or below). You can help to cool a child with a very high fever by sponging him with tepid water or placing him in a tepid bath. Do not use alcohol; the vapors can be harmful. Cold water or ice is unnecessarily drastic and painful.

For Further Reading

Kavaler, Lucy Estrin. *A Matter of Degree: Heat, Life & Death.* New York: Harper & Row, 1981.

Sore Throat: Often Trivial, Sometimes Serious

Sore throat, one of the most common health complaints, is also one of the most frequently mistreated. A sore throat is not a disease, but a symptom. To say your throat is sore is no more informative about its cause than if you complain of a pain in your stomach or head.

The cause of a sore throat can be as trivial as having talked too loud and long or smoked too much or as serious as leukemia or tuberculosis. Sore throat may be a symptom of a serious bacterial infection, infectious mononucleosis, sinusitis, syphilis, or a tumor. But by far the most common cause is a minor viral infection, for which time is the only cure.

When to Call the Doctor

Lest a sore throat with a serious and treatable cause be overlooked, it is important to know when to consult a doctor and when you can safely rely on home remedies to relieve your discomfort and time to heal you.

Any one of the following circumstances warrants a prompt call to a physician:

- If the sore throat is severe or has lasted longer than a week.
- If it is accompanied by a cough, hoarseness, difficulty in breathing, or a temperature over 100 degrees Fahrenheit.
- If similar soreness has recurred several times in recent weeks.
- If the patient has ever had rheumatic fever.

These circumstances do not necessarily mean that the sore throat is caused by a serious illness, but they could be signs of conditions that warrant medical attention.

Is Strep Throat the Cause?

The most common *serious* cause of sore throat, particularly in children, is a bacterial infection by *beta hemolytic streptococcus,* or strep for short. Unlike viral sore throats, strep throat can be cured by appropriate antibiotic therapy, and also unlike the situation with a virus infection, failure to treat strep throat adequately can sometimes lead to rheumatic fever and permanent damage to the heart or kidneys.

If sore throat is associated with a high fever, headache, and swollen glands in the neck, the chances are that it is a strep infection. The pain of strep can be so mild that it is hardly noticed or so severe that it interferes with swallowing. Strep is a more common cause of sore throat in late winter and early spring.

A diagnosis of strep throat should be based on a throat culture — a swab of the throat that is smeared on a special laboratory dish and incubated overnight — and an examination by a physician. Even the most astute clinician is likely to be wrong half the time in trying to diagnose a strep throat without a culture. Rarely, even though the culture is negative, the physician, on the basis of a physical examination, has strong reason to suspect strep as the cause.

If the diagnosis is strep, it should be treated with ten days of penicillin or a suitable alternative (such as erythromycin, not tetracycline or sulfa drugs) in the case of penicillin allergy. The penicillin may be administered as a single injection that is effective for ten days or as oral capsules or liquid doses if the patient will reliably take them for the ten-day schedule. It is crucial not to stop taking the antibiotic when the symptoms disappear; the therapy should always be continued, as prescribed, for the entire ten days. A repeat culture is advisable after therapy has been completed, to be sure the infection has cleared.

Doctors often recommend that young children who are in close contact with a patient with strep should also have a throat culture. Some doctors prescribe penicillin for five days as a preventive for such exposed youngsters even before an infection develops.

However, it is unwise to give antibiotics if strep (or some other bacterium) is not the cause of a sore throat. These otherwise miraculous drugs do no good against viral infections and may do harm. Antibiotics, much abused in modern medicine, can cause serious side effects, including allergic reactions and the emergence of infectious bacteria that resist antibiotic treatment. Some doctors are all too quick to hand the patient a prescription for an antibiotic, and some patients are not satisfied unless the doctor writes such a prescription. Your doctor may well be practicing the best medicine if all you're told is to rest, gargle, and take aspirin.

Treating Viral Sore Throat

Most sore throats are minor, uncomplicated viral infections (usually a part of the common cold) that clear up within five days without specific treatment. Whereas the symptoms of strep tend to come on suddenly, viral sore throats usually start slowly, often as a feverish feeling, with headache, loss of appetite, runny nose, and dry cough as accompaniments.

One viral sore throat that may be confused with strep is known as herpangina, a rather common summertime illness in children. Temperatures may soar to 105 degrees Fahrenheit. The patient has little energy and very painful raised sores in the back of the mouth. Symptoms usually disappear by the fourth day.

Although there is no cure for viral sore throat, various measures — which, as one doctor put it, "keep the patient busy while he is getting well" — can relieve the soreness. The best of these is gargling every few hours with half a teaspoon of salt in a glass of warm water. Half a teaspoon of hydrogen peroxide or a teaspoon of molasses or corn syrup can substitute for the salt. The gargle helps to wash away irritants and mucus.

It is also helpful to drink lots of warm liquids (the warmth increases the blood flow to the throat, bringing the body's natural defenses to the site of the infection). A humidifier or vaporizer may be used, especially in the bedroom. In fact, adding moisture to the air you breathe may help to prevent wintertime sore throats since the heated, dry indoor air dries the mucous membranes and paralyzes the cilia (hairs) that line the respiratory tract, two natural defense mechanisms that protect against invading organisms. [See chapter on humidifiers, page 372.]

Most doctors recommend against prolonged use of medicated lozenges because they may mask the symptoms of more serious illness. Sucking on a hard candy works just as well to keep the throat moist. It is also a good idea to avoid irritants, such as smoking or spicy foods, until a sore throat heals.

Some youngsters who suffer from severe, repeated infections of the tonsils (chronic tonsillitis) and, as a consequence, have little energy and poor appetites and fail to gain weight, may benefit from tonsillectomy and adenoidectomy — surgical removal of the tonsils and adenoids. Although this procedure is helpful for the small percentage of children with severe, recurrent tonsillitis, doctors today generally recommend against it as a treatment for recurrent colds or other respiratory infections. [See chapter on tonsils and adenoids, page 306.]

Cough:
A Lifesaving Reflex

Coughs break the silence between scenes of a play and movements at a concert. They punctuate the smoke-filled air at the rear of airplanes. They compete with the teacher in an elementary school classroom and keep concerned parents awake at night. In a year's time cough is responsible for some 30 million doctor visits.

The cough is an extremely common, yet physically remarkable and potentially lifesaving reflex in which a powerful rush of air is expelled from the respiratory tract with a velocity of up to 500 miles per hour. The usual purpose of a cough is to clear the airways of an irritating or obstructing substance that can damage the lungs or interfere with the smooth exchange of oxygen and carbon dioxide. People who are unable to cough — for example, those under general anesthesia — are in danger of serious disease and death because they cannot protect their lower respiratory tracts from noxious insults.

A cough can also be an annoying and debilitating symptom, especially common in the winter months, when millions of Americans breathe dry, heated indoor air and spread respiratory viruses. For that pesky "cough due to the common cold," American pharmaceutical companies offer a wide array of cough preparations, both single drugs and combinations of ingredients, few of which have been shown to be any more effective than Father Time in curing a cough.

For a chronic, persistent cough, treatment with an over-the-counter cough remedy rarely brings lasting relief unless it is combined with therapy for the underlying cause of the cough. And if the underlying cause is properly treated, symptomatic treatment of the cough is rarely necessary. In fact, by masking the symptom with a cough suppressant, you may delay proper diagnosis of a serious condition.

Anyone who has had a cough for more than three weeks should be seen by a physician, who may in turn suggest an examination by a specialist in respiratory disease. Call your doctor immediately if you are coughing up thick, foul-smelling mucus that is yellow or green in color, or if your cough is accompanied by a fever over 102 degrees, or if you've had a fever of over 100 degrees for more than four days.

Because of the power and persistence of a cough (pressures in the respiratory tract can reach 300 millimeters of mercury), coughing can cause problems of its own, including insomnia, exhaustion, loss of appetite, fractured ribs, ruptured abdominal muscles, and, rarely, loss of consciousness.

Causes

A cough is not a disease, but a symptom — a sign that something is wrong in the body. The underlying cause may be as insignificant as a cold virus or, rarely, as serious as lung cancer. Other cough-inducing conditions include chronic bronchial irritation from cigarette smoking, postnasal drip caused by chronic sinusitis or nasal allergy, exposure to cigarette smoke among those with asthma or allergies, a foreign body lodged in the airway, hairs tickling the eardrum, asthma, bronchitis, pneumonia, tuberculosis, enlarged adenoids or tonsils, and heartburn. In some cases chronic cough is a psychogenic — mind-induced — condition that gets worse during times of stress.

By far the most common type of cough is the one associated with the common cold. The mucous secretions, postnasal drip, and stuffy nose and ears trigger the cough receptors in the upper respiratory passages. According to Dr. Sidney S. Braman, respiratory disease specialist at Rhode Island Hospital in Providence, these virus-induced coughs are nearly always self-limited — that is, they go away in a few weeks even if you do nothing at all.

If after a week or two of coughing you succumb to the pharmaceutical pitchmen selling over-the-counter cough preparations or you visit your doctor, who prescribes a more costly but probably no more effective cough remedy, the cough is likely to subside. But in all probability the same improvement would have occurred had you done nothing at all.

Cough Medicines Are Questionable

The usual cough remedies contain an expectorant, intended to liquefy the secretions in the bronchial tubes and make them easier to expel by coughing, and/or an antitussive, intended to suppress the cough by quieting the cough receptors. Dr. Richard S. Irwin, an expert on coughs at the University of Massachusetts Medical Center in Worcester, points out that the combination preparations are probably counterproductive, since one ingredient loosens secretions that you want to cough up and the other ingredient inhibits coughing. Suppressing a productive cough (one that brings up mucus) is undesirable and may actually be harmful for some patients.

"I never use these medicines," Dr. Irwin said, adding that if they don't cancel one another out, it's because neither ingredient probably does what it is purported to do. The most popular expectorant, glycerol guaiacolate (guaifenesin), was found to be ineffective in a controlled study, and its competitors (including ammonium chloride, terpin hydrate, camphor, and menthol) are also of unproven effectiveness. The most popular antitussive, dextromethorphan, has not been subjected to any good studies that showed it works, he noted. However, if it should prove effective, dextromethorphan is less likely to cause sedation than codeine, a potentially addictive, albeit effective, cough suppressant that is available only on prescription.

Recommended Treatments

Over-the-counter cough remedies may do little more than soothe the cough receptors in the upper respiratory tract, an effect that can be achieved by your drinking warm or cold liquids, inhaling the steam from a vaporizer or the mist from a cold-mist humidifier, or standing in a steamy shower. For coughing provoked by an irritation in the back of the throat, drinking liquids and sucking on candies or lozenges usually provide relief.

For a cough fed by the congestion and postnasal drip of a cold, it would make more sense to take a decongestant, Dr. Irwin believes. If a bad cold is accompanied by a bad cough that hangs on for many weeks after the cold abates, an asthmatic type of sensitivity in the lower respiratory tract is usually the cause, and medications that dilate the bronchial tubes can bring relief, Dr. Braman said. In some people, an asthmalike bronchial sensitivity may persist for two months after a viral respiratory infection, and coughing may be readily provoked by exposure to irritants like cigarette smoke.

More than 70 percent of the patients who are referred to Dr. Irwin because of a persistently troublesome cough turn out to be suffering from a form of bronchial asthma and/or postnasal drip. The latter is commonly caused by allergies (for which antihistamines are useful) or chronic sinus infection (treated with antibiotics, decongestants, and perhaps an antihistamine).

The rest of Dr. Irwin's chronic cough patients have bronchitis caused by cigarette smoking. In nearly all persons with a smoker's cough, the cough will essentially disappear within four weeks of quitting smoking, he has found. [See chapter on quitting smoking, page 256.]

Itch:
A Perennial Plague

Itch — the very word is enough to start fingers scratching. For we all itch somewhere for some reason virtually every day of our lives. In winter, dryness is the most common cause of itchy skin. In summer — thanks to sun, water, plants, insects, heat, and humidity, among other factors — itch takes on epidemic proportions.

Though no one escapes being plagued by this four-letter word, many of us have limited knowledge of what to do about it. Some of the most popular remedies only aggravate the problem. Others are just a waste of money and effort.

Beware Mistreatment

Old-fashioned home remedies — cold compresses and calamine lotion — are often the most effective way to relieve itching. Heat makes matters worse. Antihistamines have direct benefit for allergy-caused itches that involve a release of histamine in the skin; otherwise, they are useful only for their sedative effect. The new topical cortisone creams, ointments, and lotions that are now available over the counter may be very useful to combat itching caused by a mild allergic or inflammatory response, but they can make an infection worse.

Medications with ingredients or names that end in the suffix "dryl" or "caine" should be avoided since they commonly cause a secondary allergic reaction that aggravates the situation. And scratching that abominable itch can lead to complicating infections.

In all cases, warns Dr. Sidney Rogers, a dermatologist at Downstate Medical Center in Brooklyn, New York, the bottom line is this: If the itchy lesion is raw, oozing, wet, red, or angry-looking, or if whatever you do makes the situation worse or does not bring distinct relief within a week to ten days, see a physician (a dermatologist, if possible). Do not attempt further self-treatment.

The Common Causes of Itch

Here is a guide to common itchy afflictions, how to prevent them (if possible), and what to do to relieve them. In addition to those listed, there are itchy problems like irritations of the vaginal area (aggravated by wearing tight pants, pantyhose, and nylon underwear and relieved by not wearing them); nickel dermatitis (a reaction to cheap jewelry), which may be brought out by the warm moist environment that is characteristic of human skin in summer; and sensitivity to soap or laundering agents.

Prickly heat. This itchy rash results from a temporary blockage of the sweat pores when the skin gets "waterlogged" with sweat. The pores

506

swell, and sweat behind them can't get out. Instead, it breaks through the walls of the pores and creates pinhead-sized pimples or tiny blisters that itch and burn. Prickly heat tends to occur where skin surfaces are close together or constricted by clothing. Plump babies and overweight adults are especially vulnerable. Heat and moisture make the condition worse.

Treatment involves keeping the skin cool and dry by bathing often in cool water, changing frequently to dry clothes that are lightweight and loose-fitting, using baby powder, limiting activities that provoke sweating, and, if possible, spending time in air-conditioned areas.

Athlete's foot. Myths abound about this vexing condition, a combination fungal-bacterial infection that causes redness and cracks between the toes that itch and burn, peeling skin, and sometimes blisters on the sole of the foot.

First, you don't have to be an athlete to get it, though athletes who spend many hours in sweaty socks and shoes are particularly vulnerable. Secondly, you don't really "pick it up" from swimming pools and locker rooms, though the wetness of your feet in these areas can precipitate an attack. Apparently people are susceptible to athlete's foot or they're not (some, in fact, get it on one foot but not the other). Thirdly, boiling your socks, wearing white socks, treating your shoes, or swishing your feet in a chlorine bath at pools is not a preventive.

What *does* prevent athlete's foot is to keep your feet dry, especially between the toes. Avoid medications other than a very light dusting of powder (plain talcum or an antifungal powder). Ointments can make matters worse by holding moisture. Wear absorbent cotton or wool socks, and change them several times a day. Whenever possible, keep your feet bare or in open sandals.

Jock itch. This is a close relative of athlete's foot, and like the former, it is not restricted to "jocks" or even to men, although those who exercise strenuously in hot, humid weather are more susceptible, as are obese people. Jock itch, an itchy, burning eruption in the groin area, can actually be any one of several infections — a fungus, yeast, or bacterium, or a combination of them — or it can be an allergic or inflammatory response to chemicals in clothing, irritating garments, or a result of drugs you take.

The classic fungal infection is often spread from the feet, which should be checked for signs of athlete's foot. It also helps to avoid chafing by wearing loose-fitting garments and underwear and to keep the groin area as dry as possible. Treatment should be geared to the cause, making it difficult for the layman to know what to do. If self-treatment with an antifungal powder or cream does not bring relief, consult a physician.

Poison ivy, oak, and sumac. From 25 to 60 percent of Americans are allergic to the sap of these plants (and anyone can eventually become sensitive), which cause a red, blistering, burning, itching, swelling rash, sometimes with fever and headache. The rind of mangoes contains a related substance that can produce a poison-ivy-like reaction on the mouth and hands.

Prevention involves learning to recognize and avoid contact with the offending plants. Don't touch shoes or clothing that may be contaminated with the sap. Should you touch the plants or contaminated articles, wash promptly with soap and water. Mild cases can be treated with calamine lotion or a poultice of baking soda or Epsom salts. More severe outbreaks need a doctor's attention. [See chapter on poisonous plants, page 409.]

Insect bites and stings. The six-legged critters that can turn a beautiful summer outing into an itchy nightmare include the ubiquitous mosquito, biting flies, caterpillars, and chiggers (which are tiny red mites). Mosquitoes and flies are attracted to dark colors, warmth, and moisture, so wearing light-colored clothing may help. Repellents containing the ingredient deet (for diethyl-meta-toluamide) are among the most effective. Be sure to reapply them after swimming. Once you've been bitten, cold compresses (water, ice, alcohol, or witch hazel) and calamine lotion can bring relief. [See chapter on insect pests, page 412.]

Some people are allergic to caterpillar hairs and react with intense itching to caterpillars that fall from trees onto the neck or shoulders. Antihistamines as well as cold compresses and calamine may be helpful here.

Chiggers hide out in fields and weedy areas. For protection, use a chigger repellent on your clothing and exposed skin, tie your pants at the cuffs and shirts at the wrists, and don't sit on the ground. After the fact, a long bath with sulfur soap and scrubbing with a brush may help. Try cold compresses and calamine for the itch, but don't scratch. [See chapter on insect stings, page 412].

Swimmer's itch. The culprit here is a bird parasite called a cercarial schistosome that lives part of its life in snails in freshwater lakes. Though it cannot grow in human skin and eventually dies there, that doesn't stop it from invading. It causes intensely itchy pimples that resemble insect bites. Surefire prevention means no swimming in lakes known to be infested. If you should bathe in an infested lake, shower and dry yourself with a towel immediately after coming out of the water. There is no specific treatment, just applications of cold and calamine. In severe cases a sedative such as an antihistamine may help you sleep.

Sunburn. Prevention involves staying out of the sun or using a sun-blocking agent. Before you buy, check the label for effectiveness in preventing sunburn. If you get a rash from the sun block, try a brand with different ingredients. In the early stages of sunburn, calamine and aspirin are useful. When the blisters dry and burned skin begins to peel, the maddening itch may be relieved by a lubricating lotion.

Low Blood Sugar: Often Misdiagnosed

Growing thousands of Americans have been told or have convinced themselves that they have a disease that, in fact, doesn't exist. The "disease" is hypoglycemia, literally "low blood sugar," which isn't a disease at all but is a possible sign of a number of different underlying health problems.

In recent years hypoglycemia has become the catchall diagnosis for all the mystifying ills of modern men and women, ranging from asthma to schizophrenia. It is said to be the underlying cause of many undiagnosed or misdiagnosed ailments, including chronic fatigue, migraine, inability to concentrate, alcoholism, anxiety, and sexual problems.

Yet real hypoglycemia is a rare problem. Experts on sugar metabolism estimate that it is only one-tenth to one-twentieth as common as diabetes, not several times more common, as contended by others. And the usual causes are not unexplained abnormalities of blood-sugar metabolism. They are such real and sometimes serious problems as misuse of diabetes drugs that lower blood sugar, previous stomach surgery, pancreatic tumors, alcoholism, liver disease, serious hormonal disorders, and the beginnings of diabetes. Most of these causes are extremely rare, and many can be corrected to eliminate the low blood sugar problem.

The vast majority of patients who go to medical specialists with a presumed diagnosis of hypoglycemia do not have low blood sugar at all. On the other side of the coin, many normal people who have no symptoms that can be related to hypoglycemia develop surprisingly low levels of blood sugar when given the kinds of tests commonly used to diagnose hypoglycemia.

How To Tell What You Have

People arrive at the conclusion that they have hypoglycemia by any of several routes. They may have read popular articles or books and found the very things that plague them among the catalogue of symptoms attributed to hypoglycemia. Or an acquaintance may have suggested that hypoglycemia is the cause of the litany of woes, or a doctor may have made the diagnosis because the patient's blood sugar, in response to a laboratory test, dropped to seemingly abnormal levels.

The test, a five-hour oral glucose tolerance test, involves serial measurements of a person's blood sugar (glucose) levels after he or she has drunk a highly concentrated sugar solution. In true hypoglycemia the individual's blood sugar drops precipitously several hours after drinking the test solution and *at the same time* the patient develops symptoms of hypoglycemia. The blood sugar drops because the patient's body overshoots in sending out insulin to clear the blood of excess sugar. With too

509

much insulin circulating, too much blood sugar is metabolized, and the sugar level drops below normal.

In one type of hypoglycemia, symptoms may include shakiness, weakness, sweating, rapid heartbeat, and faintness. They are a result not of the low blood sugar, but of an outpouring of the adrenal hormone epinephrine, which is sent to signal the liver to start making more glucose. Some patients get a different set of symptoms, indicating a shortage of glucose available to the brain. These include headache, mental confusion and dullness, visual disturbances, muscular weakness, and personality changes. In severe cases, convulsions and coma may result.

In arriving at a diagnosis of real hypoglycemia, blood sugar specialists insist that at least three conditions be met: The patient should indeed have a low blood sugar level at the time the symptoms are felt, the symptoms should be characteristic of low blood sugar, and the symptoms should be readily relieved by giving the patient some form of sugar. To help confirm the diagnosis, some doctors also examine insulin levels to determine if they are high when blood sugar is low.

It is incorrect, the experts say, to diagnose hypoglycemia merely on the basis of a test-related drop in blood sugar and some vague feelings of discomfort.

In fact, the best test for hypoglycemia is based not on the unnatural conditions of a glucose tolerance test, but on the effects of a patient's ordinary meals. Many doctors advise those who suspect they have hypoglycemia to come in for a measurement of blood sugar when they are experiencing the symptoms they attribute to low blood sugar. Far more often than not, low blood sugar is *not* found.

One reason for the frequent misdiagnosis of hypoglycemia is that many doctors don't realize how common it is for low blood sugar levels to develop in normal people following a glucose tolerance test. Even after ordinary meals, one study showed, 23 percent of the normal people developed blood sugars of less than 50 milligrams per 100 milliliters, a level many doctors mistakenly label hypoglycemic. Another study showed that 43 percent of normal people without symptoms may develop such low levels of blood sugar.

Types and Treatment

There are two basic types of hypoglycemic reaction. One, reactive hypoglycemia, occurs about two to four hours after eating, especially if the meals are high in carbohydrates. The usual symptoms — sweating, tremor, rapid heartbeat, dizziness — reflect the effects of epinephrine. People in the early stages of diabetes may have this type.

The second type, called fasting hypoglycemia, develops more slowly as the blood sugar gradually drops lower and lower. It commonly produces central nervous system symptoms, and its causes can be serious underlying disorders, for instance, tumors that produce insulin. Diabetics who take too much insulin for the amount of food they eat may experience the symptoms of fasting hypoglycemia.

Treatment of hypoglycemia should involve a correction, if possible, of its cause in the fasting type, or more careful attention to diet and eating patterns in the reactive type. People prone to reactive hypoglycemia are commonly advised to eat frequent meals and snacks, six or more times a day, that are high in protein, relatively low in fat, and very low in carbohydrates. However, newer studies show that diets high in fiber and complex carbohydrates (starchy foods) can effectively control reactive hypoglycemia without introducing the coronary risks of a diet high in fatty proteins. In either type of diet, sweets, pastries, such caffeine-containing drinks as coffee, tea, colas, and cocoa, and alcoholic beverages should be avoided since they can precipitate reactive hypoglycemia in susceptible people, especially if they are consumed before or between meals.

XII.
Pesky Health Problems

Many common medical problems, though rarely serious threats to life, nonetheless can take the joy out of living and sometimes make you downright miserable. Yet chances are you'll hesitate to bring these problems to medical attention, resorting instead to self-treatment that may actually make matters worse. In other cases, when you do seek medical aid, you may receive inappropriate care or be dismissed as a complainer. The nagging problem lingers on, sometimes for years, with little or no relief.

Aching head and back, sore feet, allergic sniffling and sneezing, itchy hemorrhoids, sleeplessness, minor infections, even jet lag are among the many pesky health problems that can be minimized if you understand their causes and appreciate the various approaches to prevention and treatment.

513

Colds and Flu:
Nothing to Sneeze At

As you read this, some 30 million Americans are sneezing, coughing, blowing, shivering, or otherwise enduring the miseries of our species' most common illness, the cold. If you don't already have one yourself, odds are three in four that you will within the next twelve months. Even if you escape a cold, you may not be so lucky when it comes to the flu, which attacks fewer people but usually hits with greater severity.

Colds and influenza constitute the vast majority of what are known as acute respiratory infections. The American Medical Association has put a $5 billion price tag on colds alone, counting lost productivity as well as medical costs. Americans spend more than half a billion dollars just on over-the-counter nostrums — not including aspirin — in an attempt to relieve the distress of colds and flu.

The Causes

Colds and influenza are viral infections. Although both tend to be catchall diagnoses for a variety of related symptoms, they are actually distinct ailments. Colds can be caused by any of perhaps 150 kinds of viruses; that is why a person can get several colds every year, year in and year out, and why no effective cold vaccine has ever been developed. With each cold, you develop an immunity, often short-lived, to the particular causative virus, but you may still be susceptible to dozens of other cold viruses going around.

Influenza, on the other hand, is caused by relatively few virus types — all are variants of two major subtypes, A and B — and reasonably effective vaccines have been developed against certain flu viruses. However, flu viruses tend to change genetically through the years and resurface in forms that people are no longer immune to. Hence, the same person who gets two or three colds every year may get the flu only once in four or five years.

Young children are most susceptible to new variations of influenza viruses. Sick children expose their teachers and parents, who in turn transmit the virus to their colleagues and friends as well as to strangers encountered at meetings and on public transportation. The flu virus is spread through the air by coughs, sneezes, laughs, and even normal conversation, and newly infected victims can transmit the infection at the very start of their illness before they know what's wrong.

The Symptoms

Colds usually start gradually with a runny nose and sneezing and a feeling of chilliness (although fever is rare in adults and tends to be low-grade in children). Cough, headache, sore throat, malaise, loss of appetite, and sense of smell are common accompaniments. In the later stages, nasal discharges become thick and stuffy. Symptoms typically last three days to a week, but sometimes complications like sinusitis, ear infection, laryngitis, or bronchitis lead to a more prolonged illness.

Flu, on the other hand, starts abruptly, usually with a high fever (up to 103 in adults, higher in children), a dry cough, and often a headache. Influenza A is more likely than B to result in serious complications and deaths.

No matter which variant of the flu virus you happen to contract, the spectrum of symptoms is pretty much the same. The typical flu victim feels sick enough to stay in bed and has aches and pains in his or her muscles and back. The nose may be congested, throat sore, and eyes sensitive to light. Nausea and vomiting may accompany flu, but diarrhea rarely does. There is no such thing as "intestinal flu" — the vast majority of diarrheal illnesses are bacterial infections.

Flu symptoms generally persist for a week to ten days, followed by a week or two longer of feeling tired and possibly depressed.

Some people have such mild cases of flu that their symptoms are indistinguishable from a cold. Others, particularly those with chronic respiratory or heart diseases, are prone to serious complications following flu, including pneumonia, bronchitis, and even death.

Prevention

Despite their commonness, colds are actually quite difficult to catch. According to Dr. Elliot C. Dick, professor of preventive medicine at the University of Wisconsin, it takes a rather severe cold and many hours of close contact to transmit a cold to susceptible persons. Even within families, only half the susceptible people (that is, those lacking antibodies to the particular cold virus involved) are likely to catch a cold from another family member who lives in the same home.

Studies have shown that cold viruses are naturally transmitted through nasal discharges, which are heavily laden with viruses. Coughs and sneezes apparently rarely spread colds. Rather, finger contact with nasal secretions from nose blowing, rubbing, or sneezing seems to be the more common way that the virus is spread around. To reduce spread, wash your hands often, use absorbent handkerchiefs or disposable tissues (cold viruses die rapidly in these), and avoid rubbing your eyes and picking your nose.

Flu, on the other hand, is a more generalized infection — large amounts of virus can be found in secretions from the nose and throat — and spreads much more easily than a cold. In a family setting, Dr. Dick found, nearly all members not immune to the particular flu virus will catch it from one sick member.

Whereas someone just coming down with a cold usually doesn't shed the virus until a runny nose develops, in the early stages of flu the moment the victim starts to cough the virus is being spread. Therefore, it is much harder to avoid catching the flu from a sick relative or associate. The colleague who comes to work with flu symptoms is not doing co-workers any favors. It is better to avoid even casual personal contacts for the first three or four days of the illness. The usual incubation period — the time from exposure to the virus to onset of illness — is two days.

Both cold and flu viruses are more easily spread in places where large numbers of people congregate indoors, such as schools and camps. Young school-age children, in fact, are the prime spreaders of these viruses since they are exposed daily to organisms to which they lack immunity. Young children typically get seven or eight colds a year, and the parents of young children get five or six, but as the children and parents age, the frequency of colds drops — down to about two or three a year by age forty-five.

Most colds occur between September and May, with the peak in winter, when people spend more time indoors and when heating dries the air and the protective mucous membranes in the nose and throat. It is healthiest to keep home temperatures in the 60's during the day, and it may help to humidify the air if it drops below 20 to 30 percent relative humidity. [See chapter on humidifiers, page 372.]

516

Contrary to popular belief, studies have shown that exposure to cold weather, being in a draft, or getting chilled does not cause colds or make them worse. However, doctors suspect that fatigue, undue stress, and poor diet increase one's susceptibility to colds and flu, though the influence of these factors has not been systematically studied.

Some evidence suggests that large daily doses of vitamin C may have a slight preventive effect in warding off colds and flu, but according to Dr. C. Gordon Douglas, Jr., head of the Infectious Diseases Unit at the University of Rochester, the effect is too small to warrant large-scale use of a substance with possible adverse side effects and long-term hazards that are not known. [See chapter on micronutrients, page 42.]

The best flu preventive, short of becoming a recluse for the entire flu season, is annual vaccination, which is 70 to 80 percent effective in protecting against flu. The vaccine is changed annually to accommodate the new season's likely flu virus variants; it takes effect within ten days.

However, since the vaccine can produce significant side effects — including flulike symptoms for two or three days — it is not recommended for general use by healthy, young individuals. Rather, only those who are most likely to suffer serious and potentially fatal complications from a bout of flu are advised to obtain the vaccine. Included are all individuals over age sixty-five and people of all ages with chronic heart or lung disease, kidney disease, diabetes, chronic severe anemia (such as sickle cell disease), and immunological deficiency diseases, as well as people being treated with immunosuppressive drugs.

Others who might consider vaccination — after weighing benefits and risks — are people who work with patients in medical care facilities and those who provide essential community services, such as police and fire department personnel. Because the vaccine is prepared in eggs, it should not be taken by anyone with an allergy to egg white. To reduce the risk of side effects, a special vaccine is used for children under thirteen.

Treatment

Let's start with the bottom line: Despite the 50,000 or more different products Americans dose themselves with, there is no cure for the common cold or for influenza. Nor do these "remedies" shorten the duration of respiratory illness.

At best, if used wisely, some treatments may make it easier to endure the siege. The trick is to select products that can best relieve your symptoms and to avoid drug combinations that are irrational and possibly hazardous.

For example, while antihistamines, which are widely used in cold remedies (their names often end in the suffix -amine), may relieve symptoms of runny nose and sneezing, they may also increase and thicken the mucus in your lungs and set the stage for bronchial complications. Tablets containing potent drugs that constrict blood vessels, such as epinephrine, should also be avoided. Studies have not shown that large doses of vitamin C can abort a cold or flu.

People with diabetes, high blood pressure, heart disease, or thyroid problems or those already taking a prescription drug should check with their doctors before dosing themselves with any cold remedy.

Because colds and flu are viral infections, antibiotics (which attack bacteria and fungi) are worthless and may actually be dangerous since they cause side effects of their own. Antibiotics are useful only if you develop a secondary bacterial infection, such as an ear infection, sinusitis, or pneumonia.

Then what *should* you do for a cold or the flu? The old home remedy of rest, warmth, fluids, and aspirin is still your best bet. Lots of fluids — hot or cold — help to loosen the secretions in your respiratory tract and thus decrease the chances of complications like bronchitis, ear infection, and sinusitis.

Rest is somewhat harder to justify. But if you are tired or taking drugs that make you drowsy or you have a bad cough, which can be aggravated by your breathing cold air or running around, it may be best to stay home and rest for a few days. Dr. Douglas says the decision to stay home should be based on the severity of your symptoms; if your fever is over 100, if you have any severe symptoms, such as a bad cough or muscle aches, or if you feel you can't work, stay home. To reduce chances of relapses or complications of flu, it's best to take a couple of extra days to recover at home.

For victims of the A type of influenza who have severe symptoms, as well as those who face a high risk of flu complications, Dr. Douglas recommends a prescription drug — amantadine (Symmetrel) — which can diminish the severity and length of illness and the chances of complications. However, because of side effects, this drug is not recommended as a flu remedy for otherwise healthy people.

Call a doctor if you start to cough up blood, if you have a high fever that doesn't respond to aspirin, if you develop an earache, or if you have severe symptoms that persist beyond a week.

Otherwise, the best you can do is self-treat your symptoms. Consumption of a great deal of liquids of all kinds (except alcohol) is perhaps the single most important remedy. It replaces fluids lost through sweating and helps to keep bronchial secretions moist, warding off secondary infections. Aspirin or acetaminophen can relieve headache and muscle aches and reduce fever. [See chapter on aspirin, etc., page 463.] Gargling with warm, salty water can relieve a sore throat, and use of a cold-mist humidifier or steam vaporizer will help a cough. If you have a dry, unproductive cough, a cough suppressant may relieve it, but drinking lots of liquids and breathing moist air is the preferred treatment. Expectorants, which are intended to help you bring up thick mucus in your chest, are of questionable value. [See chapter on coughs, page 503.]

518

Nasal sprays or drops containing decongestants can relieve nasal and sinus stuffiness (be sure to stick to the recommended dose, and don't use them longer than three or four days at a time). However, oral decongestants, antihistamines, and combinations thereof are not generally recommended by infectious disease experts. For the minimal relief they may give, they're not worth the risks they entail.

A safer approach would be to follow the lead of a British medical officer who said he never takes medicine: "If I get a cold, I treat it with the contempt it deserves." And if mental ostracism doesn't do the trick, time will.

For Further Reading

Bennett, Hal Zina. *Cold Comfort.* New York: Clarkson Potter, 1979.

Headache:
Not Just a Pain in the Head

A headache is more than just a pain in the head. It's a temper shortener, a thought disrupter, a sleep disturber, and a joy stealer. Tolerance of frustration, noise, even light may disappear under the throb of a headache. Occasionally a headache portends a life-threatening illness. [See, for example, the chapter on strokes, page 637.] Headaches that suddenly become more frequent or more severe should be brought to a doctor's attention without delay.

However, most headaches — regardless of how painful — do not reflect serious health problems. Too often, though, people reach for a pain-killer to treat the symptom but never get to the cause. When headaches are caused by sinusitis or allergies, treatment of the underlying problems is needed to bring lasting relief. [See chapters on sinusitis, page 300, hay fever, page 542, and food allergies, page 548.] When muscular tension is the cause, as is the case in most garden-variety headaches, techniques for reducing or avoiding undue tension can often abort the problem without pills. Even many migraine headaches can be prevented once their cause is properly understood.

Tension Headaches

A young attorney had been suffering from recurrent headaches ever since graduating from law school. Most often, it seemed, the headaches occurred on Sunday when he should have been enjoying a day off and relaxing in anticipation of the workweek to come. But what he was really doing on Sunday was worrying about his ability to perform well in court, where he had to appear nearly every Monday. His anxiety caused him to tense the muscles in the back of his neck and scalp, precipitating one of America's most common afflictions, a tension headache.

This is the most common headache that afflicts nearly all of us now and then, often at a time of unusual emotional or physical stress, such as when we are anxious about a pressing deadline or have to drive for hours through heavy traffic. Unconscious tensing of head, face, and neck muscles in response to the stress results in pain, known technically as a muscle contraction headache. The muscle spasms may in turn constrict blood vessels, contributing to the discomfort.

Mild, occasional tension headaches usually are relieved by over-the-counter analgesics like aspirin or acetaminophen. But for many victims, tension headache is a chronic, severe, long-lasting phenomenon that is untouched by simple pain-killers. The headache may last for hours, days, weeks, even months on end.

Though migraine headaches receive more attention, perhaps because of their dramatic nature and strong familial tendencies, tension headaches are far more common and can be equally devastating. About 60 to 80 percent of people who suffer frequent headaches are victims of tension headaches. Many suffer needlessly for years, unaware that lasting relief may be possible, sometimes from relatively simple therapies. Too often people with chronic tension headaches become pill poppers, with self-prescribed medication actually contributing to, rather than alleviating, the problem. The longer a person suffers with tension headaches, the worse they are apt to get; the fear of the pain serves to exaggerate it.

Contrary to popular assumption, the pain of a tension headache is

519

not "all in the mind." Though emotional factors are frequent precipitants of tension headaches, the pain has a definable physical basis and is not imaginary.

Symptoms. In most cases tension headache is a dull, steady ache or a feeling of tightness or pressure on both sides of the head. The symptoms may be felt in the back of the neck and head, in the forehead, in the temples, or as if there were a too-tight band circling the head. A furrowed brow or stiff set of the head (as if trying to withdraw into a shell) may be the victim's frequent posture. In about 10 percent of cases the tension headache is combined with a migrainelike vascular headache that throbs and causes nausea and a sensitivity to light.

Contraction of muscles is a natural response to stress, both emotional and physical. If the contraction is not soon relieved by relaxation, the resulting muscle spasm may become painful. Tense muscles in the neck, head, and face may also constrict blood vessels in the scalp and inhibit the removal of toxic substances produced by the muscles. The tight muscles may be tender to the touch or feel as if they have knots in them.

Characteristic victims. Those who suffer from frequent muscle contraction headaches have a tendency to repress anger, frustration, and anxiety and to find many aspects of daily life stressful. They may be highly competitive, constantly racing against the clock, doubtful about their abilities, angry at their bosses or spouses, frustrated by their jobs, and unable to relax. Some are chronically depressed; others have frequent bouts of anxiety.

Instead of expressing these feelings openly and constructively and thus dissipating them, they tense their head and neck muscles, precipitating a headache. Often the headache greets them upon awakening in the morning, after the unconsciousness of sleep has permitted buried conflicts to surface.

For others, frequent headaches result from a bad habit of unconsciously tensing muscles when under pressure, such as when concentrating intensely while driving, working, or even cooking or playing a game. In some cases clenching of the jaw or grinding of the teeth at night is a clue to headache-causing muscular tension. Other possible precipitating factors include eyestrain, poor neck posture (when asleep or awake, for example, while reading, watching television, typing, or talking on the phone), and arthritis of the vertebrae in the neck. For some people, excessive consumption of caffeine — in coffee, tea, or soft drinks — causes muscle tension.

Treatment. Treatment of tension headaches should start with a careful history, including a psychological inventory, and a physical examination to determine sensitive muscle areas and possible underlying physical causes. X rays of the head and neck may be done, but rarely are more elaborate tests needed. Many patients with periodic headaches are helped by keeping a headache diary in which they record the times, places, and circumstances that may be related to their pain.

Drugs are only a temporary solution to tension headaches. For some patients, weaning from heavy doses of strong pain-killers, such as those containing narcotics, is the first crucial step in effective treatment since prolonged use of these drugs can result in a reduced tolerance to pain and may cause other health problems. Antidepressants or antianxiety drugs are among the most effective drug therapies; muscle relaxants are also often used in conjunction with pain relievers. Soaking in warm water, using a heating pad, doing exercises to stretch and loosen muscles in the neck, and massaging tense muscles may also bring temporary relief.

More permanent remedies include simple psychotherapy (often just talking with a physician) to uncover emotional triggers, find better ways of resolving stress, and learn to make things easier on yourself by not setting unreasonable goals, demanding perfection from yourself and others, and overcrowding your schedule. [See chapter on stress, page 138.]

Biofeedback, in which a machine is used to help teach you to relax the responsible muscles, and relaxation exercises, which may be just as effective as, and less expensive than, biofeedback therapy, are also useful and potentially long-lasting therapies. An excellent description of self-treatment through relaxation can be found in *Headache*, a paperback book by Dr. James W. Lance, an Australian neurologist (see "For Further Reading and Information," page 523). Others are best helped by an instructor trained in relaxation techniques. Check the local Y or community health facilities or school-based adult education programs for courses on relaxation exercises.

Migraine Headaches

The Union Army Camp, several miles from Appomattox Courthouse, April 8, 1865: "I was suffering very severely with a sick headache," Ulysses S. Grant wrote in his memoirs. "I spent the night in bathing my feet in hot water and mustard and putting mustard plasters on my wrists and the back part of my neck, hoping to be cured by morning."

But the next day, as General Grant pressed for Robert E. Lee's surrender, the headache persisted. Toward the end of the day an officer brought a note from General Lee declaring his willingness to discuss surrender. "When the officer reached me, I was still suffering with the sick headache; but the instant I saw the contents of the note, I was cured."

Ulysses S. Grant had migraine. Not unlike the cases of many of the 25 million Americans who currently suffer from this affliction, emotional tension helped to precipitate his attacks of "sick headache." Other famous migraine sufferers included Sigmund Freud, Charles Darwin, Thomas Jefferson, and George Bernard Shaw. Lewis Carroll is said to have created the bizarre sensations and distorted characters in *Alice's Adventures in Wonderland* during the auras that preceded his migraine attacks.

According to Dr. Arnold Friedman, neurologist and headache specialist at the University of Arizona in Tucson, "Most migraine sufferers are worthwhile people," an observation that is small comfort to the victims of these often incapacitating headaches. The pain of migraine can be so intense that sufferers are sometimes convinced that a life-threatening condition, like a brain tumor or stroke, must be the cause. Only rarely is there a malignant reason for the discomfort, but when migraine appears for the first time in older people, the possibility of a cerebral aneurysm or other serious underlying disorder should be checked out.

Characteristics. Migraine results from contraction followed by rapid expansion of cranial blood vessels, which painfully stretch the artery walls and cause them to throb with every beat of the heart. The severe, dull, pulsing pain usually starts in the center of the forehead or over one eye, but may spread to other parts of the head. It may last for hours or days. The pain is often accompanied by loss of appetite, nausea, or vomiting, hence the popular name of sick headache.

But migraine actually begins before the pain —- with sensory, motor, or mood disturbances, called auras, that may occur hours or minutes before an attack. There may be ringing in the ears, tingling or numbness or weakness of a limb, extreme sensitivity to light, vertigo, visual blurring, distorted depth perception, nausea, or unaccountable emotional changes.

Aura is uncommon in one type of migraine, the cluster headache, which causes such intense pain that it is sometimes called the suicide headache. Striking nine men for every woman and usually starting during sleep, cluster migraine can drive its victims to bang their heads against the wall, seeking relief. Each headache lasts five to ninety minutes and may occur nightly for up to five or six weeks, then disappear for months or years (hence the name cluster).

For migraine, generally, approximately two-thirds of adult sufferers are female, but in children migraine is two times more common in boys than in girls. Migraine usually begins during the teen or early adult years but may be heralded during childhood by motion sickness or cyclic vomiting.

Causes. Migraine tends to run in families. Two-thirds of victims come from families in which others had migraine. If both parents are migraine sufferers, three-fourths of the children are likely to develop the problem. If one parent has migraine, half the offspring will, too. The children are believed to inherit an instability of the cranial blood vessels that causes the vessels to contract and expand inappropriately in response to various stimuli.

Headache specialists have observed that the typical migraine sufferer is an unyielding perfectionist, a meticulous, methodical, compulsive person with rigid behavior standards who suppresses anger and resentment of authority.

Although migraine may result wholly or in part from a reaction to emotional stress, it is a physical, not a psychiatric, illness. Its victims cannot "will away" a migraine attack any more than a person with epilepsy can decide not to have a seizure. However, migraine frequently can be controlled — its attacks reduced in number or eliminated entirely — by the victim's avoiding or learning to overcome some of its causes. To achieve this, each person must decipher the factors that trigger his migraine attacks.

Many migraine headaches are precipitated by allergies, or supersensitivities, to certain odors, foods, or inhalants. Common triggers include molds and dust; the odors of tobacco smoke, paint thinner, perfumes, aerosols, and traffic fumes; and such foods as milk, chocolate, cola, corn, garlic, onions, eggs, pork, legumes (peas, beans, and peanuts), cinnamon, bay leaf, citrus fruits, wheat, coffee, and apples. Some people with migraine are extremely sensitive to beverages containing alcohol or caffeine. Wine-sensitive patients may also get headaches from raisins, grapes, or grape juice.

Avoiding exposure to the triggering substances is the best way to control attacks of migraine (desensitization shots may themselves start the headaches), but avoidance can sometimes be difficult.

Nonallergic triggers of migraine include premenstrual tension; oral contraceptives; menopausal estrogens; such physical factors as exposure to bright light, heat or cold, motion, noise, or viral infections; and psychic stress. Often the best way to pinpoint the cause of migraine is to keep a diary, recording the circumstances or substances that precede each attack.

Prevention and treatment. Prevention of migraine attacks often involves the use of a drug, such as Sansert, to suppress attacks. Recently some doctors have successfully used biofeedback techniques to train patients to abort their headaches. If migraine results from psychic tension, psychotherapy often helps by enabling the patient to recognize the emotional triggers and learn to avoid them or relieve them in other ways.

Treatment of the acute attack may involve, in addition to lying in a dark, quiet room, use of a drug called ergotamine tartrate.

For Further Reading and Information

Brainard, Dr. John B. *Control of Migraine.* New York: W.W. Norton, 1977.
Lance, James W. *Headache.* New York: Scribners, 1975.
Rose, F. Clifford, and M. Gawel. *Migraine: The Facts.* New York: Oxford University Press, 1979.
Saper, Dr. Joel R. and Dr. Kenneth R. Magee. *Freedom from Headaches.* New York: Fireside/Simon & Schuster, 1981.
Star, Cima. *Understanding Headaches.* New York: Monarch Press, 1977.

For additonal information about migraine headaches, write the National Migraine Foundation at 2422 West Foster Avenue, Chicago, Illinois 60625.

Backaches:
Preventable Plague of Millions

You lunge for a tennis ball, stoop to pick up a child, lean over to make the bed, reach for something on the back seat, push the car out of a snowdrift, and ow! you can't get up. Something has "snapped" in your lower back. Or you awake in the morning, stand after a long plane ride, or come to the end of a car trip and find your back stiffened with pain.

Next to headache, low back pain is the most common painful affliction of Americans, striking with no consideration for sex, social status, or educational achievement. It is also one of the nation's most expensive health problems, rivaling the cost of heart disease but receiving only a fraction of the research dollars it deserves.

Nonetheless, much is now known about how to prevent back problems, and new approaches to treatment promise more lasting results with less risk of damaging side effects. Since recent studies indicate that back pain is primarily a disease of living — in particular, American-style sedentary living — prevention and treatment are now being focused on life habits that protect or stress the back. This means that the patient, not the doctor, holds the key to a healthy back. Accordingly the latest approach to recurring or chronic low back pain is the "back school," in which patients learn how to sit, stand, work, play, and relax in ways that help, rather than hurt, their backs.

Some 20 million visits to doctors each year are prompted by back problems, and four in five Americans experience back pain at least once in their lives. Most victims recover in a few days or weeks with conservative treatment. But the chances are pretty good that once a person has had a severe backache, attacks will recur repeatedly.

More often than not, victims of back trouble are sedentary individuals with sagging guts, twenty or more extra pounds on their frames, and poor posture, who suffer a temporary lapse of good sense or a stroke of bad luck. With their bodies unprepared for the stress, they overdo, straining or spraining the muscles or ligaments that support the spine or sometimes injuring a disk between two vertebrae.

Yet, experts estimate that perhaps 80 percent of backaches can be prevented by learning and applying a few simple back-sparing tips.

The Mechanics of the Back

To appreciate the importance of these measures, it is helpful to understand the mechanics of the human back. Many people blame our high incidence of back problems on the fact that the spinal column originally evolved to support animals that maintain a horizontal posture (standing on four legs). While modifications evolved to adapt the spine to an upright two-legged stance, there is decidedly more strain on the human back when you sit or stand than while you lie down. When you bend over to reach the floor and lift a heavy object, the pressure on parts of the spine may reach 900 pounds.

The spine consists of bones called vertebrae — twenty-four separate ones and nine fused ones at the "tail." A channel through the bones houses the spinal cord and nerves. Between the nonfused vertebrae are pads of collagen — a very tough fibrous protein — called disks, which act as cushions separating the bones. When a disk ruptures ("slipped disk" is a misnomer), it may press on spinal nerves and cause intense pain in a leg — the pain of sciatica. The vertebrae in the lower back are where most back pains originate.

The lower spine is supported by muscles and ligaments in the back

EXERCISES TO PROTECT YOUR BACK

Most people could benefit from strengthening the muscles that act as guy wires for their backs. Three exercises are ideal:

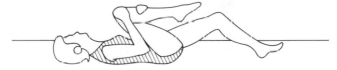

Lower back stretch. Lie on your back with both knees bent. Grasp one knee, and bring toward your chin. Hold for ten counts; then release. Repeat up to ten times for each leg.

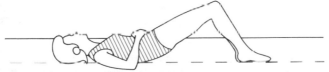

Pelvic tilt. Lie on your back with your feet on the floor and knees bent. Suck in your gut so that the small of your back presses hard against the floor. Then, tightening your buttocks, lift your hips off the ground. Hold for ten counts; then release and rest for a count of five. Repeat up to twenty times.

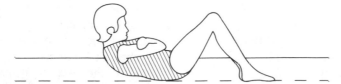

Bent-leg sit-ups. Lie on your back with your feet on the floor and knees bent. Tuck your chin to your chest, and fold your arms across your chest, placing one hand on each shoulder. Then raise your trunk about thirty degrees off the floor, and return to starting position. Repeat in a smooth rocking motion, starting with ten and gradually working up to fifty a session.

Caution: Exercises should be started slowly, and the number of repetitions should be gradually increased. Stop any exercise that causes or increases pain.

and abdomen which act as guy wires. If those wires are weak, their hold on the spine is not sufficiently protective, and an injury may occur. A New York study of thousands of back sufferers indicated that four out of five backaches are due to muscle weakness. Contributing to this weakness and strain on the back are a sedentary life-style (particularly when punctuated by occasional bursts of activity), poor posture, improper shoes, overweight, poor mattress and sleeping position, and improper lifting of heavy objects.

In addition to injuries, the causes of backache include congenital deformities; osteoarthritis; spinal tuberculosis; pain "referred" to the back from diseased kidneys, pancreas, liver, or prostate; and psychological factors. Emotional tension — repressed anger, resentment, anxiety — can cause muscular tension and backache. Persons with psychogenic backache often experience strange pains that move up and down the back and experience pain when doing activities not ordinarily stressful to the back.

How to Protect Your Back

The goal of prevention is to avoid undue stress on injury-prone back tissues and to strengthen the muscles that support those tissues. Many of the following suggestions come from an excellent booklet called "Back Aches" (see "For Further Reading," page 529), one of a series of family health guides prepared by the Tufts-New England Medical Center.

Weight control. Overweight is one of the most common causes of back pain; it greatly increases the stress on soft back tissues. Three-fourths of those with chronic back pain are obese. An orthopedist who treated me for back pain told me, "You can never be too thin for your back." For maximum back protection and surest weight loss, combine calorie control with exercise (see page 525).

Standing. Swayback, or lordosis, which exaggerates the curve in the lower back, causes abnormal pressures on soft back tissues (muscles and disks). So does a protruding abdomen and wearing high-heeled shoes. But having a firm, flattened abdomen and holding your stomach in when you stand and sit will tilt the pelvis toward the back and provide crucial support for the lower spine. When standing for long periods, you can tilt the pelvis back and flatten lordosis by placing one foot on a stool, chair railing, or other object about four to six inches off the floor.

Sitting. Sitting is far more stressful to the back than standing. Avoid prolonged sitting: On car trips, stop often to stretch and walk about; on airplanes and in theaters, request aisle seats that enable you to get up often; if you work at a sedentary job, be sure to take a stand-up break every hour.

The chair you sit in can make the difference between a healthy and a sick back. Avoid soft, cushiony seats that you sink into, stools from which your legs dangle, and chairs with no support for the lower back. The ideal chair tilts and swivels, has an adjustable height so that you can sit with your feet flat on the floor and your knees slightly higher than your hips, has enough seat room to allow you to shift your weight, curves into the lower back, and has arm rests (these reduce stress while you sit and when you get up). If necessary, place a support under your desk or table on which to rest your feet, or cross your legs to tilt the pelvis back.

Car seats are notoriously poorly designed for backs, with bucket seats being the worst. An exception is the Volvo seat, the design of which is based on the Swedish company's extensive research on backs. When driving, place a towel roll or small pillow behind the lower back, and rest your right arm on something. Keep the seat forward so that your knees are raised to hip level; your right leg should not be fully extended.

Sleeping. Always sleep on a firm mattress (a half-inch-thick plywood bed board under the mattress is helpful), on your side with your knees bent at right angles to your torso or on your back with a pillow under your knees. Lying on your stomach exaggerates lordosis and stresses your back. Use just enough pillows to keep your head in line with your body; your neck should be straight, not bent forward or to one side.

Since lying down is by far the least stressful posture for your back, use it whenever possible instead of sitting, such as when reading or watching television.

Lifting and bending. Never bend over from the waist, not even to pick up a piece of paper. Squat close to the object you want to lift, bending at the knees with back straight and stomach muscles tensed. Stand up slowly, holding heavy objects close to your body.

When working at home or on the job (sweeping, gardening, filing, etc.), stand with back straight and knees slightly bent.

Exercise and sex. Good muscle tone, especially of the abdominal muscles, is vital to a strong back. Accordingly, any activity that tightens these muscles and straightens out lordosis can be helpful. See the drawings on page 525 for a series of back exercises that strengthen supporting muscles without stressing the back.

Never do toe touches, sit-ups, or leg raises with knees straight or raise your legs or chest while lying on your stomach. The guiding principle of all exercise should be: If it causes back pain or makes it worse, don't do it. Also, don't stop your back exercises when your pain disappears. A back once injured is likely to go out again; back-strengthening exercises are a crucial preventive that should be continued for life.

Sports that involve sudden starts and stops, twists and turns, falls, or collisions with other players place the spine at risk of injury. Among them are racket sports, baseball, football, golf, and downhill skiing. However, many of these activities can be enjoyed by people with back problems if they take proper precautions (learning, for example, how to

527

place the ball on the tee or how to pick up a tennis ball without bending). "Safe" sports include swimming (but not the breaststroke since it sways the back), cycling in an upright posture, walking, and jogging (preferably not on concrete).

Back pain need not bring sexual activity to a halt. Find positions (for example, lying on your side or with the partner who has the stronger back on top) that do not strain your back. Sexual problems you can't solve on your own might be brought to the attention of a sex therapist.

Conservative Treatment is Usually Best

Before a backache is treated, a diagnosis of the probable cause is important. The doctor should take a careful medical history and do a thorough physical examination, the most revealing test. A series of back X rays is typically taken when a sudden incapacitating injury occurs, but they usually show nothing. That doesn't mean your pain is imaginary. CAT scans — special computerized X rays — may be more revealing, but they are also much more expensive and involve a lot more radiation.

Myelograms, hazardous X ray tests involving injection of a dye into the spinal column, are not done unless surgery is anticipated. Dye may also be injected directly into a disk in a test called a discogram. An electromyogram, measuring the response of muscles to an electrical current, may be done to assess nerve damage.

For most patients, bed rest in a comfortable position, local heat, massage with linament, and aspirin are curative. Damage to muscles or ligaments as a result of flabby muscles or muscular tension and the psychological stress that often precipitates it is the most common cause of back pain, especially in people under 50. Such soft-tissue injuries do not show on an X ray. Structural problems like herniated ("slipped") disk, arthritis, bony abnormalities, etc. account for at most 20 percent of problems. Thus, the treatment emphasis is now on strengthening weak muscles (especially in the abdomen), and learning how to relax tense muscles and how to avoid undue muscular tension.

Acute back pain with or without sciatica (pain or numbness radiating down the leg) is treated with complete bed rest (twenty-two hours a day or more in the positions described above) until the muscle spasms have largely subsided (anywhere from two days to six weeks). Applications of heat and aspirin to relieve pain and relax muscles are also helpful. If you are in severe pain, if the pain is getting worse, if leg symptoms are increasing, or if your pain has not subsided substantially in two or three days, see a doctor, preferably an orthopedist.

Stronger pain-killers, muscle relaxants, and anti-inflammatory drugs (if, for example, arthritis is a cause) may be prescribed for a limited time when needed, but their use on a long-term basis is not safe. Some drugs have harmful side effects, and some patients become addicted to the drugs and subconsciously hang on to their pain as a means of justifying continuing drug use.

Only about 1 percent of patients require surgery. These are people with progressive nerve damage, or chronic symptoms that interfere with life and don't respond to conservative treatment, or acute disabling symptoms that don't improve after four to six weeks in bed. Beware of doctors who are too quick to recommend surgery.

Treatment with the enzyme chymopapain, believed to relieve pain by dissolving part of a protruding disk, is still experimental in this country, though it is approved for use in Canada and is used in some states here. The enzyme has long been the subject of controversy among back experts, with some saying it is worthless and others saying it could eliminate two-thirds of back surgery.

Biofeedback, hypnosis, meditation, yoga exercises, and other techniques to promote muscle relaxation are effective in some patients with persistent or recurring back pain. Sometimes injections are used to destroy "trigger points" — isolated spots of weak muscle tissue that continue to trigger pain long after the initial injury.

Studies comparing chiropractic manipulation to massage, physiotherapy, corset, and aspirin have shown that manipulation may speed up initial recovery but that it offers no long-term benefit. Since manipulation can occasionally make a back injury worse, some doctors advise against it. At the least, prior to manipulation, a medical doctor should establish a diagnosis.

529

Even if nothing at all is done, 90 percent of low back pains go away within two months. Although herniated disks do not go back to their normal positions, the body usually makes some accommodation that relieves the pain. However, in more than half of cases, the pain will recur within a year, unless preventive steps are taken. Exercises to strengthen abdominal muscles, reduce lordosis, and tilt the pelvis back should be started as soon as pain allows. Too often patients are handed a sheet of exercises without proper instructions on how and when to do them.

In the small but taxing group of patients who develop chronic crippling back pain, psychological and family counseling is often needed to counter emotional factors that perpetuate the pain. Some must be weaned from the "rewards" they get for their pain — such as being the center of attention or relieved of onerous chores. Many have to be weaned from drugs and alcohol which they used habitually to control pain. Such patients often benefit from treatment at a pain clinic, where the various approaches to relieving chronic pain are applied in a coordinated fashion. [See chapter on pain, page 486.]

For Further Reading

Belkin, Stuart C., M.D., and Henry H. Banks, M.D. "Back Aches" (a Tufts-New England Medical Center Family Health Guide). Providence, R.I.: Arandel Publishing (55 Dupont Drive, Providence, R.I. 02907),1978.

Cyriax, James. The Slipped Disc. New York: Scribner's, 1980.

Linde, Shirley. *How to Beat a Bad Back*. New York: Rawson, Wade, 1980.
Stoddard, Dr. Alan. *The Back: Relief from Pain*. New York: Arco, 1979.
Zauner, Renate, and Albert Gob, M.D. *Speaking of: Back-Aches*. The Medical Adviser Series. New York: Delair/Consolidated, 1978.

Hemorrhoids: A Historical Hurt

Although to most victims they are a pedestrian, albeit embarrassing and painful, ailment, hemorrhoids have the unusual distinction of having helped to change the course of history. Napoleon is said to have delayed his attack at Waterloo because he was temporarily incapacitated by painful hemorrhoids. He lost the battle and the war, and his dream of a grand European conquest was brought to an end.

Many modern-day sufferers will readily attest to the power of hemorrhoidal pain. In 1979 desperate Americans spent more than $85 million on over-the-counter hemorrhoidal ointments and suppositories. But in contrast with Napoleon's time, there are now a number of relatively simple treatments, and it is probably possible to prevent the development of most hemorrhoids by proper diet and bowel habits.

Cause and Prevention

Hemorrhoids are overly stretched veins in the rectum, comparable to varicose veins in the legs. They are extremely common — 50 to 70 percent of adult Americans have them — and in most cases they cause little or no discomfort most of the time. They result from excessive pressure within the abdominal veins into which the veins in the rectum must drain.

Many situations contribute to this excess venous pressure, the most common being straining to pass the stool. Thus, hemorrhoids frequently occur among people who are chronically constipated or who have hard stools. Other causes include pregnancy, which puts direct pressure on the rectal veins; cirrhosis of the liver, which leads to increased pressure in the veins that carry blood from the intestines to the liver; heart failure, which also increases venous pressure; and tumors in the intestines or abdomen. Even the pressure caused by coughing and sneezing may contribute to the development of hemorrhoids.

In 1970 a British physician, Dr. Denis Burkitt, pointed out that native populations that regularly consume large amounts of fibrous foods rarely have problems with hemorrhoids, among other ailments he relates to a sluggish colon. In parts of Africa, for example, the diets contain up to seven times more fiber than the typical British or American diet, and the Africans pass much larger, softer stools than their frequently constipated counterparts in Western cultures.

530

Dietary fiber, or roughage, as our grandparents called it, is found in substantial quantities in whole grains (for example, rolled oats, whole wheat breads, and cereals), bran (the fibrous outer shell of grains), fresh fruits, and vegetables. Fiber passes through the human digestive tract untouched by digestive enzymes. It has the capacity to absorb many times its weight in water. Once in the colon, it helps to make the stool large and soft. [See chapter on dietary fiber, page 36.]

This greatly facilitates passage of the stool without straining, and thereby probably reduces the chances that hemorrhoids will develop. The word "probably" is used because no one has yet proved in a scientific experiment that eating fiber prevents hemorrhoids, but proctologists agree that once hemorrhoids develop, a high-fiber diet is useful in relieving the pressure and the discomfort that hemorrhoids can cause.

It's important to be gradual about increasing the fiber in your diet. Too rapid an increase can cause gas, abdominal cramps, or diarrhea. Some increase in intestinal gas is common at first even if you start slowly, but it usually disappears in a few weeks as your system and the bacteria that inhabit your colon adjust to the new diet.

Be sure to drink lots of fluids if you add foods like whole grains or bran to your diet (fruits and vegetables come naturally packaged with water). Otherwise, these fibrous foods may actually cause constipation. Also, stay away from breads containing wood fiber. This is high in a type of fiber (lignin) that can be constipating.

Severe constipation problems can also be treated temporarily with a type of laxative known as a stool softener. Your pharmacist can recommend one of several brands. Examples include Metamucil and Effersyllium. Be cautious about the laxatives that act on the muscles of the colon and rectum, such as Ex-Lax; prolonged use can cause permanent malfunction of the bowel. Prolonged use of mineral oil can interfere with the absorption of several essential vitamins that instead wash out of the body with the oil.

As part of prevention (as well as treatment of existing hemorrhoids), don't try to move your bowels unless you feel the urge to do so, and don't spend any more time on the toilet than it takes to defecate without straining. It has been suggested that squatting is a more natural position than sitting for moving one's bowels, but unfortunately Western toilets are not designed to make this possible for most people.

Diagnosis and Treatment

The most common symptom of hemorrhoids is bleeding. Since other more serious conditions, such as colitis and colon-rectal cancer, can also cause bleeding, this symptom should be looked into promptly. A proctosigmoidoscopic or colonoscopic examination of the colon and rectum and, in patients over forty or forty-five, a barium enema followed by X ray are advised, to be sure hemorrhoids are the real and only cause of bleeding. [See chapter on detecting colon cancer, page 652.]

There are two types of hemorrhoids: external and internal. External hemorrhoids are seldom painful, but sometimes pressure will cause them to enlarge suddenly and become filled with clots. They may bleed and cause severe pain for about three to five days, after which the clots are absorbed, leaving behind a skin tag. Sometimes the tag is bothersome or itchy, but it is otherwise harmless.

Internal hemorrhoids can cause bleeding without pain. However, they may sometimes protrude through the anal opening and become enlarged and painful.

In most cases conservative treatment with frequent sitz baths or other forms of moist heat, compresses soaked in witch hazel, stool softener, high-fiber diet, bed rest, and pain medication is all that is needed to get rid of the discomfort. Instead of using toilet paper, cleanse the anal area by washing with a warm, soapy cloth or cotton, and then rinse thoroughly. You should also avoid heavy lifting, and be sure to get exercise daily to relieve some of the pressure on hemorrhoidal veins caused by standing and sitting. Avoid sitting and standing for long periods.

However, prolonged use of over-the-counter hemorrhoid preparations is not advised. Those containing ingredients ending in the suffix –caine should be avoided, since they can further irritate the anal area and may cause an allergic reaction. A national advisory panel recommended that hemorrhoidal suppositories and ointments be used for no longer than seven days without medical supervision. They may cause allergic reactions and delay the diagnosis and cure of the real problem. Also, those that claim to "shrink" hemorrhoidal tissue provide only temporary relief. Hemorrhoids that develop during pregnancy usually disappear in three to six months after delivery without special treatment.

More involved therapy may be needed for hemorrhoids that don't clear up on their own and that bleed enough to cause anemia, or that cause disabling pain or intolerable itching. In recent years, doctors have developed a number of new treatments for hemorrhoids that avoid prolonged, costly hospital stays and the many complications and pain which have been associated with surgery for hemorrhoids.

The most popular of these new approaches is the painless rubber band technique, which can be done in a doctor's office without anesthesia. It cuts off the blood supply to the hemorrhoid, causing it to shrivel. Several treatments may be necessary to get rid of multiple hemorrhoids. The patient is able to return to work the day after treatment. Improvement in symptoms occurs gradually over a period of about two months. Complications are infrequent when the doctor is experienced in the technique.

Another new procedure involves cryosurgery — freezing the hemorrhoidal tissue. This, too, is painless and can be done in a doctor's office without anesthesia. Other treatments include anal dilation, popular in Britain, which requires anesthesia and incapacitates the patient for a day or two. Internal hemorrhoids are sometimes treated with an injected chemical, but this technique is said to offer no advantage over the rubber band approach.

In some cases, however, more involved surgical techniques that require general anesthesia and hospitalization for a week or longer are necessary. Surgery is usually reserved for patients who are not helped by other, less involved treatments. Even surgery has recently been improved: A technique called closed hemorrhoidectomy requires only about four days in the hospital and is associated with less pain and fewer postoperative complications than the old, notorious open method.

For Further Reading

Wanderman, Dr. Sidney E., with Betty Rothbart. *The Hemorrhoid Book.* New York: Grosset & Dunlap, 1981.

Flatulence and Belching: Painful and Embarrassing

533

"It is universally well known, that in digesting our common food, there is created or produced in the bowels of human creatures, a great quantity of wind." — Benjamin Franklin, who proposed that this "wind" be rendered less offensive by consumption of an agreeable scent along with one's food.

Gas may be in short supply as a source of energy, but not in the intestinal tracts of Americans. Whether it merely causes private pain or is the source of significant public embarrassment, intestinal gas is a vexing problem for millions of people. Although not yet a topic for cocktail party conversation, the recent fiber revolution and the growing reliance on vegetable sources of protein have helped to make intestinal gas a matter of widespread concern.

Few sufferers realize that gastrointestinal gas is often a self-created problem and is usually curable by a change in habits or diet. Gas is a normal constituent of the human digestive tract, and most of the time in most people it causes no problems. But under some circumstances and in some people, abnormal amounts of gas accumulate or normal amounts produce abnormal discomfort.

Sometimes the distress masquerades as symptoms of a serious illness, like the agonizing chest pains of angina, gallbladder disease, or ulcer, and may lead to a mistaken diagnosis and unnecessary treatment. At other times the symptoms of intestinal gas conceal a more serious underlying disorder that may be overlooked.

Causes of Gastrointestinal Gas

The two main causes of distressing gas are:

● Excessive swallowing of air, a correctable habit that usually results in belching and may also contribute to intestinal distention and discomfort. The usual source of swallowed air in people plagued by chronic belching is belching itself.

● Consumption of foods — such as beans, bran, and broccoli — that provide intestinal bacteria with a hearty meal of carbohydrates that the human digestive tract cannot completely digest. The bacteria ferment the undigested carbohydrates and produce gas, most of which emerges as flatus.

Sometimes a gastrointestinal disorder, such as celiac disease or lactase deficiency (intolerance of milk sugar), results in failure to absorb carbohydrates that the body normally would digest. Instead, these nutrients are used by gas-producing intestinal bacteria. [See chapter on food allergies, page 548.] In other people, spasms in the intestinal tract slow the movement of food and gas and cause painful pockets of gas, even when the total amount of gas is normal. Eating while under stress or eating too much at one time can cause or aggravate the problem of a sluggish digestive tract.

Swallowed air, however, is the most common culprit, causing an estimated one-half to two-thirds of problems with excessive gas. If you eat while anxious or under stress, if you eat or drink too fast and don't chew thoroughly, if you slurp or talk with your mouth full, you're likely to increase significantly the amount of air you swallow with your food.

Even without eating, anxiety, stress, and pain increase swallowing and add extra air. Gum chewing, sucking on candy, excessive smoking, and postnasal drip may have a similar effect. Consumption of carbonated beverages, including beer, also creates gas in the stomach. As the drink warms inside you to body temperature, the carbon dioxide comes out of solution and fills you with gas.

Chronic Belching, a Self-Created Problem

Normally excess stomach air is released by a belch. A single belch, maybe two, will usually accomplish the release. However, some people acquire the habit of repeated belching and in the process create the very problem they think they're trying to relieve. Chronic, or forced, belching starts with an aspiration of air into the esophagus (you can usually see the Adam's apple moving up and down), most of which is quickly released again through the mouth.

But every forced belch adds more air to the stomach than it removes, according to Dr. Michael D. Levitt, a gastroenterologist at the Veterans Administration Hospital in Minneapolis who is an expert on intestinal gas. The treatment for this problem is simple: Just stop belching, and the extra gas will soon be dissipated.

The extra air that doesn't go up the digestive tract goes down into the intestines, to be absorbed into the bloodstream and released through the lungs or to be passed through the rectum as flatus.

Food Is Main Source of Flatus

Analyses of the gases in flatus have shown that it most often results from bacterial fermentation of food. Aside from nitrogen, which may come from swallowed air, the predominant gases in the bowel — hydrogen, methane, and carbon dioxide — are odorless; they acquire their scent from other constituents of the diet and from digestive wastes.

Some foods are infamous for their ability to induce gassy intestinal cramps and flatulence. Beans, for example, contain two nonabsorbable carbohydrates, raffinose and stachyose, that are readily fermented by bacteria living in the colon. Soybeans are about the worst offenders. However, fermented soy products, such as tofu and tempeh, have already had their carbohydrates broken down before you eat them and so provide no meal for colonic bacteria.

Other vegetables, such as cabbage, spinach, cauliflower, broccoli, brussels sprouts, and eggplant, also commonly cause flatulence. Diets containing large amounts of fibrous foods, such as fruits and bran, increase the amount of fermentable carbohydrates that reach the colon and therefore can result in flatulence. Even ordinary baked products made from white wheat flour may increase flatulence in a large percentage of people, recent studies indicate.

There's no permanent cure for flatulence other than eliminating the offending foods from the diet, says Dr. Allen S. Levine, a food scientist who works with Dr. Levitt. He tells of one twenty-year-old man who suffered for five years from excessive belching and flatulence. Finally, a lactose tolerance test revealed that he was unable to digest milk sugar, but avoiding the offending dairy products only partly solved his problem. He then systematically stopped eating one food after another — testing more than 130 foods — until he came up with a diet that resulted in no more gas than other people normally produce.

In addition to milk, his diet eliminated onions, dried beans, celery, carrots, raisins, bananas, apricots, prune juice, pretzels, bagels, wheat germ, brussels sprouts, pastries, potatoes, eggplant, citrus fruit, and apples, but he can eat some of these foods in moderation without aggravating his problem.

Although the foods that bothered this man are among common offenders, each person has his or her own sensitivities, which would have to be discovered through trial and error. Occasional use of activated charcoal — available over the counter in pharmacies in tablet or capsule form — to adsorb excess gastrointestinal gas is OK, but frequent use may lead to deficiencies of certain mineral nutrients, which also become adsorbed on the charcoal.

535

Most people can prevent the release of flatus for a time. But it can build up and cause pain and eventually must be released. Sometimes flatulence that is normally well controlled passes at embarrassing moments. This results from a relaxation of the rectal muscles, such as may occur during sexual excitement. Dr. Gerald M. Feigen, a proctologist at Mount Zion Hospital in San Francisco, suggests that the problem may be resolved by the expulsion of the gas in a bathroom or with the use of a minienema with a baby syringe prior to sexual activity. Eliminating gas-producing foods from the diet may also help, he says.

Trapped Gas

Some people have the opposite problem: They fill up with gas that they can't release. The gas forms a froth in their digestive tract and can't be passed. Such cases may respond to treatment with an antifoaming agent, simethicone, some studies indicate. Simethicone is available as a prescription drug and as an ingredient in several over-the-counter antacids.

A sluggish digestive tract in which food and gas become painfully trapped can often be stimulated by exercise (a brisk walk, jogging, or swimming aids the release of trapped gas), increased consumption of fresh fruits and vegetables and whole grains, and drinking plenty of fluids throughout the day.

Vaginitis: An Ecological Disturbance

The large array of "feminine hygiene" products on drugstore shelves speaks in part to the widespread nature of the problem. Vaginitis, an inflammation of the vagina, is the most common health complaint brought to gynecologists. At least 20 percent of women get it, and for many it becomes a persistent or recurring problem. Its various symptoms — among them, heavy discharge, maddening itch, burning irritation, unpleasant odor — have prompted some women to renounce their gender temporarily. Yet simple precautions can often prevent it.

Vaginitis is, for the most part, an ecological disturbance. Normally there is a natural balance of microorganisms that live in the vagina, kept in check by one another and by the environmental conditions of the healthy vagina. When something upsets this natural balance, however, one or another organism may proliferate.

Oral contraceptives, antibiotics, nylon underwear, pantyhose, and tight pants are among the factors that may disrupt the vaginal ecological balance and that have been blamed for the alarming increase in vaginal infections in recent years. Other precipitating factors include a decline in a woman's overall resistance to disease, excessive douching with irritating solutions, unusual emotional stress, diabetes or prediabetes, foreign objects that irritate the vagina, and even colored or perfumed toilet paper.

Common Causes

Vaginitis can afflict females of all ages — from early childhood to old age, but it is most common among sexually active women. The microorganisms that cause vaginitis may also infect a woman's sexual partner without his realizing it, and unless both partners are treated at the same time, they may pass the infection back and forth. During therapy it is best to abstain from intercourse or use a condom.

The common infectious causes of vaginitis, their symptoms, and usual treatments include the following:

Candida albicans, a fungus (also called monilia), produces a thick white discharge resembling cottage cheese and has a yeasty odor. It may start suddenly, cause intense itching, and make intercourse painful. Because it prefers a warm, moist environment, it is particularly common in summer. Diabetes, oral contraceptives, and pregnancy also predispose one to it. It is usually treated with an antifungal cream (nystatin or candicidin) or gentian violet.

Trichomonas vaginalis, a protozoan, produces a profuse, foamy, greenish white, foul-smelling discharge. Itching and burning commonly flare up during or shortly after menstruation. It may also cause a urinary tract infection. Trichomonas likes an alkaline environment that may occur when antibiotic therapy (for example, tetracycline) incidentally destroys the vaginal bacteria that normally keep the vagina acidic. About 25 percent of women harbor this protozoan but have no symptoms.

Treatment of trich, as it is often called, is a mixed blessing. The most effective drug, Flagyl, causes genetic damage (and should not be used orally during pregnancy) and cancer in laboratory animals. An acid vaginal jelly or a couple of tablespoons of plain yogurt (it contains acid-forming bacteria) applied vaginally or douching with a solution of one to two tablespoons of vinegar in a quart of water can bring relief.

Haemophilus vaginalis, a bacterium, produces a creamy white or grayish foul-smelling discharge, burning, and itching. Mixtures of bacteria may also cause vaginitis, as may gonorrhea bacteria. Women with bacterial vaginitis are usually treated with sulfa drugs or other antibiotics in a vaginal suppository or cream; men are given antibiotics by mouth. Gonorrhea is treated by injections of penicillin. [See chapter on venereal disease, page 188.]

Noninfectious causes of vaginitis include mechanical irritation and postmenopausal changes in the vaginal wall. Women past menopause with symptoms of vaginitis may benefit from estrogen therapy. [See chapter on menopause, page 229.]

537

Before vaginitis is treated, it is important for the doctor to make a definite diagnosis of the causative agent by means of a wet smear and culture. A Pap smear, pelvic exam, and urine test are also advised. Don't self-treat symptoms of vaginitis for more than two or three days.

Prevention and Control

The following measures have helped many women to prevent vaginitis or get rid of a persistent or recurring case:

● Wear cotton underpants or at least those with a cotton crotch. Even pantyhose can now be obtained with a cotton crotch. Avoid wearing tight pants, wear knee-high stockings rather than pantyhose under slacks, and sleep in a nightgown without underpants, rather than in pajamas.

● Wash or bathe at least once a day, using your own towel and washcloth and a mild, nonperfumed soap. Change underwear daily. Have your partner wash his genital area before intercourse. Wipe the anus from front to back to avoid contaminating the vaginal area.

● Avoid unnecessary antibiotics, but if you must take them, try eating yogurt (or inserting some plain yogurt into the vagina) to help restore the bacterial balance.

● Keep down your consumption of sugar, which encourages the growth of undesirable vaginal organisms.

● Avoid sitting around in a damp bathing suit. After swimming, put on a robe or skirt, and slip off your suit.

● If your vagina is dry and easily irritated during intercourse, apply a sterile, water-soluble lubricating jelly (not petroleum jelly or oil) before sexual activity. Contraceptive jellies and creams are acidic and may help retard the growth of vaginitis organisms.

● Don't use irritating sprays, soaps, or powders in the vaginal area. So-called feminine hygiene sprays have been associated with hundreds of reports of vaginal irritation and infection. Bubble baths are also a problem for some women.

The value of douching in preventing vaginitis is highly controversial. Some doctors insist that you should cleanse the vagina regularly, just as you do your mouth. Others say that nature does this job adequately and that regular douching disrupts the balance of nature and may precipitate vaginitis.

If you douche, observe these precautions: Hang the douche bag no more than two feet above your hips. Don't use a bulb syringe or compact douches. Don't douche during menstruation or pregnancy. Keep your douching equipment clean, and don't let anyone else use it. Use plain lukewarm water, or a tablespoon of vinegar in a quart of water, or a doctor's prescription, and recline at a forty-five-degree angle.

Urinary Tract Infections:
Conquering a Stubborn Problem

The doctor, grinning knowingly, called it honeymoon cystitis. To the twenty-six-year-old bride of six months, it was no honeymoon. Nor was it anything to smile about. She retorted angrily, "If this doesn't get cleared up, it will soon be *divorce* cystitis."

The problem of urinary tract infections is known only too well to millions of American women and a lesser number of men. For many, it is a chronic or recurring problem that is physically and emotionally debilitating and highly disruptive of normal living. The difficulties in getting rid of it once and for all lead many to question the wonders of modern medicine and the competence of their physicians.

An understanding of how and why the disease strikes and how it should be diagnosed and treated, plus the observance of some simple preventive measures, can go a long way to protect against future difficulties. Stubborn recurrent infections can now be prevented in most cases. It also helps victims to know that they have not been singled out to suffer — perhaps as punishment for some immorality — but that many other "innocent" people share their misery.

Causes

Urinary tract infections usually result from bacterial colonization of all or part of the body's liquid waste disposal system: the urethra, which carries urine from the bladder to outside the body; the bladder, which stores urine for excretion; the ureters, which carry urine from the kidneys to the bladder; and the kidneys, which extract liquid wastes from the bloodstream. The most common types of infection are urethritis, involving the urethra, and cystitis, involving the bladder. If the infection ascends to the kidneys, it's called pyelonephritis.

Bacteria are normally present in the urethra and sometimes even in the bladder. Ordinarily most bacteria are washed out by urination and don't have the opportunity to establish colonies in the urinary tract. However, if something interferes with this natural defense mechanism, such as an obstruction that prevents complete emptying of the bladder, the bacteria can multiply and cause an infection.

Conditions that can set the stage for urinary tract infections include irritation and swelling of the urethra or bladder as a result of sexual intercourse, pregnancy, and bike riding; the use of irritants like bubble bath, feminine hygiene sprays, douches, or the diaphragm; urinary stones; enlargement in men of the prostate gland; vaginitis; strictures or other abnormalities of the urethra; and psychological stress and fatigue.

Women are highly susceptible to urinary tract infections (UTIs) because their urethras are only about 1.5 inches long, compared with 8 or 9 inches in men. The short urethra allows easy migration of bacteria to the bladder. Also, the urethral opening in women is near anal and vaginal sources of infectious organisms, and women lack the antibacterial action of prostatic fluid.

By far the most common cause of UTI is the bacterium *Escherichia coli,* a normal inhabitant of the human intestinal tract which is readily transferred from the anus to the urethra of women.

UTIs occur in about 1 to 2 percent of infants usually because of congenital abnormalities that may require surgical correction. Thereafter it becomes almost nonexistent in young males but increases in prevalence by about 1 percent per decade of life in females. In middle age 5 to 10 percent of women have UTIs, often precipitated by postmenopausal dryness and atrophy of the vagina, which can be relieved by estrogen supplements or, more safely, by the use of water-soluble lubricants. Because of prostate and other problems, UTIs become almost as common in elderly men as in older women.

In young women the most common — and most distressing — precipitant is sexual activity. Women may develop UTIs when they first have sexual intercourse, when they acquire a new sexual partner or resume sex after a long interval, or when the frequency of intercourse increases significantly.

Prevention

Women can help protect themselves against UTIs by observing the following preventive measures:

● Drink lots of liquids throughout the day, every day — at least five or six glasses and preferably enough to necessitate voiding every hour or two.

● Be sure to void frequently to cleanse out the urinary tract.

● Always wipe from front to back to prevent contamination of the urethra from the vagina and anus.

● Wash the genital and anal area with mild soap and water often.

● Don't use bubble bath, feminine hygiene sprays, or scented douches.

● Be certain to empty your bladder before and immediately after intercourse. An empty bladder is less likely to be injured during sex, and any infectious organisms that might already be there or that might be introduced during sex will be washed out. In one study, women who postponed voiding for more than fifteen minutes after sex were more likely to develop a UTI.

Many women find it helpful to drink cranberry juice daily (and several times a day when an infection is present or threatening). Women prone to UTIs who use the diaphragm might consider switching to another contraceptive since the ring of the diaphragm may press against and irritate the bladder. It may also help to avoid sex positions in which the penis presses on the belly side of the vagina, where the bladder rests. The role, if any, that oral-genital sex may play in precipitating UTIs is not known, but if it is a factor, washing the genital area and emptying the bladder before and after sexual activity should greatly reduce the likelihood of infection. If irritation occurs during intercourse, it may help to soak in a hot tub for about fifteen minutes afterward.

Diagnosis and Treatment

An analysis and culture of the urine are necessary before diagnosis of a UTI and choice of treatment are made. A "clean-catch" urine specimen is usually obtained: After washing the genital area, the woman voids in three separate portions, discarding the first and the third and catching the second in a cup for analysis.

The doctor can check the specimen immediately under the microscope for the presence of bacteria and pus and should send part of it to a laboratory, where the number and type of contaminating organisms and their antibiotic sensitivities can be identified. Some patients develop symptoms of UTI, perhaps caused by lesions that irritate the urethra or bladder, but actually have no infection.

If an infection is confirmed by the culture, treatment usually involves at least a week and often two on an appropriate drug, usually an antibiotic or sulfa drug or a drug like nitrofurantoin or methenamine mandelate. For some drugs the urine should be kept quite acid, so cranberry juice or vitamin C tablets may also be prescribed. Be sure to complete the full course of treatment; even though the symptoms may disappear after a day or two, the infecting organisms take much longer to be killed.

A newer approach to treatment involves a single injection or one large oral dose of an antibiotic mixture — trimethoprim and sulfamethoxazole (TMP-SMX). This treatment is not appropriate for persons who are sensitive to sulfa drugs.

To relieve the discomfort of a UTI, the doctor may prescribe an analgesic (the most commonly used one turns your urine bright orange), a smooth muscle relaxant, or a barbiturate. Drinking water continuously and sitting in warm baths or using a heating pad will also bring relief. While you are battling an infection, it's best to avoid coffee, tea, alcohol, and spicy foods since these irritate the urinary tract. Some doctors recommend sexual abstinence during treatment, but others say that sex is OK after the symptoms subside.

Following completion of treatment, the doctor may want to do another culture. If the infection recurs — and some four out of five do within eighteen months — a new culture is necessary; the results may suggest that a different drug should be used. After several recurrences the patient should be seen by a urologist, who should do a kidney X ray and may examine the bladder through a cystoscope. If an obstruction or

541

structural abnormality is found, surgery may be necessary to prevent further UTIs and head off kidney damage.

In the absence of an obstruction, persistent recurrent infections can usually be prevented by your taking a single dose of antibiotic either nightly or immediately after sexual intercourse, depending on the drug regimen the doctor chooses. Low doses of nitrofurantoin or TMP-SMX have proved most effective in preventing recurrent infections.

Sometimes, rather than produce intense discomfort, a UTI will cause minimal or no symptoms and instead smolder for months or years and perhaps eventually damage the kidneys. Thus, it's a good idea to have a urine culture (not merely a urinalysis) done whenever you have routine physical or gynecological exam.

Hay Fever, Etc.:
What to Do About Seasonal Allergies

Many of the nation's 35 million allergy sufferers are, in a sense, lucky. They're sensitive to a substance, such as cat dander, that they can quite easily avoid. But for nearly 15 million Americans, the source of distress is in the very air they breathe. They are allergic to one or more of the pollens from trees, shrubs, grasses, and flowers and/or the spores from ubiquitous molds that live on dead and decaying organic matter. They are the victims of hay fever (a misnomer, since it is neither a fever nor caused by hay), which allergists prefer to call allergic or seasonal rhinitis.

Short of moving to a desert or snowcapped mountaintop or living in an air-conditioned, hermetically sealed, dehumidified room twenty-four hours a day during the allergy season, there is no surefire way to avoid these irksome microscopic substances. However, once you know what you're dealing with, it is possible to reduce your exposure to the offenders and to limit the severity of your allergic response.

Contrary to popular belief, hay fever is not merely a phenomenon of late summer, when ragweed, the principal culprit for most victims, sheds a quarter of a million tons of pollen grains that are blown across the eastern and central states. For many Americans, such as those living in the southern states, hay fever begins in January or February, when the local trees bloom, and may not end until November, when the ragweed finally dies back.

In the Northeast and Middle West, the sneezing season starts in March and ends in October, and in the Rocky Mountain states it extends from April to October. In the Northwest, where there is no serious ragweed problem but where grasses shed pollen for six months, the hay fever season lasts from March to November. "Rose fever" commonly strikes at midsummer, the result of pollinating grasses (not roses).

Mold allergies have even greater longevity. Because molds are not killed by frost, they can form and shed spores at any time of year that the weather happens to warm up, and thus, they may precipitate winter or year-round hay fever in susceptible people. Sometimes seasonal allergies are caused not by plants, but by insect dust.

What Is an Allergy?

An allergy is an overreaction of the body's immune defense system to a substance that would otherwise be harmless. Instead of ignoring the substance, the body produces immunological weapons that turn your innards into a battlefield. In the case of ragweed pollen, the main hay fever culprit, a group of antibodies called IgE are formed when the pollen is inhaled. The antibodies attach themselves to immune cells, which in turn release histamine and other symptom-provoking substances into the respiratory tissues. Histamine causes the runny nose, sneezing, itchy eyes, and wheezing breath classically associated with hay fever.

Other *allergens*, as substances that trigger allergic reactions are called, produce similar symptoms; among them are animal dander (scales from hair, feathers, or skin), grass or tree pollen, house dust, and mold spores. In some cases, such as in allergy to penicillin or insect stings, the reaction is widespread and sometimes life-threatening. In food allergies the reaction may disrupt the normal workings of the digestive tract or have distant effects on other organs, such as migraine headaches. [See chapter on food allergies, page 548.]

What Is the Cause?

A proper diagnosis of the allergy and its likely cause or causes is critically important. Too often, says Dr. Peter Kohler of the University of Colorado Medical Center, "allergy is a wastebasket diagnosis" in which all kinds of symptoms are blamed on allergies to all sorts of substances. The allergist's best weapon, he and other allergy experts agree, is a careful history and physical examination. What symptoms occur and under what circumstances? In some cases the patient may be asked to keep a diary of symptoms.

This is followed by skin tests, in which a tiny amount of various suspected allergens are applied to the skin and the reaction observed. If a hive or redness appears at the site, an allergic sensitivity is present. However, not all substances to which a person shows an allergic reaction on a skin test actually produce symptoms in the course of natural exposure.

If too much of the allergen is used in the test, almost everyone will seem to be allergic to it. Dr. Kohler cautions patients to be suspicious of tests that show them to be allergic to lots of different substances. In addition to potential allergens, a skin test should be done on the substance used to dilute them, since some patients react to it, producing misleading results.

Some allergists now use a simpler and probably more accurate diagnostic technique called RAST (for RadioAllergoSorbent Test). It is a blood test that measures the IgE antibody, thus determining what the patient is allergic to and the degree of sensitivity.

Symptoms of Seasonal Allergies

The symptoms of pollen allergies are all too familiar: sneezing fits, itchy and swollen eyes, stuffed and runny nose, tickly throat, and fullness in the ears and head. Some victims cough and wheeze, especially at night, interfering with a good night's sleep. In mold allergies, asthmatic types of symptoms — dry cough, shortness of breath, and wheezing — are more common, but sometimes all the sufferer has are nasal symptoms. Those who suffer on days when the pollen count is low probably have mold allergies as well.

Seasonal allergies can lead to a number of more generalized symptoms, including fatigue, headache, lethargy, irritability, and gastrointestinal upsets. Some victims develop secondary infections in congested sinus cavities.

Weather, as you might have guessed, has a lot to do with the extent of seasonal allergy symptoms. Hot, sunny, windy days send pollen counts soaring, whereas cool, rainy days often bring relief. Lots of rain, however, is a great stimulus to mold growth. Symptoms are also likely to be aggravated by rapid changes in temperature and barometric pressure.

How to Minimize Symptoms

While there is little you can do about the weather, you can, if you are sensitive to pollen and mold spores, try the following:

● Avoid treks through the woods and fields during the season of your discontent. One solution is to stay in the city since urban pollen counts are nearly always lower than those in rural areas.

● If tree pollen, the first to cause seasonal distress, is your problem, avoid landscaping your home with the common offenders: elm, maple, birch, poplar, ash, oak, walnut, sycamore, or cypress. Those with ragweed allergy should avoid such ragweed relatives as chrysanthemums, dahlias, daisies, cosmos, zinnias, golden glow, and goldenrod. Mold sufferers should avoid potted African violets and geraniums since mold frequently grows around them.

● Pets are another source of trouble. Chances are that anyone allergic to pollen or molds already is or will become sensitive to animal dander and feathers, further aggravating the problem. According to allergists, the only acceptable pets for the allergy-prone are fish and reptiles.

● Plan your vacations carefully. According to *Patient Care*, a medical magazine, the safest time in the Northeast is in late July or early August. Europe has little or no ragweed. But eastern ragweed sufferers who try to escape to the West Coast may find themselves afflicted with grass pollen allergies in August. Generally moving to another part of the country is not recommended because new allergies are likely to develop in the new locale. [See map below.]

　● As much as possible, stay indoors in an air-conditioned room on days when the pollen count is high. To keep from making matters worse, the room temperatures should not be more than 10 degrees colder than the outdoor temperature. Don't drink very cold liquids.

　● Keep your bedroom free of dust, and avoid exposure to such irritants as perfumes, tobacco smoke, and chemical vapors, any of which can aggravate your allergic reaction. If you must be in dusty areas, wear a

THE HAY FEVER MAP

ZONE	TREES	GRASSES	RAGWEED
1	March to June	May to August	August to October
2	March to June	May to October	August to October
3	January to May	April to October	July to December (except Florida)
4	February to May and September to January	April to November	August to December (except in the West)
5	March to June	May to October	August to October
6	March to July	May to November	August to December (except in high mountains)
7	April to June	May to September	July to October
8	March to May	May to November	Not serious at any time
9	February to June	May to November	June to November

Based on data from Allergy Foundation of America

545

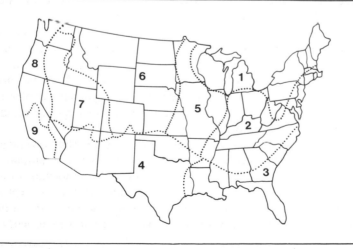

good nose mask. An air cleaner to purify the air might also prove helpful in your bedroom.

• Avoid fatigue, overwork, overheating, strong drafts, and alcoholic drinks (these cause further swelling of mucous membranes).

• To reduce exposure to spores, mold sufferers should discard old, damp items like furniture, pillows, carpets, and paper, keep their basements dry with a dehumidifier, use antimildew sprays in damp areas, stay away from damp woods and shores, avoid seaside and country summer cottages, and use Dacron-filled sleeping bags.

• Those allergic to animal dander should avoid furry or feathery pets and feather pillows.

If these measures fail to bring adequate relief, treatment with antihistamines and decongestants and possibly eye drops can help a great deal. There are four different classes of antihistamines sold (and many different drugs within each class), so if one does not do an adequate job or causes too many side effects, another may be better. Some antiallergy drugs (usually combinations of antihistamines and decongestants) are sold over the counter, but the more potent ones can be obtained only with a doctor's prescription.

The side effects of antihistamines include drowsiness, loss of alertness, and coordination problems. It's best to avoid driving a car or operating machinery while you take them. Decongestants help to counter the sleep-inducing effects of antihistamines as well as to relieve allergy symptoms. Antihistamines should not be taken by persons with glaucoma or prostate inflammation, and the decongestants ephedrine or pseudephedrine should not be used by those with high blood pressure. Seasonal respiratory allergy may also be safely relieved by a steroid nasal spray (beclomethasone of flunisolide), but continuous use of high doses should be avoided.

Allergy Shots, a Solution for Some

If drug treatment is not sufficiently effective or if the side effects are intolerable and the allergy is long-lasting and seriously interferes with the person's life (for example, prevents sleep, work, or study), immunotherapy to desensitize the sufferer can be tried.

In a nation where miraculous preventives administered through hypodermic needles are well known, it's not surprising that some 6 million Americans choose shots as the solution to their allergies. But allergy shots are not the simple preferred solution that many people think they are. While they are often highly effective in relieving the symptoms of a well-defined allergy, they rarely "cure" the allergy or suppress all its symptoms. In a significant number of people they don't work at all, and for many kinds of allergies they are wholly inappropriate. In a few rare cases the shots themselves can be dangerous. Furthermore, they are very expensive and bothersome and require continued treatment for an indefinite period of time — years in most cases.

Yet, when appropriately used, desensitization through allergy shots can make the difference between a distressing affliction that interferes with work and learning and a comfortable, productive existence.

Desensitization is a medical procedure in which the allergic person's immune system is made more "tolerant" of the allergen. Tiny doses of the allergen — so small that they produce no allergic symptoms — are injected into the patient, and the doses are gradually increased over a period of days, weeks, or months. Instead of producing the troublesome IgE antibodies, the body makes a protective blocking antibody called IgG, which combines with the allergen and blocks the release of histamine.

Eventually, if the therapy is done properly, a dose is reached at which the patient now experiences many fewer symptoms when exposed to the allergen in the course of daily living. In the case of ragweed hay fever, this generally takes twelve to fifteen weeks of injections, usually starting in April to protect against the next hay fever season. To maintain the immunity, regular booster shots are needed every three to six weeks throughout the year. Sometimes, when rapid protection is needed, a faster treatment involving several shots a day or daily shots several days in a row can be used.

It may take two or three years to obtain the maximum benefit from desensitization. The immunization program should be started by a qualified allergist, but often the family doctor can take over the frequent injections, with only occasional visits to the specialist.

Generally allergy shots are highly specific. Treatment with ragweed pollen offers no protection against grass or tree pollen or mold spores. Some patients who obtain little benefit from ragweed desensitization may actually have a number of other allergies as well.

Ragweed desensitization brings substantial relief in about 80 percent of people who give it enough time. Insect venom therapy is also highly effective. [See chapter on insect pests, page 412.] However, the treatment agents used for other allergies are still far short of ideal, and the results are less good.

The main risk of immunotherapy is triggering an allergic reaction. If the proper doses are used and administered in slowly increased amounts, this should not happen. If an allergic response does occur, the time between doses or the amount of allergen used may have to be adjusted. Very rarely a severe and potentially life-threatening reaction may occur. Therefore, anyone administering allergy shots must have proper emergency equipment on hand and know how to use it. For these reasons, administering immunizations at home is not advised.

For Further Information

To assure the best results, make sure you are treated by a qualified specialist. Ask your family physician for a recommendation, or contact your local chapter of the Asthma and

Allergy Foundation of America. The national office is at 19 West Forty-fourth Street, New York, New York 10036 (212-921-9100).

Food Allergies: Often Misdiagnosed

A boy coughs and wheezes every time he eats peanuts. A man breaks out into hives immediately after eating strawberries. A woman gets severe migraine headaches hours after consuming corn products, which are "hidden" in hundreds of processed foods. Another woman develops intestinal cramps and diarrhea the day after eating soybean products.

All will tell you, "I can't eat that. I'm allergic to it." Bad reactions to foods are quite common, but recent studies indicate that allergies are often blamed for symptoms they do not cause. As a result, many people needlessly deprive themselves of various foods they think they are sensitive to, and some "allergic" children are placed on such restricted diets that they fail to grow normally.

Food allergy has become a "wastebasket" diagnosis used to explain a wide range of symptoms which may or may not have something to do with what the patient eats. Popular books have improperly blamed foods for everything from fatigue and nervousness to painful menstrual cramps and bed wetting, says Dr. Zack H. Haddad, who heads the Department of Pediatric Allergy and Immunology at the University of Southern California in Los Angeles.

However, careful studies show that:

● Not all bad reactions to foods are allergic reactions.

● Many persons, including children, who think they have food allergies really don't.

● Foods are often blamed for reactions that are actually due to other causes, including work stress.

● Children often outgrow sensitivities to certain foods.

● Even when a food allergy exists, consumption of that food in small amounts may not cause symptoms.

In other cases food may be overlooked as a possible cause of a distressing symptom because of a time lag between eating the food and experiencing the reaction. Or the food may be consumed so often that the relationship between it and the resulting symptoms is not noticed.

What Is a Food Allergy?

An allergic reaction has a specific definition: When exposed to the substance in question, a person who is allergic to it produces antibodies to that substance that ultimately result in the appearance of certain symptoms. Classic symptoms of food allergy include severe abdominal pain, diarrhea, hives, swellings, wheezing, violent vomiting, hayfever types of symptoms, eczema, and even shock or loss of consciousness. Milder forms of these symptoms may also occur, Dr. Haddad says. For unknown reasons, the same food may provoke different allergic symptoms in different people — for example, asthma in one, hives in another, cramps and diarrhea in a third.

The foods most commonly incriminated in food allergy are milk, eggs, and peanuts, followed by wheat, corn, fish, shellfish, berries, nuts, peas and beans, and some spices.

People who are allergic to certain foods may be able to consume them in limited amounts without difficulty, but some people are extraordinarily sensitive and suffer violent reactions to the smallest amount of the food. They must be extremely careful not to eat the food in question; that may mean avoiding all processed foods and not dining out. Currently there is no cure for food allergy other than not eating the food responsible for the symptoms. One drug being studied in Europe, cromolyn, an asthma medication, may be able to block reactions in some patients with food allergy.

Many people produce antibodies to certain foods that do not actually make them sick. For example, they may have a positive skin test to an extract of the food or they may have antibodies in the blood serum. But when the food is disguised and then consumed, no symptoms result. Such individuals may be sensitive to that food immunologically speaking, but they do not have allergic symptoms when they consume it. Thus, a positive skin test or blood test alone is not enough to diagnose a food allergy.

In studies at the National Jewish Hospital-National Asthma Center in Denver, Dr. S. Allan Bock and his colleagues could not confirm the existence of food allergy in 60 percent of children examined who were said to be allergic to certain foods and who showed positive skin tests to those foods. The Denver physicians tested for allergic response by disguising the foods in capsules so that child, parent, and doctor were unaware of which capsules were given at which time. These blind challenges removed the possibility that emotional factors would affect the response. Only two in five tested in this way were found to be truly allergic to foods.

Another approach to allergy diagnosis involves the elimination diet. When suspected foods are not eaten and the symptoms disappear, only to reappear when the incriminated foods are reintroduced, allergy is often assumed to be the cause of the symptoms. The trouble is, people who are convinced they are allergic to foods may have psychologically induced reactions that result in the symptoms, even when a true allergy doesn't exist. Here, too, a blind test — reintroducing the suspect food in disguised form unbeknownst to the patient — may give a more accurate diagnosis.

However, Dr. Bock notes, if an elimination diet does not get rid of the symptoms, "it's probable that the suspected foods are not the cause of the problem."

In cases of severe allergic types of symptoms that are difficult to diagnose, the patient — infant or adult — may be sustained entirely on a liquid food called Vivonex (originally developed by NASA for astronauts but later abandoned by the space program), which is nutritionally balanced and free of allergy-producing substances. After about a week the suspect foods are introduced one by one, and the patient notes the appearance of any symptoms.

Nonallergic Reactions to Foods

In addition to allergic reactions, there are other causes of adverse reactions to foods. They include:

● Sensitivity to a natural toxin or a contaminant of the food, such as penicillin in milk (as a result of antibiotics given to the cows) or red tide contamination of seafood. Dr. Haddad notes that the tyramine in cheese and milk can provoke migraine in some people.

● Enzyme deficiencies, such as an insufficiency of lactase, the enzyme that digests the milk sugar, lactose. Those with lactase deficiency commonly develop abdominal cramps, flatulence, and diarrhea when consuming lactose-containing dairy products or processed foods to which milk or milk solids have been added. Varying degrees of lactase deficiency are quite common, particularly among blacks, Orientals, and persons of Eastern European descent.

Many lactose-intolerant people are able to consume hard cheeses, cultured dairy products (yogurt, buttermilk, and sour cream) in which much of the lactose is predigested, and even small amounts of ordinary lactose-containing milk without difficulty. For those who are highly sensitive, specially prepared lactose-reduced milk or pretreatment of milk at home with the enzyme LactAid (available at pharmacies and some health food stores) are helpful.

● Psychological reactions, such as a person's belief that he "can't eat eggs" because they make him or her very sick. Dr. Bock found chocolate to be the food most frequently incriminated incorrectly. In studies of 300 allergic children, he has yet to find one who is truly allergic to chocolate.

In a number of "allergic" children studied, emotional problems were found to be at the root of their difficulties, especially for a symptom complex known as tension-fatigue syndrome. Psychological counseling and slowly convincing the child he can safely eat the foods in question often bring relief, Dr. Bock reports.

Young children who are found to have food allergies should be re-tested every three to six months because they often outgrow them, Dr. Bock says. However, allergies acquired as adults seem to last indefinitely.

Foot Problems:
How to Care for Your Feet

Millions of Americans who might otherwise heed the advice of health experts to let their feet, rather than their fingers, do the walking are discouraged from doing so by aches, pains, and other discomforts in those lowermost appendages. "My feet are killing me" may well be the most common health complaint.

Feet are the most used and abused parts of the human body. According to a study conducted by the Pennsylvania College of Podiatric Medicine, the average American walks 115,000 miles — the equivalent of more than four times around the world — in a lifetime. With each step, minor abnormalities in foot structures and/or shoes that don't fit right can result in such distressing ailments as corns, calluses, bunions, and hammertoes. An estimated 87 percent of Americans suffer from one or another foot problem.

Though these problems are not a direct threat to life, their presence can take the joy out of many life-enhancing activities and make others impossible. In summer, when warm weather and vacations prompt more walking than usual, foot problems are likely to become painfully apparent. They are also troublesome in winter, when feet are usually confined in closed shoes and boots.

The constant introduction of foot-distorting shoe styles for women and the fitness craze that has millions of American feet jogging, running, dancing, and jumping have greatly swelled the ranks of podiatric and orthopedic patients. In addition, disorders like diabetes, obesity, and circulatory abnormalities predispose their victims to foot problems that require professional attention.

Those who try to cope with foot problems on their own often throw good money after bad with successive purchases of inappropriate over-the-counter medications and appliances. In some cases improper self-treatment can make matters worse.

Yet many painful afflictions of the feet can be avoided entirely, or their more serious consequences averted, by simple preventive measures and daily attention to these usually neglected (until they hurt) parts of our anatomy.

Select Sensible Shoes

"If the shoe fits, wear it." While few would argue with such sage advice, if we judge from what many people, especially women, put on their feet, a more accurate description of the situation is: "If the shoe doesn't fit, wear it anyway."

The human foot is an intricate structure well designed for supporting a two-legged animal that walks and sometimes runs. But if any of its twenty-six bones are put in an unnatural position by the shoe that was intended to protect it, the balance and function of all the other bones are disrupted. The joints are then unable to function properly, and the result can be contracted and deformed toes, osteoarthritis, weakness of the foot muscles, misdirected tendons and ligaments, and strain on supporting tissues in the leg and back.

From infancy onward the "common knowledge" on how — and when — to select a pair of shoes is riddled with myth and misconception. As a result, people waste extraordinary amounts of money, and cause themselves much needless discomfort, by buying the wrong kinds of shoes. Podiatrists and orthopedic surgeons around the country offer the following guidelines on foot care and shoe selection.

Bare feet. Bare feet are highly desirable for babies who cannot yet walk and all right for people of any age who trek on sand and soft, unpolluted earth or grass. Everyone else should have some kind of covering to support the foot in its battle against cement and to protect it from injury by obstacles and debris.

552

Dr. Alexander Hersh, chief of the foot service at the Hospital for Special Surgery in New York City, even advises against bare feet at home, where slivers of glass and pins and needles can stab the unprotected foot, and toes can be stubbed and even broken on furniture and miscellaneous objects left lying about.

Babies' shoes. Babies do not need to wear shoes of any sort until they begin to walk. Even then the only reason for the shoes is to protect their feet from injury and keep them warm. Shoes place restrictive forces on the growing bones in a baby's foot. "Most people put shoes on a baby long before they need to," notes Dr. René Cailliet, head of physical medicine and rehabilitation at the University of Southern California at Los Angeles. "Baby shoes are mainly for the psychological benefit of the parents and for warmth."

Corrective shoes. There is no such thing as a corrective shoe for children. Such shoes merely support and guide the foot to prevent an abnormality from getting worse, but they cannot undo the problem. Thus, you may be able to buy special shoes to accommodate and support feet that toe in or are extremely flat, but don't expect the problem to be corrected by the shoes, says Dr. Paul Scherer, dean of the California College of Podiatric Medicine in San Francisco.

For adults with foot abnormalities that cannot be corrected surgically and that prohibit wearing ordinary shoes, molded shoes can be made to order from a cast taken of their feet. These cost anywhere from $100 to $350.

Sneakers. Despite everything your parents or grandparents may have told you, sneakers are not bad for your feet. In fact, foot specialists say, the flexibility of sneakers makes them ideal for young children, most of whom can wear them all the time with no adverse effects. In one study children who wore sneakers 85 percent of the time over a ten-year period did not develop flat feet or fallen arches. Sneakers permit the foot to spread out, yet they can be laced tightly for support and their rubber sole give good traction and a sure step, Dr. Cailliet says. They should be made of a fabric that breathes, not of plastic or artificial leather.

Only children with severely flat or very highly arched feet should not wear sneakers, Dr. Hersh says. The rest do fine in sneakers that have a little arch pad in them. Sneakers are best worn with absorbent socks,

HOW TO BUY SHOES THAT FIT

● Shop for comfort, not fashion. If you have normal feet, you should not have to buy ugly, clumsy-looking shoes to get ones that fit. But you do have to pay careful attention to factors other than style.

● Buy at the end of the day. Foot specialists routinely advise that you never buy shoes in the morning. Even if you walk nowhere, your feet swell during the course of the day, and the shoes you buy should fit comfortably at the end of the day, when your feet are largest.

● Buy at a reputable store that carries a wide variety of sizes. The store should be willing to take the shoes back if after trying them on at home, you find them uncomfortable.

● Buy only leather or fabric shoes, not man-made materials that don't breathe. Ideally the soles should be leather as well, since the bottoms of your feet sweat more than the tops. Sweating in shoes can cause infections, blisters, shriveled skin, and bad odors.

● Never buy shoes that you have to break in. Shoes should not be a little uncomfortable when you buy them. Don't accept a salesman's statement that the shoes will feel better after you've worn them a few hours.

● Don't buy size. Buy fit, no matter what the numbers say. One manufacturer's 7-B may be another's 6½-C. Instead of asking for your size, the salesman should measure your foot when you are standing.

● Always fit the larger foot, and if necessary, use an innersole to improve the fit on the other foot. No two people have the same feet, and no person has the same two feet, Dr. Hersh points out.

● The end of your longest toe should be a thumb's width away from the end of the shoe while you are standing. You should have enough room across the widest part to be able to pinch the leather. As a test, stand barefoot and compare the width of your forefoot to the width of the shoe in which that foot must fit. Chances are your foot is bigger than the shoe; that means it will be unnaturally and perhaps painfully squeezed across the toes.

● If your feet are wide in front but narrow in the heel, Dr. Joseph Seder, podiatrist at the Cleveland Clinic, says you'll do best with a combination last (the last is the foundation of the shoe). The size would say something like 7AA-B, meaning a double A heel width and B width across the ball of the foot. However, combination lasts are now very hard to get. As an economy move in recent years, manufacturers have greatly reduced the choice of widths. If you cannot fit both forefoot and heel, fit the forefoot and use padding (for example, a half innersole under the ball of the foot) to improve the heel grip.

containing at least 40 percent cotton or wool.

High heels. The higher the heel, the more weight is thrust upon the ball of the foot. This pressure eventually produces a callus and then a painful corn within the callus. The large toes are also painfully jammed into the end of the shoe, and the front of the foot is crammed into the narrow tip, producing hammertoes. The muscle in the calf and the tendon behind the heel become shortened, causing pain and possibly tearing when the high heels are removed.

High heels also throw you off-balance and cause unsteadiness, increasing the likelihood of twisted ankles and strained backs. Dr. Scherer says he and his colleagues treated a tremendous increase in injuries related to dancing in high-heeled disco sandals, including broken ankles and torn ligaments. If foot specialists had their way, no heel would be higher than an inch above the forefoot.

Negative heels. Despite claims to the contrary, scientific studies have shown no special advantage to having the heel lower than the forefoot. The real benefit of these shoes is their wide front, which leaves plenty of room for the ball of the foot.

In fact, for people with short, tight ankle tendons or calf muscles, the negative heel can cause considerable pain, possible injury, and backaches. To avoid undue strain, those who switch to very low or negative heels should do it gradually, wearing the shoes for only a few hours at a time at first and taking two or three weeks to work up to an entire day.

Platform soles. These are in competition with high heels for causing the worst foot and ankle injuries. Wearing a shoe with a sole two or three inches off the ground is like walking on stilts. Your center of gravity is thrown off, and your foot is deprived of its normal flexibility, greatly increasing the chances that a misstep will produce a painful twist, tear, or break.

Clogs can cause similar problems. If your heel slips and you land on the edge of the shoe, the sole, acting as a lever, can produce enough force to break bones.

Boots. Unless they have high heels, are too tight, or are made of synthetic materials that don't breathe, there is no harm in wearing boots all day, foot specialists say. Boots that have been treated with silicone to waterproof them don't breathe and are best removed indoors.

Sandals. Low-heeled sandals are all right as long as they are well fitted with straps and the foot can grip them firmly. The main hazards are stubbed toes and tripping when the tip of the shoe gets caught on an uneven surface.

Coping with Common Foot Disorders

Once you've bought comfortable and practical footwear, you can further reduce the chances of problems by changing your shoes and socks daily. Feet should be cleansed once or twice a day, dried carefully, and dusted with foot powder. A ten-minute soak in warm water, with or without two teaspoons of Epsom salts or table salt, is a treat as well as a treatment for tired feet. Severe foot pain can be relieved by ice compresses to reduce swelling and inflammation. Here's what to do about other common foot problems.

Corns and calluses. These, the most frequent foot mishaps, are composed of layers of dead skin cells and result from repeated friction or pressure against parts of the foot. They represent the body's attempt to protect sensitive tissue. Hard corns are usually found on the tops of toes, where skin rubs against the shoe. Sometimes a corn will form on the ball of the foot beneath a callus, resulting in a sharp localized pain with each step. Corns are cone-shaped, with the tip pointing into the foot. When a shoe exerts pressure against the corn, the tip of the cone can hit sensitive underlying tissue, causing pain.

Self-treatment can be risky since the chemicals used to soften corns also damage healthy tissue. Follow the directions carefully, and limit self-treatment to five applications. People with poor circulation, such as diabetics, should seek professional help. Never try to remove corns with a razor blade. Hard corns are best prevented by protecting any rubbed area with a stick-on nonmedicated corn pad or horseshoe-shaped piece of moleskin or foam rubber and by not wearing the shoes that are the culprits.

Soft corns, which are rubbery, form between toes where the bones of one toe exert pressure against the bones of its neighbor. To help prevent their formation, use lamb's wool or cotton between toes that rub together. Once established, they are best treated professionally.

Calluses form over a flat surface and have no tip. They usually appear on the weight-bearing parts of the foot — the ball or heel. Each step presses the callus against underlying tissue and may cause aching, burning, or tenderness. Calluses may result from the friction of loose-fitting shoes or the pressure of shoes that are too tight. Women who wear high-heeled shoes are especially vulnerable to calluses. People with high arches are also vulnerable since the heel and ball of the foot bear all the weight. Arch supports may help to relieve the pressure and cause the callus to disappear slowly. Cushioned innersoles may also help prevent calluses.

Calluses can be gradually eliminated at home if you rub the callused area with a pumice stone after soaking or bathing has softened the dead skin. Then apply a moisturizing lotion. Do not try to remove too much of the callus at one time. Diabetics should consult a professional rather than attempt self-treatment.

Bunions. These swollen, inflamed protrusions occur on the side of the foot at the joint of the big toe. A similar swelling can develop at the outside of the foot, where it's called a bunionette. The usual cause is the persistent wearing of shoes that are too tight and short. Not surprisingly bunions and bunionettes are four times more common among women, many of whom wear high-heeled, pointy-toed shoes that cause the big toe to bend inward. In some cases bunions result from an inherited misalignment of the bones in the foot.

Bunions cannot be self-treated, and only surgery can correct the problem. However, considerable relief may be obtained through more conservative measures: using devices in the shoes that change the weight balance of the foot and wearing shields to protect the bunion from friction against the shoe.

Many podiatrists today operate on bunions under local anesthesia in their offices. However, the bunion may recur if the bones in the foot are misaligned. Podiatrists trained in ambulatory surgery correct such problems through office procedures that involve tiny incisions. However, other experts say that when realignment of the bones, muscles, or tendons is needed, the operation is best done in a hospital by an orthopedic or podiatric surgeon.

Hammertoes. As with bunions, this problem can result from wearing high heels or shoes that are too short. The usual victim is the second toe, which in most people is longer than the big toe. The middle joint on a hammertoe bends the wrong way, causing the segment of the toe nearest the main part of the foot to stick up. People with high arches are more likely to develop hammertoes. Sometimes, if caught in time, the problem can be remedied by splints and exercises, but a long-standing, rigid hammertoe requires surgery.

Ingrown toenails. In this misnamed condition, the nail doesn't really grow in; rather, the surrounding soft tissue presses against the edge of a nail that has been cut too short. The big toe is most often involved. The problem is prevented by cutting toenails straight across, rather than in a curve, and by leaving a piece of "white" nail on either side. If there is no evidence of infection (such as red, swollen, pus-filled tissue), you may treat ingrown toenails at home by forcing a tiny piece of absorbent cotton under the nail. This allows the nail to grow out without digging into sensitive soft tissue. Replace the cotton twice daily, perhaps first dipping it into an antibiotic solution, such as gentian violet.

Blisters. These commonly appear where a shoe rubs against skin that is unprotected by a corn or callus. Ease the friction with moleskin padding, wear socks, and change shoes. Don't pop blisters because they may then become infected. If a blister breaks on its own, apply an antiseptic and keep the area covered with a sterile bandage. Remove the bandage at night to promote healing.

"Falling" arches. Feet that feel tired and achy after prolonged standing may be suffering from strained arches. Get off your feet, soak them in warm water, and massage them for relief. If the problem occurs frequently, arch supports may be needed. In special cases these can be custom-designed, but much less expensive ready-made supports help many people. The problem is often averted by wearing shoes with low heels and strong, supportive arches.

For Further Reading

Arnot, Michelle. *Foot Notes.* New York: Doubleday/Dolphin, 1980.
Roberts, Elizabeth H., D.P.M. *On Your Feet.* New York: Pyramid, 1975.
Schneider, Myles J., D.P.M., and Mark D. Sussman, D.P.M. *How to Doctor Your Feet Without the Doctor.* New York: Scribner's, 1980.

Insomnia: Curable Without Pills

Tonight tens of millions of Americans will lie awake for hours, wondering and worrying whether they'll be able to get a good night's sleep. They are the victims of insomnia, which afflicts some 25 million Americans all the time and millions of others some of the time.

The Hazards of Sleeping Pills

Well over $100 million a year are spent on prescription sleeping pills alone to try to counter insomnia, which ruins both the nights and the days of its sufferers. Yet, according to experts on sleep disorders, most of these prescriptions are a total waste of money, and in many cases the drugs actually cause rather than cure insomnia. An expert panel of the National Academy of Sciences concluded in 1979 that sleeping pills are potentially dangerous and largely ineffective and more often than not aggravate the very problem they are supposed to be solving.

Doctors at the Sleep Disorders Clinic at Stanford University report that about 40 percent of patients who complain of insomnia actually lose sleep because they have become dependent on the drugs they were taking to "treat" their insomnia. When these patients are gradually withdrawn from the drugs — one dose at a time every five or six days — they sleep on the average 20 percent more than they did with the drugs, and many have no symptoms of any sleep problems.

The expert panel concluded that sleeping pills should be prescribed in only very limited numbers of pills for only a few nights at a time in especially stressful circumstances, such as during travel or following the death of a loved one. Sleeping pills should never be given to patients with respiratory problems, mental depression, or addiction to other drugs, including alcohol, the panel said. They should be prescribed with great caution for patients "who are or who may become pregnant, who operate machinery, who have kidney or liver disease or who are old."

What Is Insomnia?

Insomnia can take different forms and have many causes. People who have trouble falling asleep may lie awake for an hour or more after going to bed. They may wake up one or more times during the night and have difficulty going to sleep. Or they may wake up very early in the morning and lie in bed for hours, trying to go back to sleep.

None of these sleep patterns is really a problem unless it is chronic and interferes with life during the day, leaving the victim sleepy, fatigued, depressed, or anxious. Insufficient sleep for one or two nights is not debilitating, according to Dr. Sidney Cohen, a psychiatrist at the University of California at Los Angeles. "The major debilitating factor," he says, "is related to the worry about not having slept."

One of the most common causes of insomnia is no cause at all. The person simply thinks he or she has insomnia, but in fact, all-night recordings of sleep cycles show no problem. The treatment in these cases is education and reassurance. Pseudoinsomnia, as this condition is called, may result from ignorance of the fact that sleep requirements normally diminish with age. A newborn baby sleeps eighteen hours a day, young adults need to sleep an average of seven to eight hours, and elderly people require only four and a half to six and a half hours of sleep. Thus, as people get older, they may continue to go to bed at the same time and lie awake for hours, or else they may wake up in the wee hours of the morning and be unable to go back to sleep, simply because they have slept all they need to.

Sleep specialists report that patients complaining of insomnia often overestimate how long it takes them to fall asleep or how long they are up during the night, and thus, they underestimate how much sleep they actually get. This can be documented by recording the person's sleep pattern for one or more nights in a laboratory. Reassuring such patients that their sleep is normal is usually all the treatment necessary. Prescribing sleeping pills for patients with pseudoinsomnia is useless and may actually be harmful, leading to drug tolerance, escalating dosages, and drug-induced insomnia.

Causes of Sleeplessness

Real, chronic insomnia may be caused by a variety of medical disorders, psychological problems, or behavioral factors, such as drinking large amounts of caffeine-containing beverages.

Insomnia may be secondary to sleep-disrupting diseases like asthma, ulcers, or the pain of arthritis, migraine, or angina. In these cases the underlying cause must be treated to cure the insomnia. Perhaps 20 percent of insomnia patients are afflicted with so-called primary sleep disorders — problems that happen only in relation to sleep.

One of these is sleep apnea, a potentially life-threatening condition in which the victim stops breathing during sleep, snores and snorts raucously in a vain attempt to get air into the lungs, and finally awakens to breathe, usually not knowing the reason for awakening. The problem can result in dangerously high blood pressure. It can often be relieved by weight loss, but severe cases may require surgery to create a breathing hole through the trachea (the hole is closed during the day to allow normal speech).

Sometimes an insomniac's sleep is disturbed by muscular twitching in the legs called nocturnal myoclonus, a condition that only the sleeping partner is usually aware of. Other insomniacs have restless leg syndrome — a crawling feeling inside their legs that disappears with motion and often forces them to get up and walk around many times a night. There are no established treatments for these problems, but several possibly useful drugs are under study.

Some patients have disturbances in their biological rhythm, finding themselves wide awake at bedtime and sleepy when it's time to get up — a kind of permanent jet lag. If such people cannot adapt their lives to when their bodies want to sleep, it may be possible to reprogram the body, one hour at a time, to a more normal daily rhythm. Such reprogramming has been tried successfully in a few cases in sleep clinics.

Anxiety and depression are probably the most common psychiatric causes of sleep loss, and in severe cases antidepressant medication or a sleeping pill may be prescribed until psychotherapy takes effect. About 20 percent of insomniacs need psychotherapy for emotional problems, Dr. William C. Dement, director of the Sleep Disorders Clinic at Stanford University, estimates. Depression is one of the most common causes of insomnia in the elderly; prescription of sleeping pills for such persons can actually make their depression worse and compound the problem.

Home Cures and Medical Therapy

For garden-variety uncomplicated cases of insomnia, many of the time-honored remedies remain the best. Get some exercise during the day on a regular basis. Refrain from caffeine-containing beverages (coffee, tea, colas, and other soft drinks) after noon. Just before bedtime take a relaxing hot bath, engage in sexual intercourse, drink a glass of warm milk (the tryptophan in milk actually has sleep-inducing properties), read a difficult or boring book, or count sheep.

Whatever you do, don't try to fall asleep. Dr. Peter Hauri, who heads the sleep laboratory at Dartmouth Medical School in Hanover, New Hampshire, says the harder you try to sleep, the more aroused you become and the less likely you'll be to fall asleep.

Dr. Hauri finds that internal conditioning is usually successful in countering the try-to-sleep syndrome. People with this problem usually have no trouble falling asleep when they're doing something else, like watching television or reading. "So we tell them to stay up and do something to keep their minds off trying to fall asleep," Dr. Hauri says. One activity he has found very effective is a relaxation exercise in which the person relaxes all the muscles in his or her body one by one, starting from the toes and working up to the top of the head. Counting sheep has a similar distracting effect but lacks the muscle-relaxing component.

Biofeedback techniques have also helped some insomniacs. Those who are physically tense benefit from biofeedback training that teaches them to relax certain muscles. Other biofeedback techniques involve stimulating an increase in certain brain waves that are prominent during sleep and in short supply in many insomniacs. But, Dr. Hauri emphasizes, before biofeedback training is tried, "you should know what's wrong, what's missing," as determined by brain wave studies.

Some patients create their own insomnia by learning the habit of not sleeping. They take their worries to bed with them and keep themselves awake. Or they become anxious about an occasional night of insomnia. They start to think of their bedrooms as places of sleeplessness, and this becomes a self-fulfilling prophecy. For such patients, behavioral therapy to recondition them to associate the bedroom with sleep can be very effective. Exercise, relaxation techniques, meditation, and self-hypnosis are often helpful.

Dr. Richard P. Bootzin, a psychologist at Northwestern University in Chicago, has devised an effective reconditioning program. The person is told to go to bed only when tired. If sleep doesn't come within ten minutes or so, the person is to get up, leave the bedroom, and do something else until sleep again seems imminent. This process is repeated — all night long if necessary — and even if the person has slept little or not at all, he or she must get up in the morning at a preset time. Naps during the day are forbidden. Eventually, in three or four weeks, the vast majority of people with this problem finally learn to associate their bedrooms with sleep and overcome their insomnia.

Dr. Hauri has found that most insomniacs stay in bed too long. Thinking it will take a long time for them to fall asleep, they go to bed hours before they're really ready to sleep.

Beware of Alcohol and Drugs

Alcohol is a mixed blessing as a sleep inducer. While it helps some people relax, sleep after drinking is "shallow with many awakenings," Dr. Hauri says. A far better remedy, his studies show, is aspirin, possibly because it enhances the passage of tryptophan into the brain. Dr. Hauri also believes a chronic insomniac should have a few sleeping pills in the house to take no more often than once or twice a week. "Just knowing that the pill is there and can be taken if sleep eludes him for several nights in a row helps to relieve the panic associated with not sleeping night after night."

In any case, experts agree, an automatic prescription of a sleeping pill to the millions of Americans who complain of insomnia is highly inappropriate, often self-defeating, and sometimes even dangerous therapy. Furthermore, the vast majority of sleep-inducing drugs lose their effectiveness within two weeks. Only one, flurazepam, marketed under the trade name Dalmane, remained effective for four weeks in a study of ten patients with severe insomnia. Barbiturates can produce a tolerance, which means that increasingly larger doses may be needed to induce sleep. Eventually, the sleep-inducing dose may match the lethal dose, especially if the patient also consumes alcohol.

For Further Reading and Assistance

If your physician is unable to diagnose the cause of your insomnia or treat it effectively, you may benefit from referral to a sleep disorder clinic. The address of the nearest clinic can be obtained by writing to the American Association of Sleep Disorders Centers, Sleep Disorders Program, State University of New York at Stony Brook, Health Sciences Center, Stony Brook, New York 11794.

Many books have been written about insomnia and other sleep problems. Good ones include the following:

Goldberg, Philip, and Daniel Kaufman. *Natural Sleep (How to Get Your Share).* Emmaus, Pa.: Rodale Press, 1978.

Hales, Dianne. *The Complete Book of Sleep.* Reading, Mass.: Addison-Wesley, 1981.

Hartmann, Ernest, M.D. *The Sleeping Pill.* New Haven: Yale University Press, 1978.

Langen, Dr. Dietrich. *Speaking of: Sleeping Problems.* The Medical Adviser Series. New York: Delair/Consolidated, 1978.

Maxmen, Jerrold S., M.D. *A Good Night's Sleep.* New York: W.W. Norton, 1981.

Trubo, Richard. *How to Get a Good Night's Sleep.* Boston: Little, Brown, 1978.

561

Varicose Veins: A Disease of Affluence

Animals that walk on four legs don't get varicose veins, but people do. The upright human posture places great demands on the vessels that must transport blood against the pull of gravity back to the heart, sometimes over a distance of nearly five feet.

Nonetheless, varicose veins are not an inevitable consequence of standing upright. In fact, they are uncommon among people living in developing countries. But many factors in our society can make the task of the veins especially difficult, among them tall stature, lack of exercise, excess weight, confining clothing, sitting in chairs, and a diet of highly refined foods. The net result is that approximately one in five American women and one in fifteen men have veins in their legs that are stretched and swollen. Actually more men may have them than statistics indicate, but men are much less likely than women to notice bulging veins unless they cause discomfort.

In most people, varicose veins are only a cosmetic problem, resulting in unsightly bluish, bulging lines down the legs. However, millions do suffer, typically with a feeling of heaviness, aching, and fatigue in the legs, especially at the end of the day or if they've been standing a lot. The ankles may swell, and pain may extend down the leg along the vein.

Sometimes scaly, itchy skin develops over the affected area. Night leg cramps, leg ulcers, phlebitis (inflamed veins), and clots may also result.

Why Varicosities Develop

Unlike arteries, which have thick muscular walls, veins are relatively thin. Their job is to carry "used" blood back to the heart, which sends it on to the lungs to be reoxygenated. The blood must go in one direction only, and to assure this, the veins are lined with one-way valves that normally prevent backflow. As pressure builds up behind each valve, it opens, lets the blood through, then closes again.

In most parts of the body this occurs millions of times throughout life with no problem. In the legs, and sometimes in the arms, the process may be disrupted. Pressure on the leg veins may interfere with the normal flow and cause the veins to become stretched. The valves then fail to close properly, allowing the blood to seep back and form pools that stretch the veins even farther. Varicosities most commonly develop in the outer veins that run down the leg just under the skin.

Although experts still are not agreed on the precise causes of varicose veins, the following facts are important clues:

• Varicose veins run in families. Some people may inherit a weakness in the vein walls or valves or a reduced number of valves. In others the familial pattern may reflect common environmental causes, such as obesity or diet.

• Female hormones, especially those released during pregnancy, play a role in producing noticeable varicose veins in susceptible women. Varicosities that develop during pregnancy often recede after delivery. Varicose veins often appear in the first months of pregnancy, suggesting that the weight of the fetus is less a factor than the hormones. However, pregnancy in and of itself appears not to cause varicose veins. As Dr. Denis Burkitt, the renowned British surgeon, points out in his book *Eat Right* (New York: Arco Publishing, 1979), in developing countries, where the birthrate is very high, varicose veins are far less common than in Western countries, where the women have many fewer pregnancies.

• Several physicians, Dr. Burkitt among them, have noted that varicose veins are rare among people who live on high-fiber diets, but very common in Western countries where the diet is low in roughage. Dr. Burkitt explains that the hard stools that result from a low-fiber diet and the straining applied to excrete them put enormous pressure on the leg veins. Prolonged sitting on the toilet, which cuts off circulation along the back of the legs, further intensifies the problem.

• Varicose veins are aggravated by standing or sitting in one place for too long. The muscles in the calves act as an auxiliary heart; when the legs are in motion, the muscles contract, helping to pump blood in the large veins deep in the leg up toward the heart. This creates a negative pressure in the veins in the outer reaches of the body, allowing them to deliver their blood to the main route. The process is similar to what happens when a highway traffic jam clears; cars from side roads are then able to feed in.

● Constriction or compression of the legs by tight knee-high boots, garters, girdles, overly tight pantyhose, or crossing the legs while sitting can aggravate varicose veins, notes Dr. Howard C. Baron, a surgeon at New York University College of Medicine.

How to Prevent Them

To reduce the chances of developing serious varicosities, then, it would seem wise to eat lots of fiber (found in fruits, vegetables, whole grains, and beans); keep your weight down; stop reading on the toilet; get adequate leg exercise through walking, jogging, cycling, or swimming; move about often on long trips; avoid standing still (Dr. Baron suggests wriggling your toes frequently and periodically rising up on your toes if you are stuck in one spot for long); wear elastic support stockings throughout pregnancy and support hose at other times if you must stand a lot; do not wear binding garments around the groin or below; keep your legs uncrossed, and put your feet up whenever possible.

Treatments: From Stockings to Surgery

The first line of treatment for uncomplicated varicose veins should be elastic stockings, to the knee or above, which act like muscles to aid blood flow through the veins. If these do not bring adequate relief, surgery to tie off and remove the offending veins is recommended. This usually involves two or three days in the hospital and two weeks to recover, although some surgeons do the procedure without overnight hospitalization. Once the damaged veins are removed, other healthy ones take over their job without harm to normal circulation.

Another treatment approach, popular in Britain and increasingly so

563

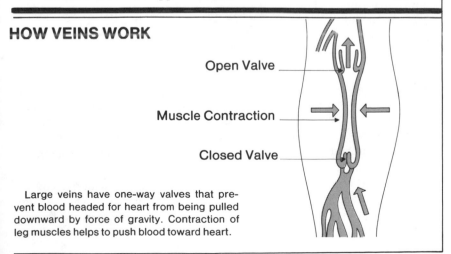

HOW VEINS WORK

Open Valve

Muscle Contraction

Closed Valve

Large veins have one-way valves that prevent blood headed for heart from being pulled downward by force of gravity. Contraction of leg muscles helps to push blood toward heart.

here, involves injecting a chemical into the veins to close them off. With the injection methods currently used, complications rarely occur, and for small and moderate-sized uncomplicated varicose veins, results are as good as those following surgery. Patients can continue with their normal activities while injection therapy is in progress. The injection technique is commonly used to get rid of cosmetically objectionable but medically insignificant spider veins, those sunburstlike patches of tiny surface veins.

For Further Reading

Baron, Dr. Howard C. *Varicose Veins.* New York: William Morrow, 1979.

Lice and Mites: Afflictions of Rich and Poor

Robert Burns was aghast at seeing a louse "On a Lady's Bonnet at Church":

564

> *Ye ugly, creepan, blastet wonner,*
> *Detested, shunn'd, by saunt an' sinner,*
> *How daur ye set your fit upon her,*
> *Sae fine a Lady!*
> *Gae somewhere else and seek your dinner,*
> *On some poor body.*

As the poet Burns so aptly noted, lice and mites are not confined to the poor and unkempt but also readily invade the well groomed and well-to-do. Each year well over 3 million Americans are invaded by these people-loving parasites, which are spread by direct body contact with infested persons or with contaminated articles of clothing, toiletries, bedding, or furniture. The recent upsurge in victims (ten years ago scabies was practically nonexistent, and only a few hundred thousand Americans contracted lice) has been variously attributed to communal living, sexual permissiveness, longer hairstyles, and lapses in personal hygiene.

While ordinarily not dangerous (diseases spread by body lice do not occur naturally in the United States), infestations by lice and mites can result in secondary infections if scratched hard and long enough, and severe infestations can produce lethargy, swollen glands, headache, and fever. Although some people infested with lice have no symptoms, most experience itching of varying intensity caused by the irritating excrement of the organisms.

To prevent infestations, avoid borrowing or lending combs, brushes, or hats or using towels or bed linens used by others. And, as one lice expert put it, "maintain good hygiene and have commerce with people of like taste." Since it takes awhile for a louse to become attached or a mite to burrow, prompt bathing after possible exposure can also help.

The Culprits

Understanding how lice and mites live — and die — can help you protect yourself and your family against infestations and promptly cure those that may occur. A description of the most common parasites in this country follows. All these organisms need to spend some time on humans to complete their life cycle; they live only a short time away from their two-legged hosts.

Head lice (*Pediculus humanus capitis*). The adult head louse is a mere two to three millimeters long and has a preference for the hair behind the ears and at the back of the head. The adults are few in number and hard to see, especially because they usually assume the color of the host's hair. They move about and occasionally wander to the beard and eyebrows.

During her thirty-day life-span the adult female lays 50 to 150 eggs, cementing each to a hair shaft near the scalp. The eggs, or nits, are whitish and transparent, more firmly attached than dandruff and easily seen with an ordinary magnifying lens.

Although head lice neither jump nor fly, they can crawl very quickly and pass easily from one child to another with a single scratch of the head or a friendly tussle. They can also be transmitted via a borrowed comb or brush; by a hat, hood, headband, or ribbon; by a loose strand of hair that harbors a nit; by exposure to contaminated furniture or car seat; or even by standing near an infested person combing his or her hair.

Poor personal hygiene is *not* a necessary condition for infestation, although frequent shampooing with hot water may help to squelch it (the creatures don't like to be hot). Children are the most frequent victims, and epidemics of head lice frequently force school closings.

Many parents react to the discovery of head lice on their well-cared-for offspring with disgust and shame, keeping the matter to themselves and thereby encouraging the spread of this annoying scourge. You may clear up the case or cases at home and fanatically clean everything in the house that might be contaminated, only to have your child become reinfested through contact with another louse-ridden child. Since an in-

HEAD LOUSE

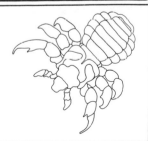

Magnified 200 times.

festation can go undetected for weeks or longer, it's easy for the tiny insects to spread from head to head before anyone knows they are about. Once they're detected, however, it's important to uncover all active cases among school acquaintances and friends and get them treated at the same time.

As a general precaution, it's wise to check your child's head carefully for nits, perhaps once every week or two. Other telltale signs are itchy scalp and red, rashlike marks on the scalp. If lice are discovered, inform the school and the parents of your child's friends. Also check others in the household, including adults and baby-sitters.

Body lice (*Pediculus humanus corporis*). This organism, somewhat larger than the head louse, lives permanently next to human skin, usually in the seams of clothing. Its predilection is for the waist, armpit, crotch, neck, and shoulders. An invasion of body lice, nearly always the result of poor personal hygiene, is common among dirty, neglected people, vagrants, and those with inadequate sanitation. The adult female lays several hundred eggs during her month of life, attaching the nits to body hairs and clothing fibers. The bite of the adult leaves a small, red, intensely itchy lesion.

Pubic lice (*Phthirus pubis*). Smaller and squatter than the head and body louse, the pubic louse looks crablike under the microscope (hence the popular designation "crabs"). Its usual habitat is the pubic hairs of men and women, and its usual mode of transmission is sexual contact. But infested clothing, bedding, towels, and, rarely, toilet seats have also been implicated as sources of crabs. The adult pubic louse is sedentary, but vigorous toweling may move it to other parts of the body, such as the armpit or chest hairs. Children may get crabs on their eyelashes, resulting in an inflamed crusting of the lids.

Adult pubic lice, few in number and difficult to see, may look like rust-colored specks after their meal of human blood; the whitish, oval nits, visible with a hand lens, are hard to remove from the hairs they are attached to.

Scabies (*Sarcoptes scabiei hominis*). This tiny mite — a mere third of a millimeter long — has felled armies, among them Napoleon's troops who laid down their arms to scratch until they bled. Scabies is spread by intimate contact with an infested person, bedding, towels, or clothing. The female itch mite burrows under the skin, usually between the fingers, on the backs of the hands, elbows, armpits, groin, breasts, navel, buttocks, or small of the back. There she lays her eggs, and the larvae that hatch may make burrows of their own. The irritating excrement of the mite causes blistering of the skin and intense itching.

What To Do for Infestations

A suspected attack of lice or mites should be promptly seen by a physician and vigorously treated. Other people who may have been exposed, including all family members, should also be examined and possibly treated as a preventive. Don't be so embarrassed that you and your family suffer needlessly. Lice can happen to anyone, even the doctor. If you are certain of the diagnosis, you can treat infestations on your own.

Treatment of lice and mites is simple. One application of a lotion, cream, or shampoo containing the insecticide gamma-benzene hexachloride (lindane, sold under the trade name Kwell and available only by doctor's prescription) or of pyrethrins with piperonyl butoxide (A-200 Pyrinate and others, available over the counter), is usually adequate. For heavy infestations, a second application is recommended twenty-four hours or a week later. If desired, the nits can be removed with a fine-tooth comb, but once they've been properly treated with insecticide, they are dead and cannot start a new invasion.

It's important not to exceed recommended doses of Kwell (lindane) because it can be absorbed through the skin and may produce convulsions if too much is left on for too long. Consumers Union, raising questions of possible hazard, has asked the Food and Drug Administration to review the safety of lindane.

To avoid reinfection, anyone who has intimate contact with an infested person should be treated simultaneously, and all possibly contaminated clothing, bedding, and towels should be dry-cleaned or machine-washed in very hot water and ironed or dried in a hot dryer. Upholstered furniture and car seats should be thoroughly vacuumed. Disinfect combs and brushes by washing them with the insecticide shampoo. You might also use an antilice insecticide spray on furniture that cannot be washed or dry-cleaned. But the value of such sprays has not been clearly established.

Acne:
A Psychosocial Disease

Acne is a problem that more teenagers have in common than probably anything else, yet each one tends to think of himself or herself as a specially afflicted victim, alone in his or her ugliness. Teenagers commonly share their trials and tribulations over schoolwork, girlfriends and boyfriends, parents and teachers, but rarely do they commiserate with one another on the agonies of acne.

Yet if they did discuss this "unmentionable" affliction, they might find that the comfort, support, empathy, and sympathy of their friends would go a long way to relieve their emotional discomfort, improve their self-images, and help to dispel the many widely believed myths about the causes and treatment of acne.

At least four out of five teenagers have acne. It is so common, in fact, that many doctors consider it a "normal" feature of adolescent development. Acne may be a problem for only a year or two or, more commonly, for ten or twenty years, into the early twenties. Rare cases continue throughout most of adult life.

Since it is so common and results in no serious physical illness, some doctors — and parents — fail to take acne seriously. But it is a condition that needs prompt, sympathetic medical care to prevent permanent scarring of the skin and the psyche. Acne can turn a happy, sociable child into a miserable, lonely, outcast adolescent and aggravate tensions between parent and child.

Many of these tensions stem from misunderstandings about what acne is and what the sufferer can and should do about its causes. Parents may blame their children for having acne, charging that it is due to the fact that they sleep too much, sleep too little, eat nothing but junk food, don't eat enough, eat too much, don't bathe often enough, bathe too often, are too interested in the opposite sex, don't take an interest in dating. The truth is, acne has nothing to do with any of these situations.

However, heredity has a lot to do with acne, and it would be far more accurate for children to "blame" their parents for an acne problem.

The Real Causes of Acne

Acne results from the effects of androgens — the male sex hormones — produced in increased amounts by both males and females (in the testes, ovaries, and adrenal glands) when puberty begins. Androgens stimulate the sebaceous (oil) glands of the hair follicles. These glands are largest and most numerous on the face, upper parts of the chest and back, and shoulders — just where acne is most likely to develop.

In response to androgens, the sebaceous glands produce a fatty substance called sebum, which travels to the opening of the hair follicle and produces oily skin. In acne, this passageway becomes plugged with sebum mixed with scales from the follicle walls and sometimes bacteria and other microorganisms that can grow in the "fatty soup."

The blackheads of mild acne form when sebum becomes oxidized and mixed with skin pigments in the plugged pores. Blackheads are not caused by either dirt or bacteria. Sometimes the follicle becomes so stuffed with sebum and scales that it closes off, forming a whitehead at the skin surface. In the more severe forms of acne, as pressure builds in the sealed-off follicle, some of the "gunk" may leak into the surrounding skin layers, bacteria may invade the wound, and the result is a painful boil. If such lesions are untreated, some may leave permanent scars.

Careful studies have shown that counter to widespread beliefs, such teenage dietary favorites as chocolate, nuts, cola, pizza, potato chips, and shellfish do not cause acne. However, about 1 in 100 acne sufferers finds that a particular food seems to make his or her acne worse and is best not consumed. Acne may also be worsened by emotional stress and by hot, humid weather (warm, dry sunshine or sun lamps can help combat acne). Many girls find that their acne flares up before, during, or just after their menstrual period.

How to Treat Acne

While acne is not caused by dirt, poor hygiene — failure to keep the skin clear of oil and the pores open — can certainly aggravate it. In fact, the main treatment for acne — and often the only one necessary for less severe cases — is good hygiene: keeping greasy hair off the face, thoroughly cleaning the face with soap two or three times a day, and shampooing the hair twice a week. No special soap is necessary. Since the bacteria in acne pustules are below the skin surface, antibacterial soaps have little, if any, effect on them.

The goal in cleansing is to keep the skin dry and tight, but not so dry that it becomes red, abraded, and sore. Between thorough washings, alcohol swabs or acne wipettes can be used to remove excess oil from the face. Oil-based makeup should not be used, but numerous over-the-counter acne lotions, creams, and makeup can help to dry the skin and partially conceal blemishes. Different ones seem to help different people.

According to an expert panel convened by the Food and Drug Ad-

ACNE BLEMISHES

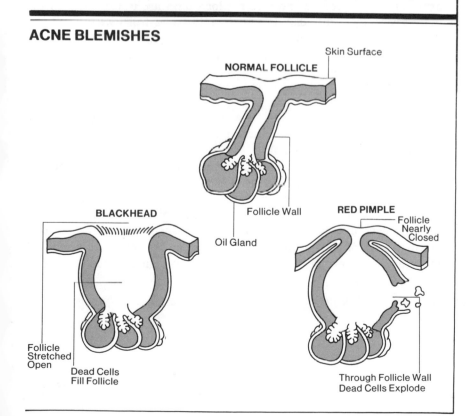

ministration and an independent evaluation by Consumers Union, the most effective over-the-counter acne products contain benzoyl peroxide, which helps to prevent the formation of new acne lesions. The most effective products are in gel form. Sulfur medications help to heal existing lesions but do not prevent the formation of new ones. But alcohol cleansers and medicated soaps are no improvement over ordinary soap.

For those not adequately helped by such conservative measures, the family physician or a dermatologist can frequently provide relief through prescriptions for peeling agents, vitamin A acid (resorcinol) cream, and antibiotics applied to the skin or taken by mouth.

Antibiotics do not cure acne, but combined with good hygiene, they can go a long way to control the development of inflamed pus-filled lesions. Oral antibiotics — particularly tetracycline — have been used to treat acne ever since their introduction to medicine. Treatment may continue for months or years. The antibiotic is usually started at its normal full dose for about three weeks and gradually reduced to a maintenance level of a quarter dose. Periodically the drug should be discontinued for several weeks to see if the acne has cleared up on its own.

An expert committee of the American Academy of Dermatology has reviewed the best available studies, concluding that tetracycline drugs are both effective and safe for long-term use in treatment of the more severe forms of acne. Fewer than 10 percent of patients had unwanted side effects (the most common was a vaginal infection called candidiasis), and those that occurred were usually minor and short-lived.

An improvement over antibiotic therapy for severe cases of acne may be the oral drug 13-cis-retinoic acid, a cousin to vitamin A (which itself is too toxic to be taken in large doses). Responses to treatment, which should be administered by a dermatologist, have been dramatic and complete or nearly so, with acne remaining suppressed even after the therapy has been discontinued.

To prevent scarring as an aftermath of acne, do not squeeze or pick at pimples and blackheads. Blackheads can and should be removed with a specially designed extractor by a physician or trained family member. In the worst cases of cystic acne, the dermatologist may repeatedly have to lance each cyst to prevent scarring. The unsightliness of scars that occur in spite of such preventive measures can be significantly reduced by dermabrasion (professional skin planing) once the acne has subsided.

For Further Reading

Flandermeyer, Kenneth L., M.D. *Clear Skin.* Boston: Little, Brown, 1979.

Hair Loss:
What Can and Can't Be Done

Baldness undoubtedly contributed to the success of actors Yul Brynner and Telly Savalas and the high-fashion model Pat Evans. But somehow the glamour of their gleaming pates hasn't caught on with the average man or woman. While many are content merely to lament the gradual loss of their straight or curly locks, others squander millions of hard-earned dollars in a frantic and fruitless search for ways to halt the inexorable passing of hair follicles.

Short of castration, there is currently no safe and effective way to prevent or cure the most common kind of baldness that afflicts humankind. It is programmed by the genes and triggered by hormones that few would part with. No lotion or drug, no amount of massaging, oiling, brushing, or washing, no vitamins or minerals or protein supplements can halt or reverse the loss of hair as we get older.

But there are now various ways to camouflage hereditary baldness as well as to prevent or correct other causes of hair loss. You *can* avoid unnecessary damage to your hair, and you *should* avoid unscrupulous "hair specialists" (trichologists) who may promise you a Samson mane but succeed only in emptying your pocket.

Hair and Its Growth

Normal hair growth depends on certain vitamins and minerals and adequate protein in the diet. But this does not mean that extra amounts beyond the normal daily requirements of these nutrients can halt or reverse hair loss.

A healthy head of hair holds some 100,000 to 150,000 individual hairs. It also loses, on the average, 30 to 60 hairs a day. On some days only a few hairs may be lost, but then on others 100 or more may fall out. This is perfectly normal. You would have to lose as many as 40 percent of your hairs before the thinning would be evident.

A normal hair goes through a typical life cycle. For two to six years it grows out of its follicle at a rate of about half an inch a month. Then the hair enters a resting stage, lasting about three months, during which it stops growing and starts separating from its root. Ordinarily at any one time 15 percent of your hairs are in the resting stage.

The scalp end of the resting hair becomes club-shaped, and it is easily dislodged. Although washing, brushing, or combing may seem to cause many to fall out, such hair loss occurs at most a few days sooner than it would had you done nothing to your hair. After a varying interval a new hair will grow out of the follicle to replace the one that was lost.

After the mid-twenties, virtually everyone's hairline starts receding, and the hair begins to thin. The growth rate of some follicles shortens, and after a while these aging follicles revert to producing the tiny, fuzzy hairs typical of prenatal life. Despite claims to the contrary, these deceased follicles cannot be rejuvenated.

Follicular senescence results from the effects of androgens, the sex hormone abundant in men and present in smaller amounts in women. High doses of the female sex hormone estrogen could counter this effect in men, but the hormone has undesirable and sometimes dangerous side effects. In women, hormone treatments seem to have no significant effect on hair loss.

How much of your hair will stop growing and your pattern of loss are determined by your genetic background. Both your mother's and your father's sides of the family contribute equally to your baldness tendencies. The condition, called male (or female) pattern baldness, is a common one. Cosmetically significant hair loss occurs in 12 percent of men aged twenty-five; 37 percent of those aged thirty-five; 45 percent of those aged forty-five, and 65 percent of those aged sixty-five. In women, actual baldness is uncommon, but with increasing age significant thinning of the crown hairs occurs in many, often starting after menopause.

Common Causes of Hair Loss

Aside from male (or female) pattern baldness, there are other causes of hair loss, most of them reversible. One is a condition called alopecia areata, which produces patchy hair loss at any age and occasionally affects the whole head. It usually reverses with time or sometimes responds to cortisone treatments.

Other factors that may cause hair loss (usually reversible when the cause is eliminated) include:

● Permanent waving, straightening, or excessive bleaching. These procedures may damage the hair shaft and result in breakage of the hair near the scalp. Permanents should not be done on already damaged (overly bleached or brittle) hair, and in using home permanents, be sure to read and follow the directions carefully. Avoid the use of hot combs to straighten hair.

● Tight hairstyles. Ponytails, pigtails, and tight buns pull on hairs in the front of the scalp. The tension damages the follicles, and the hairs may fall out.

● Rollers and clips. To prevent damage, use foam-rubber rather than brush rollers, winding the hair tightly around the roller but loosely between the roller and the scalp. Use bobby pins with rubber tips.

● Heat. High heat softens hair, so use your dryer on medium heat, and don't overmanipulate your hair when it is hot. Hold the dryer six inches or more from your hair, and keep it moving. Be sure the dryer has the Underwriters Laboratories (UL) seal, which means it should shut off automatically if it exceeds a certain temperature. Don't use electric curlers more than a couple of times a week.

● Vigorous toweling or brushing and teasing (back-combing). Pat, rather than rub, your hair dry to avoid tangling and breakage. Use a soft, natural-bristle brush (nylon bristles have rough ends), and don't brush excessively — no 100 strokes a day. Teasing can also cause tangling and breakage. If your hair gets tangled, brush it first at the ends, and gradually move toward the scalp. Wet hair is best groomed with a wide-toothed comb rather than a brush.

● Pregnancy and oral contraceptives. During pregnancy and the pseudopregnancy associated with the pill, fewer hairs enter the resting stage. After childbirth or after the pill is stopped, however, the hairs make up for lost time, and a lot of hair may be lost at one time.

● Illness, injury, and drugs. Reversible hair loss can result from high fevers, inflammatory skin disorders, sudden and extensive weight loss, severe anemia, intestinal disorders, X ray therapy of the head, general anesthesia, and certain drugs, among them cortisone, blood thinners, amphetamines, antithyroid and anticancer drugs. Burns and lacerations of the scalp may damage hair follicles.

It also helps to know what hair loss is not caused by. It is not the result of ordinary dandruff or too frequent shampooing, unless you use soap or such a strong shampoo that your hair becomes overly dry and tangles easily. Contrary to the claims of some trichologists (hair specialists), baldness is not caused by bacteria or by a loss of circulation in the scalp. Even pulling out hairs will not stop healthy follicles from producing new ones.

What to Do About Thinning Hair

If your hair is thin, there are several things you can do to make it

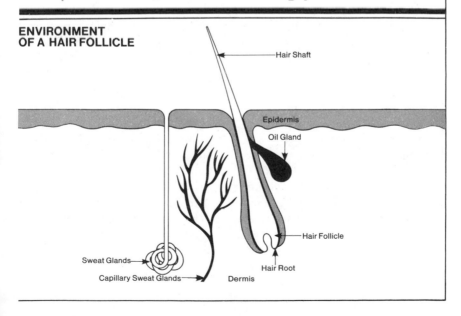

ENVIRONMENT
OF A HAIR FOLLICLE

Hair Shaft

Epidermis

Oil Gland

Hair Follicle

Sweat Glands

Capillary Sweat Glands

Hair Root

Dermis

look fuller. The market is glutted with products that can condition your hair and give it more body. As with beer and egg shampoos, protein conditioners coat the hair shafts and make the hairs appear thicker. Conditioners and cream rinses also reduce tangling and thus help to prevent breakage. These are only temporary measures that wash out with your next shampoo. Since hair is dead tissue, there is nothing you can put on your hair to "feed" it permanently.

Proper styling can make a big difference to someone with thin hair. A layered cut can make your hair look thicker, and short thin hair looks more substantial than long thin hair. Cutting does not make your hair grow faster, but it can get rid of split and straggly ends that make your hair less attractive.

For the more obvious problems of a receding hairline or actual bald spots, there are a number of alternatives once you can no longer attractively style your hair to cover the empty places. Some of the alternatives are less desirable medically and socially than others, so you should have a clear idea of what's involved before you make your choice.

Hairpiece or wig. Aside from doing nothing, filling in for nature with a manufactured substitute of natural or synthetic hair has long been the most popular and least traumatic approach to baldness. There are many kinds of hairpieces, and they range in price from about $15 to more than $600 each.

Those made of real hair cost more to start with and must be redyed every six months or so. Those mounted on a plastic hard top hold their shape longer, but they don't "breathe" well and can be uncomfortable in hot weather. Other hairpieces have a soft mat that is more comfortable, and some have a mesh in front that helps to create a more natural-looking hairline.

The biggest disadvantage of hairpieces is their impermanence and the possibility that they will flip off at embarrassing moments. However, it is possible to purchase ones that can be worn when swimming or showering — even scuba diving. If a quality product is purchased from a responsible purveyor of hairpieces, you should be able to wear it twenty-four hours a day.

If you wear a hairpiece, you will probably eventually want to have at least two — one to wear while the other is being cleaned and styled. Before you buy a hairpiece, shop around and compare prices, quality, and service. Ask your friends for recommendations, and call the Better Business Bureau to check out the establishments.

Hair weaving. This is a process of braiding your remaining hairs to create an anchor for a hairpiece to keep it from falling off. There are several disadvantages to weaving. The tight braids create tension on your hairs and may cause what little hair you have left to start falling out. As your hair grows, the braids move away from your scalp, and the hairpiece moves with them, necessitating a retightening every month or two.

It is also very difficult to clean properly under the hairpiece, especially around the braids.

The initial weave costs several hundred dollars, and the retightening may run around $35 a visit. If you are considering a hair weave, first check out the agency with the Better Business Bureau. You might also ask to talk with other customers.

Hair implants. This involves stitches or wire anchors implanted in the scalp to hold a hairpiece or tufts of hair. The body often tolerates these anchors poorly, and they may cause redness, soreness, and infection. An unpleasant odor may develop. Some people have continual discomfort from implants; others experience pain only when the hair is gently tugged, such as when turning in bed. Also, the stitches tend to pull out in a year or so.

Implants of synthetic fiber are a disaster, causing severe scalp swelling, infection, and pain. Nearly all the implanted fibers fall out within ten weeks.

Hair transplants. According to Dr. Herbert S. Feinberg, a New Jersey dermatologist who specializes in hair transplants, about a million people have had healthy hair follicles transplanted from one part of the scalp to another. It is usually done in a doctor's office under a local anesthetic. Tiny plugs of scalp, each containing ten to fifteen active hair follicles, are removed with a punch, and similar plugs of bald scalp are removed.

The hair-containing plugs are then properly aligned and inserted in the holes, with clotting blood acting as the natural sealer. There is little or no pain afterward. Between 10 and 40 plugs can be safely transplanted at one time. Since 100 to 200 plugs are usually needed for a good cosmetic result, several sessions a month or more apart are needed to complete the process.

It takes two to six months for new hairs to grow from the transplanted plugs. Nine months to a year after transplantation you can expect to see the final result. The part of the scalp that donated the plugs for transplantation will never again grow hair, but if the donor plugs were properly selected, surrounding hairs should cover the area adequately.

Hair transplants are not suitable for everyone with hair loss. The doctor must be able to tell which part of the scalp will not become bald so that a good site for donor plugs can be chosen since the transplanted follicles will follow their original genetic destiny regardless of where they are put. Enough hair should have been lost to make the procedure worthwhile. The hair in the donor area should not be too thin, and the person should not have unrealistic ideas of what a transplant will do for him or her. People in poor health or those who scar abnormally should not have hair transplants.

Transplants are commonly priced by the plug, ranging from about

$7.50 to as high as $35 a plug. Thus, a complete transplant could easily cost between $1,000 and $3,000. The main advantages of a hair transplant are that the person has his or her own hair that lasts a lifetime, and the costs are one-time.

It is very important that the procedure be done by a physician expert in the technique. Beware of bargain clinics and doctors who recommend transplanting flaps or strips of scalp. This technique is subject to complications and has a high failure rate. Ask the local medical society or a reputable dermatologist to recommend a qualified doctor. Be sure to see before-and-after pictures of the doctor's patients, if not the patients themselves.

For Further Reading

Feinberg, Herbert S., M.D. *All About Hair.* Alpine, N.J.: Wallingford Press, 1978.
Schoen, Linda Allen, in consultation with the American Medical Association's Committee on Cutaneous Health and Cosmetics. *The AMA Book of Skin and Hair Care.* Philadelphia: Lippincott, 1976.

Mononucleosis: A Great Masquerader

A high school basketball player developed a severe sore throat, swollen glands, and a bad headache. A college student had a rash all over her body, swollen lymph nodes under her arms, and a low-grade fever. A businessman was bothered by a recurrent sore throat and became so fatigued that he could hardly do his work, let alone play squash at lunch or go out in the evening. A young mother developed severe abdominal pain and was too exhausted to keep up with her housework and two children.

Although their symptoms varied, tests showed that all had infectious mononucleosis, a pesky, debilitating virus infection better known as mono or glandular fever. Each had symptoms that could easily have been confused with some other disease, such as strep throat, German measles, gallbladder disease, or even leukemia. For mono is a great masquerader, and the symptoms of many victims mimic those of more or less serious diseases. Because the infection involves nearly every organ of the body, the symptoms tend to be varied and confusing.

Yet if the doctor recognizes the possibility of mono and does a quick, simple blood test, in most cases the correct diagnosis can be made readily and the patient spared many more costly, hazardous tests and inappropriate treatment.

Symptoms and Consequences

The classic symptoms of mono include sore throat, enlarged lymph nodes around the neck, fever, puffy eyes, headache, and extreme fatigue.

Victims sometimes walk around with vague complaints and marked, unexplained fatigue for weeks before becoming sick enough to seek medical attention.

Mono is most commonly diagnosed in teenagers and young adults. However, recent studies indicate that most people actually become infected by the mono virus during childhood. A study of West Point cadets, for example, showed that more than two-thirds already had antibodies to the causative virus by the time they entered college, indicating that they had been infected sometime in the past. A single infection seems to confer lifetime immunity.

In most cases in youngsters the infection is mild and short-lived; it usually passes without any specific diagnosis being made, or it is mistaken for a cold, the flu, or an ordinary viral sore throat. The disease is more serious in older people, and in adults the symptoms are likely to be varied and bizarre, such as abdominal pain or a strange type of pneumonia. On college campuses mononucleosis seems to peak during fall and early spring, but experts say it is really a year-round phenomenon that attracts greater attention when it interferes with exams and project deadlines.

As infectious diseases go, mono is not very contagious and victims do not have to be isolated. The virus can be found in the throats and saliva of patients and is most commonly spread by mouth-to-mouth contact. Although sometimes jokingly referred to as the kissing disease, after its reputed mode of transmission, mono — its victims will tell you — is no laughing matter. Its debilitating effects can hang on for months, sometimes for as long as a year or more, and keep the sufferer from fully resuming his or her normal activities. Some students are forced to drop out of school temporarily.

Mono can also lead to serious complications, including bacterial infections of the throat, diphtheria, liver inflammation and jaundice, and, less commonly, rupture of the spleen (a potentially fatal complication), meningitis, encephalitis, inflammation of the heart, severe anemia, and respiratory problems.

The Epstein-Barr (EB) virus, which was shown a decade ago to cause mono, stimulates the infection-fighting white blood cells — called lymphocytes — to increase in number and become greatly enlarged and less able to fight off other infections. Although some have referred to mono as a self-limited leukemia, there is no evidence that it can develop into cancer. However, about 90 percent of patients show abnormalities on liver function tests, and one in ten develops jaundice.

Diagnosis and Treatment

Mono is diagnosed by a blood test that can be completed in a few hours in a doctor's office or commercial laboratory. The test detects the presence of an antibody peculiar to mono that can clump horse red blood cells. If the doctor is uncertain of the diagnosis, a more complicated test for EB virus antibody can be done.

There is no specific treatment to kill off the mono virus. The key to a rapid recovery is rest — bed rest for a week or two during the more severe phase of fever and extreme fatigue, followed by restricted activity until all the symptoms disappear.

"Your body will tell you very well what you can do," says Dr. Richard H. Meade, chief of pediatric infectious diseases at Boston Floating Hospital. "Pay attention to what your body tells you," he advises mono victims. "When you feel able to do something, there's no harm in it."

But, the expert adds, "There *is* harm in doing what you feel compelled to do even though you're really not up to it." Those who overdo before they are well enough may experience a recurrence of symptoms that lands them back in bed. One sixteen-year-old developed a sore throat whenever she became fatigued for a year after she had recovered from the acute phase of mono.

Other aspects of therapy include aspirin, salt-water gargles, and drinking lots of fluids. Hospitalization is usually not necessary unless the patient develops serious jaundice or difficulty in swallowing or breathing. Antibiotics are useful only if a secondary bacterial infection develops, and ampicillin should not be used in mono patients because it can cause a bad toxic rash.

If the spleen is enlarged, Dr. Paul G. Quie, professor of pediatrics at the University of Minnesota, rules out all sports that may involve bodily contact, such as football and basketball, because of the danger of rupturing the spleen.

In selected cases, some doctors prescribe steroids — prednisone — to relieve symptoms. However, Dr. Meade emphasizes that since the steroids themselves can produce serious reactions, they should be reserved only for those cases in which it is vital for the patient to be able to function well for a few days, such as to get through final exams.

Jet Lag:
Readjusting Body Rhythms

A half century ago, when jet travel was not even an aviator's dream, Wiley Post, who piloted his monoplane around the world in eight days, had already discovered what we now call jet lag. Mr. Post recognized the disruption of body rhythms caused by rapidly changing time zones and worked out a program to counter the deleterious effects of altered sleep-wake cycles on flying efficiency.

Nowadays every year tens of millions of people — most of them passengers rather than pilots — cross four or more time zones in a matter of hours. Watches are easily reset to local time, but bodies tend to lag behind. For days, multitime-zone travelers are likely to find themselves getting hungry and sleepy at the wrong times.

A Hundred Rhythms Disrupted

While virtually all travelers are aware of the effects on sleeping and eating patterns, few may realize that in abruptly changing multiple time zones, they throw more than 100 different bodily functions out of whack. Normal rhythms for a host of biological activities are no longer in synchrony. Included are not only the accustomed times to sleep and eat but also such less obvious cycles as those for body temperature, breathing, heart rate, hormonal output, urine and blood constituents, and the chemical activities of the kidneys, liver, digestive tract, and central nervous system.

The disruption of the body's many internal clocks can detract from the joy of a vacationer and the wits of a negotiating executive as well as the physical prowess of a competing athlete and the expertise of a pilot. It pays, therefore, to know the possible effects of jet lag and how they may be mitigated or at least accommodated.

Studies of people subjected to real and laboratory-created phase shifts, as disruptions of circadian rhythms (or daily body cycles) are called, have revealed that decrements occur in mental alertness, reaction time, short-term memory, grip strength, ability to solve simple mathematical problems, and performance of complex psychomotor tasks (such as piloting a flight simulator). These diminished abilities may last for two or three days after a flight across several time zones.

Biological functions vary in the length of time it takes for them to adapt to a time change of four or more hours. Whereas a person may adjust in a few days to a new sleep-wake and eating cycle, daily rhythms in hormones and body temperature may take a week or longer before all the disrupted rhythmic functions become resynchronized. In general it takes one day to adapt for each time zone crossed.

According to one study, body temperature readjusts in eleven to twelve days after a westerly flight across six time zones, and fourteen to fifteen days after an equally long easterly flight. Reaction time takes six days to return to normal after the westward trip, but nine days after the eastbound return. For reasons not well understood, it seems easier for people to adjust to a flight in a westerly direction, in which the traveler lands at an earlier time than his biological clock says it is, than to flights going east. People have less trouble staying up a few hours later than usual (as would happen going west) than arising a few hours earlier (as occurs after an eastward flight).

There is also a great deal of individual variation in sensitivity to time zone changes. Whereas some people experience little or no disturbances or become quickly resynchronized, others can be severely impaired. The older you get, the more difficult it seems to be to reset your biological clock rapidly.

How to Minimize the Effects

Although there is no way to prevent the disruption of your body rhythms short of flying only directly north or south, studies of jet lag have revealed ways to mitigate the symptoms. They include the following:

● Preadapt your body rhythms to the time zone of your destination. Starting several days before departure, gradually change your eating and sleeping schedule. If you're going to be flying west, go to bed an hour later each day (and sleep later in the morning). If you're flying east, go to bed and arise earlier each day.

● If you're just crossing one or two time zones and will be gone only a few days, keep your watch — and your schedule — on home time.

● For longer trips, be sure you are well rested before starting out. Avoid eating heavy meals or drinking alcoholic beverages just before or during the flight. The combined effects of alcohol and altitude greatly enhance fatigue, and two or three drinks consumed at 5,000 feet (the altitude to which the cabin is pressurized) have the physiological effect of three or four drinks at sea level.

● Similarly, avoid smoking during flight. The accumulation of carbon monoxide in your blood combined with the effects of altitude of 5,000 feet is equivalent to the fatigue from lack of oxygen experienced at 10,000 feet.

● Schedule your flight so that you arrive as close to your regular bedtime as possible. Then go to bed, and try to sleep through to a reasonable waking hour at your destination. If you're flying eastward and will be arriving at midday local time (bedtime on your body's clock), don't schedule any demanding activities or a night on the town for the remainder of that day. Instead, eat a light meal, and go to bed "early."

● If you have trouble falling asleep, take a warm bath, get some exercise (run around the room if need be), or read a boring book. But avoid tranquilizers, sleeping pills, and alcohol. These can further interfere with sleep patterns that are already disrupted.

● If you're traveling on business and must have your wits about you, go a day earlier than necessary. Whether traveling for business or pleasure, if you're going a great distance — say, from New York to Tokyo — schedule a day or two of rest in Honolulu instead of making a direct flight.

Dr. Morton S. Buchsbaum of the National Institute of Mental Health reports that a number of psychiatric drugs may prove useful in countering jet lag, particularly for people like pilots. Included are lithium, which appears to slow the biological clock, and imipramine, which speeds it up. Alcohol also slows the clock, so if you insist on drinking while flying, try to limit it to westbound flights.

For Further Reading

Goeltz, Judith. *Jet Stress: What It Is and How To Cope With It.* Huntington Beach, Calif.: Institute Publishers, 1981.

Traveler's Diarrhea: It Can Happen Anywhere

The name varies, depending on the country of origin. In Mexico travelers know it as *turista*, Montezuma's revenge, and the Aztec two-step. In the Middle East, you'll hear such euphemisms as Gippy tummy, Aden gut, and Basra belly. In North Africa it goes by Casablanca crud; in India, Dehli belly and Poona poohs; and in the Far East, Hong Kong dog and Tokyo trot.

Despite the amusing epithets, traveler's diarrhea is funny only to those who don't have it. As the most common ailment among travelers to other countries, striking a third or more of tourists in some areas, it has ruined or at least taken the edge off many an otherwise exciting trip.

With growing millions of Americans traveling to ever more exotic places, traveler's diarrhea has become an increasingly important health problem. In one study of healthy American students summering in Europe, nearly half had attacks of diarrhea, the attack rate being twice as high for Mediterranean countries as for northern Europe. In another series of studies of American students in Mexico, one-quarter to one-third got *turista* within ten days of their arrival.

Fortunately, as doctors have begun to understand more about the disease, methods have been developed that can help to prevent it or ameliorate its symptoms. The disorder strikes usually within ten days of arrival in a foreign port. In addition to frequent, watery stools, the symptoms may include nausea, vomiting, headache, abdominal cramps, and sometimes fever. They usually last one to three days.

The Causes

After much speculation about causes — ranging from the stress of travel, new climate, strange foods, strong spices, and food poisoning to the chilling effect of cold drinks and irritation of the gut by sand and dust — it now appears that almost all cases are caused by variants of a commonplace bacterium naturally present in virtually everyone's gut. This organism, *Escherichia coli* (*E. coli*, for short), comes in a variety of forms, called serotypes, some of which can produce toxins that are extremely irritating to the unaccustomed bowel. Natives who have been exposed for years to the toxins of the local *E. coli* serotypes probably become immune to their effects, but visitors have no such immunity.

While traveler's diarrhea is most common in tropical and subtropical areas where sanitation and personal hygiene may not be the best, it also occurs quite often among travelers to such relatively "clean" countries as the United States. Mexicans who travel to California are known to suffer from an identical ailment they call San Franciscitis. This probably happens because people from other countries are not accustomed to the particular serotypes that are native to us. They may be exposed to our indigenous organisms through the inevitable occasional slips in personal hygiene, techniques of food preparations, and public sanitation that can and do occur anywhere.

E. coli is not the only cause of diarrheal disease among travelers. Some cases, usually the more severe ones, result from a bacterium called shigella. Sometimes a virus such as those that cause "intestinal flu" back home may be the cause. Food poisoning by the salmonella bacterium is an infrequent cause. The parasite that causes amebic dysentery is an occasional problem, and rarely *Vibrio comma*, the cholera bacterium, is responsible. Among the cases that occur after the return home, an infectious protozoan called *Giardia lamblia* is commonly the culprit.

Diagnosis and Treatment

Whereas "ordinary" traveler's diarrhea caused by *E. coli* is a short, self-limited illness, some of the other causative organisms can produce severe, prolonged symptoms. If the stool contains blood or mucus or the patient develops a fever of over 101 degrees or shaking chills, a physician should be consulted immediately. Symptoms that persist for more than a few days or severe vomiting or diarrhea (more than ten loose bowel movements per day) that can result in dehydration or that occur in infants or persons who are aged or have other illnesses should also be brought to a doctor's attention.

Otherwise, treatment is simple: Don't eat solid foods or drink milk or take drugs (other than what a doctor has prescribed) until the symptoms abate. It's critically important, though, to replace lost fluid and electrolytes (sodium, potassium, and chloride that are dissolved in the body fluids). *Emergency Medicine,* a magazine for physicians, recommends such beverages as orange, apple, or other fruit juice, laced with honey or corn syrup (half a teaspoon in eight ounces of juice) and a pinch of salt, alternated with a glass of bottled carbonated or boiled water to which a quarter teaspoon of baking soda is added. In addition, tea made with boiled water and bottled carbonated beverages may be consumed.

Before leaving home, you can have your pharmacist prepare individual packets of glucose and salts that can be mixed with boiled water to restore body chemicals lost during an attack of diarrhea. Or you can mix your own — one-half teaspoon salt plus one-half teaspoon baking soda and four tablespoons sugar, which should be added to one quart of water that has been boiled for fifteen minutes. In many countries you will be able to purchase an electrolyte replacement solution under the brand name ORS or Oralyte.

Over-the-counter drugs like Kaopectate are of little help, and prescription drugs for diarrhea (Lomotil and others) can prolong the illness if it is caused by bacteria other than *E. coli*. A drug called Entero-Vioform, which may be sold without prescription in some countries, should not be taken; it can cause severe nerve damage.

Preventive Measures

Although there are no guarantees, the chances of getting traveler's diarrhea can be significantly reduced by observing the following precautions:

● Unless you are sure the water is chlorinated, don't drink it or brush your teeth with it — and don't use ice cubes — unless you boil the water first for fifteen minutes. (The water supply is usually safe in large hotels that cater to American tourists.) Only chlorinated water provides real protection against infectious viruses and bacteria that are spread through water, as *E. coli* is, and even chlorination does not kill the parasites that cause giardiasis and amebic dysentery.

● Stick to drinks that are made with boiled water or that come in — and are served in — bottles and cans. (Glasses may have been washed in contaminated water.) And dry the tops of cans before opening them. Bottled carbonated drinks are safe because the carbonation makes the water too acid for bacteria to survive.

● If unchlorinated water is your only choice, sanitize it by adding a 2 percent tincture of iodine to the water (five drops to a quart of clear water, ten drops for cloudy water) or by adding liquid laundry bleach (two drops per quart of clear water, four for cloudy water).

● If the drinking water is not chlorinated, chances are the swimming pool isn't either, and since few bathers can avoid getting pool water in their mouths, it may be best to stay out of the water altogether.

● Avoid uncooked vegetables, fresh fruits that have no peel, and salads. Eat only those vegetables that are cooked and served hot and fruits that you peel before eating.

Recently researchers at Johns Hopkins University showed that an antibiotic called doxycycline, taken once a day, can greatly reduce the risk of traveler's diarrhea. The drug provides 60 to 90 percent protection against the disease and remains effective for about a week after it is stopped. Doxycycline, a tetracycline, is recommended only for those who cannot tolerate even a brief illness. The drug is not recommended for prolonged use (more than a month or so), nor should it be taken by pregnant women or children under eight years old, because it may permanently stain their teeth. It may also cause a skin rash in some people following exposure to sunlight.

According to another study, large doses of Pepto-Bismol, an over-the-counter suspension, taken as one 240-milliliter (about an eight-ounce) bottle per day, can reduce the incidence of traveler's diarrhea by about 60 percent. This medication can also relieve symptoms, should diarrhea develop. However, Pepto-Bismol contains large amounts of an aspirinlike chemical, salicylate, and should not be used by anyone already taking large daily doses of aspirin or other salicylates for arthritis and those taking anticoagulant drugs, the gout medications Benemid or Anturane, or the anticancer drug methotrexate.

Cold Hands and Feet: Victims of Raynaud's Disease

Although often the butt of jokes in and out of the bedroom, cold hands and feet are not funny to millions of people — most of them women — who suffer from a circulatory problem known as Raynaud's disease. When temperatures drop both indoors and out with the arrival of winter weather and energy-saving thermostat settings, the fingers and toes of Raynaud's sufferers often turn white with cold.

For most sufferers the condition, best defined as a hyperreaction to the cold, is an annoyance that doesn't seriously disrupt their lives. Outdoors they may have to wear warm mittens, perhaps over wool gloves, and lined, weatherproof boots over warm socks; indoors they may wear socks and gloves to bed. This strategy, incidentally, could help anyone who is plagued by cold hands or feet, even if they are not due to Raynaud's.

For those with severe symptoms of Raynaud's, the resulting crippling pain, lost dexterity, ulcers, and even gangrene may cause serious disability. No matter how warmly dressed, they may be unable to go out in winter without making the condition worse. They may be awakened in the middle of the night by a painful attack triggered by moving onto a cold part of the bed. Some must wear mittens to take food out of the refrigerator.

No one knows how frequently Raynaud's disease occurs. One estimate indicates that the milder forms affect about 20 percent of the female population. The disorder affects four to five times more women than men. (Other disorders involving the blood vessels in the outer regions of the body, such as migraine headache, also occur more often in women.)

Many Possible Causes

Raynaud's-like symptoms may result from a variety of underlying physical problems, among them a connective tissue disorder called scleroderma, the aftermath of frostbite, obstructions of the arteries, damage to the outlying nerves, thyroid deficiency, or the long-term effects of continuous pressure, such as from a jackhammer, typing, or piano playing. When the disorder is the result of other problems, it is called *Raynaud's phenomenon.* It usually starts abruptly late in life, affects men as well as women, and may involve the fingers on only one hand. Emotional factors are rarely involved. Treatment is usually directed at the underlying condition.

Primary Raynaud's disease has no known physical cause, and emotional stress frequently contributes to attacks. It is much more common among women, often starting in the late teens and affecting both hands and sometimes both feet. The small arteries in the fingers and toes go into spasm in response to cold, cutting off circulation and turning the digits white and numb. The temperature of the fingertips quickly drops to that of the surrounding air or the object in hand. Emotional factors — such as anger, fear, and anxiety, which lower hand temperature in everyone — can increase susceptibility to the cold in a person with Raynaud's disease.

Many Treatments, Too

Although the disease was first described more than a century ago (in 1862 by Maurice Raynaud), it has thus far defied a precise explanation. In addition to arterial spasms, it often involves an abnormal thickness of the blood and abnormal amounts of protein circulating in the blood.This has led to such treatments for severe cases as a steroid drug that breaks up blood clots and increases blood flow to the hand, surgery that severs the nerve center involved in arterial spasms, and replacement of the patient's own blood plasma with plasma from a blood bank. Treatment with an ointment called glyceryl trinitrate may also reduce the frequency and severity of attacks.

Biofeedback appears to have long-lasting effects, according to Dr. Edward Taub, psychologist at the Institute for Behavioral Research in Silver Spring, Maryland. Dr. Taub has used it mainly for primary Raynaud's disease, but others have reported success with Raynaud's phenomenon that results from scleroderma. In biofeedback the temperature of the patient's fingertips is recorded and amplified electronically, and the results are displayed visually so that the patient can detect tiny increases in finger temperature that normally would escape notice. Within a short time the patient learns how to control voluntarily a response that is not normally subject to voluntary control — in this case, finger temperature.

In Dr. Taub's institute patients are trained for one hour at a time once a week for three to four months. Some get a home trainer to practice on once or twice a day between formal training sessions. In this way they learn to raise finger temperature under a variety of different circumstances until they can call upon the response whenever they go out in the cold or feel an attack coming on.

Dr. Taub reports that on the average, biofeedback patients experience a 60 percent reduction in Raynaud's attacks, with some completely rid of the problem and others showing no response. Patients are brought back for a refresher training session once a year — in November — which seems to last through the winter.

Before seeking formal therapy, patients with Raynaud's attacks might try to abort them with an arm-whirling technique proposed by Dr. Donald R. McIntyre of Rutland, Vermont. While standing with fingers outstretched, swing your arms briskly in a circle (about eighty revolutions per minute) in the direction that a softball pitcher would — downward behind the body and upward in front. Gravity and centrifugal force move blood into the fingers. It is not a treatment, however, for persons with bursitis or back trouble.

Other home remedies that have proved helpful to many include keeping warm all over (including your head), avoiding consumption of caffeine-containing beverages (coffee, tea, colas, etc.) and drugs, and stopping smoking. Caffeine and cigarette smoke cause constriction of blood vessels in the outer reaches of the body and thus interfere with natural warming of fingers and toes. Before you go outdoors in the cold, it may also be wise to avoid consuming alcohol, which creates only a temporary feeling of warmth; it ultimately causes a loss of internal body heat and results in chilling.

XIII. Common Serious Illnesses

Some of our most common health problems are neither minor nor usually life-threatening. But they are nonetheless serious. Often they are chronic in nature (for example, arthritis, osteoporosis, epilepsy, and intestinal disorders) and have far-ranging effects on our overall ability to function. Sometimes, as with pneumonia or intestinal parasites, they can threaten survival.

Despite their commonness, myths and misunderstandings about many of these ailments prevail and compound the grief they cause. In other cases thoughts about causes and treatment have changed in recent years, but the knowledge of patients and sometimes of doctors as well has not kept up with the latest developments.

In most cases the toll these diseases exact can be greatly minimized through an understanding of their causes and effects and the pursuit of proper preventive measures and treatment. Is surgery really necessary to treat gallbladder disease? If so, when? Can ulcers be cured through diet, or are drugs necessary? Can the crippling effects of arthritis be prevented? What can you do to prevent the softening of bones that is responsible for so many fractures in older people?

Ulcers:
New Thoughts about Causes and Cures

True or false?

- The typical ulcer patient is an ambitious executive with many responsibilities and little time to relax.
- Milk is the ideal food for ulcer patients.
- Surgery is the only way to cure an ulcer.
- Although coffee is bad for ulcers, decaffeinated coffee is all right.
- To prevent a recurrence, ulcer patients must stick to a bland diet and stay away from spicy and fatty foods, citrus juices, and alcohol.
- Ulcers can lead to stomach cancer.

Recent studies indicate that all the above are false. There are perhaps more myths about ulcers than about any other common chronic disease. Much of the misinformation results from the fact that experts themselves are unsure of how or why ulcers occur and how best to treat them. In the last decade or so, virtually every assumption about the causes and cure of ulcers has been called into question. At the same time new facts have come to light that should help ulcer patients and their families cope more easily with the disease.

Who Gets Them and Why?

About 1 person in 10 will get an ulcer sometime in his or her life. While some reports suggest that ulcers are becoming less common among Americans, others indicate the opposite. One trend is certain, however: Ulcers today are far more common among women than they used to be. In decades past, only 1 in 20 ulcer patients was female; today nearly 1 in 2 is.

The reason for this shift can only be guessed at. One possibility is the rising use by women of cigarettes and alcohol, which irritate the lining of the gastrointestinal tract. So far there is no scientific evidence to suggest that the emotional and occupational stresses of women's liberation are factors.

Experts also now know that ulcers more commonly affect children than most people realize. Many a child's chronic stomachache, so readily dismissed by parents and physicians alike as merely an excuse to avoid school, may actually be the symptom of an ulcer.

Peptic ulcer, as this disease is properly called, is an open sore that results from the eating away of a spot in the lining of the stomach or small intestine by the stomach's highly acid digestive juices. The stomach normally secretes hydrochloric acid and pepsinogen, which is converted to the enzyme pepsin, which digests protein. The acid secretions are controlled by the vagus nerve. This nerve connects the stomach to the brain and stimulates the release of a hormone, gastrin, which in turn triggers the acid secretions.

Most ulcers occur in the duodenum, the part of the small intestine closest to the stomach; these are called duodenal ulcers. Gastric ulcers, only one-tenth as common, occur in the stomach. They seem to have different causes. Duodenal ulcers are associated with excessive production of stomach acid, which probably breaks down the resistance of the intestinal wall; gastric ulcers are usually associated with normal amounts of acid but may result from an inherent weakness in the stomach wall.

Factors known to increase the flow of stomach acid, possibly causing an ulcer, include alcohol, coffee, aspirin, and emotional stress. Yet, for unknown reasons, many people who chronically produce large amounts of acid or take sixteen aspirin a day for years never get an ulcer.

Heredity definitely plays a role. Ulcers are three times more common among blood relatives of ulcer patients than in the general population, and persons with type O blood are more likely than others to develop ulcers. But the influence of environmental stress is not as simple as is generally believed.

Seemingly calm, relaxed people are as prone to ulcers as the hard-driving, high-pressure kind. Ulcers occur as often in bus drivers, farmers, and construction workers as in business executives and writers with deadlines. It is not the existence of stress, but how a person reacts to stress, that seems to make the difference. A stress that is harmful to one person may be stimulating and healthful to another. [See chapter on stress, page 138.]

Although there is no clear-cut ulcer personality, there is no doubt that emotional tension, acting through the vagus nerve, can precipitate an ulcer. A person who is under constant strain, who is anxious, worried, frustrated — regardless of his or her station in life or apparent demeanor — is more apt to develop an ulcer.

Ulcers most often occur for the first time between the ages of twenty-five and forty, but they have been diagnosed as early as fetal life and as late as the tenth decade. The peak age for ulcers in children is seven to nine. Once ulcers develop, they tend to recur months or years later.

Symptoms and Diagnosis

The usual symptom of an active ulcer is pain, variously described as a gnawing or burning or hungry sensation, usually in the area just above the navel. The pain commonly occurs half an hour to two hours after eating and sometimes awakens the person during the night. It is frequently relieved by eating or taking an antacid. In children, however, eating may not bring relief. Other complaints, including headache, may accompany the stomachache in children.

An X ray taken after barium has been swallowed is the usual way an ulcer is diagnosed. A gastroduodenoscope — a long, flexible, lighted tube inserted through the mouth — may also be used to allow the doctor to view directly ulcers that may be missed by an X ray. If the apparent ulcer is in the stomach, the scope should always be used and a biopsy taken to be sure it is not a cancer masquerading as a gastric ulcer. However, ulcer patients are not more likely than others to develop gastrointestinal cancers.

Rather than a person's living with the discomfort of a tempestuous digestive tract for months or years, perhaps gulping over-the-counter antacids to soothe it when it acts up, it is important to get the condition diagnosed and treated by a physician. Ulcers can lead to serious, even fatal complications. An intestinal obstruction may develop. The ulcer may cause bleeding from small blood vessels, eventually resulting in anemia. If it eats into a major blood vessel, it can cause a severe internal hemorrhage. Or an ulcer may eat a hole into another organ or into the abdominal cavity, allowing the caustic contents of the stomach to spill out and cause life-threatening peritonitis. More than 8,000 Americans die each year from the complications of ulcers.

Treatment

With treatment, most ulcers heal in two to six weeks. But the approach to treatment is going through a number of changes, especially with regard to diet. A bland diet is usually recommended for about a week, until symptoms subside. After that, however, most doctors now advise avoiding only those foods that cause distress. Ulcer patients are usually told to avoid coffee (both regular and decaffeinated have been shown to stimulate stomach acid), tea, cola, and cocoa, and to drink alcoholic beverages only with food and in moderation, if at all. Aspirin should also be avoided; acetaminophen should be used for pain relief, instead, since this does not irritate the gastrointestinal tract. [See chapter on aspirin, page 463.]

Many doctors recommend eating frequent small meals, rather than three large ones, so that there is usually food in the stomach to absorb the acid. But milk, the traditional balm for ulcer, has been shown to stimulate stomach acid secretion and to have only a brief neutralizing effect on the acid. This has raised doubts about the usefulness of milk in treating ulcer patients, although many doctors say milk's soothing effects make it still worthwhile for some patients.

Another study showed that ulcers are least likely to develop in people who drink one to four glasses of milk a day. This finding may mean that milk protects against the effects of stomach acid or that those people who drink milk are less likely to drink alcohol or coffee or smoke cigarettes, which may promote the development of ulcers. Smoking also delays healing of ulcers, so the doctor may urge you to quit (a good idea whether you are told to or not).

Treatment is also likely to include antacids (aluminum hydroxide alone or with magnesium hydroxide), taken hourly at first and gradually tapered off. Antacids relieve symptoms and, studies indicate, promote the healing of ulcers. The liquid form is more effective than the tablets, although less convenient. But do not dose yourself with bicarb (sodium bicarbonate, or baking soda) because this can lead to kidney damage. People using large doses of antacids for long periods should supplement their diets with phosphorus-rich foods, among them milk, fish, nuts, beans, peas, whole wheat, and egg yolk, to prevent softening of the bones.

The current rage in ulcer therapy is a drug called Tagamet (cimetidine), which blocks production of stomach acid for four to six hours and, in doing so, relieves ulcer pain and speeds healing. The drug is taken four times a day, with meals and at bedtime. It is usually taken for a period of six to eight weeks. It does sometimes produce side effects, including dizziness, muscle pain, diarrhea, and skin rash, and thus should not be casually prescribed.

Other drugs may also be prescribed, including anticholinergics to delay the emptying of the stomach (especially useful at bedtime); antispasmodics to relax the muscles of the stomach and intestines; sedatives to relieve anxiety and tension.

When ulcers occur in children, psychotherapy or family counseling may be needed to help the youngsters deal with the stressful causes. All patients can benefit from practical advice on coping with stress. At any age, regular exercise or participation in sports helps to relieve the tensions that stimulate stomach acid.

Surgery may be necessary if an ulcer recurs repeatedly despite medical treatment or if a life-threatening complication develops. A portion of the stomach may be removed, and parts of the vagus nerve cut to reduce acid secretions. After surgery 90 to 95 percent of ulcers do not recur, but because the operation can cause chronic complications, it is best avoided as long as possible.

For Further Reading

Eisenberg, M. Michael, M.D. *Ulcers.* New York: Random House, 1978.

Intestinal Disorders: Secret Suffering

The symptoms of bowel disease are familiar to more of us than are likely to admit it: abdominal cramps, gas, or diarrhea alternating with constipation. They are so little talked about and so poorly understood that many people suffer needlessly for years, often compounding their problem by worrying and by the remedies they choose.

Sometimes the symptoms signal a serious underlying disease that, if neglected, can cause irrevocable damage and even death. Other times the symptoms merely mimic those of serious disorders and cause more emotional distress than the actual physical situation warrants. More often than not, however, prompt and accurate diagnosis and proper treatment can reduce greatly the mental and physical anguish and halt or even reverse the underlying disorder.

The symptoms reflect disorders in the intestinal tract — the twenty-foot-long small intestine and the five-foot-long large intestine, or colon, where digestion of food is completed, the resulting nutrients are absorbed, and the dietary wastes prepared for excretion. When the intestines malfunction, the body's ability to derive essential nutrients from foods may be impaired, leading to problems that affect other organs.

To make an accurate diagnosis of bowel disease, doctors must take into account the patient's symptoms and what may precipitate them as well as the results of a thorough intestinal examination with a proctosigmoidoscope (a foot-long tube inserted through the rectum) or a colonoscope (a six-foot-long flexible tube similarly inserted) and an X ray following a barium enema.

The more common intestinal disorders that afflict Americans include the following:

Irritable Bowel Syndrome

592

Also called spastic colon, this most common of gastrointestinal problems is considered a disorder of civilization, reflecting the stresses and strains of the American way of life. Although it may cause severe pain and alternating diarrhea and constipation, the condition is not associated with any underlying organic disease of the colon. Rather, it is a functional abnormality. The symptoms are real enough, and the discomfort can certainly disrupt the ordinary course of life; but the colon is not physically damaged, and the condition is not serious. Worrying about it, however, can make it worse.

Diagnosis of irritable bowel syndrome, which afflicts up to half of all patients with abdominal disorders, is made when the symptoms indicate a bowel disorder but a thorough examination of the colon and the stool reveals no evidence of disease.

Victims of irritable bowel syndrome tend to be tense, anxious, emotionally mercurial people, often leading hurried lives with irregular meals and inadequate sleep. Attacks are usually triggered by emotional stress but may also be precipitated by such drinks and foods as coffee, alcohol, spices, salads, raw fruits and vegetables, milk, very hot or very cold foods (which irritate the colons of sensitive individuals) as well as by infections or even a change in the weather.

The resulting spasms of the colon may cause sharp, knifelike pains or deep, dull pains, which may be relieved by manual pressure or heat. Constipation — more common than diarrhea in this disorder — should be treated with physical activity and possibly more roughage in the diet, rather than with laxatives, which can aggravate the problem.

Some patients are helped by mild sedatives or antispasmodic drugs. Changes in life-styles to relieve stress are also helpful, but psychotherapy rarely is. [See the chapter on stress, page 138.] The disorder may disappear entirely when a person's life circumstances change.

Diverticulosis

This is another disorder of civilization, but in this case the highly refined diet of affluent countries is the probable cause. Diverticula are sacs of tissue that protrude through the muscle wall of the colon. A third of all Americans over forty-five and two-thirds of those over sixty (more women than men) have these outpouchings.

Sometimes the pouches become infected and inflamed, a potentially serious condition called diverticulitis. The pouches of diverticulosis, the noninfected state, are believed to result from excessive pressure of gas and food on weak spots in the intestinal wall. A principal cause of this pressure is probably straining to move the bowels, with laxatives and enemas contributing to the problem.

The disorder is rare among peoples who live on diets high in fiber (roughage). Studies in several countries have shown that a high-fiber diet, plus lots of liquid, can both prevent the problem and help to correct one that already exists. Fiber — as found in fresh fruits and vegetables and whole grains — is not directly absorbed as a nutrient (hence it contributes few calories) but, rather, passes undigested into the colon, where it helps to make the stool soft, bulky, and easy to pass. [See chapter on dietary fiber, page 30.]

People with diverticulosis should avoid foods containing small seeds, such as figs, raisins, strawberries, and tomatoes, or hard particles, such as cracked wheat, and foods that produce intestinal gas (beans, cabbage, spinach, carbonated drinks, and the like). The infected state, diverticulitis, is generally treated with antibiotics and a low-roughage diet. Sometimes surgery is needed to treat complications.

Inflammatory Bowel Diseases

These disorders — regional enteritis (also known as ileitis or Crohn's disease) and ulcerative colitis — are among the most serious and life-disrupting of the gastrointestinal diseases. They afflict more than 2 million Americans, including 200,000 children. Neither a cause nor a cure is known, but most patients can be helped to live reasonably normal lives through treatment with drugs and/or surgery. Unfortunately delay in obtaining a correct diagnosis often leads to complications that could have been avoided and sometimes to irrevocable damage to the intestinal tract.

The symptoms associated with these diseases include bloody diar-

593

rhea, fever, abdominal blockages, pain, loss of weight, anemia, and malnutrition. Liver and kidney diseases, arthritis, and inflammation of the eye may also develop as complications.

Ileitis is an inflammation of the ileum, or lower section of the small intestine; colitis is an inflammation of the large intestine. The diseases vary greatly in severity from patient to patient, and the symptoms often disappear for long periods, then reappear.

Inflammatory bowel diseases most commonly afflict young adults, and 75 percent of cases occur before the age of 40. In about 10 percent of cases the disease involves an hereditary factor and more than one member of a family is affected. Emotional factors are also thought to predispose certain people to inflammatory bowel disease.

Patients with ulcerative colitis have a higher than normal risk of developing cancer of the colon or rectum. They should be examined regularly to detect early curable cancers, should they arise. [See chapter on detecting colon cancer, page 652.]

Treatment may involve rest; a mild sedative or antispasmodic drug; a bland diet high in protein, calories, and vitamins (but low in roughage); antibiotics; and corticosteroid drugs. The adverse side effects of the steroid drugs may be reduced by their being administered as rectal suppositories. Severe cases may require surgical removal of part or all of the diseased portion of the intestine; in some cases this necessitates an opening on the abdomen to collect body wastes. Surgery to remove the colon can cure ulcerative colitis, but it is considered a treatment of last resort.

594

For Further Reading and Information

Erlich, David, with George Wolf. *The Bowel Book: A Practical Guide to Good Health.* New York: Schocken Books, 1981.

Vernace, Salvatore J., M.D. *Living with Your Digestive System.* New York: E.P. Dutton, 1981.

The following organizations can supply free information on bowel and other digestive diseases:

● American Digestive Disease Society, Suite 1712, 420 Lexington Avenue, New York, New York 10017.

● National Foundation for Ileitis and Colitis, Inc., 295 Madison Avenue New York, New York 10017.

● National Institute of Arthritis, Metabolism and Digestive Diseases, Bethesda, Maryland 20014.

In addition, an excellent free pamphlet, *Inflammatory Bowel Diseases,* is available from the Gastrointestinal Research Foundation, University of Chicago Medical Center, Chicago, Illinois 60637. Patients or their families may also want to subscribe to a newsletter, *Crohn's Colitis Update,* published quarterly by Educational Insights, Inc., 150 West Carob Street, Compton, California 90220.

Gallbladder Disease:
Trouble from a Defunct(?) Organ

Each year Americans pay about $1 billion for the care of a body part they apparently can live very well without: the gallbladder. This three-inch pear-shaped organ is the storage depot for bile, a substance produced by the liver that is essential for the digestion and absorption of fats. A reservoir holding a ready supply of bile may have been very useful for those predecessors of modern man who lived a feast-and-famine existence and who gorged periodically on a fatty kill. Today, however, food is consumed on a more regular basis, and having a storehouse full of bile is unnecessary.

In the gallbladder, bile is chemically changed and concentrated about tenfold. When stimulated by the presence of food in the digestive tract, the gallbladder contracts and squeezes the bile out into the small intestine. In the absence of a gallbladder, the liver secretes bile directly into the intestine.

Since people who have their gallbladders removed have no problem digesting their meals, it seems that nowadays the gallbladder does little except cause trouble. It can get inflamed, stop working, and become filled with stones that can obstruct the flow of bile. The result can be agonizing pain, nausea, chills, fever, and prostration.

Gallstones, which form from natural constituents of bile, are the most common cause of gallbladder distress. In the United States 16 million people — 12 million women and 4 million men — have gallstones, although half of them have no symptoms. Each year some 800,000 new cases are diagnosed and 500,000 people have their gallbladders surgically removed. This operation, called cholecystectomy, is the most common form of abdominal surgery in adults in this country.

If research on the subject continues to show promise, in the near future many of these operations may be avoided by drugs that can dissolve the most common type of gallstones, those made mainly of cholesterol. At the same time, however, a growing number of surgeons are arguing that people with gallstones should have their gallbladders removed even if they cause no symptoms.

When symptoms do occur, they are often vague and easily confused with other conditions, such as appendicitis. Therefore, before any surgery is considered, a careful diagnostic work-up must be done. It may include a repeated X ray or an X ray combined with an ultrasound examination.

Causes

Gallstones are extremely common in societies like ours, where the diet is high in calories and cholesterol. The stones result from a chemical derangement in the liver that produces a high concentration of cholesterol in the bile. (A far less common type of gallstone is formed from hemoglobin pigments.)

Other factors that contribute to an increased risk of gallstones include the use of such drugs as oral contraceptives, menopausal estrogens, and clofibrate; intestinal disorders that interfere with the absorption of bile; diabetes; and probably pregnancy and obesity.

The risk of developing gallstones increases when an obese person starts losing weight. This is one reason why the obese should avoid repeated weight losses and gains but should try, instead, to lose the undesirable weight once and for all. [See chapter on permanent weight control, page 72.] There is some evidence that those who consume a diet high in fibrous foods, such as wheat bran, are less likely than others to develop gallstones. [See chapter on dietary fiber, page 36.]

Symptoms

The notion that people with gallbladder trouble develop indigestion, flatulence, and bloating in response to eating a large fatty meal has been dispelled by controlled studies. Patients who say they cannot tolerate fatty foods report no symptoms when given a meal in which fat is concealed, and patients with X ray signs of gallbladder disease do not suffer more indigestion than those with normal gallbladders.

Rather, the symptoms of gallbladder disease are commonly pain and tenderness in the upper right abdomen. The symptoms are most often the result of a stone's becoming lodged in the duct that transports bile to the intestine. More than 60 percent of patients with gallstones experience no attacks or only one attack. Most of the rest have pain as their only symptom. But some can become seriously ill, developing severe infections and potentially life-threatening complications, with little or no advance warning.

Among those with "silent" gallstones, between a third and a half eventually develop symptoms or complications. In 10 to 20 percent of the cases these complications are serious. About half the patients sooner or later have their gallbladders surgically removed.

Treatment: Surgery, etc.

Because serious complications can sometimes develop suddenly and because younger, healthy people face less risk from surgery, some surgeons believe the gallbladder should be removed as soon as gallstones are discovered even if they are causing the patient no trouble. Other physicians reply that operating on that group of people, half of whom will never encounter any problems from their condition, results in a great deal of unnecessary surgery.

If surgery is recommended for a gallbladder problem, it's wise to get opinions from two or more physicians, including an internist who specializes in gastroenterology as well as one or more surgeons. As with any operation, gallbladder surgery carries a risk of serious complications and death. The risk of death from the operation exceeds 1 in 1,000 in the best of circumstances. As currently practiced, in patients under fifty years of age, the death rate from surgery is less than 5 per 1,000; in those fifty to sixty-four years old, it is 1 per 100, and in those over sixty-five, it may be as high as 5 per 100. The surgery is not a guarantee of cure; 15 percent of patients still have symptoms afterward.

For some, there may be an alternative to surgery. In twenty-five countries around the world a drug called chenic acid (short for cheno-deoxycholic acid) — a natural component of bile — has been licensed as effective in dissolving cholesterol gallstones. The drug, not yet approved for United States marketing by the Food and Drug Administration, has undergone a two-year national test in this country that showed it was effective in about 40 percent of patients. Thin people and those with small stones had the best response.

However, in patients whose stones do not respond to the treatment, the drug does not significantly alter pain caused by gallstones or eliminate the need for surgery, the study indicated. In some patients the stones re-form after the drug has been discontinued. The only side effect noted has been mild diarrhea in some patients. A second drug, ursodeoxycholic acid, also a natural component of bile, has been found to be as effective as chenic acid in preliminary studies abroad. Apparently this substance does not bring on the side effect of diarrhea. However, little is known about the long-term effectiveness and possible hazards of either drug.

Another new method for treating gallstones involves the use of a flexible scope that can be inserted through the digestive tract. Without surgery or general anesthesia, stones can be grasped and removed from the bile duct. The procedure, called endoscopic papillotomy, was developed by German and Japanese researchers, and as of 1982 relatively few American physicians had learned it.

Intestinal Parasites: They Occur Here, Too

Americans, including American physicians, tend to think of intestinal parasites as problems of poor people living in underdeveloped, tropical countries. Indeed, that is where such parasites most commonly cause illness and death. But as millions of dismayed Americans discover each year, we have them, too. Many parasites are native to this country — you can get them without ever leaving home — and they often have little respect for socioeconomic status. In addition to the native sources of infection, which can include household pets and sexual partners as well as contaminated soil, food, and water, Americans who travel out of the country may be exposed to both exotic and common parasites.

The parasites themselves range in size from a microscopic single-celled protozoan to a worm that may exceed 30 feet in length. Infections, usually acquired by ingesting the egg, cyst, or larva of the parasite, are often spread by people, such as food handlers, who don't even know they have them.

Detection and Prevention

Because the signs and symptoms of intestinal parasitic infections are often vague and confusing and because many physicians in this country are not familiar with them, a victim can suffer for weeks or months and undergo many needless tests and treatments before the proper diagnosis is made. One woman suffered for ten months with recurrent bouts of diarrhea, nausea, and vomiting; underwent a series of gastrointestinal X rays, numerous blood tests, and doctor visits; and ran up a $1,000 bill before she was finally diagnosed as having a parasitic infection called amebiasis, or amebic dysentery.

Today treatment for the usual causes of parasitic infections in this country is much simpler and more effective than it used to be. Therefore, it pays to know something about these problems, when to suspect them as well as how to prevent them.

Prevention requires careful attention to personal hygiene: Always wash your hands after using the toilet and before eating. When traveling to areas where such parasites are common, don't eat foods that are served raw (such as salads) or that may have been handled after they were cooked. Stick to fruits that must be peeled before eating. If you become ill after traveling abroad, be sure to tell the doctor where you've been.

If you develop a diarrheal illness that does not clear up in a few days, parasitic infections should be suspected and a stool sample examined by a competent laboratory. If your regular physician cannot solve the problem, it's wise to see a gastroenterologist, preferably at a university medical center. If possible, in cases that prove difficult to diagnose, try to see a specialist in tropical medicine.

In all cases of intestinal parasites, follow-up examinations after treatment is completed are important to establish whether the treatment worked and to check on the possibility of reinfection.

The Common Offenders

Pinworms. Some 20 million Americans, most of them children between the ages of four and twelve, are infected with these half-inch-long worms each year. Most people with pinworms have no symptoms. The most common symptom is itching around the anus, particularly at night when the female worms crawl out of the rectum to lay their eggs on the skin. Members of the most fastidious of households can become infected.

The parasite is spread not just by contact with infected clothing, bedding, and toys but also by an infected child, who may carry the eggs on his or her fingers or under his or her nails and spread them to others directly or through the air.

Pinworms are best detected by examining the anal area for the tiny white worms at night about two hours after the sufferer has gone to bed. Cellophane tape placed around the anal opening in the morning can pick up the eggs, which are visible under a microscope.

Treatment often involves the whole family. One dose of the drug pyrvinium pamoate eradicates the parasite in about 90 percent of cases. In addition, in the week following treatment, bed linens should be changed daily and cotton underpants should be worn day and night (changed twice a day) and sterilized in a clothes dryer or with a hot iron. Hands should be washed, fingernails scrubbed often, and the toilet seat washed frequently. The sleeping area should be thoroughly dusted and vacuumed, and the floor scrubbed.

Amebiasis (amebic dysentery). This is contracted by ingesting the cyst of a protozoan, a microscopic single-celled organism. As with pinworms, most people who carry this infection have no symptoms. Those with symptoms may have mild to severe diarrhea and/or abdominal cramps.

Health officials in New York, San Francisco, and a few other cities have noted an increase in detected cases of amebiasis among homosexual men, who apparently spread it to one another through anal-oral contact. It may also be spread through food or water contaminated by an infected food handler or by soil containing human feces. According to the Centers for Disease Control in Atlanta, "Although the number of persons infected [with amebiasis] is small, the potential for complications and death is great for the patient with undiagnosed infection."

Diagnosis is made through a stool test by a laboratory that is expert in detecting parasitic diseases. The proper diagnosis is sometimes missed because of a falsely negative lab test. The disease can be confused with a variety of intestinal disorders, including colon cancer, leading to many unneeded and costly tests.

Drug treatment lasts about ten days, after which the stool test should be repeated and a second course of treatment given if needed.

Giardiasis. Although not long ago considered a disease contracted only by travelers to the Soviet Union, this protozoan infection is now known to be present throughout the United States. It has caused community-wide outbreaks in some places where the water supply is chlorinated but not filtered. The organism also infects beavers and dogs, which may contaminate reservoirs with their feces. It is also a common cause of traveler's diarrhea. [See chapter on traveler's diarrhea, page 581.]

Typical symptoms involve diarrhea, abdominal pain, and weight loss. Giardiasis is diagnosed by a stool examination. It is treated for a week to ten days with quinacrine, an antimalarial drug, or metronidazole (Flagyl), both of which may cause gastrointestinal and other disturbances.

Roundworms. More than 1 million Americans are believed to harbor the giant roundworm, *Ascaris lumbricoides*, which may reach fourteen inches in length. It is relatively common in the southern United States but can also be found in New York City and other northern regions.

The disorder is contracted by ingestion of eggs. Because the larvae migrate through the lungs, the first symptoms are of a pneumonialike illness, with cough, wheezing, and fever. Later, after being coughed up and swallowed, the adult worm develops in the small intestine, causing abdominal cramps, mild diarrhea, and sometimes intestinal obstruction. The infection is usually diagnosed by the finding of eggs in the stool and is treated with drugs for one or two days.

People may also contract roundworms from pet dogs or cats. Dr. Peter Schantz, a veterinarian with the Centers for Disease Control, says that more than 80 percent of puppies born in this country are infected with roundworm. Children who handle the animals and put their hands in their mouths are especially prone to becoming infected. [See chapter on dog bites and other pet-caused diseases, page 416.]

600

Dr. Schantz urges that all puppies be treated for worms by or in consultation with a veterinarian beginning at the age of three weeks. By the time most puppies are brought in for their shots the whole household may be infected.

In people, the dog roundworm causes confusing symptoms that may be hard to recognize, including swollen liver and pneumonialike symptoms. The eye may become invaded, causing partial or complete blindness. The infection can be diagnosed by a blood test and cured by drug treatment.

Other roundworms, in addition to pinworm, that infect people include whipworm, threadworm, and hookworm. All prefer a warm, moist climate, such as is found in the southern United States; all cause abdominal pain and (except for hookworm) diarrhea; and all are diagnosed by a stool test. The larval forms of hookworm and threadworm invade through skin that contacts contaminated ground.

Tapeworms. Tapeworms can be acquired by the eating of raw or inadequately cooked beef, pork, or fish that is contaminated with tapeworm eggs. The eggs are destroyed by proper cooking.

The beef tapeworm is common in Africa, the Middle East, Eastern Europe, Mexico, and South America. It also occurs in California and New England. Pork tapeworm, rare in this country, is common in Asia, Eastern Europe, and Latin America. Fish tapeworm is found in freshwater fish in Scandinavia, Japan, Africa, South America, and Canada, and in Florida and the north-central states.

Human infection by fish tapeworm usually results in no or mild gastrointestinal symptoms, but beef and pork tapeworm can cause more serious illness. Tapeworms are diagnosed by finding eggs in the stool or around the anus.

Arthritis:
Controlling a Costly Crippler

Arthritis is truly a universal illness. Virtually all of us, if we live long enough, will develop arthritis in one or more of our joints. The disease has been around at least as long as Neanderthal man; the one nearly complete specimen of a Neanderthal spine is deformed by arthritis, creating the misimpression that all such early humans walked in a bent posture.

Today arthritis in one of its myriad forms afflicts some 31 million Americans seriously enough to require medical treatment. More than 1 in 10 arthritis victims are severely affected and unable to carry out normal activities. In one form arthritis is the most common cause of pain and stiffness in people over fifty; in another, it afflicts a quarter of a million children under age sixteen.

Despite its frequency, arthritis is subject to serious public misunderstanding. As a result, many victims become needlessly crippled because, thinking nothing can be done, they delay proper treatment. Others are improperly treated, and even more disregard established treatments to pursue quack remedies that only waste precious time and money. Nearly $1 billion is squandered each year on unproved arthritis treatments, ranging from copper bracelets and snake venom to Chinese herbs and fad diets. None has been proved to be any more effective than the ancient remedy of stewing patients in a brew made by the boiling of whole wolves in oil.

At the same time few patients and their families fully appreciate the role they can and should play in preserving normal joint function. While arthritis is still incurable, many more people could avoid its crippling effects than now do. Currently the average victim of arthritis waits four years after symptoms begin to seek medical help. For some this delay results in irreversible crippling. To avert disability, avoid quackery, and obtain the best available care for patients, it is crucial to understand the nature of the diseases called arthritis and how they can be treated.

What Is Arthritis?

Arthritis means "inflammation of the joints." The most frequent forms of arthritis are osteoarthritis, a wear-and-tear disease that becomes increasingly common with age, and rheumatoid arthritis, a more severe disorder that can strike at any age, even during infancy. In both disorders symptoms tend to wax and wane; they are usually worse in the morning, may be worse some days than others, and may even completely disappear for a time, only to flare up again days, weeks, or months later. It is important for family and friends to realize this and not to assume arthritis patients "conveniently" develop symptoms to avoid unpleasant tasks.

Osteoarthritis. This is a degenerative, rather than an inflammatory, disorder, which afflicts 40 million Americans, 16 million of whom require medical care. It usually results from a wearing down of the cartilage in the joints. The pads of cartilage at the ends of the bones become frayed and rough instead of smooth. Bony spurs may develop, preventing normal movement of the joint, and the joint begins to grate like a rusty gate instead of operating smoothly like a well-oiled machine.

Osteoarthritis most often affects the large weight-bearing joints — knees and hips — as well as the spine, and it usually begins in the fifties or later. Bony growths in the outermost finger joints may appear even earlier.

Overweight individuals are more likely to get osteoarthritis, and weight loss is an excellent way to relieve symptoms even after the disease has occurred. Osteoarthritis can also follow injury to or repeated abuse of a joint, such as often happens to athletes. Thus, arthritis of the knees forced Willis Reed to retire from basketball, and an arthritic elbow ended Sandy Koufax's baseball career. It is not known why many people who subject their joints to constant abuse escape from arthritis while others succumb.

Pain and stiffness are the most common symptoms; they usually are noticeably worse in the morning and sometimes in wet or cold weather. (However, moving to a warm, dry climate does not necessarily provide lasting relief. Before you pack up your household, it's advisable to live in your chosen area for several months or longer.) Sometimes affected joints become tender and swollen.

Diagnosis is based primarily on symptoms and physical and X ray examinations. Laboratory tests, such as those for white blood count, sedimentation rate, and rheumatoid factor, are usually normal.

Rheumatoid arthritis. Unlike osteoarthritis, which usually affects a few joints, rheumatoid arthritis is a systemic, or whole-body, disease. In addition to stiff, hot, painful, inflamed joints, many patients experience overwhelming fatigue, weakness, fever, malaise, muscular stiffness, loss of appetite, anemia, and weight loss. Damage may also occur to connective tissues and organs throughout the body, including the heart, lungs, nerves, and eyes.

Although the precise cause or causes is unknown, rheumatoid arthritis acts like an autoimmune disease, in which the body attacks its own tissues. There is often a hereditary predisposition, although the disease itself is not inherited. It can strike at any age — from infancy onward.

Joint damage results from an inflammation of the synovium, a thin membrane in the joint that produces the fluid that lubricates the joint. Prolonged inflammation destroys the cartilage, weakens the ligaments of the joint, and may damage the tendons. Attached muscles weaken and may develop painful spasms. The joints most commonly affected are those at the base and middle of the fingers, the base of the toes, the wrists, and the knees. Shoulders, hips, elbows, and ankles may also be involved. In severe cases joints become grotesquely twisted and useless.

While clearly more severe, fortunately this is a less common disease than osteoarthritis. Of the 6.5 million Americans with rheumatoid arthritis, about a third have intermittent symptoms, sometimes with long periods during which symptoms disappear. In most, however, the disease persists and may become progressively worse. Still, through early, skilled treatment crippling disability can be prevented in the vast majority of patients. More than two-thirds of children with rheumatoid arthritis recover by the time they reach adulthood. In all cases the sooner effective treatment is begun, the less likely crippling deformities will occur.

Diagnosis of rheumatoid arthritis is based on symptoms, physical and X ray exams, and laboratory tests showing such abnormalities as the presence of rheumatoid factor and a high white blood cell count. A firm diagnosis can sometimes take weeks.

For unknown reasons, women are three times more likely than men to develop rheumatoid arthritis. Although emotional distress can precipitate a flare-up, there is no particular arthritis personality common among victims.

Preventing Arthritis

As doctors have gained a more complete understanding of arthritis, it has become apparent that many cases of osteoarthritis can be prevented. Interestingly prevention involves regular use — although not abuse — of your joints. In his excellent book *Arthritis: A Comprehensive Guide* (see "For Further Reading," page 607), Dr. James F. Fries, director of the Stanford University Arthritis Clinic, emphasizes the importance of daily exercise. He writes: "For arthritis prevention, you need strong bones, strong supporting ligaments, and healthy cartilage. Exercise is the way to get these."

Dr. Fries recommends walking, biking, and swimming; if you're in shape, jogging, tennis, handball, soccer, and basketball are good. But he advises against weight lifting, push-ups, and other such activities and against football and baseball as arthritis preventives. Strive for twelve to fifteen minutes of steady exercise each day, at least five days a week.

Maintaining a normal body weight is also an important part of arthritis prevention. Overweight places excessive stress on weight-bearing joints and interferes with the smooth functioning of tendons, ligaments, and muscles.

Protect your joints from degenerative decay by maintaining a proper posture while sitting and standing. Sleep on a good bed, and wear good shoes. Learn the proper way to perform physical activities, and listen to your body's pain messages. Do not exercise a joint that is injured or inflamed. Increase the strenuousness and extent of your activities slowly. Warm up your muscles and joints prior to vigorous activity.

When to See a Doctor

In view of the importance of prompt and proper treatment to prevent arthritic crippling, it is critical to heed symptoms that could represent one or another form of arthritis. See your doctor if you experience any of the following:

- Pain, tenderness, swelling, or redness of one or more joints.
- Persistent pain and stiffness after you wake up in the morning.
- Joint pain at night severe enough to interfere with sleep.
- Inability to move your limbs properly or do normal activities.
- Any worsening or recurrence of joint symptoms or involvement of additional joints.
- Tingling sensations in the fingertips, hands, and feet.
- Joint symptoms associated with unexplained weight loss, fever, weakness, or fatigue.

If arthritis is diagnosed or suspected, you may wish to be referred to a specialist in rheumatic diseases for confirmation of the diagnosis and outline of a comprehensive treatment plan.

Treating Arthritis

Even without the discovery of a cure, the major crippling forms of arthritis would disable far fewer people than they now do if not for three obstacles:

1. Many victims self-treat or ignore their arthritic symptoms for years before seeking medical assistance, and as a result, they suffer irreversible joint damage.

2. Too often the treatment prescribed is not sufficiently comprehensive, relying almost entirely on drugs and neglecting physical and occupational therapy, emotional needs, and life-style changes that could greatly improve the success rate of treatment.

3. Even when appropriate treatment is prescribed, many patients fail to follow their doctors' advice and therefore reap only partial benefits. Some take their medication irregularly or at less than optimal doses — enough to stop the pain but not enough to suppress the joint-damaging inflammation. Others take the medication but fail to do the prescribed exercises. Still others abandon established treatments in favor of quack remedies of no known benefit, except to the purses of the purvey-

ors. The Arthritis Foundation estimates that for every dollar spent on legitimate arthritis research, $25 is squandered on quackery. It would be far better if victims donated these dollars toward the search for a cure.

There are today so many effective drug therapies for arthritis that there is something to help nearly every victim. If one drug brings little or no improvement or produces intolerable side effects, another can be tried — and another, and another, until one is found that is both effective and reasonably safe. In addition, there are many simple do-it-yourself treatments that can greatly ease symptoms and help to ward off permanent, crippling joint damage.

Your success in living with arthritis depends largely on your willingness to obtain and follow a comprehensive treatment plan and maintain a positive outlook. A woman I know has been seriously afflicted with arthritis for twenty years but is determined not to be defeated by it. She has taken her medication faithfully, adhered to the prescribed program of daily exercise and rest, and today, with the occasional aid of a cane, is still able to conduct a reasonably normal life of shopping, cooking, housekeeping, church, and community affairs. Her husband developed the same disease — but the opposite response — ten years after she did. He retired from his job, took to his favorite chair and stayed there, becoming more and more crippled until today he can hardly move and is in constant pain.

The goal of arthritis therapy is to relieve pain and stiffness, stop destructive inflammation, and maintain joint mobility. Because comprehensive treatment is needed, you are best cared for by a rheumatologist (a doctor specializing in arthritis) or at an arthritis center. Here's what you should know about current arthritis treatments:

Drug therapy. Believe it or not, aspirin remains the first choice therapy for both rheumatoid and osteoarthritis. It relieves pain and reduces inflammation with the least hazard to patients. Only if aspirin produces intolerable side effects (or is dangerous for a particular patient) or has been tried and found wanting should stronger medications be used. [See chapter on aspirin, page 463.]

However, unlike the occasional use of aspirin to treat a headache or muscle pain, in arthritis therapy aspirin should be taken two or three tablets at a time three or more times a day every day, whether joints hurt or not. This is to achieve and maintain the blood level of aspirin needed to suppress inflammation. Although pain and stiffness may disappear at low doses, inflammation does not, and it is the inflammation that causes crippling. The doctor will prescribe the maximum amount of aspirin your body can handle.

To reduce stomach irritation, aspirin can be taken after meals, with a full glass of water, or as coated tablets that do not dissolve in the stomach. However, buffered aspirin does not contain enough buffer to be much help, and so-called extra-strength and specially formulated aspirin offer no particular pain-relieving advantage and cost considerably more than the equivalent dosage of ordinary aspirin.

All other antiarthritis drugs are available only on a doctor's prescription. They include — in the order in which they are commonly tried — nonaspirin salicylates, nonsteroidal anti-inflammatory drugs (naproxen, tolmetin, and sulindac are some), pyrazolones (phenylbutazone), indomethacin, gold salts, and penicillamine. The drugs toward the end of the line are more toxic and therefore reserved for cases resistant to milder therapy. Corticosteroids (cortisone, prednisone, etc.), which are potent anti-inflammatory agents once thought to be the long-awaited miracle cure for arthritis, produce side effects that greatly limit their usefulness.

Whichever drug you are given, it is critically important to take it as prescribed. Don't stop or reduce the dosage when you feel better. But do tell the doctor if you are bothered by side effects. In the treatment of arthritis it often takes weeks or months to see significant improvement. Stick with the prescribed treatment for as long as your doctor recommends before trying something new.

Exercise and rest. Daily exercise is crucial to maintaining mobility of arthritic joints. If joints are not used, they tend to stiffen up, the cartilage deteriorates, and the nearby muscles atrophy. Exercise maintains the health of cartilage and strengthens muscles, tendons, and ligaments, which enable them to support your joints. Exercise also helps you to achieve and maintain a normal body weight, and it has decided psychological benefits, producing relaxation, alleviating depression, and enhancing self-image.

Swimming and walking are among the best overall activities for arthritis patients; in addition, specific exercises for particular problems may be prescribed. The doctor may recommend that you work with a physical therapist.

In treating arthritis, exercise must be balanced with rest — sometimes complete body rest and sometimes rest only of affected joints. This is needed to reduce inflammation. Daily exercise and rest programs should be individually designed for each patient. Many arthritis patients find an afternoon nap greatly enhances their ability to get through the day.

Maintaining correct posture when sitting, standing, or lying down is also important to preserving joint mobility. Women should not wear high heels, which distort posture and place unnatural stresses on joints.

Heat, sex, diet, and other aids. Heat, especially moist heat, is ideal for relieving pain and easing motion of arthritic joints. It is especially useful prior to exercise sessions. Try soaking in a warm bath or standing under a hot shower. Or apply hot washcloths or Hydrocollator packs (obtainable at pharmacies), or use a heating pad.

Too often arthritis needlessly brings a couple's sex life to a close. Yet sexual activity actually helps to relieve arthritic symptoms. Any form of sexual arousal — with or without a partner — is helpful. If you are unable to devise comfortable positions and techniques on your own, a qualified sex counselor can be a great help.

A nutritious — balanced and varied — diet that will enable you to achieve and maintain a normal weight can greatly ease the strain on arthritic joints. However, fad diets, megadoses of vitamins and minerals, and other food supplements are of no known benefit to arthritis patients. The value of special diets for arthritis is currently unconfirmed by proper scientific study.

Many gadgets (such as a long-handled toothbrush) or rearrangements of items at home and at work can greatly simplify life for arthritis patients and enable them to maintain their independence and jobs. A wide variety of aids and techniques are described and depicted in an excellent new book, *Overcoming Arthritis* (see "For Further Reading" below), by Dr. Frank Dudley Hart. Your local chapter of the Arthritis Foundation can provide several booklets (some are free) describing home care and self-help techniques.

Surgery. This is reserved for cases of badly damaged joints that cannot be helped by more conservative therapy. In cases of rheumatoid arthritis, inflamed synovial tissue may be surgically removed. Joints rendered useless can be replaced with artificial joints, including hip, knee, and finger joints and sometimes elbow, ankle, and shoulder joints.

Experimental therapies. Periodic blood filtering and low-dose radiation treatments are among treatments under test that have shown early promise. However, they should be used only as part of approved experimental programs. Another experimental remedy, DMSO, has not been shown to be either safe or effective in treating arthritis. It can have dangerous side effects, including chemical burns and possibly damage to the eyes.

For Further Reading

Carr, Rachel. *Arthritis: Relief Beyond Drugs.* New York: Harper & Row, 1981.

Freese, Arthur S. "Arthritis: Everybody's Disease." Public Affairs Pamphlet No. 562. Available for 50 cents from Public Affairs Pamphlets, 381 Park Avenue South, New York, N.Y. 10016.

Fries, James F., M.D. *Arthritis: A Comprehensive Guide.* Reading, Mass.: Addison-Wesley, 1979.

Hart, Frank Dudley, M.D. *Overcoming Arthritis.* New York: Arco, 1981.

Partridge, Raymond E.H., M.D. *Arthritis and Rheumatism.* Tufts-New England Medical Center Family Health Guide. Providence, R.I.: Arandel (55 Dupont Drive, Providence, R.I. 02907), 1978.

Various pamphlets are available from the Arthritis Foundation. Contact local chapters or write to the national office, 3400 Peachtree Road, NE, Atlanta, Georgia 30326.

Gout: No Longer
a Disease of Gluttony

Although for centuries gout has been sneered at as the "rheumatism of the rich" and depicted in caricatures of nobility, gout is no laughing matter to those who have it. As one victim put it, "It hurts like hell, and I didn't do anything to deserve it." Nor is it a disease limited exclusively, or even primarily, to the upper classes, although certain excesses among the nobility of yore could have precipitated its occurrence in susceptible individuals.

Gorging on food and drink was once a common entertainment of the rich, and when you look at the menu of a typical feast, it's no wonder it took a toll. Samuel Pepys, himself a sufferer, described the menu for his dinner party for nine: fricassee of rabbit and chicken, leg of boiled mutton, three carps, side of lamb, roasted pigeons, four lobsters, three tarts, lamprey pie, a dish of anchovies, and several kinds of wine. And this was light fare compared to the dinners of kings and queens.

Today gout is a far more democratic disease. With outright gluttony now an uncommon practice, excesses of diet and drink play a less important role in precipitating it. Gout does, however, show an unexplained predilection for intelligent, hard-driving, socioeconomically successful men.

Gout has been recognized as a disease since antiquity. Egyptian papyri referred to it as "arthritis in the toe." Its victims have included Kublai Khan, Leonardo da Vinci, John Milton (whose suffering with gout is said to have contributed vivid imagery to his portrayal of hell in *Paradise Lost*), Alexander the Great, Isaac Newton, Martin Luther, Henry VIII, Charles Darwin, and Benjamin Franklin.

In centuries past, it was common to see important personages afflicted with gout being carried on litters or sitting with their painfully swollen feet resting on gout stools. Indeed, many regarded "the gout" as a status symbol.

Gout, however, is a serious and potentially crippling form of arthritis. It is also the one type of arthritis that can be totally controlled in the vast majority of cases. Through modern methods of treatment the agony of recurring attacks can be largely prevented, those attacks that do occur can be relieved quickly, and the permanent crippling that once afflicted many can be avoided.

Approximately 1 million Americans currently have gout, and nearly 90 percent of them are male. The 10 to 15 percent of cases that afflict women occur mainly after menopause. The disease usually shows up during the middle years, although it can also occur in young men.

The Causes

Most cases of gout are caused by an inherited metabolic defect that results in an overaccumulation in the blood of uric acid, which the body manufactures normally from substances called purines. While they are found in many foods — including all organ meats, meat extracts, bouillon, beer, anchovies, and sardines — most purines found in the body are made there from other substances.

Uric acid is only slightly soluble in blood, and above a certain concentration it tends to precipitate out as microscopic crystals of sodium urate. These sharp crystals lodge in joint tissues, their favorite resting place being the big toe, with lesser affinity for the ankles, insteps, knees, elbows, wrists, and fingers.

In two out of three cases of so-called primary gout the victim's body manufactures excessive amounts of uric acid; in the remaining one-third there is a defect in the body's ability to get rid of sodium urate in adequate amounts. There is no evidence that gouty patients of today habitually consume foods high in purines.

Heredity plays a role that has not yet been clearly defined. Some 10 to 20 percent of patients with gout have one or more relatives with the disease, and 15 to 25 percent of a victim's close relatives have abnormally high levels of uric acid in their blood. Gout may also develop as a complication of some other disorder, such as leukemia, diabetes, or lead poisoning. Certain drugs, such as penicillin, insulin, thiazide diuretics, and low doses of aspirin, can precipitate gout by interfering with the excretion of uric acid.

Oddly the majority of people who have above-normal blood levels of uric acid never develop gouty symptoms. Those who do can often relate the onset of an attack to a particular event. Precipitants of symptoms include surgery, injury, infection, overindulgence in food or alcohol, very low-carbohydrate (ketogenic) diet, ill-fitting shoes, fatigue, emotional stress, strenuous exercise, or even the minor stress of excessive walking.

Symptoms and Diagnosis

Symptoms result from a vicious cycle starting with the formation of microcrystals in the joints, followed by an invasion of white blood cells to attack and remove the crystals, followed by the precipitation of more crystals and the invasion of more white blood cells. The result is an extraordinarily painful inflammation. In 90 percent of patients the big toe is the primary site of attacks. The crushing, throbbing pain can begin suddenly, often during the night. The affected joint becomes swollen and tender, and the surrounding skin gets hot and tight and turns dusky red or purplish. Other symptoms may include fever, rapid heartbeat, chills, and malaise. Some gout sufferers develop deposits of a chalky white derivative of uric acid. These deposits, called tophi, commonly occur in or near the joints, around the elbow, or in or near the ear rims.

Diagnosis of gout is generally based on these telltale symptoms, supplemented by a blood test for uric acid and possibly the finding of urate crystals in the fluid in the affected joint. Rapid relief (within twelve to forty-eight hours) from a drug called colchicine is also considered diagnostic of gout.

Even without treatment, symptoms usually subside within a week or two. But unless treated by medication, attacks of gout tend to become more severe and more frequent. Eventually they can lead to kidney damage from kidney stones or deposits of urate and to permanent damage to the joints.

Treatment, but No Cure

There is no cure for gout, but there are a number of drugs that can treat the acute attack and some that can prevent future attacks when taken regularly. Each of the drugs has undesirable side effects, and a certain amount of trial and error may be necessary to find the right therapy and dose for a particular patient. The drugs include colchicine; an anti-inflammatory drug called phenylbutazone; probenecid, which increases excretion of urate; and allopurinol, which reduces the body's production of uric acid.

An acute attack can often be aborted if the proper drug is taken at the first twinge. During an attack it is important to rest and keep weight off the affected joints. Consumption of large amounts of water (three quarts a day) helps dilute the urate in the kidneys and prevent dehydration.

Following a rigid low-purine diet has been found to be of little help in preventing attacks, but the doctor may advise avoiding certain foods heavily laden with purines as well as excessive indulgence in alcohol, which can diminish the kidneys' ability to get rid of urate. Obviously gout patients should avoid any particular stress, food, or drink that has been found to precipitate an attack. If the victim is obese, weight loss helps to prevent recurrent attacks.

Osteoporosis: Bone Loss Is Preventable

"Dowager's hump," hip fractures, shortened stature — these hallmarks of late-middle and old age are the result of a common disorder, osteoporosis, a progressive loss and weakening of bone.

Although long regarded as an inevitable and irremediable consequence of aging, especially in women past menopause, recent studies suggest that osteoporosis may be largely preventable and partly treatable. The protein- and mineral-rich foods you eat and the amount of exercise you get may make the difference between a lifetime of healthy bones and progressive skeletal deterioration.

The studies indicate that one major cause of osteoporosis is a chronically inadequate consumption of calcium, the mineral that joins with phosphorus to form the rigid crystalline structures that give your bones their strength. According to the findings, the amount of calcium currently recommended for adults — 800 milligrams a day, the amount in about 21 ounces of milk — is at least 50 percent lower than it should be to maintain strong healthy bones and teeth throughout life.

At the same time calcium in the diets of most adults in this country is below even the 800-milligram level and has been dropping for years, along with a decline in consumption of milk and other calcium-rich dairy products. The average woman over forty-five consumes only 450 milligrams of calcium daily. Further, the rising popularity of foods rich in phosphorus — such as meats, poultry, fish, and many processed foods — may impair the body's ability to use what calcium it does get.

Each year 6 million Americans, most of them white postmenopausal women, suffer bone fractures as a result of osteoporosis, which afflicts one in two elderly women and one in eight elderly men in this country. Hip fractures alone cost the nation about $1 billion a year and are frequently the start of invalidism and sometimes the precipitant of death among the elderly. Collapse of the vertebrae in the spine, resulting in low back pain and loss of height (as much as an inch and a half each decade after menopause), is a frequent result of the problem.

When and Why Bone Loss Occurs

While osteoporosis is commonly considered a disease of old age, in fact, it usually begins decades earlier. A ten-year survey of healthy Americans by Dr. Anthony A. Albanese and colleagues at the Burke Rehabilitation Center in White Plains, New York, showed that as early as age twenty-five, 10 to 15 percent of Americans already show reduced bone density.

Some bone loss with age is considered normal. After menopause, bone loss in women speeds up apparently because the decline in estrogen impairs the ability of a woman's body to absorb dietary calcium and incorporate it into her bones. The loss of bone is accelerated by nervous tension. Cigarette smoking also increases the risk.

Women are also more susceptible to osteoporosis because their bones start out less dense than men's, in part because women tend to be less active physically. Studies of athletes have shown that exercise and muscle development lead to denser bones. Some researchers have used exercise to slow the bone loss of osteoporosis. As little as one hour of mixed exercises repeated three times a week can slow or stop bone loss, one study indicated. Another showed that a daily hourlong walk was effective.

Dr. Albanese points out that the calcium demands of childbearing and breast-feeding can take their toll on a woman's calcium stores unless she consumes sufficient extra calcium to meet her own and her baby's needs. In addition, women are forever going on diets, and bone is lost when weight is lost. Finally, women live longer, increasing their chances of suffering the consequences of bone loss.

Contrary to what most people believe, bones are fluid, not solid, immutable structures. Bone minerals, especially calcium, are continually being removed from and added back to bones throughout the body under the influence of an elaborate network of hormones that includes an activated form of vitamin D. Bones serve two essential functions: They provide structural support, and they are a storehouse for calcium, which is required in tiny amounts by cells throughout the body.

When the blood level of calcium falls below normal (perhaps because inadequate amounts are present in the diet), some calcium is removed from the bones to make up the difference. When your diet provides a surfeit of calcium, more is absorbed through the intestinal tract and some is added back to the bones. However, a prolonged deficiency in absorbed calcium can lead eventually to a net loss of bone calcium and consequent weakening of the bones, making them susceptible to breakage. In some elderly people the bones have become so thin that the stresses of normal walking can cause a fracture. A deficiency of as little as fifty milligrams of calcium a day over a twenty-year period can lead to osteoporosis.

Studies show that the high-protein diet common among Americans can reduce the amount of calcium absorbed. Although diets high in fiber (roughage from grains, fruits, and vegetables) had been thought to interfere with calcium absorption, recent research by the United States Department of Agriculture has shown otherwise.

Treating Bone Loss

Most of the treatments for osteoporosis are still experimental. In postmenopausal women, estrogen replacement therapy can often reduce bone loss. But the hormone treatment may also cause uterine cancer and is usually reserved for women known to face a high risk of bone loss. [See chapter on menopause, page 229.]

Several researchers have reported good results in many, but not all, patients, using a combination of calcium, vitamin D, and fluoride supplements. This treatment is too hazardous to attempt without the guidance of a knowledgeable physician. Fluoride helps to strengthen bones as well as teeth, and osteoporosis is less common in areas where the water is naturally fluoridated. However, fluoride is also a poison, and its use in treating osteoporosis often causes unpleasant side effects. Vitamin D is also poisonous in large doses, and vitamin D supplements should not be taken without medical guidance.

More promising is treatment with the still-experimental activated form of vitamin D known as calcitriol. The body's ability to manufacture this hormone declines with age, particularly after menopause. Treatment with the hormone increases the amount of calcium that can be absorbed from the diet and become incorporated into the bones. A related approach, using phosphate salt and calcitonin, a naturally occurring hormone, also increased bone formation in a preliminary study of women who had suffered fractures as a result of osteoporosis.

Prevention Through Diet and Exercise

After significant bone loss has occurred, it's unlikely that any treatment will be able to restore the bones to their normal density, although some remineralization may be possible. Therefore, prevention is the most effective approach to osteoporosis.

Calcium-rich foods, such as milk (whole, low-fat, skim, or powdered), yogurt, hard cheese, sardines and canned salmon (with bones), and leafy green vegetables, should be a regular part of your diet from youth onward. A quart of milk a day would provide the amount of calcium recommended for adults by osteoporosis researchers. Milk also contains vitamin D and the sugar lactose, which enhance calcium absorption. For those unable to digest milk, fortified soy milk can be a good calcium source, but most tofu (bean curd) available in the United States is not.

CALCIUM-RICH FOODS

Item	Serving size	Calcium (in milligrams)
Sardines, with bones	3 ounces	372
Skim milk	1 cup	296
Whole milk	1 cup	288
Yogurt	1 cup	272
Swiss cheese	1 ounce	262
Cheddar cheese	1 ounce	213
American cheese	1 ounce	198
Oysters	¾ cup	170
Salmon, canned with bones	3 ounces	167
Collard greens	½ cup	145
Cottage cheese, creamed	½ cup	116
Spinach, cooked	½ cup	106
Ice cream	½ cup	97
Mustard greens, cooked	½ cup	97
Corn muffin	2 medium	90
Cottage cheese, dry curd	½ cup	90
Kale, cooked	½ cup	74
Broccoli, cooked	½ cup	68
Orange	1 medium	54

Source: Based on data in Agriculture Handbooks Nos. 8 and 456.

Calcium is absorbed best if consumed in small doses throughout the day. Calcium pills are far less effective than food in increasing your body's calcium supply. Regular exercise throughout life is another important factor in maintaining strong bones.

Asthma:
It's Not Psychosomatic

Known since ancient times, asthma today afflicts at least 9 million Americans of all ages. Yet it remains a remarkably misunderstood ailment, and common misconceptions often stand in the way of a successful battle against this respiratory disorder.

Myth: Asthma attacks can be held in check only by powerful drugs.
Fact: In many cases attacks can be prevented by treatment of the allergies or infections that trigger them. Other harmless treatments, such as biofeedback and breathing exercises, can sometimes head off or lessen the severity of asthma attacks.

Myth: People with asthma cannot exercise.
Fact: Exercise is as important to the asthmatic as to any person, and many athletic activities can be safely pursued. In the 1972 Summer Olympics five gold medalists in swimming events were asthma victims.

For some sufferers asthma is severely disabling, resulting in many lost hours of school or work and frequent hospitalization. But thanks to a better understanding of the disease and improved methods of diagnosis and treatment, today the majority of asthmatics need not be seriously limited. In fact, most asthma victims can lead quite normal lives, and very few become lifelong invalids.

Causes and Prevention

Asthma, a term first used by the Greek father of medicine, Hippocrates, is characterized by attacks of breathlessness that result from one or more of the following conditions: contraction of the muscles, or spasms, in the respiratory passages (tubes) called bronchioles; swelling of the membranes that line the bronchioles, and plugging of the bronchial tubes by excessive amounts of mucus.

These abnormalities reduce the flow of air into and out of the lungs, causing shortness of breath, coughing, wheezing, whistling, and rattling noises as the asthma victim struggles to get air through openings the size of a pinhole. During an attack air enters the lungs more easily than it can be expelled, resulting in a buildup of stale air in the lung sacs, which overstretches them. Untreated attacks may last for minutes, hours, days, or weeks. Over a period of many years overstretched air sacs may lose their elasticity and be rendered useless, resulting in emphysema and chronic shortness of breath.

All asthmatics have what is called a hypersensitive bronchial tree — that is, the network of respiratory tubes tends to overreact to substances or conditions that are innocuous to other people. Among the factors that commonly trigger asthmatic attacks are pollen; mold spores; house dust; animal hair and skin; feathers; insects (including cockroaches); cigarette smoke; household and industrial chemicals; metallic dust; flour; drugs (like aspirin); infections of the nose, throat, and sinuses; certain foods; exercise; exposure to cold air; and emotional distress.

Asthmatics may inherit a predisposition to developing the condition, but environment plays an equally important role. Allergy to one or more substances is the most common cause of asthma in children. In infants food allergy can precipitate asthma, and many specialists urge that children born into allergic families should not be fed anything but breast milk (or soy milk formula) for their first six months of life. Early feeding of solid foods can trigger allergic reactions in susceptible infants.

Children with hay fever seem particularly prone to later developing asthma, and allergists recommend either avoiding exposure to the allergy-provoking pollen (for example, by spending hay fever season on a mountaintop or other pollen-free location) or undergoing desensitization treatments (allergy shots) to prevent the allergic reaction. [See chapter on hay fever, page 542.]

615

Preventing and Treating Attacks

For those who already have asthma, it is essential to be under the care of a physician who is well versed in its management. The doctor's first task is to take a careful history and perhaps to do skin tests to identify the triggering factors. If possible, the patient should avoid exposure to such triggers. Someone whose asthma is triggered by exposure to cold air or exercise may benefit from wearing a cold-weather or surgical mask over the mouth and nose. If an adult becomes sensitive to a substance used at work (such as happened to a baker who developed an asthmatic reaction to flour dust), a job change may be necessary.

For unavoidable inhaled substances like pollen, mold spores, or house dust, allergy desensitization shots over a period of months or years can solve the problem in some cases. If a bacterial infection is the trigger, antibiotic treatment or vaccination may eliminate the problem.

The home of an asthmatic should be kept as free of provoking substances as possible. Residents should avoid smoking indoors. Pets with fur, feathers, or hair are not recommended even if the animal always stays outside. Fish, turtles, lizards, frogs, and snakes, however, are usually OK. The bedroom of an asthmatic should be cleaned regularly and have no dust catchers like drapes, venetian blinds, and knickknacks. Avoid rugs, woolen blankets, bedspreads, feather or kapok-filled pillows or quilts, horsehair mattresses, upholstered furniture, and stuffed animals. Synthetic fabrics and foam are not likely to cause trouble.

An asthmatic should stay away from people with colds and be sure to get the flu vaccine each fall. Aspirin and aspirin-containing drugs are best avoided. Regular balanced meals, lots of liquids, and adequate rest should be a daily routine. Six to eight glasses of water a day can help keep bronchial secretions loose and replace lost fluids.

Daily exercise is very important. Short bouts of exercise (one to two minutes at a time) actually help to open the airways. Swimming is especially encouraged for asthmatics, but football, basketball, tennis, or sprinting may also be possible. If breathing difficulties develop during exercise, the asthmatic can rest until the symptoms subside and then resume the activity. Use of a bronchodilator or an inhaled drug called cromolyn before vigorous activity can often prevent an exercise-induced attack.

Many drugs are available to treat attacks that cannot be prevented. Asthmatics can carry inhalers that stop an attack before it becomes serious. However, these medications should be used only under the guidance of a knowledgeable physician. Misuse or overuse can cause more problems than the drugs solve and may render them useless.

Biofeedback training, in which the patient learns to relax the muscles that cause spasm of the bronchioles, and daily breathing exercises are useful adjuncts to asthma therapy for many patients.

Experts caution against overprotecting asthmatic children or treating them with kid gloves to avoid conflicts. Asthma should not be used as an excuse to skirt household duties and discipline for misconduct, lest the asthmatic child turn into a petty tyrant with serious emotional problems. At the same time a child whose athletic or academic accomplishments are unavoidably limited by asthma should be encouraged to develop other talents or excel in other activities. Psychotherapy may be recommended for families in which emotional problems contribute to or have resulted from asthma.

For Further Reading and Information

Lane, Donald J., and Anthony Storr. *Asthma: The Facts*. New York: Oxford University Press, 1979.

Nolte, Dietrich, M.D. *Speaking of: Asthma*. New York: Delair, 1980.

The Asthma and Allergy Foundation of America, at 19 West Forty-fourth Street, New York, New York 10036, is an excellent source of pamphlets and other information about asthma and its treatment.

Pneumonia: When Respiratory Defenses Are Down

"Don't go out like that, you'll get pneumonia," the concerned mother shouted as her daughter left for school one cold December morning with her coat unbuttoned and her hair wet. The basis for the mother's concern actually is an old wives' tale. Although many things increase one's susceptibility to pneumonia, wet hair, open coats, and cold winds are not among them.

But the mother certainly chose the right season to be thinking about pneumonia. From December through March cases of pneumonia and pneumonia deaths reach an annual peak. For those who, because of age, illness, or other factors, are especially susceptible to pneumonia, this is also the time to get the vaccine that protects against the most common deadly types of bacterial pneumonia.

In winter and early spring people congregate indoors, and viral infections such as colds and flu spread easily from person to person. These infections may impair the normal defenses of the respiratory tract and allow infectious organisms to sneak through and establish residence in the lungs. The result: pneumonia.

Causes: Breaking the Respiratory Barriers

Pneumonia is an infection of the air sacs of the lung. Infected sacs fill with fluid and white blood cells in an attempt to fight the invading microorganisms. Fluid-filled sacs are unable to function properly, and cough and shortness of breath may result.

About three-fourths of pneumonia cases are caused by viruses; most of the rest are bacterial infections. Other types of microorganisms, including mycoplasmas, rickettsiae, and fungi, can also cause pneumonia.

Normally the lower respiratory tract — the bronchial tubes and their branches and the lungs — is protected from invasions by infectious organisms by a variety of defenses. The first line of defense is the epiglottis, the flap of skin that closes off your windpipe each time you swallow and whenever something other than air tries to get into your breathing passages. Next are the mucous secretions and the hairs, or cilia, of the cells lining the respiratory tract. The mucus traps microorganisms, and the cilia sweep them back up into the throat. The normal coughing reflex helps to expel invaders from the bronchial branches. Finally, if all else fails and organisms find their way to the air sacs, they are attacked by macrophages — scavenging white blood cells that gobble up the invaders and carry them off through the lymph system.

Many situations can interfere with these defenses. Mild viral infections of the upper respiratory tract — the nose and throat — can cause large amounts of thin mucus carrying infectious organisms to leak past the epiglottis and down into the lungs. Upper respiratory infections and cigarette smoking also partially paralyze the cilia, impairing their natural cleansing activity. Other factors that interfere with natural defenses in the respiratory tract and increase the chances that invading organisms will reach the air sacs include heavy alcohol intake, surgical anesthesia, large doses of drugs like barbiturates or immune suppressants, and prolonged bed rest.

In addition, some people have chronic health problems that make them especially susceptible to pneumonia. These include persons who have had their spleens removed and those with congestive heart failure, chronic bronchitis, emphysema, asthma, diabetes, cancer, sickle-cell anemia, and immune deficiency diseases. Infants and elderly people are also at a higher than normal risk of developing and dying from pneumonia.

Viral Pneumonia: Usually Mild

Viral pneumonia is more common and usually less serious than bacterial forms of the disease. The exception is when the cause is the influenza A virus, which can result in a severe pneumonia and death, particularly among those who are old or ill to begin with. The best preventive is for high-risk persons to take influenza vaccines each fall. Although imperfect, the vaccine usually protects about two-thirds of those who receive it against the flu viruses that are likely to be around that winter. [See chapter on colds and flu, page 514.]

Most viral pneumonias are mild and often go undetected. They are the usual cause of what is popularly known as walking pneumonia in people who think they have a prolonged cold and cough and may feel very drained of energy but not sick enough to compel them to stay in bed or see a doctor. Even in mild cases a doctor can detect signs of lung congestion through the stethoscope and by tapping on the chest wall, and an X ray would show patches in the lung where air sacs are filled with fluid and debris instead of air.

There is no specific treatment for viral pneumonia except bed rest, a light diet, lots of fluids, oxygen if needed, and small doses of codeine to relieve a severe or painful cough. Most cases heal themselves in time. In all pneumonias it's important to remain at home and in bed for two or three days after fever has completely gone.

Pneumonia caused by mycoplasmas is most common among children and young adults and may cause epidemics in boarding schools and military camps. But the illness, characterized by fever, headache, malaise, chills, and cough, is usually quite mild and rarely causes death. Antibiotics are used to treat those who become severely ill.

Bacterial Pneumonia, a Potential Killer

Bacterial pneumonia is another story. Although the infection is nearly always curable by antibiotics, a patient may die from the cascading effects of the disease anyway, especially if it is not treated promptly or if the individual was in poor health to begin with.

Four out of five cases of bacterial pneumonia are caused by *Streptococcus pneumoniae*, also called the pneumococcus, which comes in eighty-three varieties. A vaccine that has been prepared is effective against the more common strains of this bacterium, which together cause 80 percent of cases of pneumococcal pneumonia.

It takes two weeks to develop an immunity after you receive the vaccine, which can be administered any time of year. The vaccine is not universally recommended for healthy people, even those over sixty-five, but it should be obtained by all people past the age of two who have chronic health problems that increase their susceptibility to pneumonia or death from pneumonia. The vaccine is ineffective in very young children.

Bacterial pneumonia can strike at any time of year. It is more common during flu epidemics because it occurs as a secondary infection in people already weakened by the flu. Typically the disease starts with an attack of shaking chills that last for minutes or hours, although sometimes the onset is less dramatic. Temperature rises rapidly and may reach 105 degrees Fahrenheit or more. Pulse and respiration are usually rapid, and the skin feels hot and dry. Cough, which is often painful, is at first dry but then bloody or rust-colored sputum is raised. Headache, nausea, and vomiting may also occur, and the patient may show signs of oxygen shortage, such as blue lips or nails.

If a doctor suspects bacterial pneumonia on the basis of a physical examination, a bacterial culture of the sputum and blood should be done, and antibiotics (penicillin or a substitute, but not tetracycline because many of the bacteria are resistant to it) should be started immediately. The antibiotic may have to be changed once the culture results are available. The patient should be isolated at first. Complete bed rest is essential, and hospitalization, at least for a few days, is usually advisable. With proper treatment 95 percent of patients recover.

Hernia:
Don't Put Off Repairs

It was moving day at the office, everything was out of place, and Alfred got impatient waiting for the porters to position the desks properly. So he moved them himself. He felt a wrenching pain in his groin, followed a few days later by a distinct bulge. His physician confirmed his suspicions: Alfred had a hernia — his second one — and like the first, it had to be surgically repaired.

A hernia — popularly but inaccurately called a rupture — is a bulge of tissue through a weak spot in a layer of muscle or other tissue. Although repair of hernias is second only to the D and C (dilatation and curettage, in women) as the nation's leading surgical procedure, many people walk around for years with hernias that could at any time become a life-threatening emergency. They "know" they should get them fixed, but somehow the time is never right to give up a month or more of their lives.

Yet hernia repair today can be a simple procedure, done under local anesthesia with only a day or two spent in the hospital and only a few weeks' absence from normal routine. After the hernia repair has healed, there is no restriction in activity. In one type of operation, developed in Toronto, the patient actually participates during the surgery by helping the surgeon test the strength of the repair while there's still an opportunity to improve it.

However, different surgeons have different views about how a hernia operation, called a herniorrhaphy, is best done. Many, for example, prefer general anesthesia, although this can be more hazardous and debilitating for the patient. Some doctors restrict patient activities for many weeks after surgery. It's up to the patient with a hernia to learn about the various alternatives and to discuss the advantages and disadvantges of these choices with the doctor before surgery.

Kinds and Causes

Inguinal, Umbilical, and Femoral. By far the most common type, called an inguinal hernia, occurs in the groin in the muscle wall that encloses the abdominal cavity. It afflicts many more men than women. The weakness is commonly present at birth, but the actual bulging through of underlying tissue may not occur for years. During prenatal development the muscle wall above the spermatic cord may not close tightly, and years later a sudden strain may cause it to give way. Lifting or moving very heavy objects is a frequent precipitant. A hernia can also develop gradually as a result of constant or repeated straining, as in straining to move the bowels.

In some cases boys are born with an inguinal hernia (often a double hernia, one on each side of the abdomen) that necessitates surgery during the first year or two of life.

Other types of hernias include umbilical hernia, which results in a protruding navel in children; femoral hernia, in the upper thigh just below the groin, which is more common in women; and hernias in scar tissue, such as along the suture line of a previous operation.

An inguinal or femoral hernia is a potential hazard whether it hurts or not. A piece of intestine can get trapped — doctors call it incarcerated — in the bulge. If the opening tightens on the loop of intestine, the blood supply can be cut off, causing strangulation and death of the tissue. This is as dangerous as a ruptured appendix. Without immediate surgery, death of the patient can follow. It is far better to repair a hernia on a nonemergency basis.

Hiatal. Hiatal hernia results from a gap in the diaphragm that permits the stomach, intestine, or other abdominal organ to push up into the chest. There is no outwardly visible bulge. The first symptom is usually heartburn that is worse after you have eaten heavy meals or when you lie down or bend forward. Eventually there may develop more severe pain that is aggravated by the consumption of irritating foods and drinks.

The condition, which must be diagnosed by X ray, is very common (20 percent of people over fifty are believed to have it) but usually causes no symptoms. Unlike an inguinal hernia, most cases of hiatal hernia can be treated without surgery — by your eating frequent small meals of bland foods, taking antacids between meals, losing excess weight, avoiding bending forward, and sleeping with the head elevated. Surgery may become necessary, however, if the symptoms cannot be controlled by such conservative measures or if the hernia results in chronic bleeding or hemorrhage.

A free pamphlet, "Person to Person about Hiatal Hernia," is available from the American Digestive Disease Society, Suite 1644, 420 Lexington Avenue, New York, New York 10017.

Treating Inguinal Hernias

Surgeons warn that the wearing of trusses — once a common practice among those who wished to avoid surgery for an inguinal hernia — is of little help and can cause real harm. As Dr. Marvin Reingold, surgeon at Kingsbrook Jewish Medical Center in Brooklyn, New York, explained, a truss may cause symptoms to subside, but the hernia can get progressively larger, and complications can still develop. The prolonged pressure of a truss can lead to pressure sores and breakdown of the underlying tissues, making it impossible later to repair the hernia surgically.

Dr. Reingold is among about 3 percent of American surgeons who routinely perform the Canadian operation, developed at the Shouldice Clinic in Toronto, where 5,800 hernia operations are done each year, about half on Americans. Local anesthesia is used; the patient is awake throughout and can leave the same or the next day. The operation itself involves many layers of tissue, which are sewn together in overlapping fashion. According to Dr. Reingold, this creates an extremely strong repair and reduces the chances that the hernia will recur. The patient begins an exercise program right after surgery, which speeds recovery and diminishes pain and swelling.

Other surgeons object to this operative approach because it violates the natural anatomy, attaching layers of tissue that ordinarily don't go together. With the more traditional operations, surgeons tend to be more cautious about exercise soon after surgery, although nearly all patients walk around the next day. Regardless of the type of operation, local anesthesia can be used, and more and more surgeons are now doing so and sending their hernia patients home within twenty-four hours of surgery.

Warding Off Hernias

While it really isn't possible to prevent a hernia — even a sneeze or cough can theoretically cause a weak spot to give way — certain precautions that are sensible for many parts of the body, especially the back, may forestall trouble.

● Don't plunge right into heavy work. Condition your body slowly to heavy work loads, allowing your muscles to build up strength over a period of weeks.

● Carry heavy objects on your shoulders rather than support them at your hips. Avoid reaching over your shoulders for heavy objects.

● When you must lift something heavy, squat with bent knees and a straight back and with your feet about a foot apart and close to the object. Then lift the object close to your body and, holding it against you, stand up by straightening your knees. If possible, have someone help you lift heavy things, or use a mechanical device.

● Avoid constipation and straining to move the bowels. Include fibrous foods — whole grains and fresh fruits and vegetables — in your daily diet. [See chapter on dietary fiber, page 36.]

Epilepsy: Most Seizures Are Controllable

Epileptics were at one time thought to be possessed by demons and were subjected to exorcisms; at another time they were considered insane or dangerous and were locked up in institutions. Although these extreme notions virtually died with the medical enlightenment of the twentieth century, the more than 2 million Americans with epilepsy are today still greatly misunderstood and often subjected to social, educational, and occupational discrimination that produces a far greater agony than their medical problem itself.

Not a few victims suffer the penalties of misdiagnosis and because of their aberrant behavior are labeled retarded, incorrigible, or mentally ill.

Through the ages a number of people have reached spectacular heights of achievement despite having epilepsy. Among them were Alexander the Great, Julius Caesar, Handel, Dante, Tchaikovsky, Van Gogh, Dostoyevsky, and Alfred Nobel. But many other epileptics have led thwarted, tainted, sheltered lives marred by irrational laws, rejection by others, and feelings of embarrassment, shame, and guilt.

As recently as the mid-1960's some states forbade epileptics to marry, and into the 1970's five states forced them to be sterilized. Even now, despite laws barring job discrimination because of a medical handicap, epileptics who admit to their condition reduce their chances of being hired, and those who lie about it can be fired if the truth is discovered.

In 1977 a special federal committee, the Commission for the Control of Epilepsy and Its Consequences, concluded that epileptics should no longer have to live as second-class citizens. Medical and social services for epileptics need to be expanded, and the public must become better informed about the condition and how to prevent it, recognize it, and treat it. Still, little progress has yet been made.

The Seizures

Epilepsy is a symptom, not a disease. It is the result of an electrical instability of some cells in the brain, which sometimes triggers an "electrical storm" that spreads through part or all of the brain. This results in a seizure, which can take one of many forms. Most patients have only one type of seizure, but nearly a third may experience two or more types.

The so-called *grand mal* seizures are the most common. They typically last two to five minutes and sometimes begin with a mood change or an aura (strange sensations that warn of an impending attack) and an outcry. The victim may fall to the floor and lose consciousness. Muscles become rigid and then contract in a rhythmic convulsion that causes the body to shake violently. The victim may lose control of bladder and bowels and stop breathing temporarily. Afterward the victim may feel sleepy and headachy, but usually will have no memory of the attack. There is no pain, unless the person gets hurt during the seizure. But the dramatic attack leaves a painful impression on anyone who witnesses it.

Far less noticeable are the *petit mal* seizures, which occur mainly in children. There are no convulsions. Rather, there is a lapse of consciousness characterized by blank staring and a lack of responsiveness lasting about ten to thirty seconds. Such attacks can happen many times during a day, especially when the child is sitting still, and can lead to serious learning difficulties if not recognized and treated.

Both the petit and grand mal seizures involve a sudden electrical discharge through the entire brain. Other seizures, called *partial*, involve only certain areas of the brain and may result in staggering, purposeless movements, twitching of part of the body, mental confusion, verbal outbursts, angry attacks, lip smacking and chewing, sudden headaches or abdominal pains, visual or auditory delusions, and dizziness. The seizure lasts usually for a minute or two but sometimes for several hours, during which time victims are out of touch with their surroundings and may resist aid.

623

Many Cases Are Preventable

Epilepsy will develop in 1 to 2 percent of people during their life-time, with 75 percent of the cases arising before age eighteen. It can re-sult from many causes, including a brain injury before or at the time of birth, very high fevers during early childhood, a head injury at any time of life, certain infectious diseases, poisons, nutritional deficiencies, chem-ical imbalances, and brain tumors.

Experts estimate that a quarter to a half of all cases could be pre-vented. The preventive approaches outlined by the federal commission include the following:

• Preventing pregnancy in teenagers, who have an increased risk of bearing children with epilepsy.

• Immunizing children against measles, mumps, and diphtheria, which can sometimes cause brain damage and seizures.

• Preventing head injuries by using lap and shoulder seat belts in cars; wearing helmets while riding motorcycles, mopeds, and bicycles; observing the fifty-five-mile-an-hour speed limit; and not driving under the influence of alcohol.

Another preventive involves the use of phenobarbital, a sedative drug, for a year or so in small children who have had a convulsion dur-ing a high fever and in anyone who suffers a serious head injury or un-dergoes brain surgery. However, many specialists now question whether febrile convulsions do carry any long-term risk and believe that in chil-dren the disadvantages of the drug's side effects may outweigh its poten-tial benefits.

Heredity is believed to play a minor role in epilepsy, serving mainly to enhance (or diminish) a person's susceptibility to developing seizures. Although many people with epilepsy have close relatives with epilepsy, only about 2 to 5 percent of the children of epileptics develop the condi-tion.

Controlling the Seizures

In about half of patients seizures can be totally eliminated by cur-rently available treatments. In another 30 percent the frequency of sei-zures can be greatly reduced. Occasionally the condition can be "cured," for example, when an operable tumor or a correctable chemical imbal-ance is the cause. About half of children with seizures outgrow them, usually when they reach puberty.

Treatment nearly always involves the continuous use of anticonvul-sive drugs — either one or several at a time. More than a dozen such drugs are available, and several different ones or different combinations and varying dose levels may have to be tried before the best treatment is found for a particular patient.

As part of the diagnostic work-up, some patients with seizures will be given a CAT scan, a special brain X ray that may reveal the cause to be a small tumor that can be removed surgically. Whatever the cause, it is especially important that epilepsy be properly diagnosed and treated early in the disorder because when therapy is delayed, seizures tend to become harder to treat and more frequent.

Overcoming Psychosocial Problems

It is far more difficult to prevent and treat the social and psychological consequences of epilepsy than the symptom itself. Many families would benefit from counseling. Most children with epilepsy can and should be educated in regular classrooms, but some teachers resist having a child in class who may have a seizure. In most cases it is not necessary to curtail a child's participation in athletics. In fact, physical activity helps to reduce the frequency of seizures.

On the other hand, the frequency of seizures is likely to be increased by stress, economic and social frustrations, and an irregular daily life. This is a "Catch-22" in the life of an employable epileptic who is unable to get a job. Every state has an office of the Department of Vocational Rehabilitation to help those who need job training. For epileptics able to work, the State Employment Service can assist in finding suitable jobs. Those unable to work at a regular job may benefit from employment in sheltered workshops that exist in many cities.

FIRST AID FOR EPILEPTIC SEIZURES

The Epilepsy Foundation of America recommends the following first-aid measures if you witness someone having a grand mal seizure:

1. Keep calm. Do not try to restrain the person, but ease him or her to the floor, and loosen his or her collar.

2. Clear the surrounding area of hard, sharp, or hot objects on which the seizure victim may get hurt.

3. Do not force anything between the teeth. If the victim's mouth is already open, you might place a soft object, such as a folded handkerchief, between the side teeth to keep the person from biting his or her tongue.

4. If you can, turn the person on the side or turn the head to one side so that saliva may flow out of the mouth, and place something soft under the head.

5. Following the seizure, let the person rest. However, if the seizure lasts beyond a few minutes or if seizures occur one after another, call a doctor immediately.

There is nothing you can do for petit mal seizures, which are characterized by vacant staring. For partial seizures that involve movements, keep dangerous objects out of the person's way. But don't try to restrain him or her unless the person is heading for a hazard. Restraint may cause the person to struggle or lash out and hurt you.

Remember that behavior during a seizure is unconscious and that once a seizure has begun, there is nothing you can do to stop it.

For Further Reading and Information

Sands, Harry, and Frances C. Minters. *The Epilepsy Fact Book*. New York: Scribner's, 1981.

The Epilepsy Foundation of America has chapters in every state that can provide information and guidance for epileptics, their families, and prospective employers. Among the foundation's services are counseling, referrals for professional help, job assistance, medical services, patient advocacy services, and educational programs for teachers. Members can benefit from reduced rates for drugs and can purchase life insurance through the organization. The foundation's main office is at 1828 L Street NW, Washington, D.C. 20036.

XIV. Common Killers

From time to time you've probably worried or at least thought about the major lethal diseases that strike Americans. But there is almost an inverse relationship between the level of concern people have about killers like heart disease and cancer and what people do to protect themselves against them. Yet, for the big killers in particular, prevention is not only the best medicine but often the *only* medicine. Frequently the way you live determines how you die and how healthy you'll be in the later decades of your life. Herein lies the secret to prolonging useful, pleasurable life.

When a potentially lethal disease strikes, the way it is treated also can make a big difference in the outcome: whether you live or die and, if you live, what the quality of your life will be. Life-threatening diseases are just that: They are not automatic death sentences. Rather, they are challenges to surmount the obstacles of illness. How much you know about them can determine how well you meet that challenge.

627

Preventing Heart Disease: It's in Your Hands

The doctor's voice was stern: "You're twenty pounds overweight, your blood pressure is too high, and so is your cholesterol level. Your weekend golf game hardly counts as exercise, and the two packs of cigarettes a day — I guess I don't need to tell you about *that*. If you want to live to see your family grow up, you're simply going to have to take better care of yourself. On the other hand, if you want to drop dead of a heart attack before you're fifty, you can continue as you are."

Jack was forty-three years old and a little scared by the doctor's no-nonsense tone and harsh warning. He began to mourn the "good life" he was going to have to give up: the eggs and bacon he loved for breakfast; the hamburgers, french fries, and beer for lunch; the two martinis before dinner; and the big juicy sirloins that followed. And the cigarettes — he really needed those cigarettes to relieve the tensions of selling advertising. And exercise, when was he going to squeeze that into his already frenetic schedule?

The "cure" seemed worse than the disease. And what was this disease anyway? He felt perfectly fine. The doctor hadn't found anything wrong with his heart, had he? Why should he sacrifice all these things he enjoyed to prevent something that only *might* happen at some future date?

Reduce Your Risk Factors

Growing numbers of Americans of all ages and both sexes are today grappling with similar choices. If not confronted by their doctors, they get the message from friends and spouses, newspapers and magazines, radio and television: If you want to preserve your heart and prevent premature death, you must reduce your coronary risk factors. Many studies have shown that people who suffer heart attacks tend to have a disproportionate number of these risk factors, including elevated blood pressure and cholesterol, cigarette smoking, obesity, poor blood sugar control, and stressful lives but sedentary life-styles.

The landmark Framingham Heart Study, in which thousands of adults in one town were periodically examined and followed for more than twenty years, showed that the more risk factors a person has, the greater his or her chances of developing premature heart disease. But many Americans remain unconvinced by such circumstantial evidence. It is easier, less painful, and certainly less life-disrupting to stick to their falsely secure attitude that "it can't happen to me; anyway, we all have to die of something sometime."

Hidden Damage

A team of cardiovascular specialists at the University of California School of Medicine at Davis has shown that even before you suffer a heart attack, your coronary risk factor score can reveal just how much hidden damage your heart and its blood vessels may have already suffered. Following a thorough examination, the team assigned a risk factor score to each of 158 patients aged thirty-eight to sixty-one who were complaining of chest pains. All the patients then had the status of their coronary blood vessels evaluated by following the progress of an injected dye on an X ray movie.

Patients who were found to have atherosclerosis blocking 75 percent or more of any major artery feeding the heart turned out to have risk factor scores that were 50 percent higher than patients whose coronary arteries were free of major obstructions. Those with two arteries that were significantly blocked had higher risk factor scores than those with only one blocked artery, and the scores were even higher if three arteries turned out to be obstructed.

Thus, the authors concluded, a person's risk factor score is a good indication of what is happening unseen to his or her heart even before a heart attack occurs.

Why is all this important? Because in 25 percent of cases the first outward sign of heart disease is sudden death from a heart attack, and 60 percent of heart attacks end in sudden death. Some 600,000 Americans die of heart attacks each year — and 160,000 of them are below the age of sixty-five. Your risk factor score may be the only warning you get of the damage being done to the crucial blood vessels that feed your heart. When a blood vessel is three-quarters blocked by atherosclerosis, all it takes is a small clot or spasm to close it off completely and — boom — you have a heart attack.

So Jack's doctor was not talking tough for nothing. He was trying to get Jack to change his habits while there was still time to prevent or reverse the damage to his coronary arteries.

What You Can Do

Cardiologists who specialize in the prevention of heart disease recommend that every person — male and female, young and old — adopt the following goals to control the major risk factors:

Blood pressure. The blood pressure of the average American rises with age, but studies among populations in which heart disease is rare show that this is not natural, inevitable, or desirable. It is best to keep your blood pressure throughout life down around 120/80 or lower. If it rises above 140/90, treatment to lower it can be lifesaving. Weight loss and reduction of salt in your diet can help prevent the development of high blood pressure and lower pressures that are already too high. Drugs may also be used if these measures are not adequate. [See chapters on high blood pressure, page 631, salt, page 66, and permanent weight control, page 72.]

Blood cholesterol. The average cholesterol level of middle-aged American males is 225 milligrams percent. But "average" in this country is neither normal nor healthy. It is too high. In countries where heart disease is not the epidemic it is here, "average" is more like 160 or 180, but certainly below 200 — which is where yours should be throughout life. You can usually accomplish this by keeping your average daily intake of cholesterol below 300 milligrams and restricting your consumption of saturated (animal) fats, which tend to raise blood cholesterol levels. A diet that emphasizes grains, beans, fruits, and vegetables and deemphasizes meats, dairy products, and egg yolks (the yolk of one large egg has 250 milligrams of cholesterol) can be satisfying and delicious as well as healthful. [See the chapters on protein, page 8, and fats and cholesterol, page 14.]

Smoking. In short, *don't.* Cigarette smokers have a 70 percent greater chance of developing coronary heart disease than persons who don't smoke. In fact, the decline in smoking by American men is thought to be the main reason behind the recent decline in coronary deaths. [See chapters on smoking risks, page 251, and quitting smoking, page 256.]

Obesity. Keep your weight within five pounds of ideal, according to up-to-date height and weight charts. Forty percent of all Americans are twenty or more pounds overweight; this excess weight fosters the development of fat-clogged arteries and high blood pressure. [See chapter on permanent weight control, page 72.]

Blood sugar. If you have diabetes or tests show that your blood sugar gets too high, keep your weight down and increase your physical activity. Complex carbohydrates — unrefined cereal grains, dried peas and beans, and other starchy foods that are rich in natural fiber — should be a major part of your diet, but keep down the amount of sugars, fats, and cholesterol you eat. [See chapter on diabetes, page 660.]

Exercise. Put motion into your life on a regular basis — if not jogging, swimming, or tennis, then brisk walking or jumping rope. Regular exercise helps to increase the amount of work your heart can do efficiently and without excessive strain. Exercise also helps you to control your weight and relieve your tensions. [See the section on exercise, page 85.]

Stress. Although its relationship to heart disease is not entirely clear, undue emotional tension is hardly desirable for your cardiovascular system or for you in general. Eliminate unnecessary sources of anxiety in your life, and try activities like meditation, tennis, running, dancing, yoga, or karate to relieve those tensions that are inevitable. [See chapters on stress, page 138, and Type A behavior, page 142.]

Millions of Americans who have tried it will tell you that living a low coronary risk life is hardly joyless. On the contrary, it helps you to feel good about yourself, work more efficiently, and probably live longer to enjoy life's more lasting pleasures. Try it, and you just might find that you like it.

For Further Reading

Aegerter, Dr. Ernest, *Save Your Heart*. New York: Van Nostrand Reinhold, 1981.

American Heart Association. *Heartbook*. New York: E.P. Dutton, 1980.

Blakeslee, Alton, and Jeremiah Stamler, M.D. *Your Heart Has Nine Lives*. New York: Pocket Books, 1966.

Cope, Lewis. *Save Your Life*. Minneapolis: Minneapolis Tribune, 1979.

Dietrich, Edward B., M.D. *Heart Test*. New York: Cornerstone, 1981.

Duke University Medical Center. *The Heart Book*. New York: Delair, 1981.

Farquhar, John W., M.D. *The American Way of Life Need Not Be Hazardous To Your Health*. New York: W.W. Norton, 1979.

Havas, Stephen, M.D. *Exercise and Your Heart*. Washington, D.C.: U.S. Department of Health and Human Services, 1981. Single copies are available free from the Consumer Information Center, Pueblo, Colo. 81009.

Mulcahy, Risteard, M.D. *Beat Heart Disease!* New York: Arco, 1979.

Nora, James J., M.D. *The Whole Heart Book*. New York: Holt, Rinehart & Winston, 1980.

High Blood Pressure: It Starts in Childhood

About 60 million adult Americans have high blood pressure, a major cause of premature death and disability in this country. Most people think of high blood pressure as a disease of old age, but doctors now realize that the problem actually has its roots in childhood.

Thanks to genetic inheritance, diet, weight, living habits, responses to stress, and probably other as yet unidentified factors, 15 percent of American children are destined to develop high blood pressure; by age sixty-five, half of us have this silent killer.

For some, abnormally elevated blood pressures may start as early as the first year of life. For others, late childhood or adolescence marks the beginning of a significant blood pressure problem. But since few children ever have their blood pressure taken and even fewer have it taken regularly, the matter of high blood pressure — and the possibility of preventing it from becoming a serious health problem — are completely overlooked in routine pediatric care.

Causes and Effects

In very young children, high blood pressure may result from an underlying and possibly correctable disorder, such as kidney disease or a defect in the aorta, the body's main artery. More often high blood pressure, or hypertension, as it is called medically, has no apparent cause. It may develop in a setting of a high-salt diet or obesity, but the underlying abnormality is not known.

Hypertension is an insidious problem that may cause no symptoms for decades. But left untreated, it greatly increases the risk of developing three of the nation's leading killers and cripplers — heart disease, stroke, and kidney failure. If you have high blood pressure, your heart has to work harder than it should to pump blood, your kidneys have to work harder to try to regulate your blood pressure, and your arteries undergo excessive wear and tear and accumulate abnormally large fatty deposits that reduce their ability to transport blood.

A person with so-called mild hypertension has twice the average risk of dying before age sixty-five, and a person with moderately severe hypertension is three times more likely to die before age 65 than someone with normal blood pressure. Children are just as likely as adults to suffer damage caused by hypertension, and the earlier in life that the problem starts, the more severe the consequences.

However, in nearly all cases the risk can be greatly reduced by effectively controlling high blood pressure through a combination of diet, weight loss, exercise, and, if necessary, drugs. While there is no surefire way to prevent hypertension, experts believe that by identifying hypertension-prone youngsters at an early age and instituting simple adjustments in life-style, many cases of high blood pressure would never develop.

632

Dr. Jennifer Loggie, professor of pediatrics at the University of Cincinnati, says that every child over the age of three should have his or her blood pressure taken once a year and at every visit to the doctor during adolescence and adulthood. To get a reliable reading, the child should be at ease and the surroundings quiet. In suspicious cases in which adequate calm cannot be achieved in the doctor's office, the parent may be told how to take the child's blood pressure at home.

Measuring Blood Pressure

Blood pressure is measured by an instrument called a sphygmomanometer and is recorded as two numbers, in the style of a fraction: the arterial pressure when the heart beats (the systolic pressure) over the arterial pressure between heartbeats (diastolic pressure).

To get an accurate reading in children, the doctor must use a blood pressure cuff that is the right size for the child's arm (there is a standard-sized cuff for adults). It should cover two-thirds of the upper arm, and the inflatable portion should meet but not overlap. To determine the normality of a blood pressure reading in a child, the doctor should plot it on a curve that describes the normal distribution of blood pressure for children of the same age. A reading of 120 over 70 would be considered normal for an adult but is high for a four-year-old, whose pressure should be about 105 over 60.

At least three measurements should be taken at three separate visits before the doctor decides whether a person has abnormally high blood pressure. A single reading is totally unreliable. If a child is found to have high blood pressure, other members of the family should be checked as well. When the parents have high blood pressure, the doctor should be certain to check the children's pressures regularly.

If blood pressure is found to be abnormally high on several separate readings, the doctor should look for possible underlying causes by doing a thorough physical examination and a variety of lab tests. A kidney X ray may be recommended. The doctor should also take a careful family medical history to determine whether there is a high risk of hypertension-related diseases.

Treating Essential Hypertension

In most cases no underlying cause will be found for elevated blood pressure — which is then called essential or primary hypertension. To treat and to prevent this condition, the following factors should be taken into account:

Controlling weight. Dr. Sidney Blumenthal, who directs a task force on hypertension in children for the National Heart, Lung and Blood Institute, points out that at any age there is a close relationship between overweight and high blood pressure. In children, excess weight need not mean gross obesity to cause an abnormal rise in blood pressure. Maintaining a normal body weight is a harmless and important way to keep blood pressure low. [See chapter on permanent weight control, page 72.]

Limiting dietary salt. It may shock you to learn that salt — that is, the table salt sodium chloride — is not an essential dietary additive. Enough salt is present naturally in foods to meet body requirements for sodium. Yet Americans commonly consume three to five times more salt each day than if they just relied on the salt already in food. [See chapter on salt, page 66.]

Many Americans are resistant to high blood pressure and don't get it despite a diet high in salt and other sources of sodium. But up to half of us are not so fortunate, and it is impossible to tell in advance who these susceptible people are. In populations in which salt intake is extremely low, hypertension is a rare disease. When laboratory rats that are genetically predisposed to hypertension are placed on a high-salt diet, they develop severe high blood pressure and die at an early age. But the same genetic strain will live a full life without high blood pressure if their diets are low in salt.

Hypertension experts are especially concerned about the salt in infant foods. Cow's milk has four times the sodium content of human milk. Leading manufacturers have greatly reduced the amount of salt in prepared baby food. But Dr. Blumenthal points out that the tendency to start infants on table food early in life may defeat this measure because table food is usually salted to the family's tastes.

For adolescents, salt is a particular problem. A single commercial hamburger and a serving of potato chips contains four-fifths of the recommended daily salt intake, and that doesn't include the pickles.

Dr. Jeremiah Stamler, a cardiologist at Northwestern University, recommends that Americans should halve their regular salt intake. He suggests adding little or no salt during cooking or at the table and avoiding heavily presalted foods, such as tomato juice, canned vegetables and soups, convenience foods, salted snacks, and condiments. Instead of salt, learn to use herbs, spices, garlic, onions, and peppers to season foods.

Exercising regularly. Aerobic exercises like swimming, running, cycling, and brisk walking, which promote the use of oxygen and can be sustained for more than a few minutes at a time, help to lower blood pressure and keep it low. However, isometric exercises like wrestling, water skiing and weight lifting, which clamp down on the muscles, actually raise blood pressure and should be avoided by people prone to hypertension. [See chapter on how to choose an exercise, page 88.]

Reducing other risk factors. It is especially important for a person with high blood pressure or a high normal pressure to avoid other factors that predispose to heart disease, such as a diet high in fats and cholesterol and cigarette smoking.

Drug Therapy

Some 30 to 40 percent of children who have high blood pressure readings will outgrow the problem as they get older. Therefore, doctors are extremely reluctant to use drugs to reduce blood pressure in children, unless the child's pressure remains significantly higher than normal for his age despite attempts to bring it down using the harmless measures described above. In many people with mild to moderate hypertension, a low-sodium diet can reduce blood pressure to normal levels.

In cases where drugs are necessary, doctors start with mild ones least likely to cause long-term side effects, progressing to more potent medications only for those who need it. In adults the use of drugs to reduce even moderately elevated blood pressure has been shown to have lifesaving effects. Anyone on medication to reduce blood pressure should see to it that swallowing the pill each day becomes as routine as brushing teeth. It does no good to take the drug for a while and then to stop when the blood pressure is reduced to normal. The medication does not eliminate the cause of high blood pressure, and it works to lower pressure — and to reduce the risks associated with hypertension — only while it is being taken.

Any person — child or adult — placed on medication to lower blood pressure should be sure to report discomforting side effects to the doctor. There are more than two dozen medications that might be used, and chances are the doctor can find one that controls hypertension without causing debilitating side effects.

For Further Reading

Wolff, Hanns P., M.D. *Speaking of: High Blood Pressure*. New York: Delair/Consolidated, 1978.

Heart Attack Symptoms: Swift Action Saves Lives

In the midst of an after-luncheon speech to a large group of his constituents a New England politician in his forties developed a crushing pain in the middle of his chest and became light-headed and short of breath. He continued talking, and the pain seemed to settle in his throat. Thinking a fishbone from lunch might have lodged there, after the speech he visited an ear, nose, and throat specialist, but the doctor found no bone.

On the way back to his hotel with his aides the politician passed out and was taken to a hospital emergency room, where an electrocardiogram revealed that a myocardial infarction — a heart attack — was in progress.

Asked later about his response to his symptoms, the politician said it never occurred to him that the pain might be coming from his heart (although both his father and an uncle had had heart attacks at about his age). When no bone was found, he said he thought momentarily about his heart but quickly dismissed it because "I could not imagine it would happen to me — not in that way — in front of an audience."

Denial and Delay Can Be Deadly

This case, related by Dr. Thomas P. Hackett to a meeting of the American Heart Association, unfortunately is typical of the way most Americans deal with the symptoms of a possible heart attack: They deny that anything serious could be wrong, they attribute the symptoms to some other organ with less lethal implications than the heart, and the victim's companions share in the denial and fail to take appropriate action.

Studies of hundreds of people who suffered heart attacks revealed that on the average four to five hours elapse between the onset of symptoms and arrival of the patient at a hospital. In fact, some people walk around for days with increasingly severe symptoms of an impending heart attack and do nothing about it until they literally collapse.

This delay in making the correct diagnosis and starting life-saving medical care is believed to be responsible for the unnecessary loss of more than 100,000 lives each year and needless damage to the hearts of tens of thousands of others who survive their heart attacks. The first hour after a heart attack is the period of greatest danger — when 40 to 45 percent of deaths occur, most of which could be prevented — but the aver-

635

age patient does not come under proper care until the maximum risk has passed.

Recognizing the Signs

A major problem is that many people don't recognize the symptoms of a heart attack because these symptoms may be vague and readily ascribed to something else. Between 70 and 90 percent of patients have chest pains of sufficient intensity to stop them from what they are doing. But contrary to what many believe, a heart attack usually does not produce a giant immobilizing pain that takes one's breath away. Nor does a heart attack cause a sharp, stabbing pain.

The pain is more like uncomfortable pressure, fullness, or a squeezing sensation in the center of the chest behind the breast bone — like a sack of sand pressing on the chest. The pain may radiate to the shoulder, neck, or arms, and it may come and go, sometimes disappearing for hours or overnight. The heart attack victim may also feel weak, nauseated, or short of breath. Many patients apparently mistake their symptoms for indigestion since the most common response to the pain of a heart attack is to reach for an antacid.

It is not uncommon for the first symptoms of a heart attack to begin at a time of emotional or physical stress, such as while the person is giving a speech or playing tennis. But a heart attack can happen at any time, any place, and under any circumstances, awake or asleep.

The American Heart Association recommends that anyone experiencing chest discomfort that lasts more than two minutes should go to a hospital immediately. Once at the hospital, the patient should be treated as if he or she were having a heart attack until it is proved otherwise.

A person in the midst of a heart attack may have a normal electrocardiogram, and doctors sometimes mistakenly reassure patients that "it's not your heart" because the tracing on the cardiogram is normal. Various blood tests must also be done. It may take three days of hospital tests to rule out — or confirm — a heart attack.

One in five heart attacks is not diagnosed at the time it occurs, and many thousands of people are walking around today with damaged hearts and don't know it. These so-called silent infarcts are missed because they produce little or no pain or because they cause only brief — or no — electrocardiographic or blood changes. Sometimes the doctor simply misses the diagnosis. But by far the most common problem in missed and delayed diagnosis is denial by the patient and his or her companions that a heart attack could be occurring.

Overcoming Denial

Dr. Hackett, who is director of psychiatry at Massachusetts General Hospital in Boston, says that like the New England politician, patients commonly feel "it couldn't be happening to me." Or they don't want to "cause a fuss" or get the doctor out of bed. In one study more than 90 percent took an over-the-counter medicine or home remedy — ranging from Tums to alcohol — and half actually increased their physical activity for a while after their symptoms began.

Some knew they were having a heart attack but did nothing about it because they preferred death to what they imagined would be life as a "cardiac cripple." In fact, the great majority of people who survive a heart attack are hardly cripples. Rather, they lead full, normal lives, taking only moderate precautions to preserve their hearts.

Dr. Hackett maintains that teaching people the symptoms of a heart attack is not enough to overcome denial. Denial is also common among people who know the symptoms, such as patients who have already had one heart attack and physicians, who delay twice as long as average in responding to their own heart attack symptoms.

A person who realizes he is having a heart attack feels a sense of impending disaster, which pushes him further into denial. "Denial of peril is one of our most basic responses to danger," Dr. Hackett points out. But, he adds, it may be possible to counter it by telling people to *expect* to deny heart attack symptoms and to blame them on other organ systems.

"We should tell people that when they reach for a Brioschi to ease the pain that has been there over two minutes, they should instead reach for a phone and get to the hospital," Dr. Hackett recommends.

637

Whoever is with the patient at the time symptoms occur — spouse, business associate, friend, or passerby — is perhaps the most effective means of countering denial. (Unfortunately a wife is as likely to deny her husband's symptoms as he is.) Dr. Hackett believes if that person — called the heartsaver by the American Heart Association — takes executive action, telling the patient, "Come on, we're going to the hospital right now," the most reluctant, denying patient will go along.

For Further Reading

Halhuber, Carola, M.D., and Max Halhuber, M.D. *Speaking of: Heart Attacks.* New York: Delair/Consolidated, 1978.

Stroke: Preventing Disability

True or false?
- Strokes happen only to older people.
- They strike without warning.
- There is nothing you can do to prevent them.
- Few who survive strokes are ever normal again.

All the above statements are, as you may have guessed, false. The very myths that surround stroke — the nation's third leading cause of death — contribute to the fact that it disables so many thousands of Americans annually. The truths are that stroke can occur at any age, though it is far more common after age sixty; that many, perhaps most, strokes are preventable; and that to be most effective, prevention should start while you are young.

Furthermore, strokes often give warnings that can alert you and your physician to the need for treatments that can head off a potentially crippling attack.

Even after a major stroke has occurred, all is not lost. Though most stroke victims suffer some lasting disability, about a third recover fully, and those who do not can often regain many of their abilities through modern rehabilitation programs. Louis Pasteur suffered a stroke at age forty-six that nearly killed him, but through determined effort he returned to work, and despite lasting paralysis on his left side, he continued his pioneering work in establishing the lifesaving science of immunology. [See chapter on surviving a stroke, page 680.]

Types of Strokes

A stroke is a sudden disruption of the blood supply to a part of the brain, which in turn disrupts the body function controlled by that brain area. Without a source of fresh blood, brain cells are deprived of oxygen, which can paralyze or kill them, depending on how long the deficit lasts. Though cell paralysis is often reversible and the lost function is regained after a while, death of brain cells is permanent, usually leaving lasting disability. Sometimes, however, uninjured cells can take over the lost brain functions.

Strokes are of three major types, as follows:

Thrombotic. The most common type, it arises in arteries supplying the brain that have become partly closed by the fatty deposits of atherosclerosis. Blood flow around the obstructions is slowed so clots can form and lodge in the clogged vessel, blocking the blood supply to a part of the brain. (An identical process in the coronary arteries is the primary cause of heart attack.)

Embolic. In these cases a wandering clot becomes lodged in a cerebral artery and, as in the thrombotic stroke, blocks the blood flow.

Hemorrhagic. Sometimes, because of a weakness present from birth or as a result of uncontrolled high blood pressure, a "blowout" occurs in a cerebral artery, and a leakage of blood or a hemorrhage results. The fatality rate from this type of stroke is extremely high, and the chances of complete recovery are less than with strokes caused by clots.

Of the half million Americans who suffer strokes each year, two-thirds survive. Among the survivors a third recover fully or nearly so and are able to return to their usual activities. About half remain partly handicapped, and 15 percent are incapacitated. Nearly 3 million Americans alive today have suffered strokes.

Preventing Strokes

With or without full recovery, a stroke and the frightening damage it can induce are usually a devastating experience. Although little progress has been made in reducing the death rate among the victims of strokes, much is known about how to prevent them. The main clues to prevention reside in the factors known to increase a person's risk of suffering a stroke. Most of these factors are identical to those that increase the chances of a heart attack, so preventing one may prevent both.

High blood pressure. This silent health problem is the single most common factor associated with strokes, both the clot and the hemorrhagic types. More than half of strokes occur in people with high blood pressure. Even mild hypertension, if not adequately treated, increases the risk. Elevated blood pressure promotes clogging of the arteries and puts abnormal pressure on walls of blood vessels, possibly causing a rupture at a weak spot. Your blood pressure should be checked regularly (twice a year from mid-life on), and consistently high pressure should be treated with a low-sodium diet, weight control and, if necessary, drugs. [See chapters on salt, page 66, and high blood pressure, page 631.]

High-fat diet. The typical American diet, rich in saturated fats and cholesterol, promotes atherosclerosis, the accumulation of fatty deposits in arteries throughout the body, most critically in the arteries that nourish the heart and the brain. Lowering your blood cholesterol level (if it is above 200 milligrams per 100 milliliters) by eating less fat and fewer cholesterol-rich animal foods may reduce your risk of brain-damaging clots. [See chapter on fats and cholesterol, page 14.]

Stress. A stroke often seems to be precipitated by stress, perhaps through a direct effect on circulation in the brain or because stress raises blood pressure. Various relaxation techniques or professional counseling may help to improve the quality of your life as well as ward off a stroke. [See chapters on stress, page 138, and Type A behavior, page 142.]

Inactivity. Though the link between sedentary living and stroke is not firmly established, the potential benefits of exercise to the circulation — less atherosclerosis, larger and more numerous blood vessels — should benefit the brain as well as the heart. However, exercise should be regular and moderate; occasional bursts of vigorous activity could actually precipitate a stroke. [See section on exercise, page 85.]

Smoking. Again, although the evidence is not conclusive, most researchers believe that for men at least, stroke should be added to the list of life-threatening disorders that may be increased by tobacco smoke, probably because of nicotine's adverse effects on blood vessels. Men who are heavy smokers have nearly three times as many strokes as nonsmokers, with the effect of smoking most prominent in men aged forty-five to

639

fifty-four. [See chapter on quitting smoking, page 256.]

Obesity. This all too common health problem increases the likelihood of a person's developing high blood pressure, heart disease, and diabetes, all of which in turn increase the risk of stroke. [See chapter on permanent weight control, page 72.]

Oral contraceptives. Women who suffer migraine headaches while taking birth control pills that contain estrogen face an increased risk of stroke. The pill is also a stroke hazard to women in their forties, especially those who smoke. [See chapter on birth control, page 192.]

Heed the Warning Signs

Other factors linked to stroke, such as being male, black, or genetically prone to atherosclerosis, are not under your control. However, greater attention to life habits and underlying diseases that are also linked to stroke can reduce risk substantially.

One such problem, called transient ischemic attacks, or TIAs, actually serves as a warning sign of an impending stroke. Recognition and prompt treatment of TIAs can avert a serious stroke. A TIA is actually a ministroke caused by a temporary loss of blood supply to a part of the brain. It lasts usually for only a few minutes and nearly always less than an hour, with complete recovery within a day.

640

Symptoms are often vague and confusing, and because they are temporary, people tend to brush them off. However, any of the following symptoms, even in people as young as thirty or forty, should be brought to a doctor's attention without delay: weakness of or numbness in an arm, hand, leg, or facial muscles, usually only on one side of the body; difficulty in speaking, understanding speech, or swallowing; failing or blurry vision in one or both eyes; deafness or ringing in the ears; clumsiness or mild loss of balance; dizziness or fainting, often with double vision; sudden, unexplained headache; abrupt personality disturbances (irritability, impatience, suspiciousness); impaired judgment; or forgetfulness.

Four out of five stroke victims have a history of TIAs, and 35 percent of them suffer a stroke within five years unless treatment intervenes. Effective treatments include the use of anticoagulant drugs, small daily doses of aspirin, or surgery. Stroke-preventing operations include bypass surgery to improve circulation to an area of the brain supplied by a damaged artery and surgery to clean out the carotid arteries, blood vessels in the neck that are the main source of the brain's blood supply. Other risk factors would also be treated.

For Further Reading

Hess, Lucille J., and Robert E. Bahr, M.D. *What Every Family Should Know About Strokes.* New York: Appleton-Century-Crofts, 1981.

Sarno, John E., M.D., and Martha Taylor Sarno. *Stroke*, rev. ed. New York: McGraw-Hill, 1979.

Cancer Treatment: Lifesaving Improvements

Every year more than 800,000 Americans face a diagnosis of serious cancer. It is the disease Americans fear most, though heart disease is by far the greater killer. It is made all the more frightening by the fact that few of us face such a diagnosis more than once in our lives, and we tend to remember those cancer patients who died tragically and painfully far more readily than we recall those who fought cancer and won. In their fear and confusion many patients turn their backs on scientifically established remedies and choose instead unproved treatments that offer unjustifiable promises of cure.

A diagnosis of cancer is naturally cause for despair, but many patients incorrectly regard it as an automatic death sentence. Current data on cancer survival do not justify such a fatalistic outlook. Among patients diagnosed as having a life-threatening cancer in the early seventies, two in five were still alive five years later, with the vast majority of them having been cured of their disease.

During the last decade survival rates improved significantly for many cancers, and a number of new and better therapies which are now benefiting many thousands of patients were developed. Thus, experts believe the chances of being cured of cancer now exceed 40 percent and may even approach 50 percent. For some cancers, including several that were once almost universally fatal, 80 percent or more of patients can now look forward to a lasting cure.

Increasing the Odds for Cure

Your chances for cure depend very much on how your cancer is treated. Cancer therapy is now in a state of explosive evolution, and physicians are often hard put to keep up with the barrage of new developments. Patients, too, are often reluctant to look beyond the first doctor they see for an opinion on the best approach to treatment. As a result, many patients are not benefiting from the latest treatments that offer the best chance for cure.

Dr. Isadore Rosenfeld, author of *Second Opinion* (New York: Linden Press, 1978), points out:

> It is extremely important to get the best and most up-to-date opinion from an expert in the field about how to treat any malignancy as soon as it is discovered. If you are told that you have cancer, regardless of its type or location, no matter what outlook you are given, you must get an opinion from an expert oncologist [a doctor with special training in cancer treatment]. Your family doctor, internist, and even one cancer specialist may not be enough.

Dr. Vincent DeVita, director of the National Cancer Institute, emphasizes the importance of getting a second opinion from a qualified physician. He says, "When you face any disease that may kill you, don't rely on the judgment of a single person. A second opinion is especially important if the first doctor has a pessimistic view of your chances for recovery."

The Diagnosis

The most important first step in dealing with cancer is to be sure the diagnosis is correct. Many purported cases of cancer "cured" by vitamins, special diets, mind control, or any other unproved remedy actually involve patients who never had a proper diagnosis and more than likely did not have cancer to begin with.

A diagnosis of cancer should be based on a biopsy: Suspicious cells are removed from the patient and examined microscopically by a pathologist, preferably one who frequently deals with the diagnosis of cancer. If the cancer involves blood-forming organs (leukemia, for example), the diagnosis is based on a blood test and bone marrow sample; in the case of solid tumors (such as breast cancer), the tumor usually must be removed surgically to make the correct diagnosis. Sometimes a needle biopsy, in which a small amount of tissue is removed through a large hypodermic needle, is possible.

If you are being treated at a major teaching hospital (where doctors are trained to become specialists in various fields) or at a nationally recognized cancer center supported by the National Cancer Institute, it's safe to assume the pathologist's diagnosis is correct. However, if there is any doubt in the pathologist's mind whether the cells are truly malignant or what type of cancer it may be, then another pathologist's opinion is in order. Any good pathologist would automatically consult another expert in such a situation, but patients have a right to seek their own independent consultations.

The Treatment

After a diagnosis of cancer has been made, the doctor may try to determine if the disease has spread — metastasized — beyond the site of origin before treatment is actually begun. Special tests, such as a bone scan or X rays, may be done to search for evidence of spread before treating the main tumor. There are approximately 100 kinds of cancer, and your treatment and prognosis for cure will be based on the kind you have and whether it is still confined to one area or has already metastasized.

Once you know what you're dealing with, the next job is to be sure the doctor who is caring for you or the hospital where you are being treated has solid experience in treating that type of cancer. A doctor or hospital that treats only a few cases a year of a particular cancer may not be able to apply the best therapy. In such cases patients may want to be referred to a center with more experience in dealing with their disease. This is especially important when the cancer is a relatively rare type or one that requires highly specialized therapy.

Cancer experts now believe that for most cancers a delay of a week or two between diagnosis and treatment will not hinder chances for cure. So you have some time to look into the best place for treatment.

According to Dr. Frederick F. Becker, vice president for basic and clinical research at the M.D. Anderson Hospital and Tumor Institute in Houston, the hospital where you are treated should have on its staff a qualified oncologist who can discuss with you the overall approach to therapy. Ask about potential benefits and risks of the proposed treatment and about other possible therapies. Also, ask about adjuvant therapy — the use of cancer drugs (chemotherapy) or radiation therapy that would follow the primary treatment (surgery or radiation). If you are told that adjuvant therapies exist or are currently being tested but that the doctor does not recommend them, you might want to get another opinion from an oncologist.

In many cases involving common cancers, it's not necessary to go to a cancer center to get good treatment. They can be treated adequately in your home community if the physician is aware of the latest methods. Even if the doctor's knowledge seems up-to-date, you can call or ask that your doctor call the nearest cancer center or the National Cancer Institute's Cancer Information Service to find out what the newest treatments may be and whether they can be applied by your own doctor. The service can be reached through the following toll-free numbers: in the continental United States (except Maryland, 800-638-6694; in Maryland, 800-492-6600; in Alaska and Hawaii, 800-638-6070.

When promising new treatments are currently under test, it may be to your benefit to participate in a federally financed clinical trial — a study in which patients are randomly assigned to receive either the best therapy currently in use or a new experimental treatment that may be even better. In most such trials your medical expenses will be partly or completely covered by the funds allocated for the study. The Cancer Information Service provides information to patients and physicians about all aspects of cancer and about suitable clinical trials in your area.

Your attitude and the attitude of your family and friends are important to your fight against cancer. The will to live and the emotional support of loved ones help patients weather sometimes harrowing treatments; a positive outlook has actually been shown to increase the chances for survival. [See chapter on coping with cancer chemotherapy, page 684.] But attitude alone cannot cure cancer; properly researched remedies are needed to do the job.

Alternative Therapies

Whenever a disease is crippling or life-threatening and cure is uncertain, quackery steps in to fill the gaps, preying upon people's fears and ignorance. Nowhere is this more prominent than in cancer treatment. In recent years those offering such unproved methods of treatment as Laetrile, coffee enemas, vitamin megadoses, metabolic therapy, and mind therapy have flourished as growing numbers of Americans have become disillusioned with establishment medicine.

The sales pitch for these so-called alternative therapies is often strengthened by claims of seemingly miraculous cures that are not founded in fact. When the therapy fails, its practitioners claim that the patient's chances for cure were robbed by previous conventional therapy or that the patient simply waited too long to try the "miracle."

Needless tragic deaths have resulted when patients abandoned established remedies in favor of unproved treatments. According to Dr. Edward J. Beattie, director of Memorial Hospital in New York, the celebrated case of Chad Green, the two-year-old Massachusetts boy with acute lymphocytic leukemia, is a case in point. Chad's parents rejected the chemotherapy that would have offered the boy a 50 percent chance of permanent cure and opted, instead, for Laetrile and "nutritional therapy" at a Mexican clinic. The courts tried, without success, to bring Chad back for chemotherapy, and the boy died (in fact, some experts believe his Mexican treatment actually hastened his death). [See chapter on cancer quackery, page 655.]

[See chapter on cancer quackery, page 655.]

644

For Further Information

Beattie, Edward J., M.D., and Stuart D. Cowan. *Toward the Conquest of Cancer.* New York: Crown, 1980.

Brody, Jane E., with Arthur Holleb, M.D. *You Can Fight Cancer and Win.* New York: Quadrangle/Times Books, 1976; McGraw-Hill, 1977.

McKhann, Charles. *The Facts about Cancer.* Englewood Cliffs, N.J.: Prentice-Hall, 1981.

Morra, Marion, and Eve Potts. *Choices: Realistic Alternatives in Cancer Treatment.* New York: Avon, 1980.

Salsbury, Kathryn H., and Eleanor Liebman Johnson. *The Indispensable Cancer Handbook.* New York: Wideview, 1981.

Breast Cancer: Are You High-Risk?

People generally think of cancer as a capricious disease, one that strikes without warning or regard for the particular characteristics of individuals. However, for several major cancers, individuals can be distinguished ahead of time as facing a high risk of developing the disease.

One instance is breast cancer, and the fact that you can be determined as high risk could help to save your life. Since methods exist for detecting breast cancer at a stage early enough to cure more than 85 percent of patients (instead of the 50 to 60 percent who are currently saved), it pays to find out if you are among the high-risk group. And if you are, it pays to take appropriate advantage of early detection techniques.

The detection methods include manual examination by a physician or nurse, mammography (a breast X ray), and thermography (a heat picture), supplemented by monthly self-examination of the breasts, which every woman should do regardless of her risk. (See diagram below.) However, your risk level largely determines how often you should undergo a medical breast exam. Some high-risk women should be examined by a doctor as often as every three months. For other women an annual exam is considered adequate.

Since the most valuable detection method — mammography — involves exposure to low-dose radiation, which in itself may pose some hazard (albeit very small), it is important to know if the potential benefits of mammography would outweigh the possible risks in your case.

If, for example, you face a considerably lower than average chance of developing breast cancer, it may be best for you to avoid routine mammography perhaps until the age of fifty, when your chances of getting the

HOW TO DO A BREAST SELF-EXAMINATION

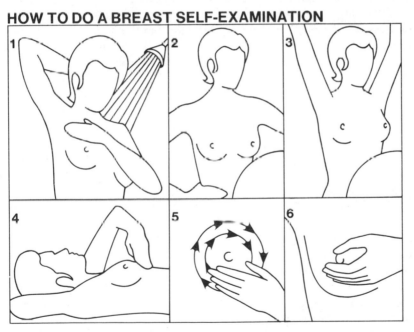

Monthly breast self-examination, best done right after menstrual period. (1) With fingers flat and together, massage in circular motion every part of both breasts, checking for lumps, hard knots, or thickenings. (2) Stand before mirror and look at breasts with hands on hips and muscles tensed. (3) Raise arms above head and check for dimpling or changes in shape. (4) Lie on back with pillow under right shoulder and right hand behind head. (5) Feel right breast gently with circular motion. Begin at outermost part of breast and, when first circle is completed, start again one inch inward. Repeat until entire breast has been covered. Repeat (4) and (5) for left breast. Finally, (6) squeeze each nipple gently and look for discharge.

disease increase by virtue of your age. But if you are among the high-risk group, annual mammography may be advisable from age thirty-five.

The Risk Factors

The average woman in the United States faces a 9 percent chance of developing breast cancer sometime during her lifetime — of every eleven newborn girls, one is destined to get breast cancer. Through extensive studies of the backgrounds of breast cancer patients in the United States and other countries, researchers have learned a great deal about which women are most likely to develop the disease. The most important factors determining the risk of breast cancer are as follows:

Family history. On the average, close blood relatives of breast-cancer patients — their daughters, sisters, maternal aunts, and nieces — are two to three times more likely to get breast cancer than women whose families are free of the disease. Breast cancer that occurred after menopause has no appreciable effect on a relative's risk of also developing the disease. However, under some circumstances, a relative may have a nearly fifty-fifty chance of getting breast cancer.

Through studies of the families of several hundred breast cancer patients, Dr. David E. Anderson, a geneticist at the M.D. Anderson Hospital and Tumor Institute in Houston, found that if a female relative had cancer in only one breast, the risk to a woman was only slightly greater than that faced by the average woman in the population. However, if the relative had cancer in both breasts, the risk to other females in the family was five and a half times higher. If the cancer was bilateral (in both breasts) and also occurred before menopause, the risk to her relatives was nine times higher than expected, giving them a nearly 50 percent chance of developing breast cancer. The greatest risk of all is faced by a woman under the age of forty whose sister and mother both had breast cancer before menopause.

Menstrual history. The earlier in life a woman starts menstruating, and the later she enters the menopause — that is, the longer her ovaries produce sex hormones — the greater her chances of developing breast cancer. Women whose natural menopause occurs after age fifty-five have twice the risk of those whose menopause starts before age forty-five. Surgical removal of the ovaries prior to menopause has a protective effect, with a 70 percent reduction in the risk of breast cancer if the ovaries are removed before age thirty-five.

Childbirth history. In general the younger a woman is when she bears her first child, the lower her breast cancer risk. Women who have borne children before the age of thirty have a lower risk than childless women or women whose first birth occurred after that age. Women who give birth to their first child before age eighteen have about a third the risk of those whose first delivery occurs at thirty-five or older. To be "protective," the pregnancy must be full-term — abortions don't count.

Contrary to popular belief, having lots of babies does not reduce your risk of breast cancer. Nor does breast-feeding your babies make any difference in breast cancer risk.

Hormonal Drugs. Although birth control pills have not been in use long enough to say with certainty that they do not increase breast cancer risk, no clear relationship has yet been found between taking the pill and the later development of breast cancer, and there is some evidence of a positive effect of the pill. However, menopausal estrogens, taken by millions of American women, have been linked to twice the expected risk of breast cancer if the hormone drug is used for ten years or longer.

Benign breast disease. Women who have a noncancerous breast disorder known as fibrocystic disease (also called chronic cystic mastitis or cystic breast disease) are about four times more likely to develop breast cancer than women without this condition. The disease, which occurs in about 5 percent of middle-aged women, gives the breasts a "lumpy" feeling and may produce no symptoms or may be accompanied by breast pain or premenstrual breast discomfort. Avoidance of all foods and beverages containing caffeine and its chemical relatives, including coffee (regular and decaffeinated), tea, colas and other soft drinks, chocolate and cocoa, may relieve the swelling and discomforts of fibrocystic disease. Treatment with vitamin E (400 to 600 international units daily) also may relieve symptoms. But it is not known whether either of these measures also protects against cancer.

Short-lived — as opposed to chronic — breast conditions associated with nursing do not increase a woman's risk of breast cancer.

Diet. In a sense every American woman is at high risk for breast cancer — compared with women living in many other countries — because the disease is linked to the regular consumption of a diet high in saturated fats. Thus, one way to reduce the risk of breast cancer may be to adopt the same type of low-fat, low-cholesterol diet advocated for the prevention of heart disease. [See chapter on fats and cholesterol, page 14.] Chronic constipation may also increase a woman's breast cancer risk, and a diet high in fiber may be protective. [See chapter on dietary fiber, page 36.]

Breast Cancer Treatment:
New Methods Are Less Mutilating

In the 1950's women, inspired by widely publicized reports of a new lifesaving technique, succeeded in changing the practice of medicine by demanding that their doctors do Pap smears to detect cervical cancer. In the 1970's women started agitating for another change in their care: the treatment of breast cancer.

An increasingly common disease that is detected in more than 111,000 women in the United States each year, breast cancer inflicts a double trauma on many of the women who get it. Not only is it a cancer that eventually claims the lives of half its victims, but its treatment also involves a direct assault on an important symbol of femininity. For some, the psychological consequences of losing a breast are almost as bad as the portents of their illness.

Armed once again with reports, both anecdotal and scientific, in popular periodicals and books, growing numbers of women with breast cancer are insisting upon a less radical approach to treatment than most American surgeons have traditionally used. To judge from national statistics on breast surgery and from the conclusions reached by a consensus committee of the National Institutes of Health, women are winning their fight. Radical breast cancer surgery is now rapidly being replaced by less disfiguring operations.

Of course, this change is not taking place merely because women want it that way. Although surgeons today are more willing to consider a woman's wishes in the treatment decision, the move away from radical surgery also reflects the fact that accumulating research has challenged the need for extensive operations in many cases, that more breast cancer patients are being diagnosed at an earlier stage of disease, and that new knowledge about the biology of breast cancer is forcing a reconsideration of old dogma about appropriate treatment.

Replacing the Radical Mastectomy

For nearly a century the standard therapy for breast cancer, regardless of how early it was detected, was the so-called Halsted radical mastectomy. It involves removal of the entire breast, the underlying chest muscles, and the lymph nodes in the armpit. Although through exercises and counseling most patients adjusted well to the radical surgery, others ended up with limited shoulder movement, swelling, and loss of strength in the arm on the side where the operation was done. After a radical, clothing choices may be somewhat limited, and breast reconstruction is difficult and sometimes impossible.

In the last few years, however, a more modified procedure has replaced the radical as the leading treatment for newly diagnosed breast cancer. The modified radical still removes the entire breast, the armpit nodes, and some muscle tissue, but it spares the major chest muscle. Other surgical approaches growing in popularity include total (also called simple) mastectomy — removal of the entire breast, but none of the muscles — with or without removing the armpit nodes, and partial, or segmental, mastectomy (also called lumpectomy) — removal of the cancerous segment of the breast, again with or without the nodes.

In addition to these surgical procedures, some physicians are using radiation therapy as the primary treatment for certain patients, usually after the tumor itself has been removed.

Lesser Surgery for Early Cancers

The National Institutes of Health consensus committee, staffed by advocates from all camps of the breast cancer treatment controversy, concluded that even the modified radical might be overtreatment for early breast cancer. According to the committee, many cases of breast cancer should be treated instead by total mastectomy and removal of the armpit nodes, preserving all the chest muscles. The committee reserved judgment on the benefits of partial mastectomy and primary radiation therapy, pending further study. The recommendations apply to women who have so-called Stage I cancer (small tumors that appear not to have spread to the nodes) and selected patients with Stage II (cancer in some nodes but no evidence of spread elsewhere in the body.)

Today, with increasing numbers of women going through breast cancer screening programs through which a cancer can be detected even before it is a lump, a larger proportion of patients are diagnosed when their disease is in a relatively early stage. For them, lesser surgical procedures may offer as good a chance for cure as radical mastectomy.

The reason for recommending removal of the entire breast, rather than just the cancerous segment, rests on the fact that in at least 13 percent of patients who have total mastectomies, microscopic study shows that the removed breast contains one or more hidden cancers in addition to the one originally detected. If the entire breast is not removed, these latent cancers may grow. Whether radiation therapy after a partial mastectomy can wipe out all such hidden cancers is not yet definitely known. How important these sites might be to the patient's future health if they are not removed is also not known. It appears, however, that in some — perhaps many — cases these microscopic cancers never develop into clinically apparent disease.

The committee also recommended that the diagnosis of breast cancer be separated from its treatment. Instead of having a woman "sign away" her breast even before the biopsy shows that she in fact has cancer, the committee suggested a two-step procedure. First a diagnostic biopsy, which usually involves surgical removal of the tumor, should be done, and the findings and treatment possibilities discussed with the patient. Then, if the biopsy shows cancer — which happens in only one of four cases — more definitive treatment is done. This means that the three in four women who undergo biopsies and turn out not to have cancer do not have to go through the trauma of signing away their breasts before the biopsy.

A number of studies here and abroad have suggested — but not proved — that for early breast cancer, it matters little to the survival of the patient which of the various treatments is used. Unfortunately most

649

of these studies have had shortcomings that make it impossible to reach definite conclusions. The most serious of these shortcomings is the relatively brief time — three to five years — that patients have been followed after the original treatment. Although the majority of patients who will suffer recurrences from breast cancer do so within three years of their initial therapy, a significant proportion of breast cancer deaths occur five or more years later.

Thus, some specialists maintain that unless patients are followed for at least ten years, no conclusions can be drawn on the differences in lifesaving potential offered by the various types of surgery and radiation. Others say, however, that the whole question is meaningless because surgery is only a local treatment and breast cancer seems to be a systemic, or whole-body, disease.

Treating Cancer Beyond the Breast

When surgery (with or without postoperative radiation) is used to treat the disease, 75 percent of patients found to have cancer in their armpit nodes when they are first treated eventually succumb to their disease. A similar fate is suffered by 25 percent of those who do not have evidence of cancer in the nodes. This suggests that in these patients — and probably many others who don't get recurring cancer — the disease has already spread to other parts of the body by the time it is diagnosed. In such cases it matters relatively little what kind of local treatment, surgical or radiation, they get. Treatments that can reach all parts of the body, such as drug or immunological therapies, must be used to eradicate the cancer.

The lymph nodes are the best clue doctors have to whether cancer has spread beyond the breast. That's in part why the consensus committee recommended that the nodes be removed and carefully studied under a microscope. Patients found to have cancer in the nodes can then be given further treatment with anticancer drugs and/or immunological agents that attack cancer throughout the body. Hormonal therapy may also be appropriate in some cases.

Unless the nodes are removed, it is impossible for the surgeon to be certain about their cancerous status. Even the best surgeons guess wrong in 30 to 40 percent of cases if all they do is a physical examination of the nodes. A disadvantage of primary radiation therapy is that the nodes are not removed for study, and so there may be no good way to tell who needs systemic treatment as well.

With the advent of drug and immunological therapies, which, incidentally, are still experimental, some women wonder why surgery is needed at all to treat breast cancer. The answer is, first, that unless the tumor is removed for microscopic study, a definite diagnosis cannot be made and, secondly, that surgical removal of the main tumor seems to stimulate the patient's natural immunity and helps to destroy any cancer cells that may be left behind in the breast region or elsewhere in the body.

It will be some years before doctors have better answers to the questions women have about breast cancer treatments, which undoubtedly will continue to change as more data from ongoing scientific studies become available. Meanwhile, it is increasingly apparent that there is no one "best" treatment approach. Rather, the treatment should be tailored to the individual patient, on the basis not only of the type of cancer, its size and location, and evidence of spread, but also on the woman's ability to cope with the consequences of treatment. Whether surgeons approve or not, some women would rather take a chance on the as yet unproved lesser surgical techniques or on radiation therapy than lose a breast.

Breast Reconstruction

For those who do undergo mastectomy and find it physically or psychologically inhibiting, plastic surgery may provide an alternative by reconstructing the missing breast. Although the cosmetic results of reconstruction are less than perfect, surgeons and patients alike report that nearly all who undergo it are more than satisfied with their surgically created breasts. The before-and-after reactions of many such women are poignantly described by Jean Zalon, herself a reconstruction patient, in her inspiring book *I Am Whole Again* written with Jean Libman Block (see "For Further Reading," page 652).

Although until recently breast reconstruction after cancer surgery was a complicated procedure the results of which rarely justified the risks and costs, today new and simplified techniques, improvements in insurance coverage, and changes in the treatment of breast cancer itself have made reconstruction a possibility for as many as 80 percent of patients. This is especially so if cancer surgery is undertaken with reconstruction in mind and if the cancer operation is planned with the consultation of a plastic surgeon.

Breast reconstruction usually involves the insertion of a specially molded half-moon of silicone gel (not the dangerous, banned injections of liquid silicone) under the skin to create a breast mound. If the woman wants it, a nipple and areola may be constructed in a second operation, using parts from the other breast or a tiny piece of the vaginal lip or the original nipple and areola that had been "banked" elsewhere on the woman's body at the time of her mastectomy.

Reconstruction is usually delayed for at least three months after a mastectomy to give the scar a chance to heal completely and to allow the skin to soften and stretch. Another three months are advised between the creation of the breast mound and the construction of the nipple and areola. A national counseling group called RENU (for Reconstruction Education for National Understanding) can be reached by calling 216-444-2900.

For Further Reading

Spletter, Mary. *Woman's Choice: New Options in Breast Cancer.* Boston: Beacon Press, 1982.

Walter, Carol, with Lenore Miller. *Moving Free: Post-Mastectomy Exercises.* Indianapolis: Bobbs-Merrill, 1981.

Watson, Rita Esposito, and Robert C. Wallach, M.D. *New Choices, New Chances: A Woman's Guide to Conquering Cancer.* New York: St. Martin's Press, 1982.

Zalon, Jean, with Jean Libman Block. *I Am Whole Again.* New York: Random House, 1979.

Colon Cancer:
Early Detection Is Lifesaving

Doctors call it "the cancer nobody talks about." Yet it is second only to lung cancer in the number of new cases that occur each year, and it claims more lives than breast cancer. It is cancer of the lower bowel — the colon and rectum, a part of the body generally not mentioned in "polite company" and a part many of us find embarrassing to discuss even with our spouses and physicians.

652

As a result of this reticence, most people fail to take advantage of simple, lifesaving tests, and many more people than need be succumb to the cancer or suffer its debilitating effects. Others ignore symptoms (among them, rectal bleeding, diarrhea, constipation) or dismiss symptoms as caused by some annoying but benign problem like hemorrhoids.

It's time more of us took to heart the admonition of an American Cancer Society ad promoting early detection of colon-rectal cancer: "Don't be embarrassed to death." This is especially important for all persons over forty and anyone at any age who, for reasons of personal or family medical history, may face an unusually high risk of developing the disease. Tests for colon cancer are also an important part of the examination of any adult with symptoms of bowel disease.

If diagnosed early, colon-rectal cancer is easier to cure than almost any other internal cancer. Cancers of the colon and rectum tend to grow slowly and silently for years, remaining localized and therefore curable for a long time. Following early diagnosis and treatment, 75 to 80 percent of patients are cured.

Several tests for early detection, including one you do yourself, are now readily available. In addition to finding curable cancers, these tests can detect trouble even before it becomes cancer. The problem is that many doctors don't include these tests as part of routine checkups, and patients rarely ask to have them included. Too many people wait until they have pronounced symptoms before they seek an examination of the lower bowel. By then it may be too late for a cure.

Who Is High Risk?

Some 120,000 Americans will be diagnosed as having colon-rectal cancer this year, and 54,900 will die of the disease. The likelihood of developing cancer in the lower bowel increases with advancing age, with the risk rising after age forty. The greatest number of cases occurs between the ages of fifty-five and seventy-five.

Most of these cancers develop in a polyp, a benign growth that may remain harmless for years. In many families there is a decided hereditary tendency to form polyps in the colon or rectum, and anyone with a personal or family history of polyps should be examined more often and more carefully, starting a decade or more before the forties. Most experts recommend removal of all polyps when they are found, thus intercepting them before they can turn malignant. Persons with such hereditary disorders as familial polyposis and Gardner's syndrome are especially vulnerable. So is anyone with a close blood relative who has had colon-rectal cancer.

One-fifth to one-third of patients with ulcerative colitis, particularly those with extensive disease that began before age twenty-five, eventually develop colon cancer and therefore should be watched carefully. Although hemorrhoids, which are overly stretched veins in the rectum, have nothing directly to do with cancer risk, too often rectal bleeding is dismissed as caused by hemorrhoids and a cancer is overlooked. [See chapter on hemorrhoids, page 530.]

In addition to rectal bleeding, symptoms that warrant a doctor's thorough examination include any change in bowel habits (diarrhea, constipation, or flatulence) that persists, abdominal pain, vague gastrointestinal symptoms, unexplained fever, or weight loss.

Recent studies have suggested that a diet high in fat and beef and/or low in fiber (roughage) may predispose to colon cancer, perhaps because potential cancer-causing chemicals can form and remain in the lower bowel for much longer periods than if a high-fiber, high-vegetable diet is consumed. [See chapters on fats and cholesterol, page 14, and dietary fiber, page 36.]

Detection Tests

There are five main techniques for picking up a possible colon-rectal cancer, and the American Cancer Society recommends the use of at least three of them as a routine part of health checkups for older adults.

Digital rectal exam. In this test the doctor inserts a gloved, well-lubricated finger into the rectum to feel for irregular or abnormally firm areas that might be malignant. About 12 to 15 percent of all colon-rectal cancers can be detected through this quick, inexpensive examination, which should be done annually on all people over forty. At the same time the doctor can visually examine the anal area for signs of abnormalities.

Guaiac test for occult blood. This recently developed do-it-yourself test, which detects hidden blood in the stool that might be a sign of cancer, has greatly simplified early detection of colon-rectal cancer. It is recommended annually for all people over age fifty. For four days, starting at least twenty-four hours before the first sample is taken, the patient is told to follow a meat-free diet that is high in fiber (fruits, vegetables, bran, corn, etc.), and to stop taking iron, vitamin C, and any aspirin-containing drugs (which can interfere with the test results). Then two tiny samples from each of the next three stools are smeared on specially prepared slides, which are delivered to the doctor or laboratory for analysis. If any of the slides show signs of blood, further checking for its source is necessary.

Proctosigmoidoscopy. The procto, as it is commonly called, has never been a popular test, though it was shown decades ago to be highly effective in detecting colon-rectal cancer even in its premalignant stages. "Maybe a procto isn't exactly a pleasure. Neither is cancer," reads another American Cancer Society ad. Prior to a procto, the patient prepares by eating a low-fiber diet and taking an enema and possibly a laxative. In the test a rigid lighted tube about a foot long is inserted into the rectum, enabling the doctor to examine the portion of the lower bowel where 20 to 25 percent of colon-rectal cancers arise. The examination takes but a few minutes. If polyps are found, they often can be biopsied or removed at the time of the examination.

The procto is recommended annually for two years for people over fifty, after which examinations can be done once every three to five years if the first two indicate everything is normal.

Fiberoptic colonoscopy. This instrument greatly extends the range of examination, permitting the doctor to look at the entire length of the large intestine. Unlike the proctosigmoidoscope, the colonoscope is narrow and flexible. The patient is usually given a sedative before the examination. Polyps can be removed and biopsies taken at the time of examination. Colonoscopy must be done by a specialist who is well schooled in the technique. Although the test is highly effective in detecting early cancer, not many doctors are trained to perform it. However, it is the preferred method and definitely worth shopping around for, especially for those with a family or personal history of polyps, since it can pick up trouble spots missed through the other detection techniques.

Barium enema X ray exam. Any patient with signs or symptoms of colon-rectal cancer should have a special bowel X ray taken, which involves a barium enema so that the bowel shows up clearly on the film. The X ray is complementary to the other tests.

654

Cancer Quackery:
Preying on the Desperate

One of the most frequent challenges presented to cancer specialists these days concerns the unproven cancer drug Laetrile. When a doctor advises a patient against taking it, the rejoinder is likely to be: "But how do you know it doesn't work? How can you be so sure?"

To answer honestly, the doctor would have to say something like this: "I cannot be absolutely sure because there is no such thing as certainty in science. But I can tell you that Laetrile has shown no anticancer activity in any laboratory animal nor in cancer patients who have participated in properly designed tests. Nearly all those patients who recovered after taking Laetrile had also received established, effective anticancer treatments, and Laetrile advocates don't bother to tell you about those patients who rejected conventional therapy in favor of Laetrile and subsequently died of their cancers."

Yet tens of thousands of cancer patients have taken Laetrile, and many more thousands are likely to do so now that state after state is voting to permit the use of this federally banned extract of apricot pits. Why, if Laetrile doesn't seem to work, do so many people continue to try it? Why do so many other quack cancer remedies persist year after year?

The Lure of Unproved Methods

The answer lies in the emotional impact of cancer. A diagnosis of cancer strikes terror in the hearts of even the most rational victims. Filled with fear and a sense of desperation, many are quite naturally attracted to something that promises to rescue them from the lion's mouth — to grant them a reprieve from the death sentence they think they have received. Their heads are easily turned by reports of miraculous cures described by members of one or another group advocating their own unconventional answer to cancer.

Unfortunately those who select the quick, easy promises of cancer quacks over the more complex therapies offered by established cancer specialists are simply hastening the end. In fact, they may be squandering their one and only chance for a real cure or long-lasting remission.

Another reason for the attraction of quack cancer remedies is the fear people have of the effects of established therapies — the disfigurement of surgery and the side effects of radiation therapy and anticancer drugs that are the hallmarks of modern cancer treatment. When faced with a choice between something like Laetrile, which is said to be harmless and produce no unpleasant side effects (although an overdose can be fatal), and a treatment — however effective — that the doctor warns in advance will cause discomfort, many opt for the painless — albeit ineffective — approach. [See chapter on coping with cancer chemotherapy, page 684.]

Each year Americans waste nearly $3 billion on worthless potions, vitamins, devices, diets, schemes, and ceremonies that are heralded as cancer cures. Many also waste their lives in the process. Others who may have exhausted all established remedies and who turn to unproved methods as a last resort waste their families' resources to obtain the worthless remedies.

Many, if not all, of a quack's claimed successes involve the treatment of patients who never had cancer in the first place. They may have had a suspicious symptom and been told by a physician to have a cancer test or biopsy or exploratory operation. Instead, they went to a quack who used a phony diagnostic test to "prove" the person had cancer, which the quack then proceeded to "cure" with his supposed therapy. [For information on proper cancer diagnosis, see chapter on cancer treatment, page 641.]

Don't let yourself or any member of your family fall into the hands of a cancer quack or any kind of quack. Quacks sell only false hopes, and the price they exact may be your life.

Recognizing Quackery

656

How can you tell the difference between the legitimate claims for effective cancer therapies and the spurious claims for the unorthodox treatments offered by self-proclaimed experts? In short, how can you recognize a cancer quack? Quacks may sport white coats, and some even bear a legitimate M.D. after their names. But they all have one or more telltale characteristics that will help the wary patient recognize and avoid them. These include the following:

● Quacks usually advocate a single approach to treating most or all types of cancer. Whatever you have — be it leukemia or lung cancer — their magic is said to cure it. Yet cancer researchers have shown that cancer is not one but 100 or more different diseases, with different types requiring different approaches to treatment.

● Quacks claim that they are being persecuted by established medicine for their unorthodox ideas and that no one will publish their findings. The reason legitimate journals refuse to publish the "findings" of cancer quacks is that they are totally unscientific, couched in terms that could fool an ignorant lay person but not a trained researcher.

Many quacks don't even seek legitimate outlets for their results. Instead, they advertise their wares through newspaper and magazine articles, broadcasts, and lectures and depend heavily on testimonials and financial support from patients and prominent persons who are neither physicians nor scientists and are not competent to evaluate the quack's claims.

● They also claim that the medical establishment — the American

Medical Association, the American Cancer Society, the National Cancer Institute, etc. — doesn't really want to cure cancer because that would put a lot of doctors and scientists out of business. Since many members of these legitimate organizations have themselves had cancer or have loved ones who are afflicted with cancer, it hardly seems likely that they would not want to see cancer cured, if that were possible.

• Quacks may call themselves "doctor," but in fact, most are not medical doctors and don't even have Ph.D. degrees in fields even remotely related to medicine. Rather, their degrees may be in physics or "naturopathy" or "metaphysics" or the like.

• The methods of producing a quack remedy are often kept a deep, dark secret by its promoters, who may protest that they can trust no one else to use it properly. They may also refuse to submit the purported treatment to an independent test because, they claim, the test wouldn't be done right by anyone else and the treatment would be labeled worthless unfairly.

Emphysema and Chronic Bronchitis: When You Can't Get Enough Air

There is nothing more frightening than being unable to get enough air into your lungs to sustain normal activities. Yet for more than 9 million Americans, shortness of breath is a chronic problem that interferes with work and play and even with such basic activities as eating and dressing.

They are victims of chronic obstructive pulmonary disease (COPD) — chronic bronchitis and emphysema, the fastest-growing causes of disability and death in the mid-twentieth century. Though currently incurable and often detected only after considerable permanent lung damage has occurred, they can be treated in ways that usually minimize the damage, sometimes partially reverse it, and always make life easier for victims and their families.

Even more important, most cases of COPD can be prevented by the elimination of cigarette smoking. According to Dr. Lewis Clayton, medical director of the American Lung Association, "If every smoker spent an hour with a patient in the throes of terminal emphysema, without doubt most would quickly become ex-smokers."

The Normal Respiratory Tree

Your lungs are remarkable instruments of air exchange. Stretched out flat, the average human lung would cover a tennis court. Air inhaled through the nose and mouth enters the trachea, or windpipe, the trunk of the tree. It then moves into two main branches, called bronchi (one to each lung), that divide into smaller branches, the bronchioles, and end in clusters of tiny air sacs called alveoli.

The thin membranes of the alveoli abut a web of tiny blood vessels, allowing an exchange of gases between the bloodstream and the lungs. In this way, inhaled oxygen is delivered to the blood and the waste gas carbon dioxide is removed from the blood to be exhaled through the lungs. When the respiratory tree malfunctions, your body is shortchanged on essential oxygen.

Normal bronchial tubes are lubricated by mucous secretions and lined with hairs called cilia that help to sweep dust, excess secretions, and other debris out of the airways. Normal air sacs are elastic; air is forced in and out of them by the automatic rhythmic motion of the diaphragm and chest muscles.

Symptoms of Airway Obstruction

The term "COPD" lumps together several diseases, the symptoms of which include coughing, bringing up mucus, wheezing, and shortness of breath. Frequently two or more such lung diseases occur in the same person. Untreated, COPD can lead to enlargement of the heart and heart failure as this master muscle struggles for oxygen.

In chronic bronchitis, the bronchi — the major breathing tubes — are inflamed and clogged with thick secretions. The typical symptom is a chronic coughing up of greenish yellow sputum. Bronchitis can occur as a short-lived infection, but when symptoms persist for three months or longer and recur at least two years in a row, the condition is chronic and indicates destructive changes in the airways. The cilia become ineffective as cleansing tools, and another major line of lung defense, infection-fighting cells called macrophages, also malfunction.

In emphysema the walls of the alveoli are damaged, and many of the air sacs become greatly enlarged and lose their elasticity. This destroys their ability to exchange gases with the blood. The breathing muscles are unable to push all the air out of the enlarged sacs, causing stale air to accumulate and diminishing the ability of the lungs to take in freshly oxygenated air. The main symptom of emphysema (the word means "inflated," referring to the trapped air in the alveoli) is shortness of breath. The chest may become barrel-shaped as a result of overexpanded lungs, and the muscles of the neck and shoulders become overdeveloped in the effort to breathe.

Causes

Chronic bronchitis and emphysema develop slowly over a period of many years, but early signs are typically ignored until permanent destruction has occurred. The diseases are typically diagnosed in people in their fifties and sixties, with men outnumbering women victims by about

658

eight to one. However, as more women are now heavy smokers, the incidence of COPD in women is increasing.

Smoking paralyzes the cilia that protect the lungs from harmful debris and infectious organisms. Cigarette smoke also causes the release of an enzyme called elastase that can digest the elastic tissue in the lung. Furthermore, smoking increases the production of alveolar macrophages, which produce digestive enzymes, and blocks the action of enzyme inhibitors that protect the lung tissue from destruction. The most important such inhibitor is alpha-1-antitrypsin, which for genetic reasons is missing in some people, making them highly susceptible to substances that destroy lung elasticity.

In addition to smoking, exposure to noxious air pollutants, such as sulfur dioxide and nitrous oxide, can cause or aggravate COPD. Exposure at work to cotton dust, fumes from welding and plastic wrap, and smelter gases, and at home to irritating aerosols and other volatile chemicals, can precipitate COPD, especially in people who also smoke.

Diagnosis and Treatment

Diagnosis is made on the basis of medical history — particularly the patterns of coughing, sputum production, and activities that produce breathlessness — a thorough physical exam, and tests of lung function (especially spirometry, which measures how much and how fast air moves out of the lungs). X rays may not show anything until the disease is far advanced.

Treatment of COPD is designed to relieve symptoms and slow the progress of disease. Antibiotics are used to clear up chronic infections. Bronchodilators (in a inhalant spray or as a pill) can help to open up the breathing passages. Corticosteroids may be used on a trial basis since they can sometimes partially reverse lung damage. Annual flu shots and a one-time pneumonia vaccine can help prevent infections that can be life-threatening to a victim of COPD; so can avoiding crowds and exposure to people with colds and other infectious diseases.

COPD victims can also benefit from instruction in slow, deep breathing and exhaling through pursed lips. This permits greater exhalation of carbon dioxide and more efficient ventilation.

The most important aspects of treatment involve self-help measures. First and foremost are giving up smoking and avoiding exposure to smoke and other noxious fumes as much as possible. Postural drainage (lying with the head lower than the chest) to help clear air passages of accumulated mucus should be done twice a day. Losing excess weight, maintaining a nutritionally sound diet, drinking lots of water (it helps to thin out and loosen mucus in the airways), and exercising daily (when muscles work efficiently, they need less oxygen) are crucial aspects of effective treatment.

Bedridden victims of COPD have been able to resume many normal activities following a program of graded exercises. COPD need not spell the end to sexual activity, either, once victims and their spouses learn some breath-conserving tricks, such as using a bronchodilator an hour before and adopting less strenuous positions, such as side by side.

The emotional consequences of COPD can be devastating. Spouses may suppress anger and resentment over being forced to reverse traditional roles. Victims typically sink into inactivity and suffer from depression, anxiety, and guilt. Counseling in a family setting is often extremely valuable.

For Further Information

An excellent resource for COPD victims and their families is a twenty-four-page illustrated book called *Help Yourself to Better Breathing*, published by the American Lung Association. Single copies are available free from local chapters or from the American Lung Association, P.O. Box 596, New York, New York 10001.

The Encyclopedia Britannica Educational Corporation (425 North Michigan Avenue, Chicago, Illinois 60611) produces a videocassette program called *Pulmonary Self-care: A Program for Patients* for use by professionals who guide self-care programs.

Diabetes:
Rapid Rise in Blood Sugar Disease

660

Marvin is a diabetic. His life has depended on daily injections of insulin for the last twenty-four years, since he was eleven years old. But few would guess he has a serious medical problem. Marvin is a snow and water-skiing enthusiast, a fixer-upper of old cars, a trustee in his church. He hasn't missed a day of work in more years than he can remember.

Henry is also a diabetic. He first discovered his problem at the age of fifty-two, through his annual physical. Henry made some changes in his diet and lost about twenty-five pounds, and his diabetes has been controlled without medication for the last six years.

Marvin and Henry are among an estimated 10 million Americans with diabetes mellitus, about half of whom don't even know they have it. The prevalence of diabetes has been increasing so rapidly in recent years that experts expect the number of Americans with diagnosed diabetes to double in fifteen years. The reasons for this increase and the underlying cause of the disease itself remain mysteries.

Modern medicine has done a great deal to forestall many of the serious and potentially life-threatening complications of diabetes and to enable most diabetics, like Marvin and Henry, to lead near-normal lives. Even the once-stringent dietary restrictions have recently been modified so that the diabetic can, with a few readily avoided exceptions, eat the same foods that other people eat, although the diabetic may have to limit the amount eaten to prevent overweight.

Types of Diabetes

There are several kinds of diabetes, ranging from very mild to very severe. Marvin is among the approximately 1 million Americans with the most severe form, called insulin-dependent, or juvenile diabetes. Despite its name, juvenile diabetes can strike at any age, but it usually first appears in childhood or early adolescence. The vast majority of diabetics develop symptoms of the disease in mid-life, as Henry did. Maturity, or adult-onset, diabetes, as it is called, can usually be controlled by diet and exercise alone, without insulin. The most common precipitant of adult-onset diabetes appears to be obesity.

Symptoms of diabetes include frequent urination, excessive thirst, itching (a persistent vaginal itch is common in female diabetics), increasing difficulties with sexual potency, blurred vision, muscle weakness, and weight loss despite an increased appetite. These symptoms primarily result from an accumulation of sugar in the blood that is the diagnostic hallmark of the disease.

Another type of diabetes involves no symptoms at all. This is called chemical diabetes, in which blood sugar may become abnormally high after eating, and a glucose tolerance test produces abnormal results. Some people develop temporary chemical diabetes, precipitated by a stressful event such as pregnancy or illness.

Causes and Consequences

Genetic factors are involved in diabetes, with some individuals inheriting a predisposition to develop the disease. There is also evidence that a virus may sometimes trigger onset of the disease. For reasons perhaps related to pregnancy, women are more likely to develop adult-onset diabetes than men are. The disease is also more prevalent among the poor and among nonwhites, possibly because obesity is also more common in these groups.

The high blood sugar characteristic of diabetes stems from an abnormality of insulin, the hormone produced by the pancreas that enables body cells to take up and use the blood sugar, glucose. In juvenile diabetes, insulin is lacking entirely or its supply is seriously deficient. But in many other diabetics, rather than a lack of insulin production, there appears to be a disruption in how the body utilizes the hormone. Either way glucose accumulates in the blood and spills over into the urine. That's why the disease is commonly discovered through a routine blood or urine analysis.

The body tries to dilute the high blood sugar by moving water out of the cells, and the kidneys work overtime to get rid of the sugar and water, causing frequent urination and intense thirst. Uncorrected, the combination of dehydration and excessive sugar in the blood can lead to a diabetic coma.

Glucose in the blood is ordinarily the main energy source for body cells. Because glucose doesn't enter a diabetic's cells normally, the body's fat cells act as if there were an inadequate supply of glucose to fill energy needs, and they respond by releasing fatty acids, an energy alternative. When fatty acids are used by liver cells for energy, substances called ketone bodies accumulate in the blood and ultimately make the blood acidic. The resulting condition, diabetic acidosis, can be rapidly fatal.

Diabetes involves more than a derangement in sugar metabolism. There is also a defect in the small blood vessels and early-in-life development of hardening of the arteries, or atherosclerosis. In fact, today the vascular complications are far more likely to cause serious illness and death among diabetics than are coma, acidosis, or insulin shock. It is uncertain whether proper control of a diabetic's blood sugar can forestall these vascular problems, though other types of complications can be avoided by controlling diabetes.

Thickening of the walls of the small blood vessels can produce complications involving the kidneys, the retina of the eye, the nervous system, and the skin. Diabetic retinopathy is a leading cause of blindness in adults. Several new approaches to treatment, including surgery to replace the fluid in the eye or the use of a laser beam, can restore or improve sight in some, but there is as yet no certain way to prevent the hemorrhages that led to visual loss in the first place. Premature atherosclerosis in the larger blood vessels of diabetics sets the stage for heart attack, stroke, and loss of circulation to the legs. Today four out of five diabetics succumb to cardiovascular diseases.

These complications can occur in any diabetic, even those with a mild form of the disease, but they tend to occur earlier and more severely in juvenile diabetics. Nonetheless, a study by the famous Joslin Diabetes Center in Boston of seventy-three patients who had juvenile diabetes for more than forty years showed that three-fourths had only mild or minor complications. Eighty-seven percent were married, and only three of the seventy-three were unable to work because of their diabetes.

Treatment

Diabetics who require insulin must take the hormone daily by injection. (Since insulin is a protein, it would be destroyed by digestive juices if taken orally.) Some insulin-dependent diabetics need psychotherapy or counseling to help them adjust to the demands of their disease. Throughout the country there is now available instruction on home glucose monitoring to enable diabetics to adjust their insulin doses and diet more precisely to meet their daily needs. Such monitoring and the "tight" control of blood sugar that makes it possible may forestall eye damage and other complications.

Those who do not require insulin can often bring their blood sugar down to normal levels by losing weight (if they are overweight to start with) and adopting a diet — appropriate for all diabetics — low in fats and rich in complex carbohydrate foods like bread, potatoes, rice, pasta, dried beans and peas, and other starchy foods.

Recently studies in the United States and England have shown that a near-vegetarian diet that is very high in fiber and complex carbohydrate foods — especially dried beans and peas and whole grains — is ideal for diabetes control. In this scheme carbohydrates account for 65 percent or more of daily calories, and fats only about 10 percent. Dr. James W. Anderson of the University of Kentucky in Lexington reports that by following this diet, many diabetics have been able to reduce greatly or eliminate entirely their dependence on insulin and other drugs to lower blood sugar.

In all diabetic diets, foods containing high concentrations of refined sugar — candy, cake, icing, gooey pastries, ice cream, soda, for example — should be avoided. Use of artificial sweeteners is controversial since the most widely used sweetener — saccharin — is strongly suspected of promoting the development of cancer. Fructose is better handled by the diabetic than ordinary table sugar. However, most nutrition experts recommend instead that diabetics wean themselves from their taste for sweets. Saturated fats and cholesterol should also be kept low in a diabetic diet since these promote atherosclerosis, a disease to which diabetics are already abnormally prone.

The American Diabetes Association and the American Dietetic Association have devised exchange lists that can help diabetics plan tasty meals covering a wide range of tastes. The "Exchange Lists for Meal Planning" can be obtained from local affiliates of these organizations for less than $1. Check your phone directory under "name-of-city" Diabetes or Dietetic Association. Please enclose a stamped, self-addressed legal-size envelope. Regardless of the diet plan followed or the need for insulin, diabetics should be certain to eat regularly, spacing out their calorie quota throughout the day and not skipping meals or delaying a usual mealtime for several hours.

Regular exercise is also extremely important to the diabetic. Exercise seems to reduce a diabetic's need for insulin as well as help him or her to reach and maintain a normal body weight and perhaps also counter the development of atherosclerosis.

In the past oral drugs were readily prescribed for diabetics who did not require insulin. However, recent national studies raised serious doubts about their value above and beyond diet modification and suggested they may actually increase the diabetic's risk of heart attack. Experts urge that the oral diabetic drugs be used only for those in whom diet alone does not work and those who need insulin but are unable to administer it to themselves.

For Further Reading and Information

The following organizations can provide further information about diabetes. Both organizations have local affiliates, which are the preferred sources to contact.

● American Diabetes Association, Inc., 1 West Forty-eighth Street, New York, New York 10020.

● Juvenile Diabetes Foundation, 23 East Twenty-sixth Street, New York, New York 10010.

There are also a number of good books and cookbooks to help diabetics and their families:

American Diabetes Association, The, and The American Dietetic Association. *The American Diabetes Association/The American Dietetic Association Family Cookbook.* Englewood Cliffs, N.J.: Prentice-Hall, 1980.

Anderson, James W., M.D. *Diabetes.* New York: Arco, 1981. This book includes a menu plan for the high-carbohydrate, high-fiber diet.

Dolger, Henry, M.D., and Bernard Seeman. *How to Live with Diabetes.* New York: W.W. Norton, 1972.

Jones, Jeanne. *More Calculated Cooking.* San Francisco: 101 Productions, distributed by Scribner's, 1981.

Kivelowitz, Terri. *Diabetes.* Englewood Cliffs, N.J.: Spectrum /Prentice-Hall, 1981.

Lauffer, Ira J., M.D., and Herbert Kadison. *Diabetes Explained: A Layman's Guide.* New York: Dutton, 1976.

Mirsky, Stanley, M.D., and Joan Rattner Heilman. *Diabetes: Controlling It the Easy Way.* New York: Random House, 1981.

Silvian, Leonore. *Understanding Diabetes.* New York: Monarch Press, 1977.

Liver Disease: Many Victims Are Young

664

Most people think of alcoholism when they hear about cirrhosis and other liver diseases. However, there are many other causes of liver ailments — among them, drugs, viruses, toxins, and hereditary defects — and many victims are too young to have ever taken a drink.

Pamela was three weeks old when doctors realized she had been born without the ducts necessary for transporting bile from her liver, where it is made, to her intestinal tract, where it is used to digest fats and absorb fat-soluble vitamins. She underwent three operations before doctors succeeded in creating an artificial pipeline for bile, and now, at age three, she is growing and living normally.

Despite the surgery, Pamela has cirrhosis of the liver that is getting progressively worse. If no way can be found to stop it, she will in all likelihood eventually succumb to cirrhosis, a scarring and shrinking of the liver that can render this vital organ useless.

More than 100 different liver diseases afflict children. Though rarely discussed, childhood liver disease is more common than many widely publicized disorders, including muscular dystrophy, cystic fibrosis, and Tay-Sachs disease.

Among Americans of all ages liver disease is the seventh leading cause of death, well ahead of emphysema and kidney disease. Its frequency is increasing at an alarming rate as a result of a rise in viral hepatitis, exposure to environmental toxins, and alcohol abuse, especially among women. Despite these facts, liver research receives a disproportionately small share of federal research money — about $10 million a year.

"Liver disease has remained essentially a hidden disease because people thought it was all caused by alcohol, so they kept it a secret," notes Dr. Willis C. Maddrey, liver specialist at the Johns Hopkins University School of Medicine. "It was often omitted from death certificates to protect the family name." As a result, occupational and other causes of liver failure often went unrecognized.

The Liver's Role

The liver is your body's largest and most complex organ. Its tasks would overwhelm the capabilities of the world's largest chemical factory. A list of its functions makes it obvious why an artificial liver has not yet been developed and probably never will be. The liver's staggering work load includes the production of clotting factors, blood proteins, bile, and more than 1,000 different enzymes; the breakdown of old red blood cells; the metabolism of cholesterol; the storage of energy (glycogen) to fuel muscles; the maintenance of normal blood sugar concentration; the regulation of several hormones; and the detoxification of drugs and poisons, including alcohol.

Unlike other parts of your body, the liver has a built-in redundancy. You may lose half or more of it, and the remaining tissue can carry out all the necessary activities. It also has remarkable powers of recuperation and can regenerate lost tissue the way a salamander regrows its tail.

Common Causes of Liver Dysfunction

Viruses. Within the next year 1 in 250 Americans will get viral hepatitis, and half of them will be children. Hepatitis A virus, the cause of so-called infectious hepatitis, is transmitted through contaminated food and water. One in 500 Americans is a healthy carrier of hepatitis B virus, the cause of serum hepatitis. Carriers can spread the virus to others through blood transfusions and intimate contact.

Although blood donor programs now routinely screen for hepatitis B virus, there are other viruses carried in the blood that cannot currently be screened out and that cause hepatitis in 5 to 10 percent of persons who receive blood transfusions.

As with many other liver diseases, hepatitis can result in jaundice, which appears as a yellow discoloration of the skin, eyes, and other tissues as a result of a buildup of bile pigments. Severe generalized itching may also occur in this and other liver diseases. Other symptoms of hepatitis resemble the flu: loss of appetite, malaise, nausea and vomiting, and fever. There is no specific treatment, but most patients recover within several months.

Alcohol. This widely consumed substance is a poison to the liver, diverting it from its normal metabolic functions. When alcohol is present, the liver uses it as its preferred fuel, instead of burning fatty acids. The result is a buildup of unused fatty acids, causing a reversible disorder called, simply, fatty liver.

Just two days of heavy drinking can produce an increase in liver fat and cell damage. In fact, liver injury can be produced by amounts of alcohol that don't necessarily cause intoxication — the equivalent of seven to thirteen ounces of whiskey consumed over a twenty-four-hour period. Many steady social drinkers who do not get drunk and may not be considered alcoholics (though their drinking is clearly excessive) nonetheless consume enough alcohol to damage their livers.

Fatty liver usually produces no symptoms and disappears if alcohol abuse ends. But heavy drinking can also cause hepatitis, a potentially fatal liver inflammation accompanied by fever, pain, and jaundice. Alcoholic hepatitis usually also disappears when drinking is stopped, but continued alcohol abuse often leads to irreversible cirrhosis. Contrary to previous beliefs, recent studies have shown that cirrhosis can develop even if the drinker is well nourished. About 10 percent of alcoholics develop it, usually after ten to fifteen years of heavy drinking.

Alcohol abuse and its resultant cirrhosis also increase the risk of liver cancer, even among alcoholics who stopped drinking years ago.

Drugs and toxins. Nearly 100 different drugs are known to be toxic to the liver. Occasional causes of damage include the tuberculosis drug isoniazid and the anesthetic halothane. Megadoses of vitamin A, nicotinamide (a B vitamin), and iron can cause serious liver damage.

Toxins that harm the liver include carbon tetrachloride, toluene, and trichloroethylene (commercial solvents); yellow phosphorus (a rat poison); copper sulfate; and plastics chemicals like vinyl chloride. Natural liver poisons include aflatoxin, a cancer-causing substance produced by a mold that grows on damp grains and peanuts, and amanita mushroom toxin.

Anyone who is treated with drugs known to harm the liver or who works with a liver toxin should be checked periodically by a physician for early signs of trouble. Symptoms of harm are often vague — weakness, loss of appetite, headache, and possibly weight loss. However, a physical examination and blood tests that reveal liver function can often detect problems before serious damage occurs.

Congenital factors. Like Pamela, some children are born with liver problems: the absence of bile ducts, neonatal hepatitis, and inborn metabolic disorders including galactosemia (an inability to process a sugar in milk), glycogen storage disease, and alpha-1-antitrysin deficiency (an enzyme lack). Though there is no known cure for metabolic disorders, early detection and treatment with special diets can often prevent the brain damage and other abnormalities that otherwise result.

Some states, including New York, now screen newborns for galactosemia, which can be controlled by avoidance of all milk products. According to the Children's Liver Foundation, it costs only 50 cents a child to test for this inherited disease, but it can cost hundreds of thousands of dollars to care for just one child brain-damaged because it was not detected in time.

For Further Information

Among organizations supplying information about liver diseases and patient and parent support groups are the American Liver Foundation, 30 Sunrise Terrace, Cedar Grove, New Jersey 07009, and the Children's Liver Foundation, 28 Highland Avenue, Maplewood, New Jersey. 07040. These groups raise funds to support research in liver disease, public and professional education, and patient and family assistance.

Kidney Disease: Treatments Extend Useful Life

Even if modern technology were up to such a task, a science-fiction-sized laboratory with 140 miles of tubing and millions of filter units would be needed to duplicate the remarkable workings of the human kidneys, which weigh only about five ounces apiece.

The kidneys, a pair of bean-shaped organs in the back just above the waist, are considered the body's master chemists, capable of filtering the entire blood supply — five to six quarts — twenty-five times a day, cleansing it of toxic wastes, and maintaining the proper balance of salts, acids, and water. The chemical wastes and excess water collected by the kidneys are delivered to the bladder for periodic excretion as urine — an average of one and a half to two quarts a day.

As a sideline the kidneys also help the body use vitamin D and manufacture two important hormones: renin, which regulates blood pressure, and erythropoietin, which aids the production of red blood cells

In short, the kidneys — like the heart and lungs — are essential to life. When they do not work properly, high blood pressure, anemia, and, most important, uremic poisoning (the accumulation of toxic wastes) are the likely results.

Symptoms of Kidney Disease

There are six warning signs of possible kidney disease. Any one of the following signs or symptoms warrants a prompt and thorough medical examination:

- Burning sensation or any other difficulty during urination.
- Increased frequency of urination, especially at night.
- Puffiness around the eyes or swelling of the hands and feet, especially in children.

• Pain in the lower back just below the ribs that is not made worse by movement.

• Passage of blood-tinged or tea-colored urine.

• High blood pressure.

The examination may include blood and urine tests, a kidney X ray, and/or an ultrasound scan of the kidneys. Even in the absence of symptoms, a urinalysis should be done at every routine checkup since it can reveal problems that may otherwise smolder untreated for years.

Without at least one functioning kidney, the best brain and strongest heart would quickly wither. Yet a person with kidney failure today is far better off than someone whose brain or heart ceases functioning, for medical researchers have come closer to replacing the essential function of the kidney with a machine than they have for any other vital organ.

Some 13 million Americans have kidney disease that could threaten their lives. Most of these millions still have enough function left to maintain reasonably normal lives for many years. But for the 17,000 who become victims of terminal kidney disease each year, the kidneys stop working, and drastic steps must be taken to prevent fatal uremic poisoning.

Lifesaving Kidney Machines

More than 50,000 Americans have their blood cleansed daily by artificial kidney machines, thanks to a development by Dr. Belding H. Scribner and associates at the University of Washington in 1964. The artificial kidney, which saved many patients suffering temporary kidney failure after it was first developed in the Netherlands in the early 1940's, could not be used continuously for patients with chronic failure until Dr. Scribner's laboratory devised a blood-vessel shunt, or bypass, that permitted the device to be reconnected to the patient's blood supply for cleansing many times a week, week after week, year after year.

Kidney dialysis, as this artificial cleansing is called, is now paid for by Social Security. Most patients go three times a week to a hospital or dialysis center, where they are connected to the complex machine for four to eight hours at a time, at an annual cost of about $25,000 each. About 10 percent of dialysis patients are treated at home, usually with the help of family members, at a cost of about $18,000. A special low-protein, low-sodium, low-fluid diet must be followed to reduce the work that must be done by the kidney machine.

With the use of a new and less costly technique called continuous ambulatory peritoneal dialysis, round-the-clock cleansing of body wastes is possible in any location without constant professional help and with few or no dietary restrictions. In this method, which does not directly involve the blood, the peritoneum — the lining of the abdominal cavity — acts as the dialysis membrane, and wastes pass across it into a filtering solution that fills the cavity. The filtering solution is delivered from a plastic bag directly into the abdominal cavity through an implanted tube; four to six hours later the fluid, with accumulated wastes, is drained back into the bag and replaced with fresh solution. This process is repeated four or five times a day.

The technique, being used by perhaps 1,000 people, gives kidney patients greater flexibility by reducing their dependence on a machine. Some researchers believe it may ward off the deterioration of blood vessels and other problems associated with prolonged dependence on dialysis, perhaps because more frequent cleansing is possible.

About a third of dialysis patients are able to live full, normal lives thanks to this lifesaving technique. But for others, dialysis and what it signifies result in emotional and family problems, loss of income, and sexual difficulties. Some of these problems may be avoided with the ambulatory technique if early indications hold up.

Kidney Transplantation

Even at its best, dialysis is a stopgap measure that can prolong life but not overcome the underlying fatal disease. Only kidney transplantation can "cure" terminal kidney disease by replacement of the diseased kidney with a healthy one. More than 10,000 Americans live with the aid of someone else's kidney, and 10,000 to 15,000 more are waiting for a suitable organ to become available for transplantation. Because of a shortage of donated kidneys, only 4,200 patients receive transplants each year.

With improvements in organ preservation and better methods of matching tissue and suppressing graft rejection, kidney transplantation is a highly successful procedure for those medically suitable. Among patients who receive a kidney from a living relative, about 90 percent are alive and well two years later and likely to go on being so. Among patients whose kidneys come from cadaver donors, 50 to 60 percent survive.

Rejection of a transplant is not an automatic death sentence since the patient can return to dialysis indefinitely or until another transplant attempt is possible.

Donating a Kidney

The ideal kidney donor is a young, healthy person who has died as a result of an accidental injury, brain tumor, suicide, or drug overdose. Under the Uniform Anatomical Gift Act, any mentally competent person eighteen years of age or older can become a potential donor simply by signing a donor card, which should be carried on the person. In most states and the District of Columbia you can also indicate on your driver's license your desire to donate organs after death. In addition, it is important to inform your family of your wish to have your kidneys used so the physicians who attend your death will be aware of it. Delay in removing kidneys for transplantation can render them useless.

669

Donor cards can be obtained from local chapters of the National Kidney Foundation, Inc., or from its main office at 2 Park Avenue, New York, New York 10016. The foundation can also provide pamphlets on various aspects of kidney disease and its treatment.

XV. Coping with Health Problems

We all know people who cave in when confronted by life's inevitable challenges and others who use them as stepping-stones to ever greater heights.

From the mixed blessings of retirement to the awfulness of serious illness and death, the way you respond to a health problem or threat to your emotional stability, and the way people who are healthy treat you when you are not, can make an enormous difference in your ability to overcome the limitations of the problem and achieve the fullest possible recovery.

Too often the story is some version of "the operation was a success, but the patient died." Modern medicine can sometimes work wonders, but unless the patient participates, the miracle can be meaningless: The survivor of a heart attack becomes an emotional cripple; the victim of a treatable cancer rejects the lifesaving effects of anticancer drugs; the stroke victim neglects rehabilitative exercises.

At least half the secret of a good life after a serious illness or emotional disturbance lies in understanding the true nature of the problem and learning, with the help of family and friends, how to confront and surmount it.

Retirement:
Preparing for the Shock

Retirement is not always the joy-filled time typical of American dreams. For some, in fact, it precipitates a life crisis that requires major readjustments in thinking, living patterns, and relationships. Many of the problems that take the pleasure out of retirement result from a lack of planning for the time when a job will no longer structure your day and define who you are and how you feel about yourself.

Example: Don had looked forward to his impending retirement and the many fishing trips it would make possible. But he wasn't prepared for his wife's reaction when he tried to put his retirement plan into action. "I don't want to go fishing, and I'm not going to be a camp cook," she told him.

Example: Margaret's life became not her own after her husband retired. Suddenly he had lots of time and little to do, and he was everywhere: tagging along to the grocery store; fussing around the kitchen while she was cooking; even overseeing her weekly card game. "It's like having another kid," she remarked.

Example: Joe wasn't prepared for the lost sense of personal identity and achievement that accompanied retirement from his job as a managerial consultant. His wife, Rowena, was even less happy about giving up her job as a social worker. In fact, for about six months — until she went back to work part time — she was quite depressed.

Recent studies belie the widespread belief that the stress of retirement often precipitates serious illness and death. And there are unquestionably many happily retired people who are doing just what they want, within the constraints of physical abilities, fixed incomes, and rampant inflation. However, researchers note that undesirable emotional consequences of retirement are common, particularly for those who failed to develop interests outside their jobs or who never discussed the details of retirement with their spouses. Retirement shock — as it is often called — is felt by blue-collar worker and executive alike.

Why the Upheaval?

"Work supplies a lot of basic psychological needs that suddenly are cut off when a person retires," notes Leland P. Bradford, who retired more than a decade ago from his job as director of the National Training Laboratories. "As a worker, you have a sense of belonging to the producing part of society. Work helps to give you an identity. It is a source of human contact. It defines your goals and gives you a sense of accomplishment and affirmation."

When you stop working, these needs do not disappear, and failure to find other ways to fulfill them can produce emotional upheaval and marital discord. Even someone as "prepared" as Mr. Bradford, a behavioral scientist, suffered severe retirement pangs, which he described (along with the experiences of others) in his revealing and informative book *Retirement: Coping with Emotional Upheavals* (see "For Further Reading and Information," page 674). In an article in the *Harvard Business Review* he wrote: "The first year was awful. The organization moved on without me. No one called for advice. I found that golf did not fill a day. The consultation and volunteer work I did was not satisfying. Life felt empty. I became uncertain of my identity. I knew who I had been, but I was not certain who I was."

Mrs. Bradford suffered, too. Uprooted from the home she loved, she was unhappy and resentful that the quality of her life hadn't been considered in her husband's retirement plans. She also felt that her turf — the home territory that she had managed for years — had been invaded by a frustrated retired executive.

For those who find no satisfying alternatives to work, health may begin to decline, notes Dr. Erdman Palmore, professor of medical sociology at Duke University's Center for the Study of Aging and Human Development. He says, "Those who retire to the rocking chair tend to find that their body atrophies for lack of exercise and they become withdrawn and often depressed. This situation probably occurs more often among less educated persons who have not developed interests or skills outside of work and also among highly work-oriented middle class persons who are so driven by their work that they have no outside interests to fall back on."

673

Preretirement Planning

Joe Alexander, who in his retirement became senior consultant on retirement planning for Career Research and Testing in San Jose, emphasizes the importance of frank discussions between spouses about retirement plans. He points out, "A husband and wife may each have a dream of what retirement would be, but those dreams don't necessarily mesh. They've got to sit down and talk — outline their activities, restructure their time, and define their territories.

"I discovered that my wife was very afraid that after I retired, she'd have to wait on me hand and foot and would lose all her freedom."

Mr. Alexander recommends starting at fifty to plan for retirement, through family discussions and development of pleasurable and rewarding hobbies. A policeman he knows began making turquoise jewelry before he retired, and now he has a little business going that gives him a sense of pride and achievement and that fills his empty hours with an activity he enjoys.

Here are some tips to help you prepare for retirement:

● Plan a variety of activities — indoor and outdoor, mental and physical, social and individual — to maintain a sense of physical and mental well-being.

• Start now to make a list of all the things you'd like to do if only you had the time. Keep a file. It can be a valuable resource for planning your life in retirement.

• While you're working develop and maintain an interest in athletics, hobbies, and/or projects (community or personal) that you can pursue after retirement.

• Practice living on a retirement budget for a month. Take a close look at your assets, and devise a plan for how you will spend your money. For those who live in a valuable asset but who have limited available cash, a reverse mortgage (in which the bank takes out a mortgage on your house and pays you monthly) may be obtainable in some areas.

• Take a trial retirement. Just stay home for a month, and try to develop new interests and work out new routines and territories with your spouse.

Many large companies today provide counseling for prospective retirees, but in most cases the focus is on practical issues: financial planning, medical care, residence, and the like. However, a growing number of job-based preretirement programs consider emotional and social concerns as well. In addition, many community and junior colleges and university-based gerontology centers now offer retirement counseling programs.

After Retirement

• Don't sit around and wait for people to call you. Initiate social contacts. Keep up friendships.

• Build up routines — times to play, times to work, times to be alone, times to do things with others.

• Find goals that will keep you active and interested. The significance of your accomplishments matters far less than the fact that you have to surmount obstacles to achieve them.

• Get involved with community work that you enjoy and that gives you a sense of purpose and satisfaction. If you choose a second career after your retirement from the first and now must retire from it as well, consider helping other elderly people make the most of their remaining years.

For Further Reading and Information

Bradford, Leland P. *Retirement: Coping with Emotional Upheavals.* Chicago: Nelson-Hall,1979.

Willins, Jules Z. *The Reality of Retirement: The Inner Experience of Becoming a Retired Person.* New York: William Morrow, 1981.

For information on where to get help with the psychosocial problems of retirement in your area, send a stamped, self-addressed envelope to Richard Knodell, Career Planning and Adult Development Network, 1190 South Bascom Avenue, Suite 211, San Jose, California 95128.

Mid-Life Crisis:
Myth or Reality?

In mid-life Paul Gauguin left his wife, family, and a staid bank job to live in the South Seas and paint. In his mid-forties Charles Dickens moved out of the bedroom he shared with his wife, took a nineteen-year-old mistress, and began acting strangely. William Shakespeare, who wrote two plays in which abrupt character transformations of middle-aged men led to their ruin, is said to have retired from marital sex before age forty-five and retired from work at forty-six.

Though the notion of a "male menopause" comparable to the hormonal changes that women experience has been soundly debunked, there is considerable evidence that many, if not most, men undergo an unsettled and often life-disrupting period sometime between the ages of thirty-five and fifty. This period, aptly dubbed a mid-life crisis, is often marked by self-doubt, marital discord and divorce, extramarital affairs, abrupt career shifts, personality changes, sexual problems, depression, and newly awakened anxieties about health and mortality.

For some men and, these days, for a growing number of women as well, mid-life is a crucial turning point that determines their future. Dr. Daniel J. Levinson, a Yale University psychologist who has studied life stages in adult men, points out that "men such as Freud, Jung, Eugene O'Neill, Frank Lloyd Wright, Goya, and Gandhi went through a profound crisis around forty and made themselves creative geniuses through it." But others, including Dylan Thomas and Sinclair Lewis, failed to weather the crisis, which led ultimately to their destruction.

This view of mid-life as a major transition point is not shared by all experts. Indeed, Dr. Paul McHugh, chief psychiatrist at Johns Hopkins University, describes the notion as "pure fiction." The tasks of mid-life may be different from previous ones, but no worse, he says. "The message that in mid-life we can expect to come apart — that we're entitled to come apart — is a myth and sometimes just a rationalization. Life is a series of difficulties and chances. However, life's obstacles are less dramatic than implied by such chronologically laid-out events as a mid-life crisis."

Yet, in a culture that values youth and beauty, there is little doubt that major disruptions can and do occur in the lives of many middle-aged Americans. Sometimes they result in family breakups (especially if one partner blames the marriage for his or her disappointments in life), alcohol or drug abuse, or even suicide. Knowing what the disruptions may be and what to do about them can help you move through this period constructively and emerge from it with a healthier perspective and a happier life. Just knowing that you are normal and not a lone sufferer through the pangs of mid-life can help you cope better with the issues and problems you must confront.

Who Is at Risk?

Those who seem most vulnerable to serious mid-life crises are middle- and upper-class professionals with high expectations for themselves and a desire to make the most out of life. But there is some evidence that blue-collar workers suffer as well when they begin to take stock of their lives or worry about how long they'll be able to continue in their jobs. The questions raised are likely to include: What have I accomplished? Is this all there is to life? What do I really want? Am I heading anywhere but the cemetery?

Various circumstances can trigger such a state. Among them are the death of a parent, the serious illness of a friend, personal illness, or signs of aging (graying hair, wrinkles, flabbiness), which stir up feelings of vulnerability and a fear of death. At work you may have failed to achieve your life's goal, been passed over for a promotion, realized you're stuck in your present position, or felt pressured by competition from younger employees. Or you may have achieved all you set out to do and now find it to be an empty victory.

At home your children may have become difficult adolescents who defy parental values. Or the children have gone off to school and seem not to need you any longer. Your wife may have given up her housewife's role and gotten a job or gone back to school. Or you may have grown apart, and your spouse now seems unattractive, boring, disinterested, or unable to understand you.

Sexual Effect

You may also be afflicted with self-doubts because your sexual performance or interest has fallen off. These problems may coincide with your wife's menopause and the physical and emotional upsets that may accompany it. [See chapter on the menopause, page 229.]

You may not even be aware of your personal anguish, which can instead manifest itself as a psychosomatic complaint like abdominal or chest pains, backaches, or impotence. In fact, sex researchers have shown that the majority of potency problems are psychological in origin, the result of misconceptions, fear or anticipation of failure, or underlying depression. Sometimes longstanding, unresolved marital problems show up as sexual problems in mid-life.

In contrast to the sharp drop in estrogen production among menopausal women, there is no sudden decline in the male sex hormone, testosterone, which instead very slowly diminishes in amount after the teen years. Rarely is impotence related to a lack of testosterone, although other hormonal derangements may be involved and should be tested for, as should possible underlying diseases. [See chapter on impotence, page 174.]

What does occur as a man gets older is a slowing of the sexual response: a greater need for direct physical stimulation to produce an erection, a diminished urgency to reach orgasm, and a longer period between orgasms. [See chapter on sex and aging, page 185.] A man who assumes that he is "washed up" sexually because of one or more instances of impotence or failure to reach orgasm is likely to fulfill his own prophecy. Or he may turn to a younger mistress in an effort to prove his potency and vitality. Similarly, a middle-aged woman may take a younger lover to boost her libido or reassure herself that she is still attractive.

Helpful Measures

Various constructive options are available to someone about to enter or already mired in a mid-life crisis. One of the best is to take inventory of your past accomplishments and future possibilities. Make a realistic appraisal of what you have done and what you might do in the years ahead. List the satisfying aspects of your present life as well as the desired goals you have thus far not obtained. Is what you want potentially within your grasp, what would it take to achieve it, and is the sacrifice worth it?

What problems are you having with your marriage or children? Might these be amenable to therapy? If so, get help, the sooner the better, from a marriage or family counselor, psychotherapist, or sex therapist. Similarly, get help if you are very depressed and unable to pull yourself out of it.

677

If you dread retirement or feel your present job is unsatisfying but you're stuck in it, explore outside activities that will stimulate your interest, gratify your ego, and fill your needs. [See chapter on how to avoid retirement shock, page 672.]

Make an appraisal of your personal habits. Are you slowly killing yourself or contributing to your own deterioration? Are you overweight? Do you smoke or drink too much? Do you take too many death-defying risks to prove your masculinity? You would do far more to boost your self-esteem, your health, and your life expectancy — and to ward off the ravages of age — by adopting sensible eating habits, exercising regularly, and avoiding dangerous substances and activities.

In other words, turn your mid-life crisis to your own advantage by making it a time for renewal of your body and mind, rather than standing by helplessly and watching them decline.

For Further Reading

Donohugh, Donald L., M.D. *The Middle Years.* Philadelphia, Saunders, 1981.
Farrell, Michael P., and Stanley D. Rosenberg. *Men at Midlife.* Boston: Auburn House, 1981.
Gray, Madeline. *The Changing Years.* New York: Doubleday, 1981.
Irwin, Theodore. "Male 'Menopause,' Crisis in the Middle Years." Public Affairs Pamphlet No. 526, 1975. Available for 50 cents from Public Affairs Pamphlets, 381 Park Avenue South, New York, N.Y. 10016.

Levinson, Daniel J., Ph.D. *The Seasons of a Man's Life.* New York: Ballantine, 1978.
Mayer, Nancy. *The Male Mid-Life Crisis.* New York: New American Library, 1978.
Rose, Louisa, ed. *The Menopause Book.* New York: Hawthorn, 1977.
Sheehy, Gail. *Passages.* New York: Bantam, 1977.

Surviving a Heart Attack: Life After Near-Death

Each year 400,000 Americans have a close brush with death when they suffer, and survive, a heart attack. Thanks to improvements in coronary care, most patients who are alive upon reaching the hospital will be discharged some weeks later on the road to recovery.

But medicine, which can perform such miracles to heal the heart, too often forgets the person who houses it. Doctors who are superb cardiologists are not necessarily experts at psychosocial rehabilitation. Patients, who may be reluctant to bother the doctor with "pedestrian" matters, often fail to ask the right questions. Instead, many assume they know the answers or they listen to the unschooled advice of friends and relatives.

A thirty-eight-year-old Massachusetts fisherman found himself unable to go to sea — and therefore unable to return to work — after recovering from a heart attack. Without apparent medical cause, he was extremely fatigued and had become sexually impotent.

The fisherman denied being afraid, but a cardiologist fitted him with a portable heart monitor to wear when he went out on his boat and discovered changes in his heart rhythm that were classic signs of fear. Counseling sessions and relaxation exercises helped the man overcome his fear that he would die at sea away from his family and enabled him to return to work. When he was relieved of fear and depression, his potency problems were also resolved.

Few patients are properly counseled about life after a heart attack and many — at least 60,000 people a year — who have physically mended hearts end up with minds that keep them cardiac cripples. Overwhelmed by a sense of vulnerability and beset by myths and misinformation about the effects of a heart attack, they are relegated to half a life. Because of fear, depression, and ignorance, they may be unable to work, unable to enjoy the activities they once loved, unable to express themselves sexually. Their lives are turned upside down, their places in the family and society disrupted. Not surprisingly the death rate from a second heart attack among such patients is much higher than among those who return to a more vigorous and fulfilling existence.

The Aftermath: Myth and Reality

According to Dr. Thomas Hackett, a psychiatrist at Massachusetts General Hospital in Boston, the problem usually begins the very day the

678

heart patient goes home from the hospital. Exhausted just by the walk from the car to the front door, the patient falsely attributes his or her fatigue to a failing heart (it is really the consequence of extended bed rest) and despairs of ever returning to a normal life.

In addition to fatigue, homecoming depression, as Dr. Hackett calls it, includes irritability, sleep changes, loss of interest in sex and other activities previously enjoyed, memory problems, recurrent thoughts of death, and guilt feelings about having brought the heart attack upon himself or herself. Typically the depression lasts for three months and then lifts. But for about 15 percent of patients, Dr. Hackett says, the depression doesn't clear, and "unwarranted cardiac invalidism" results.

Much of the problem can be avoided if patients and their families are told what to expect and prevalent myths are countered with facts, especially the following:

Excitement. Many heart patients are needlessly told not to "worry" or "get excited." They are prohibited from watching exciting sports events or driving in traffic, excluded from family arguments, and pushed into less demanding jobs. While overreactions to stress are not healthful to anyone, normal emotions and activities do not endanger the lives of heart patients. On the contrary, excluding a person from such things may deprive him or her of pleasure and feelings of usefulness.

Physical activity. A heart patient or the patient's family may assume or be told that exercise is dangerous to an injured heart. He or she may be cautioned against lifting things, raising the arms over the head, or returning to leisure activities that involve exercise to avoid precipitating another attack.

In truth, a prescribed program of physical activity geared to the capabilities of the recovering heart patient can strengthen the heart and help to protect against a recurrence. Ideally such a program should be begun in the hospital and continued afterward under medical supervision. Dr. Hackett says this is the single most effective way to lift a patient's spirits, alleviate anxiety, and restore feelings of potency about all aspects of life. Heart patients who exercise also seem better able to tolerate life stresses.

One man who had been a hockey player was told to slow down after a heart attack at age thirty-eight and he did just that: He sat around drinking beer, gaining weight, and feeling like an invalid. A running program gave him a new lease on life, and he gradually worked his way up to running a marathon.

Sexual expression. Perhaps the most common but least talked about aftermath of a heart attack is withdrawal from sexual activity, primarily because of fear on the part of the patient and/or the patient's spouse that the demands of sex are too taxing for a damaged heart.

In fact, however, sex is not that strenuous. Careful studies of heart rates reached during sexual intercourse showed that in familiar surroundings with one's own spouse, sex is no more demanding for a heart patient than climbing a flight of stairs or walking briskly for two or three blocks. A study of 5,559 coronary deaths revealed that only 18 of them were related to sex, and 14 of those involved extramarital relations. Furthermore, nearly all sex-related coronary deaths occur after heavy drinking or eating.

Heart patients and their spouses need thorough counseling about sex. In many cases couples have needlessly abstained from sexual intercourse, causing resentment and frustration in the spouse and depression and loss of self-esteem in the patient. In other cases anxiety has produced impotence, needlessly bringing an end to the couple's sex life.

Dr. Hackett, who has written a forthcoming pamphlet on sex for the heart patient for the American Heart Association, says couples should be told that in uncomplicated cases normal sexual relations can resume after about six to ten weeks or as soon as the doctor says it is all right; that no special position is needed; that at first anxiety may result in episodes of impotence or premature ejaculation; that the chest pains of angina can be prevented or treated with nitroglycerin tablets (but their occurrence should be reported to the physician); and that it would be wise to start slowly, with just caresses the first few times.

Other recommendations include avoiding sexual activity when the patient is extremely tired or under emotional strain, within an hour of a regular meal (or two hours after a big meal), and within one or two hours of drinking alcohol.

Many patients and families grappling with the emotional and physical adjustments necessitated by a heart attack can benefit from participation in a heart club. Most clubs operate in conjunction with exercise programs or other hospital-based cardiac programs. Some patient-organized self-help groups also exist, although Dr. Hackett and others believe such groups should always be run by a professional.

For Further Reading

Cohn, Dr. Keith; Darby Duke; and Joseph A. Madrid. *Coming Back.* Reading, Mass.: Addison-Wesley, 1979.
Weiss, Elizabeth. *Recovering from the Heart Attack Experience.* New York: Macmillan, 1980.

After a Stroke: Achieving Maximum Recovery

In 1964, while pregnant with her fifth child and in the middle of shooting a film in Hollywood, Patricia Neal suffered in quick succession three massive hemorrhagic strokes that nearly killed her. Thanks to emergency surgery to repair the ruptured blood vessel in her brain, she survived — only to emerge two weeks later from a coma to find herself with double vision and unable to speak or walk.

"I wanted to die," she recalled four years later. Instead, she began the long struggle back to life and health. Aided by her husband, author Roald Dahl, friends, neighbors, and professional therapists, Miss Neal learned to speak, read, and walk again. Six months after her strokes she gave birth to a healthy girl and immediately resumed the seemingly endless and exhausting rehabilitative exercises and speech lessons. They paid off. Three years later she was able to return to her demanding job of acting as the star of the movie *The Subject Was Roses.*

Miss Neal's recovery after such severe strokes is an inspiration to all, but especially to the 300,000 or so Americans who each year suffer strokes and live. Currently there are nearly 3 million people in this country who have survived one or more strokes. About 30 percent of stroke survivors recover fully and return to their normal activities, 55 percent are left partially handicapped, and 15 percent remain totally handicapped.

Full recovery is certainly not within reach of all stroke victims. While the extent of brain damage incurred at the time of the stroke determines the outer limits of recovery, how close a person comes to reaching these limits is determined as much by the attitudes and efforts of the patient and the patient's family as by the timing and quality of special rehabilitation exercises. For some patients tests that delineate the cause of the stroke can lead to delicate brain surgery or other therapy that may head off a recurrence.

The Fight Back Starts Immediately

For most, the main task in the aftermath of a stroke is a struggle to adjust to and regain lost abilities. The rehabilitation effort must start almost immediately to keep joints from becoming "frozen" and to take advantage of the responsiveness of the brain to speech therapy during its period of spontaneous recovery. The exercises must be vigorously pursued even when the effort is exhausting and seems hopeless since most patients do improve significantly through rehabilitation.

As a rule, whatever major recovery is going to take place happens during the first year after the stroke, although slight gains can still be made through continued exercises and practice. Within the limits of permanent brain damage, the more highly motivated the patient and the more understanding and cooperative the family, the more successful the rehabilitation and adjustment will be. Therefore, it's very important for all involved to know what can happen to a person following a stroke and to respond in a way that will help, rather than hinder, recovery. The following disabilities are common in the weeks or months after a stroke:

Speech and language difficulties. About half of stroke victims lose all or part of their language facilities, at least temporarily. The difficulty may involve an inability to form intelligible words or sentences, understand spoken or written language, write, name objects, and express what they mean, among other problems. Often, the patient will indicate understanding when, in fact, the message didn't get through or was garbled.

Speech therapy should start as soon as the patient is allowed up. In speaking to a stroke victim with language problems, stand on the person's "good" side; keep your sentences short and limited to one or two ideas; use your natural voice; speak slowly and distinctly, but don't shout; use everyday words and phrases, don't interrupt when the patient tries to speak; don't talk down to the patient or correct his or her mistakes; and when giving instructions, give them one at a time and keep them simple.

Partial paralysis. It is usual for a stroke patient to be partly or completely paralyzed on one side of the body — the side opposite the brain hemisphere in which the stroke occurred. Nine in ten patients who cannot walk in the aftermath of a stroke will recover that ability, although some may have to use a cane or walker. However, when an arm is paralyzed, full recovery is much less likely. Here again, starting rehabilitation as soon as possible after the stroke is crucial, as is devotion to the prescribed exercises.

Visual disturbances. About one in five stroke victims experiences such problems as double vision, rapid eye movements (nystagmus), total blindness in one eye, or a loss of peripheral vision in both eyes, making it seem as if there were blinders on. Patients may totally ignore objects on the side where vision is impaired, not even turning their heads and acting as if nothing were there. Eyeglasses cannot help in such cases. Spatial perceptions and sense of balance may also be impaired, which results in "navigation" difficulties — bumping into doorways, not knowing left from right or sitting from standing. A patient with visual or spatial problems should not be allowed to drive.

Fatigue. Although the reasons why are not clear, extreme fatigue is practically a universal occurrence in the aftermath of a stroke and sometimes lasts for a year or more. Everything seems to require an enormous effort, and once-active people may find this extremely distressing. It's best that the patient give in to the body's demand for additional rest. But make sure that the fatigue isn't being perpetuated by depression that should have professional attention.

Personality changes. This effect of a stroke is probably harder for loved ones to take than physical disability. In the weeks or months after a stroke the patient may be extremely irritable and demanding, resistant to assistance, and given to unreasonable anger and rapid mood swings. Sudden, unexplained crying jags, inappropriate bursts of laughter, and streaks of cursing are common; these nearly always disappear with time.

If the patient is apathetic and uninterested in living, it's up to family and friends to try to stimulate interests and reignite the spark of life, which is critical to successful rehabilitation. Excessive self-pity, depression, and resistance to therapy should receive professional attention.

Stroke patients should not be treated like helpless children and waited on hand and foot. Rather, they should be encouraged to do more and more by themselves. It is important to be reassuring and sympathetic, but not pitying. To help rebuild a sense of worth, let the patient know he or she is still loved and worthwhile. Be encouraging about all progress, giving positive feedback immediately after something is done correctly. But don't nag about errors. The patient is already frustrated enough.

Nutritional problems. Initially many stroke patients are unable to swallow and must be tube-fed. While some never recover the ability to eat solid foods, most can gradually resume a regular diet. When this occurs, it's important the foods served be as normal as possible — cooked fish that can be flaked, ground meat, mashed potatoes, applesauce, rather than baby foods or strained foods. To counter dryness of the mouth caused by some drugs, foods should be moistened with broth, juices, and gravies. Eating six small meals a day may be less tiring than three large one.

Learning problems. Though there is no loss of basic intelligence following a stroke, attention span and the ability to reason, render sound judgments, and remember things from moment to moment may be seriously impaired. Something learned in one setting may be quickly forgotten in another. Most patients do better if step-by-step instructions, appointments, or other important messages are put in writing. Written reminders around the house about where things are and how to use them are also helpful.

Stroke rehabilitation is a team effort. Professionals on the team include a physiatrist (physician trained in rehabilitative medicine), physical therapist, speech therapist, occupational therapist, recreational therapist, nutritionist, psychologist or psychiatrist, and a social worker. Most large community hospitals and medical centers today have special rehabilitation teams. In addition, some cities have freestanding (that is, apart from hospitals) rehabilitation centers.

If no rehabilitation facility exists in your area, you may be able to do a great deal yourself, with the assistance of friends and relatives, to aid a stroke patient's recovery, especially in the area of speech therapy. In addition, family and patient support may be available through Stroke Clubs organized under the auspices of the Easter Seal Society or the American Heart Association. Both these organizations (check your phone book for local chapters) can provide much valuable information about strokes.

For Further Reading

Adaptations and Techniques for the Disabled Homemaker. Available for $2.95 from the

Sister Kenny Institute, Chicago Avenue at Twenty-seventh Street, Minneapolis, Minn. 55407.

"Do It Yourself Again — Self-Help Devices for the Stroke Patient." A free booklet published by the American Heart Association.

Fowler, Roy S., and W.E. Fordyce. "Stroke: Why Do They Behave That Way?" A free booklet published by the American Heart Association.

Hess, Lucille J., and Robert E. Bahr, M.D. *What Every Family Should Know About Strokes.* New York: Appleton-Century-Crofts, 1981.

Mealtime Manual for People with Disabilities and the Aging. Available for $3.25 from Campbell Soup Co., Box (MM) 56, Camden, N.J. 08101.

Sarno, John E., M.D., and Martha Taylor Sarno. *Stroke: A Guide for Patients and Their Families.* New York: McGraw-Hill, 1979.

Cancer Chemotherapy: Surviving the Treatment

For growing numbers of Americans who are found to have cancer, treatment with potent anticancer drugs is being recommended as the main mode of therapy or as an adjunct to primary therapy with surgery or radiation. An artillery of some three dozen different drugs are now being used in various combinations to improve survival chances for patients with a wide range of cancers. Chemotherapy, as the drug treatment is called, has already turned around the grim prognosis for such cancers as advanced Hodgkin's disease and childhood leukemia, which previously were almost universally fatal.

Increasingly today chemotherapy is being used as a front-line weapon against common cancers, such as breast, colon, lung, and ovarian cancers, which collectively afflict hundreds of thousands of Americans each year. The drugs, used in combinations of up to five different ones, are usually given for periods of months or years soon after surgery has removed all visible cancer or after radiation has caused it to shrink.

As survival statistics are slowly being gathered, it appears that for some cancers and certain patients, at least, the drugs represent a substantially better chance for cure than has been possible with surgery or radiation therapy alone. Even for those who are not cured, chemotherapy can sometimes buy time, extending useful life by many months or years.

Misapprehensions Abound

Yet medical oncologists who administer the anticancer drugs report that many patients (and patients' families) are reluctant to accept the treatments. Myths, misunderstandings, and frank misinformation about cancer drugs often stand in the way of patient acceptance. Among the mistaken notions, according to Mary-Ellen Kulkin Siegel, a social worker at Mount Sinai Hospital and consultant to the Chemotherapy Foundation in New York City, are that chemotherapy is a treatment of last resort, that the side effects are worse than the disease, that patients can't lead normal lives while on chemotherapy, and that all cancer patients are guinea pigs on whom unproved drugs are tried.

Many patients who face the prospect of chemotherapy report that cancer doctors are insensitive to the needs and fears of patients. Doctors often fail to explain properly the potential benefits and risks of the drugs and fail to support patients and their families adequately through the rough times.

The Side Effects

No one who has been through it or who has watched anyone go through it would pretend that chemotherapy is fun. Among the possible distressing side effects of the various drugs are nausea, vomiting, diarrhea, loss of appetite, hair loss, fatigue, depression, loss of libido, and impotence. Some can cause such serious complications as heart rhythm abnormalities and a depressed ability to fight off infections.

Most of the effects, like nausea and vomiting, are temporary, lasting perhaps a day after each round of treatment. Others, like hair loss and diminished immune response, disappear after the treatment program has ended. Few patients experience all, or even most, of the possible side effects associated with a particular combination of drugs. And most patients are able to continue their usual routine — work, school, play, maintenance of a household — with only brief interruptions throughout the course of chemotherapy.

But a patient who prior to deciding on chemotherapy is asked to sign a consent form that lists only one uncertain benefit (longer life expectancy) and a dozen or more horrid-sounding side effects is likely to balk at the prospect unless someone — doctor, nurse, or counselor — takes the time to explain the realities and answer the lingering questions. And patients already on chemotherapy who are having a difficult time with the side effects are likely to stop taking the drugs unless empathy, practical assistance, and repeated bolstering are forthcoming from the medical team and others.

The Doctor's Attitude

The all too common attitude of chemotherapists — that the discomfort of anticancer drugs is a small price to pay for a chance to live longer — is of little help to the person experiencing the misery. The patient is likely to think a pleasant life now is preferable to an uncertain future promise.

When a patient asks the doctor about unproved alternative cancer treatments, like Laetrile and megavitamins, the response is often a stated or implied threat: "If you take anything like that, find yourself another doctor." Yet, as Dr. Jimmie Holland, chief psychiatrist at Memorial Sloan-Kettering Cancer Center, points out, throwing out the cancer patient who takes Laetrile is the wrong approach. She explains that cancer patients turn to such therapies because they "feel helpless, out of control of their destinies, and fear that traditional treatments will fail. They need to master their situation, and they hope for a miraculous cure." [See chapter on cancer quackery, page 655.]

Sources of Support

Dr. Holland recommends the use of support groups involving other chemotherapy patients, counseling sessions with the patient's family, and perhaps psychotherapy and psychotherapeutic drugs to relieve depression and anxiety. Those administering chemotherapy must not minimize the patient's discomfort but rather acknowledge how tough it is to have those side effects, Dr. Holland insists. "When patients feel that they are understood and not belittled, they will take almost anything," she says.

In addition to moral support, chemotherapy patients often need help with such everyday matters as how to cope with nausea, what to eat and drink, how to get help at home when they need it, and what to do when their hair starts falling out. Though they are no substitute for direct counseling, several pamphlets for patients and their families are now available to help with such matters. See "For Further Reading" below.

For Further Reading

Blumberg, Rena. *Headstrong: A Story of Conquests and Celebrations . . . Living Through Chemotherapy.* New York: Crown, 1982.

"Chemotherapy, Your Weapon Against Cancer." Published by the Chemotherapy Foundation, Inc., 2 East Eighty-sixth Street, New York, New York. 10028. Individual copies cost $2.

"Eating Hints: Recipes and Tips for Better Nutrition During Cancer Treatment." Available free from the Office of Cancer Communications, National Cancer Institute, Bethesda, Maryland 20205.

"Understanding Chemotherapy, A Guide for Patients and Families." Published by the Department of Neoplastic Diseases, Mount Sinai Medical Center, 100th Street and Fifth Avenue, New York, New York 10029. Single copies are free; additional copies cost 75 cents each.

Visiting the Sick:
What to Do, What to Say

A friend was near the end of a long battle against recurring cancer. Several times during her illness I had spoken to her and her husband about possible treatments. When I could no longer offer hope for cure, I was afraid to see her.

Here was a woman, lovely and talented, only a few years older than I, a woman with two young children and a loving husband. There, but for the grace of God, go I.

I postponed my visit until she was home from the hospital, justifying my delay with such excuses to myself as "I'm much too busy now" and "I really don't know her *that* well." When I finally went to see her, I arrived shielded by the company of my husband. On the way there I asked him, "What should I say?" It seemed to me that she would resent anything I might talk about because she was not well enough to "enjoy" such concerns.

The conversation was upbeat, centering on such "safe" topics as writing, theater, and work, topics of mutual interest when she was well. I later learned that after our visit my friend had cried because I was so full of life and energy and she was not — a natural human reaction, one I had anticipated. But I myself was so afraid that I could not head it off. In an hour's conversation we never talked about her, about what she was going through and how she felt about it.

I learned a lot from that experience about visiting the sick. Unfortunately what I learned cannot help her since she died before I saw her again.

Hesitancy Is Natural

Visiting a sick friend or relative is something most people know they *should* do, but many delay or avoid it, especially if the patient is in the hospital or is suffering from a debilitating or incurable condition. For most people the hospital is an alien, frightening environment full of suffering, strange goings-on, unpleasant sights and odors. In addition, seeing someone you know and love who is in pain, or worse, forces you to confront your own mortality, your inevitable vulnerability to illness and death. It is natural in such circumstances to feel anxious and afraid, sometimes to the point of avoiding loved ones when they most need you — when they themselves are anxious and afraid.

Benefits to Patients

There may be no scientific data to document the benefits to patients of visits from caring friends and relatives, but anecdotal evidence abounds. The patient who feels cut off from life, who thinks "no one cares," is likely to feel more pain and make less effort toward his recovery. One old man died at a nursing home after his son failed to show up on Thanksgiving Day. The autopsy revealed no physical reason for his death; he apparently died of a broken heart.

Rabbi Joseph Levine, chaplain at the Clinical Center of the National Institutes of Health in Bethesda, Maryland, and at St. Elizabeth's Hospital in Washington, D.C., says that the only hospital patients who get visited with any regularity are new mothers, probably because they are usually not very sick and because their hospital experience is a life-affirming event. Rabbi Levine, whose life's work is visiting the sick, says that most patients, "even if all they have is an ingrown toenail," appreciate the caring that a visit reflects.

"In spite of the color TV, books, magazines, or recreational therapy that the hospital provides, the patient remains hungry for the company of people from home or the office, people who care enough not to *send* the very best, but *to bring themselves* in person," Rabbi Levine wrote in an article in the magazine *Moment*. In an interview he added, "Patients often put up with hideous pain because family and friends are there and caring about them."

As the visitor you, too, can benefit from the visit, which is often a personal growth experience and helps you prepare for similar circumstances.

How to Behave

Rabbi Levine offers the following advice:

● You don't have to know the person very well to visit. If you care, go.

● Check first with a relative, the nursing station, or the patient to see if, and when, a visit would be appreciated. You may not be welcome when the office gang is there or right after the patient has gone through an exhausting test.

● Bringing a gift is all right, but it shouldn't be used as a shield to divert you from meaningful, emotional conversation. The rabbi believes that "It's best to go in 'naked,' just yourself; you are the most valuable gift."

● Sending a gift is not a substitute for a visit. It's all right for the office to send something, but if there's a real tie between you and the patient, a visit is better. Of course, if you cannot visit, a gift or card is better than nothing.

● If you don't know how to start the conversation, you can just say "Hello" or "How are you today?" or "I'm sorry you're ill." Then let the patient take the lead. Most patients give clues to what they want to talk about, and it's up to the visitor to pick them up.

● Whatever you do, don't show up prepared with a speech. Just be yourself. "You can even say, 'I feel terrible. This is frightening to me.' As long as you're genuine, it's OK," Rabbi Levine says. "Even visitors who bungle and say the wrong thing are a plus," he believes, since patients tend to ignore the faux pas.

● No matter what the circumstances, try to preserve the tone of your past relationship with the patient. You can joke, laugh, or argue. It's also all right to be silent, to speak with your heart and your eyes instead of your mouth.

● A patient who starts raging about his or her fate or talking about dying should not be interrupted with, "Don't talk that way; you'll be fine in no time." Let the patient say what's on his or her mind. Afterward you may want to discuss any misconceptions, but don't dismiss the patient's feelings. They're legitimate and need to be aired.

● It's not helpful to tell the patient about others with similar problems. To be compared to others diminishes the patient as a person.

●Don't forget the patient's family. In some cases it may be more important to visit the family or provide logistical support, such as transportation, baby-sitting, or preparing a meal. You can be sure the patient will hear about anything you do to help.

Dr. Michael A. Simpson, a psychiatrist at London University and author of *The Facts of Death* (Englewood Cliffs., N.J.: Prentice-Hall, 1979), adds to this list the importance of listening and touching. He points out that visitors often ignore a patient's references to death, suffering, anger, and despair, hoping the conversation will turn to more cheerful topics.

"The dying soon learn to be very considerate of our feelings, for they fear that we might not come back to see them at all if they upset us. So they discover that they are not allowed to talk about some of the things that worry them very much indeed," Dr. Simpson wrote.

As for touching, he said, "be ready to hold hands, to hug, to stroke." This primitive form of communication can convey feelings that go far beyond words and can comfort people who are sick beyond the reach of words.

Dr. Simpson notes that some people avoid visiting a dying friend or relative lest they be confronted with direct questions from the patient about the nature of the illness or the prognosis. When that happens, you might ask the patient what he or she knows or why he or she is asking or you might suggest that the matter be discussed with the doctor.

Dr. Simpson adds that the visitor can always offer hope — if not hope for recovery, then hope that the patient can go home again, or enjoy a good meal, watch a movie, or visit with friends or relatives who are coming from some distance.

A final note to visitors from Rabbi Levine: Don't stay too long. If the patient is obviously tired or embarrassed by discomfort or says or does something that translates into "good-bye for today," take the hint. Two short visits are better than one overly long one.

Dying: Easing the Way
for Patient and Family

Although it is often said humorously that no one gets through this life alive, few of us know how to deal realistically with this inescapable fact.

George, for example, knew that the doctors had exhausted their repertory of promising treatments and that his remaining time on earth was short. But when he conveyed this understanding to his family, they goaded him: "Come on, what are you talking about? There are plenty more drugs where those came from. You'll see, you'll be better in no time." As the days wore on and George got sicker and sicker, he became silent and depressed, unable to talk to the people he most loved because they refused to acknowledge his imminent, inevitable death.

Today experiencing the death of loved ones is a relatively rare occurrence until quite late in life. Half the population used to die before age forty. Now half lives beyond age seventy. More than nine in ten children born will still be alive at age forty. Nearly three-fourths of deaths occur in institutional settings — hospitals and nursing homes — with few, if any, family members present and with all kinds of equipment and strangers in the way.

As death becomes a more foreign experience, there is less opportunity for passing along the lessons of how to cope adequately with it, either to the person who is dying or to the family and friends who must live after. At the same time an increasing proportion of deaths occurs as a result of illnesses like cancer, in which the process of dying is prolonged and emotionally painful.

Thanatology: Understanding Dying

In the last decade studies by experts called thanatologists (from the Greek word for "death") have led to an understanding of what dying people go through that can greatly help them and their loved ones deal effectively with the situation. Thanatologists have learned that dying, like living, is a process and that while there are different styles of dying — just as there are different styles of living — there are common elements and problems present as most people prepare for death.

The researchers have also found that nearly all patients with terminal illnesses know that they are dying without being told, but when family, friends, and physicians pretend that the patient will recover, the process of dying is made even more difficult. Surveys have shown that four out of five people would want to be told if they had an incurable disease, and with increasing frequency doctors today are gathering patients and key family members together and telling them just what the prognosis is. With the air cleared, it is then easier for all to communicate honestly and prepare psychologically for death.

Harry, for example, had discussed his fatal illness openly with his family. Instead of squandering his last days in wishful thinking and little white lies, he brought his life neatly to completion: He bought a summer home for his children, made peace with an alienated sister, and took his wife to visit her birthplace, fulfilling a promise of many years. He died peacefully, knowing he had finished his life and taken care of his survivors.

The Preparatory Stages

A pioneer in understanding the psychology of dying is Dr. Elisabeth Kübler-Ross, an Illinois psychiatrist and author of *On Death and Dying* (see "For Further Reading," page 692), who identified five emotional stages that dying people typically pass through. Interestingly she found that those who will be the survivors also pass through these same stages. When the stages that the patients and survivors are in are synchronized, she showed, death is more peaceful for all concerned.

The stages of preparation that Dr. Kübler-Ross identified are:

Denial. This is the "No, not me; it can't be" stage, when the patient cannot accept the fact of his or her fatal illness. Those who die while still in this stage often leave behind much unfinished business. When family members get stuck in this stage, as happened in George's case, their refusal to accept the fatal prognosis may block the patient's own efforts to come to terms with his or her mortality.

Anger. This is what Dr. Kübler-Ross calls the "Why me?" stage. Ideally the patient should rant and rave and scream with justifiable rage over his or her impending fate. But since custom often stands in the way of this normal and healthy outlet for anger, the fury is often expressed in other ways. The patient may instead become hard to handle, critical and demanding, nasty and uncooperative. Friends and relatives may view this as an expression of ingratitude and respond by making their visits shorter and less frequent. As a result, the patient feels even more isolated and rejected and may become more unpleasant.

Bargaining. As the anger subsides and the patient begins to accept the reality of the situation, he or she may try to bargain for more time for good behavior. One woman prayed, "I'll be a good Christian if you give me one more year so I can see my son graduate from college."

Depression. This is a time of grieving for what the patient has already lost and what else he or she stands to lose. It is commonly a period of silence and withdrawal as the dying person tries to separate from all that he or she has known and loved. If you tell a person in this stage to "cheer up, everything will be all right," you are impeding his or her reconciliation with the inevitable, which is hardly "all right."

Survivors are expected to be depressed over the loss of a loved one. It should be far more acceptable for people who are dying to be depressed. They are, after all, losing everything and everyone they love. What better reason to be sad? Dying people should be encouraged to grieve.

Acceptance. This is the time when patients realize that the end is nearly here and "it's all right." It is not a happy or an unhappy time, but neither is it resignation.

Lyn Helton, a poet, wife, and mother when she died of bone cancer at age twenty, wrote during the final days of her illness:

"Dying is beautiful. Even at the ripe old age of twenty. It is not easy most of the time, but there is really beauty to be found in knowing that your end is going to catch up with you faster than you expected. And that you have to get all your loving and laughter and crying done as soon as you can. I am not afraid to die."

Not all dying people go through these stages in neat succession. Some stages may be skipped. Sometimes the patient gets stuck in a particular stage for a long time. Sometimes the patient passes back and forth through various stages several times. But in understanding what the stages are and learning how to recognize and respond to them, you can deal more effectively with a dying person and with your own reactions to the anticipated death.

When the stage of acceptance has been reached by those who are dying and by their loved ones, the process of grieving after death is usually shorter and less destructive. Accepting the impending death of a loved one does not mean you do not care. Rather, it means you care enough to make the end as pleasant as possible for all concerned, especially the person who is dying and those still living whom you will continue to care for afterward.

For Further Reading

Hendin, David. *Death as a Fact of Life.* New York: W.W. Norton, 1973.
Kübler-Ross, Elisabeth, M.D. *On Death and Dying.* New York: MacMillan, 1974.
Simpson, Michael A., M.D. *The Facts of Death.* Englewood Cliffs, N.J.: Prentice-Hall, 1979.

Senility:
Sometimes Reversible

A sixty-three-year-old man misplaced things all the time, couldn't remember anything, and became so disorganized that he was unable to do his work at the office. A doctor told him he was senile and nothing could be done, but he went to the behavioral neurology center at Boston's Beth Israel Hospital, where psychological tests and a psychiatric interview revealed that the man was severely depressed. His sadness, which he had not discussed with anyone, had taken on the mask of senility.

Counseling and treatment with antidepressant drugs resulted in a dramatic improvement in his "senile" symptoms.

Another man in his sixties became disoriented and forgetful following his hospitalization and treatment for a heart condition. Senile dementia was the suspected diagnosis, until doctors decided to try discontinuing the drug he'd been given for his heart problem. Within a day improvement was apparent, and two weeks later the man's normal mental state was fully restored.

Some 3 million Americans, most of them elderly, have symptoms of senility, and 1 million are severely incapacitated by them. As the aged population increases, so does the number of people afflicted with serious deterioration of mental faculties.

Yet, contrary to what many people think, senility is not an inevitable consequence of old age. Rather, only about 10 percent of people over sixty-five are afflicted, and many who survive into their eighties or nineties show no serious mental deterioration. And as the two patients described above clearly demonstrate, many so-called senile individuals are really not senile at all. Rather, they have underlying and usually treatable problems that cause symptoms resembling senility. Too often, however, doctors fail to look beyond the obvious, and instead, incorrectly diagnose senility. Unless the proper examinations and tests are done, a curable or treatable cause is likely to be overlooked.

Elderly people and their families, too, may assume senility to be the cause of forgetfulness, confusion, disorientation, lapses of attention, errors in judgment, irritability, and other changes in personality and behavior, and this assumption may prompt them to accept a superficial diagnosis or not even to consult a physician when such symptoms appear. Others waste their money on useless or unproved therapies, ranging from high-pressure oxygen to a variety of stimulant drugs.

Experts estimate that hundreds of thousands of otherwise useful lives are tragically wasted because senility is incorrectly assumed or diagnosed. Even for the millions who are truly irreversibly senile, much can be done to improve their lives and help their families cope. Furthermore, one common cause of true senility may be largely preventable.

Diverse Causes

About 50 to 60 percent of senile persons are suffering from a currently irreversible deterioration of the brain known as Alzheimer's disease (named for the man who first described it in 1907). It is characterized by tangled nerve fibers and plaques (deposits) in the brain and a deficiency of an enzyme called choline acetyltransferase. This enzyme is essential to the manufacture of acetylcholine, a substance that transmits nerve messages in the brain. Deterioration is progressive, and death generally occurs within ten years. It can afflict middle-aged as well as elderly people.

Studies are currently under way to determine if treatment with choline, a substance that occurs naturally in such foods as egg yolks, soybeans, meat, and fish, can reverse some of the symptoms of Alzheimer's disease. Results so far are inconclusive and suggest that if choline does work, it helps only in the early stages of the disease.

Another irreversible — but perhaps preventable — cause of senility is a series of ministrokes, or clots in the small arteries of the brain, that result in periodic deterioration of brain function. High blood pressure is the usual underlying cause, and early detection and proper treatment of high blood pressure could prevent it. About 20 to 25 percent of cases of senility are due to this problem. [See chapters on stroke, page 637, and high blood pressure, page 631.]

The remaining 10 to 20 percent of people thought to be senile actually have a condition that is mostly or entirely correctable. There are about 100 conditions that can produce symptoms of senility. Dementia or delerium can result from depression; toxic reactions to prescription or over-the-counter drugs; alcohol or drug addiction; an overactive or underactive thyroid gland; diseases of the heart, lungs, kidneys, or liver; infections (such as pneumonia and meningitis); nutritional deficiencies (such as thiamin or B_{12} deficiency or anemia); loss of vision or hearing; chemical or metal poisons; hypothermia (below-normal body temperature); severe pain; brain injury; brain tumors; and water on the brain, among other causes. In most cases treatment of such underlying conditions "cures" the senility or at least reduces the symptoms.

694

Diagnosis and Treatment

According to an expert task force sponsored by the National Institute on Aging, to diagnose properly a patient with apparent senility, the doctor should take a very detailed medical and personal history (from the patient or a knowledgeable relative or friend), including an inventory of drugs the patient takes. This should be followed by a comprehensive physical and mental examination with blood, urine, thyroid, neurological, psychological, and intellectual tests, a vision and hearing evaluation, and, if no other cause has been uncovered, a brain scan (computerized X ray of the brain). Examinations for possible senility are best done under the guidance of a physician who has a special interest in gerontology, the science of aging.

Even if no treatable cause is discovered, a senile patient can be helped by careful attention to diet (regular, well-balanced meals), daily exercise, personal hygiene, adequate rest, bright lighting, treatment of minor illnesses, continued intellectual stimulation and social contacts, and avoidance of all nonessential drugs. Frequent reminders from others as to time, place, and person help to keep the senile person oriented. Lists of daily activities, maintenance of regular routines, written safety messages posted around the house, color coding of drawers and cupboards, a readily visible calendar, and labeling of frequently used items can do a lot to compensate for memory loss and confusion. Patients should be under the care of a physician who is knowledgeable about senility and willing to devote the time it requires.

Family members can also benefit from counseling and services that relieve them of round-the-clock responsibility for someone who is senile. Many such services are now available at medical centers around the country. For example, group psychotherapy and patient and family support groups may be used to help relatives deal with their feelings and cope better with someone who is brain-impaired. Some centers offer day programs for brain-impaired people.

For Further Reading and Information

Information about family support groups, day programs, and drug research programs around the country can be obtained through the Alzheimer's Disease and Related Disorders Association, Inc., 292 Madison Avenue, Eighth Floor, New York, New York 10017, 212-683-2868, or through your local Office on Aging.

Mace, Nancy L., and Peter V. Rabins, M.D. *The 36-Hour Day: A Family Guide to Caring for Persons with Alzheimer's Disease, Related Dementing Illnesses and Memory Loss in Later Life.* Baltimore: Johns Hopkins University Press, 1982.

Disabilities: Surmounting the Obstacles

To a healthy, active twenty-four-year-old, my visit to the Sister Kenny Institute's annual art show was both a shock and an inspiration. There I met a thirty-five-year-old woman in an iron lung; paralyzed by poliomyelitis from the neck down, she was holding a paintbrush in her teeth to execute a delicate watercolor of a meadow she would never walk through again.

She spoke with humor and hope about her own and her family's acceptance of her profound disability: "We considered the alternative and decided I would rather see my children grow up, and they'd rather have me around. Actually, emotionally and intellectually, I have a lot more time for them now, and with my husband's help they've learned to be quite self-sufficient."

There are many such stories of people who have surmounted severe disabilities: writers, teachers, students, psychologists, artists, and others. Though life without an intact body and mind may seem intolerable to those who enjoy both, to the disabled the reactions of the people they meet and the obstacles created by the world they live in are often far harder to adjust to than the disabilities as such.

Aside from questions of humanity and civil rights, the sheer numbers affected demand that more attention be paid to our attitudes toward the disabled and the opportunities we allow them. Thirty-five million

Americans have activity-limiting disabilities, and half of able-bodied adults have a parent, spouse, child, or close friend who is physically, emotionally, or mentally disabled. More than 200,000 people are permanently disabled by spinal cord injuries and 10,000 join their ranks each year.

A Disability Need Not Be a Handicap

Experts like Jerome and Charlis Dunham distinguish between disability and handicap. As Dr. and Mrs. Dunham note in the *Disability and Rehabilitation Handbook* (see "For Further Reading," page 698), "a disability need not be a handicap." Nonetheless, the attitudes and prejudices of others can make it so. Too often the disabled are presumed to be unhappy and are pitied, avoided, treated as children, spoken for as if they were not there, and not "seen" as whole individuals beyond the disability.

Research findings do not support the assumption that the disabled are less happy. Dr. Nancy Weinberg, researcher and rehabilitation psychologist at the University of Illinois, comments that all people "have some deficit that they must cope with," such as shyness, clumsiness, or poor memory and that the physically disabled adjust to their limitations as others do to failings of a different nature. Dr. Weinberg, in a survey of eighty-eight people with serious physical handicaps, found that only a small minority viewed their problem as "a terrible thing" or "the worst thing that ever happened." Many, on the other hand, saw advantages to their disabilities that, they said, presented them with a challenge, goal, or purpose; made them more sensitive to and more tolerant of others; allowed them to meet a wider range of people; and gave them a greater appreciation of life.

Often, Dr. Weinberg says, the attitudes of the able-bodied are more debilitating than the physical limitations: "Although the disabled can learn to accept their physical impairments and often compensate for them by means of wheelchairs, canes, and personal attendants, the able-bodied too often treat the disabled as socially inferior and vocationally undesirable," she said.

Family Effects of Disability

To be sure, the birth of a disabled child or the development of a serious disability in a previously healthy person, young or old, throws many lives into disarray. Far more than the victim is affected. Indeed, says Dr. Carolyn L. Vash, author of an insightful book, *The Psychology of Disability* (see "For Further Reading," page 698), who became a psychologist after being disabled by polio, "disablement befalling any member of a family can have as far-reaching and intense an impact on the others as on the one who becomes disabled." A disability, she says, may alter the life-styles of family members as much as or more than that of the disabled individual, for schedules, duties, plans, and roles change. "All experience loss, which generates disappointment, frustration, and anger, as freedom and time for fun disappear," she adds.

Dr. Vash describes the many factors other than the disability itself that can make life difficult for the disabled and their loved ones: Parents may overprotect a disabled child; normal siblings may resent the time and attention paid to a disabled brother or sister; a marital relationship that depended on mutual interests in physical endeavors may be threatened by the disability of one partner.

Disability can also strengthen a marital bond. Having a disabled parent can foster independence and maturity in children. A disabled person can often do a lot more than most people realize at first; for example, a sexual relationship need not be ended. Books and therapy are available to guide the disabled to a fulfilling sex life; further information can be obtained from the Physical Disability Program in Human Sexuality at the University of Minnesota Medical School (2630 University Avenue S.E., Minneapolis, Minnesota 55414) and the Human Sexuality Program at the University of California Medical Center in San Francisco (Langley Porter Psychiatric Institute, 401 Parnassus Avenue, San Francisco, California 94143).

While physical pursuits may be limited by disability, intellectual ones need not be. People are multidimensional, and while old interests may be lost because of a disability, new ones can usually be found if people are given — and give themselves — the opportunities.

Barriers to a Fuller Life

Educationally, vocationally, and socially, the disabled could do a lot more if not for the many physical barriers to a full life: doors too narrow for wheelchairs; entrances with only stairways; transportation systems with no allowances for the disabled. Spurred by federal regulations, a good deal of progress has been made in recent years toward eliminating such barriers, but much more needs to be done. The wide range of possibilities for improving life for the disabled is detailed in *Access: The Guide to a Better Life for Disabled Americans* and in *The Source Book for the Disabled* (see "For Further Reading," page 698).

Dr. Vash insists: "If the disability cannot be changed, then it must be accepted, as must any other reality, pleasant or unpleasant, if the person is to survive and grow. What need *not* be accepted is the unnecessary handicapping imposed on disabled people by a poorly designed or unaccommodating world or by their own failures to accept what is and go on from there."

The personal discomfort of the able-bodied often stands in the way of their establishing rewarding human relationships with the disabled. Fear of saying or doing the wrong thing, a desire not to be reminded of the fragility of the body, and a lack of experience contribute to painfully

697

awkward social relationships or downright avoidance of the disabled.

Beth Larson, a Reno counselor and contributor to the syndicated column "People to People," offers these suggestions toward achieving more natural relationships:

• Look directly at and talk directly to the disabled person, not through a companion.

• If you think help is needed, ask, and if it is, find out just what the disabled person would like you to do.

• Do not try to avoid normal phrases. It is not inappropriate to talk about walking to a paraplegic or about seeing to a blind person.

• Talk normally about life, and do not make assumptions about the life of a disabled person. Many work, are married, have a sex life and children.

• Slow down and allow the extra time and space needed to be courteous to the disabled and preserve their dignity.

• Do not park in spaces reserved for the handicapped, no matter how much of a hurry you may be in. If you sit in a seat reserved for the handicapped, be prepared to vacate it if a disabled person needs it.

For Further Reading

Ayrault, Evelyn West. *Sex, Love and the Physically Handicapped.* New York: Continuum, 1981.

Bruck, Lilly. *Access: The Guide to a Better Life for Disabled Americans.* New York: David Obst Books/Random House, 1978.

Dunham, Jerome and Charlis. *Disability and Rehabilitation Handbook.* New York: McGraw-Hill, 1978.

Hale, Glorya, ed. *The Source Book for the Disabled.* New York: Bantam, 1981.

Kunc, Norman. *Ready Willing and Disabled.* Toronto: Personal Library, 1981.

Vash, Carolyn L. *The Psychology of Disability.* New York: Springer, 1981.

Rape:
Avoiding Mental and Physical Harm

Rape can happen to any woman, anytime, anywhere. Victims range in age from two months to ninety-odd years and come from all walks of life. Circumstances vary widely — the woman alone asleep in her bedroom or working in her kitchen; the patron of a singles bar who leaves with a man she just met; the late-afternoon jogger in the park; the elderly woman on her way home from grocery shopping. The very essence of rape is its unpredictability.

Example: A college student was sexually attacked by a blind date who was a graduate student at an Ivy League university.

Example: A middle-aged woman was working overtime in a New York skyscraper when a young man with a knife entered her office and raped her.

Example: A woman in her early twenties who taught in an inner-city school was raped in a car after accepting a ride from the son of her school's principal.

In one study almost half the rapes occurred in the victims' homes, and almost half the rapists had some previous acquaintance with their victims. Most of the time the rapist is of the same race as his victim.

Rape is the fastest growing violent crime in the nation — a reflection, experts believe, of both increased reporting and an actual increase in episodes of rape. In 1979 nearly 76,000 forcible rapes of women were reported to the FBI, an increase of 20 percent in just two years. A small but growing proportion of rape victims are male.

Federal experts estimate that only one-tenth of rapes are reported; this would mean that in fact, rape occurs once every two minutes in this country. The victim may not report the attack because she feels guilty or ashamed or she may think she "deserved" what she got. She may also fear retaliation from the rapist, or she may be unwilling to submit to police interrogation. When the attacker is known to the victim, such as a date or a man she met at a party, the police often discourage her from filing an official report (possibly because they don't believe it was really rape) or attempting to press charges since convictions are rarely obtained in such cases.

699

What's Behind the Attack

Contrary to what many think, rape is not primarily a sexual act. Rather, it is motivated by aggression and anger and a need to control. According to Dr. A. Nicholas Groth, director of the sex offender program for the Connecticut Department of Corrections, rapists are rarely "sex-starved," and most have regular normal sexual outlets. More than a third are married. Dr. Groth also notes that a third of rapists are sexually impaired during the rape, and it is not unusual to find no evidence of sperm in or on the victim.

Most rapes are planned, although the particular victim may be picked on the spur of the moment. Dr. Eleanor Schuker, director of the rape intervention program at St. Luke's Hospital in New York City, points out that rapists often choose victims because of some "special vulnerability," such as youth or old age, physical deformity or handicap, or because the women are overly trusting, are depressed, exercise poor judgment, or fail to pick up danger signals. About one-quarter of rape victims have been sexually attacked before.

As if the fact of rape were not awful enough, the emotional effects are often intensified by ignorance and insensitivity on the part of the victim's family, law enforcement officials, and medical practitioners. Mistaken ideas — such as the notions that most victims really ask for it or could have stopped the rapists if they had wanted to — frequently add guilt to the already severe psychic trauma and stand in the way of appropriate treatment.

Treating the Psychological Aftermath

Two types of immediate reactions to rape have been identified: an emotional outburst of anxiety, fear, anger, shame, etc., and an outward calm, cool, and controlled response. The latter is more common and is likely to give way to a delayed emotional reaction. The immediate reaction, which is similar to an acute grief reaction, is followed by a long phase during which the victim may experience nightmares and develop fears and phobias.

The amount of empathy and support a rape victim receives from her family and friends, and from those to whom she turns for treatment, can make an enormous difference to her emotional recovery. An "I told you so" attitude from parents or a husband or boyfriend who acts as if *he's* the one who's been hurt, contribute to the woman's emotional trauma and prolongs it, according to a five-year study by Dr. Ann W. Burgess of the Boston University School of Nursing and Dr. Lynda Lytle

HOW TO PREVENT RAPE

Although there is no guaranteed protection against rape, certain factors can increase your vulnerability to attack. A pamphlet called *How to Protect Yourself Against Sexual Assault* is available free from the National Center for the Prevention and Control of Rape, U.S. Department of Health and Human Services, Room 15-99 Parklawn Building, 5600 Fishers Lane, Rockville, Maryland 20857.

The following are among the preventive tips suggested in this pamphlet and by the Boston Police Department.

At home
- Keep lights on in all entrances.
- Keep your doors and windows locked. Use a dead-bolt lock on your door (don't rely on a chain lock), and check all visitors through a peephole before opening the door.
- If you move to a new house or apartment, have the locks changed.
- Don't let anyone in without first verifying the person's identity. That includes meter readers, postal workers, deliverymen, salesmen, and repairmen.
- If you keep a window open, use a lock that restricts the opening to a maximum of five inches.
- Let no one, except those you trust, know you are home alone.
- Keep your shades drawn at night.
- If you suspect someone has broken in, don't go into the house. Call the police from the nearest phone.
- Use only your last name on the mailbox and door.
- Don't hide your key near the door or in some other obvious place.

In an elevator
- If there is a lone man in the elevator who looks suspicious, don't take it.
- Stand near the buttons, and if someone bothers you, push as many as you can, including the alarm button.

Holmstrom of Boston College.

Although rape, by definition, is carried out under actual or threatened force, victims are less likely to suffer serious physical injury than severe psychological trauma. Many women are deeply scarred by the episode. They may become fearful, depressed, unable to work effectively or to enjoy normal sexual relations. Some leave their jobs or move away. Others develop marital problems. A few attempt suicide. Boston researchers found that as many as four to six years after a woman has been raped she may suffer adverse effects, including impairment of normal sexual functioning and flashbacks to the rape experience, especially during sexual activity. Experts regard rape as the ultimate attack on the integrity of a person, short of murder. The victim is left feeling vulnerable, humiliated, and out of control.

In the last few years, largely spurred by the women's movement, myths and mistreatment have begun to yield to publicity and new programs. Hospitals and community groups throughout the country have established counseling and treatment centers where rape victims can obtain confidential medical and emotional assistance from specially trained

- If you're on your way up from the first floor, don't ride with the elevator down to the basement first.

Using transportation
- Make sure your car is in good working order and has plenty of gas.
- Glance into the car, checking the seats and floor, before you get in.
- Have your keys ready before you reach the car, get in quickly, and lock the doors immediately, and roll the windows up.
- If your car breaks down on the road, tie a white rag on the door handle or aerial, and then get back into the car and lock the doors. Stay in the car even if a man offers help.
- Don't ever pick up hitchhikers.
- Park in well-lighted areas.
- On public transportation, stay out of nearly empty cars, and keep away from groups of men. If possible, sit near the conductor or motorman.

Out of doors
- Don't daydream; stay alert to suspicious-looking people.
- Don't overload your arms, rendering yourself defenseless.
- Avoid deserted streets, parking lots, parks, and shortcuts. Use well-lighted streets, and walk close to the curb, facing the oncoming traffic.
- Make sure the streetlamps on your block are kept in working order.
- Don't walk through a group of men; walk around them or cross the street.
- Don't hitchhike.
- Have your keys ready before you get to your front door.
- Carry a hatpin or stickpin in your hand.
- Carry a whistle around your wrist, and use it if you fear danger.
- Be aware of your surroundings, especially nearby footsteps and voices and cars that pull up or keep passing you.
- If you are being followed, ring the nearest doorbell.
- Dress so that you can run if you have to.

professionals and volunteers. Many police departments have set up special procedures for sensitive handling of rape victims. Some offer demonstration programs to teach women about vulnerability to rape and how best to protect themselves. In 1976 Congress authorized establishment of a National Center for the Prevention and Control of Rape to finance studies of rapists and their victims and to establish needed services.

A rape victim should receive immediate professional medical care and psychosocial counseling. Antibiotics to prevent venereal disease and hormones to prevent pregnancy may be administered. Talking with a trained counselor, professional or volunteer, can be extremely beneficial. A hospital-based rape treatment center is ideal. In many areas a volunteer rape crisis center or hot line has been established, and counseling may be available through local community mental health centers. Check the phone book under "rape," or call a local feminist organization for assistance.

If You Are Attacked . . .

You have three possible courses of action. There is no right way to respond to a rape threat. The best response depends on you and the circumstances.

1. Passive resistance

● Try to stall for time; someone may come along. You may be able to calm the attacker or persuade him not to carry out his threat.

● If you're at home, say that a boyfriend, husband, or roommate is expected home very soon.

● Try to turn your attacker off by gagging yourself to induce vomiting or by urinating. Tell him you have VD.

2. Active resistance

● Scream "fire" (not "police" since potential rescuers may avoid becoming involved in a criminal matter), and pull a fire alarm box.

● Break a window; someone may respond to the noise.

● Use your key or a stickpin, and decisively aim for the attacker's eyes, temples, Adam's apple, or ears.

● If you are trained *and proficient* in self-defense techniques, such as judo or karate, you might use them. But don't try unless you've kept in practice.

● A forceful kick in the groin, stomp on the instep, or hard chop against the front of the throat may disable an attacker long enough to permit your escape.

3. Submission

● If you think you might get hurt by defending yourself, if you're afraid to fight back, or if every defense you've tried has failed, submit. It's better than getting seriously injured or killed. Even if you do not resist at all, it is still rape and should be reported to the police.

For Further Reading

Brownmiller, Susan. *Against Our Will: Men, Women and Rape.* New York: Simon & Schuster, 1975; Bantam, 1976.

Eyeman, Joy Satterwhite. *How to Convict a Rapist.* New York: Stein & Day, 1980.

Smith, Captain James A. *Rapists Beware.* New York: Collier, 1980.

703

Index

705

707

(continued on next page)

Dairy products (continued)
in Basic Four food groups, 7
as calcium sources, 53, 613-614
cancer and, 83
fat in, 20, 22
and cholesterol, 16-17, 27
food poisoning from, 393-396
intolerance of, 534, 535, 550
salt in, 70
ulcers and, 590
vitamin-fortified, 45
"Dangers of Smoking, Benefits of Quitting," 252
Daydreams, 160-163
Deafness, 309-312
Death
breakfast and, 80
fear of, 689, 691
preparation for, 690-692
Decongestants, 546
Denial
of death, 691
of heart attack, 636-637
Dental Care and dentistry. *See* Teeth
Dentures, 290, 295-297
snoring and, 305-306
See also Periodontal disease
Depression, 136, 146-151
in adolescents, 150, 151
alcohol and, 168, 243, 248
after Caesarean birth, 223-224
as cause of senility, 692-693, 694
in children, 117, 147, 149-151
death and, 691-692
drug therapy for, 130
exercise for, 148, 167
fatigue and, 494-495
after heart attack, 679
holidays and, 166-169
after hysterectomy, 234-235
during menopause, 231-232
after miscarriage, 220-221
oral contraceptives and, 195
sleep problems and, 559
symptoms of, 126-127, 147-148
DES (diethylstilbestrol), 81, 82, 238
Desensitization, allergic, 546-547
Diabetes, 660-664
annual checkups and, 438
Caesarean birth and, 222
chromium for prevention of, 57
exercise and, 87, 116-117, 663
eyes and, 319
cataracts, 329
contact lenses, 336
glaucoma, 326

fiber consumption for, 38-39
foot problems and, 555
hypoglycemia and, 511
impotence and, 174, 176, 187
laboratory test for, 444
oral contraceptives and, 195
periodontal disease and, 293
starches and, 32, 34, 663
sugar consumption and, 33, 34, 662-663
Dialysis, 668-669
Diaphragms for birth control, 200-201,
540
Diarrhea, 515
in bowel disease, 591-594
herbal teas and, 267, 270
with intestinal parasites, 597-601
medication for, 470, 583-584
as symptom of colon cancer, 652-653
as symptom of food poisoning, 394-395
traveler's, 581-584, 599-600
Diet
cancer and, 81-84
elimination, 535, 549-550
fad, 72-73
Feingold, 171-172
high-fiber, 36-41
for hyperactivity, 171-172
low-carbohydrate, 29
low-sodium, 66-67, 69-72, 634
Recommended Dietary Allowances
(RDA) 2-7
sleep and, 141
for ulcers, 590-591
vitamin supplements to, 3, 7-8, 43, 45-
51
Diphtheria, 448, 450, 451
Directory of Medical Specialists, 433
Disabilities, 695-698
Disability and Rehabilitation Handbook
(Dunham and Dunham), 696
Diuretic(s), 227
caffeine as, 65
herbal teas as, 270
Diverticulosis, 593
Doctors. *See* Physicians
Dogs
bites of, 416-419
diseases from, 419-422
See also Pets
Douching, 538
Down's syndrome, 216, 287
Dreams, day, 160-163
Dressings, and bandages, 376
Drinking. *See* Alcohol; Water
Driving
alcohol and, 245-246

711

(continued on next page)

712

714

716

717

(continued on next page)

718

719

(continued on next page)

(continued on next page)

722

723